Pharmacology of Purine Receptors

Pharmacology of Purine Receptors

Editor: Madison Rousseau

AMERICAN
MEDICAL PUBLISHERS
www.americanmedicalpublishers.com

AMERICAN
MEDICAL PUBLISHERS
www.americanmedicalpublishers.com

Cataloging-in-Publication Data

Pharmacology of purine receptors / edited by Madison Rousseau.
p. cm.
Includes bibliographical references and index.
ISBN 979-8-88740-376-2
1. Purines--Receptors. 2. Purines--Receptors--Effect of drugs on. 3. Pharmacy.
4. Purines--Physiological effect. 5. Pharmacology. I. Rousseau, Madison.
QP801.P8 P43 2023
615.7--dc23

American Medical Publishers,
41 Flatbush Avenue,
1st Floor, New York,
NY 11217, USA

ISBN 979-8-88740-376-2 (Hardback)

Contents

Preface

The world is advancing at a fast pace like never before. Therefore, the need is to keep up with the latest developments. This book was an idea that came to fruition when the specialists in the area realized the need to coordinate together and document essential themes in the subject. That's when I was requested to be the editor. Editing this book has been an honour as it brings together diverse authors researching on different streams of the field. The book collates essential materials contributed by veterans in the area which can be utilized by students and researchers alike.

Purine receptors are a type of plasma membrane molecules found in nearly all mammalian tissues. They are classified into three categories and include P1 receptors, P2X receptors, and P2Y receptors. They all play a key role in the variety of neuronal and non-neuronal mechanisms, which comprise pain, immune responses, exocrine and endocrine secretion, platelet aggregation, endothelial-mediated vasodilatation, and inflammation. The G protein is mainly bound to the P1 and P2Y receptors. These receptors are differentiated by considering their reactivity towards particular activators. The brain, heart, kidneys, and adipose tissue all contain P1 and P2Y receptors. These receptors are responsible for various cellular functions, comprising vascular reactivity, migration and proliferation of neural stem cells, cytokine secretion and apoptosis. The study of purine receptors is helpful for developing therapeutic strategies for those disorders, which have new action mechanisms, such as pathogenic conditions, like trauma, pain, epilepsy, ischemia, drug dependence and psychiatric disorders. The objective of this book is to present advanced studies on purine receptors as well as their pharmacological applications. Those in search of information to further their knowledge will be greatly assisted by it.

Each chapter is a sole-standing publication that reflects each author's interpretation. Thus, the book displays a multi-facetted picture of our current understanding of application, resources and aspects of the field. I would like to thank the contributors of this book and my family for their endless support.

Editor

1

Who is Who in Adenosine Transport

Marçal Pastor-Anglada[1,2] and Sandra Pérez-Torras[1,2]**

[1] Molecular Pharmacology and Experimental Therapeutics, Department of Biochemistry and Molecular Biomedicine, Institute of Biomedicine, University of Barcelona, Barcelona, Spain, [2] Oncology Program, National Biomedical Research Institute on Liver and Gastrointestinal Diseases – CIBER ehd, Institut de Recerca Sant Joan de Déu, Barcelona, Spain

***Correspondence:**
Marçal Pastor-Anglada
mpastor@ub.edu
Sandra Pérez-Torras
s.perez-torras@ub.edu

Extracellular adenosine concentrations are regulated by a panel of membrane transporters which, in most cases, mediate its uptake into cells. Adenosine transporters belong to two gene families encoding Equilibrative and Concentrative Nucleoside Transporter proteins (ENTs and CNTs, respectively). The lack of appropriate pharmacological tools targeting every transporter subtype has introduced some bias on the current knowledge of the role of these transporters in modulating adenosine levels. In this regard, ENT1, for which pharmacology is relatively well-developed, has often been identified as a major player in purinergic signaling. Nevertheless, other transporters such as CNT2 and CNT3 can also contribute to purinergic modulation based on their high affinity for adenosine and concentrative capacity. Moreover, both transporter proteins have also been shown to be under purinergic regulation via P1 receptors in different cell types, which further supports its relevance in purinergic signaling. Thus, several transporter proteins regulate extracellular adenosine levels. Moreover, CNT and ENT proteins are differentially expressed in tissues but also in particular cell types. Accordingly, transporter-mediated fine tuning of adenosine levels is cell and tissue specific. Future developments focusing on CNT pharmacology are needed to unveil transporter subtype-specific events.

Keywords: adenosine, transporters, CNT, ENT, purinergic signaling

INTRODUCTION

Oscillation of extracellular adenosine levels is physiologically relevant because this nucleoside is the agonist of four P1 receptors known to modulate many biological functions (Fredholm et al., 2011; Burnstock, 2017). Indeed, adenosine concentrations in the extracellular milieu are determined by the balance between its appearance and its removal. In most cases adenosine appearance is the result of the sequential metabolic action of various ecto-nucleotidases on nucleotide precursors, ATP being the first nucleotide in this cascade (Dos Santos-Rodrigues et al., 2014; Nguyen et al., 2015; Pastor-Anglada et al., 2018). However, in particular cell types, there is experimental evidence supporting the possibility of adenosine also being released from cells (Almeida et al., 2003). Extracellular adenosine disposal is similarly mediated by either metabolism, Adenosine Deaminase (ADA) being the enzyme responsible for its conversion into inosine, or by its uptake into cells, where it is likely to be metabolized and trapped as AMP after being phosphorylated by Adenosine Kinase (ADK). The relative contribution of each particular mechanism to the oscillations of adenosine levels may be cell-specific and dependent upon the tissue microenvironment, but is not well-known, although some attempts to address this issue have been done (Nguyen et al., 2015). In any case, adenosine removal from the extracellular milieu is likely to play a major role in regulating adenosine concentrations.

Adenosine cannot freely permeate biological membranes and its transport across them occurs via selected adenosine transporter proteins. Accordingly, transport processes are key modulators of extracellular adenosine disposal. In this contribution, we plan to provide an updated and critical view on the particular transporter subtypes likely to mediate adenosine transport. Evidence supporting the link between transport processes and purinergic signaling will be also discussed.

ADENOSINE TRANSPORT MECHANISMS

All adenosine transporters identified so far belong to the SoLute Carrier (*SLC*) superfamily, in particular, to gene families *SLC28* and *SLC29* (Young et al., 2013; Young, 2016; Pastor-Anglada et al., 2018). *SLC28* genes encode three transporter subtypes known as human Concentrative Nucleoside Transporters 1, 2, and 3 (hCNT1, hCNT2, and hCNT3). The *SLC29* family has four members, thereby resulting in four transporter subtypes, known as human Equilibrative Nucleoside Transporters 1, 2, 3, and 4 (hENT1, hENT2, hENT3, and hENT4). Evidence for additional transporter subtypes, generated by mRNA splicing has been provided for hCNT3 and hENT2, in both cases leading to shorter proteins than their corresponding wild type transporters. Nevertheless, in all cases these small variants appear to be localized in intracellular compartments (Errasti-Murugarren et al., 2009; Grañé-Boladeras et al., 2016) and are unlikely to play any significant role in purinergic signaling. Nevertheless, it has been shown that hENT2 splice variants can regulate wild type hENT2 abundance and function at the plasma membrane (Grañé-Boladeras et al., 2016).

The type of translocation processes implicated in adenosine transport (i.e., "concentrative" versus "equilibrative") and the affinity binding of adenosine to its transporter proteins are key determinants of adenosine transport efficacy.

hCNTs are obligatory inward transporters which take advantage of the sodium gradient to accumulate nucleosides in the cells. Nucleosides and sodium are co-transported with translocation stoichiometry 1:1 (hCNT1 and hCNT2) and 1:2 (hCNT3). Indeed, those CNT proteins showing the ability to transport adenosine are excellent candidates to promote adenosine disposal from the extracellular milieu due to their concentrative capacity. hENTs are potentially bidirectional, vectorial transport being determined by the nucleoside concentration gradient across the membrane. Nevertheless, it is probable that in some circumstances, functional coupling of adenosine influx with its intracellular phosphorylation by ADK enables cells to trap this nucleoside as AMP thereby building up a transmembrane adenosine gradient which will favor unidirectional import of adenosine. It is not known whether adenosine release via these transporters can be explained by some sort of inefficient, not necessarily uncontrolled coupling between metabolism and transport.

As introduced above, affinity is also a critical parameter when discussing the adenosine transport capacity of each nucleoside transporter subtype. Reported physiological adenosine concentrations are very low, often below 1 μM (Fenton and Dobson, 1992; Espinoza et al., 2011; Rose et al., 2011; Westermeier et al., 2011), although under certain conditions, such as hypoxia or in tumor microenvironments where ATP levels can increase considerably, adenosine can also accumulate above normal physiological concentrations (Blay et al., 1997) reviewed in de Andrade Mello et al. (2017) and Di Virgilio and Adinolfi (2017). As shown in **Table 1**, apparent Km values for adenosine vary among transporter subtypes, although some intrinsic variability is observed for the same transporter subtype, probably as a result of the experimental set used to calculate this parameter.

Adenosine transport can be determined either by influx measurements of its radiolabeled form or, at least for CNT-type transporters, by electrophysiological means. In order to get accurate determinations of kinetic parameters it is important to overexpress a particular subtype on a nucleoside-transport null background, which indeed is very rare, although two mammalian non-commercial cell lines lacking CNT- and ENT-related activity had been engineered for this purpose (Mackey et al., 1998; Ward et al., 2000). On the other hand, determination of adenosine uptake kinetic constants of endogenous transporters is a big challenge. In general trends, most cell lines do not retain hCNT-related activity, because hCNT expression is highly dependent upon cell differentiation. Moreover, kinetic determinations in primary cells are not easy either because they co-express several transporter subtypes showing overlapping substrate selectivity.

Nucleoside uptake by each particular nucleoside transporter subtype cannot be determined directly. This is a limitation likely to result in experimental variability. CNT-mediated transport is Na-dependent, but uptake determinations in saturating sodium concentrations (normally 120 mM NaCl) incorporate CNT- and ENT-related transport as well a variable (often small) residual component likely to be associated with non-specific binding, to which even the support where the cells grow on can contribute to. Thus, uptake measurementsin the absence of sodium are required, being this cation often replaced by choline (120 mM Choline Cl). CNT-type activity can be calculated by subtracting uptake rates measured in the absence of Na from the total uptake activity measured in a Na-containing medium. Needless to say, uptake rates should be measured in initial velocity conditions for proper calculation of kinetic constants. This can be experimentally challenging, particularly when transporters are overexpressed. Under these conditions substrate uptake can be very fast and short uptake time points might be needed (seconds). As mentioned above, it is not correct to assume that endogenous ENT-type proteins are responsible for all apparent uptake activity measured in the absence of sodium. This means in practice that direct measurements of ENT-related activity cannot be performed either. Thus, ENTs must be pharmacologically inhibited to figure out their

TABLE 1 | Affinity constants of human adenosine transporters.

Gene name protein	Experimental model	Type of assay	Af. ct. (μM)	Reference
SLC29A1 ENT1	Human Erythroleukemia K562 cells.	Adenosine influx	75	Boleti et al., 1997
	Endogenous transporters.	Adenosine influx	32	Celis et al., 2017
	Human Umbilical Vein Endothelial Cells (HUVEC).	Adenosine influx	53	Casanello et al., 2005
	Endogenous transporters.	Adenosine influx	59	Muñoz et al., 2006
	Placental microvascular endothelial cells. Endogenous		61	Salomón et al., 2012
	transporters.		82	Escudero et al., 2008
	Heterologous expression in PK15NTD (Nucleoside Transporter Deficient) cells.		40	Ward et al., 2000
SLC29A2 ENT2	Human Umbilical Vein Endothelial Cells (HUVEC).	Adenosine influx	49	Celis et al., 2017
	Endogenous transporters.	Adenosine influx	102	Muñoz et al., 2006
	Placental microvascular endothelial cells. Endogenous	Adenosine influx	77	Salomón et al., 2012
	transporters.		98	Escudero et al., 2008
	Heterologous expression in PK15NTD (Nucleoside Transporter Deficient) cells.		140	Ward et al., 2000
SLC29A3 ENT3	hENT3AA, mutated to reach the plasma membrane in	Adenosine influx pH 5.5	1860	Baldwin et al., 2005
	Xenopus laevis oocytes.	Adenosine influx pH 5.5	1620	Rahman et al., 2017
	Δ36hENT3, deleted to reach the plasma membrane in *Xenopus laevis* oocytes.		1800	Kang et al., 2010
SLC29A4 ENT4	Expression in *Xenopus laevis* oocytes.	Adenosine influx pH 5.5	780	Barnes et al., 2006
SLC28A2 CNT2	Expression in *Xenopus laevis* oocytes.	Adenosine influx	8	Yao et al., 1996
		Adenosine influx	6	Che et al., 1995
		Electrophysiology	18	Larráyoz et al., 2006
		Electrophysiology	23	Li et al., 2001
SLC28A3 CNT3	Expression in *Xenopus laevis* oocytes	Adenosine influx	15	Ritzel et al., 2001
	Heterologous expression in yeast	Electrophysiology	18	Gorraitz et al., 2010
	Heterologous expression in HeLa cells	Adenosine influx	2.2	Damaraju et al., 2005
		Adenosine influx	2.4	Errasti-Murugarren et al., 2008

Interaction of nucleoside transporters with adenosine has been addressed either by determining the influx of radiolabeled adenosine into cells or, for hCNTs, by monitoring adenosine-induced Na^+ currents in Xenopus laevis oocytes expressing a particular CNT subtype protein. Apparent affinity constants (Af. ct.) are all given in μM for a better comparison among all NT subtypes. Endogenous transporters refer to kinetic determinations performed using cell lines which express hENT1 and hENT2 endogenously, being the contribution of each subtype calculated by selectively inhibiting either hENT1 alone or both hENTs, as explained in the text. Adenosine uptake by hENT3 and hENT4 can only be measured at acidic pH. Kinetic determinations using the intracellular transporter hENT3 can only be performed if the wild type protein is modified in a way that sorting signals are blocked, thereby allowing the protein to reach the plasma membrane and determine function. Whether these relatively small structural alterations can significantly impact on adenosine affinity is not known. hCNT1 is not included in the table because, as explained in the text, even though some adenosine affinity constants have been reported, its translocation efficacy is extremely poor and we think it cannot be considered an adenosine transporter in a physiological context.

contribution to the remaining transport activity measured in sodium-free medium. Indeed, both plasma membrane ENTs (ENT1 and ENT2) can be simultaneously blocked by μM concentrations of dipyridamole and dilazep, whereas ENT1 can be selectively inhibited by nM concentrations of the nucleoside analog NBMPR (Young et al., 2013; Young, 2016; Pastor-Anglada et al., 2018). Accordingly, ENT1 activity corresponds to the NBMPR-sensitive component whereas ENT2 contribution to nucleoside uptake can be calculated by subtracting the ENT1 activity from the dipyridamole-sensitive component (ENT1 and ENT2 working simultaneously). At this moment, the reader can easily understand to what extent accurate measurements of endogenous nucleoside transport activity can be challenging in primary cells co-expressing all types of transporter proteins.

As introduced above, electrophysiology might be suitable for accurate kinetic measurements taking advantage of the fact that hCNT proteins are electrogenic when they translocate nucleosides and sodium. The two-electrode voltage clamp technique has been broadly used in transporter biology for this purpose (Lostao et al., 2000; Larráyoz et al., 2004; Smith et al., 2004; Slugoski et al., 2008; Gorraitz et al., 2010). The cRNA coding for a specific transporters is injected in *Xenopus laevis* oocytes and, in normal conditions, transporter function can be assessed after 2 days. Oocytes are clamped and inward sodium currents triggered by the addition of a particular hCNT substrate are recorded. Indeed, the intensity of the applied current to compensate for the transient depolarization associated with sodium influx, reflects transport activity. In this particular set up, initial velocity conditions can be easily achieved, endogenous activity is not interfering and currents may be a more direct way of measuring hCNT transport function than when using radiolabeled adenosine influx determinations. However, the oocyte membrane might show physicochemical properties different from mammalian plasma membranes. To what extent the membrane environment of a particular nucleoside transporter determines function and, eventually, substrate specificity is not really well-known. In this regard, when studying a novel polymorphic hCNT3 variant identified in our laboratory several years ago (Errasti-Murugarren et al., 2008), we observed that hCNT3 can indeed be found in different membrane microdomains, hCNT3 proteins located in lipid rafts being more active than the ones off rafts (Errasti-Murugarren et al., 2010).

There are many experimental issues which are likely to affect hCNT-related activity measurements and this may explain published variability in substrate specificity (adenosine affinity constants). Despite all these experimental issues, in general terms, it seems that the transporter proteins showing the highest affinity for adenosine are hCNTs, in particular, hCNT2 and hCNT3. In our hands, apparent Km values for adenosine in HEK293 cells expressing hCNT3 are the lowest reported so far among all nucleoside transporter proteins, 2.4 μM. Nevertheless, what makes hCNT3 an excellent candidate to modulate extracellular adenosine levels is the fact that it shows a huge capacity to concentrate nucleosides inside cells, because of its unique stoichiometry. Nevertheless, as will be discussed below, hCNT3 is not ubiquitously expressed, meaning that in some particular cell types hCNT2 would be the one to do the job.

The role of hCNT1 in adenosine regulation requires a more detailed explanation because there has been an argument in the past about whether or not this protein is an adenosine transporter. Apparent Km values for adenosine have been calculated for rCNT1 when it was expressed in oocytes and transport assays were performed using radiolabeled nucleosides (Yao et al., 1996). In this set up, an apparent Km of 26 μM was reported and discussed to be similar to the one calculated for uridine (37 μM) (Huang et al., 1994). Nevertheless, under these conditions the Vmax for uridine was 300 fold higher than the one calculated for adenosine (Yao et al., 1996). The same laboratory reported very low, almost negligible, substrate-induced Na-inward currents when using saturating concentrations of adenosine (100 μM) in oocytes expressing the human CNT1 ortholog (Smith et al., 2004). In our hands currents were undetectable using the same experimental approach (Larráyoz et al., 2004). In summary, we believe hCNT1 cannot be considered an adenosine transporter protein. However, we generated some evidence suggesting the possibility that adenosine can instead bind to the transporter protein without being translocated. Evidence for adenosine binding is quite consistent. Most sodium-coupled transporters, among them hCNTs, show some sodium leakage in the absence of the co-substrate (a nucleoside in our case). Leakage can be similarly measured as a current and is dependent upon membrane potential. Adenosine was shown to block what are called pre-steady state and steady state currents of the transporter protein associated with sodium-leakage (Larráyoz et al., 2004). This can be understood as the consequence of adenosine binding to the transporter protein. The physiological relevance of this event is not known.

Regarding ENT proteins, most available literature points to ENT1 and ENT2 as major players in the regulation of adenosine levels. Although apparent Km values are definitely higher (even much higher for hENT2) than the ones reported for hCNT2 and hCNT3, efficient coupling with adenosine phosphorylation would contribute to generate a huge transmembrane adenosine gradient which thermodynamically would favor influx via these transporter proteins. As discussed below, ENT1 is by far the most studied member within the *SLC29* gene family and different laboratories have provided consistent evidence supporting a role for this particular subtype in adenosine signaling. ENT3 is mostly localized in intracellular compartments (probably mitochondria and lysosomes) but, in any case, its affinity for adenosine seems to be low enough as to preclude any role for this transporter protein in adenosine regulation (Baldwin et al., 2005; Kang et al., 2010; Hsu et al., 2012; Rahman et al., 2017).

Similarly to CNT1, ENT4 also requires some detailed explanations, because its role in adenosine signaling is still on debate. ENT4 is evolutionarily distant from the other three members of the family (Young et al., 2013) and, when cloned and functionally expressed it was reported to show poor affinity for nucleosides, whereas it could translocate monoamine neurotransmitters such as dopamine and serotonin (Engel et al., 2004). In fact the laboratory that generated all this information claimed ENT4 to be renamed as PMAT, from Plasma Membrane Amine Transporter. Interestingly, ENT4/PMAT shows functional similarity with organic cation transporters (OCTs), which means that this protein can act as a polyspecific OCT as the *SLC22* gene members encoding for hOCT1, 2, and 3. Some common substrate structural determinants between nucleoside transporters and OCTs can be hypothesized. Indeed the three hOCT proteins can efficiently translocate the antiviral nucleoside analog lamivudine. Moreover, they can also interact with several other nucleoside-based antiviral drugs such as zidovudine, abacavir, and others (Minuesa et al., 2009). Nevertheless, none of the OCT proteins can transport natural nucleosides. The possibility of ENT4 playing a role in adenosine transport was raised by Barnes et al. (2006) several years ago. These authors demonstrated that serotonin transport via ENT4 was not pH-dependent, whereas adenosine transport was. Apparent Km values for adenosine at acidic pH (5.5) were in the high micromolar range but still were considered to be compatible with ENT4 being an adenosine transporter protein in physiological conditions associated with acidosis.

In summary, we have briefly dissected and discussed the basic biochemical principles and events governing adenosine transport into cells, by highlighting which are the best transporter candidates to regulate extracellular adenosine levels, and therefore, adenosine-mediated purinergic signaling.

ADENOSINE TRANSPORTERS AND PURINERGIC SIGNALING

Once the plasma membrane transporters likely to be implicated in the regulation of adenosine levels have been identified, we will discuss what is the physiological evidence supporting a functional link between a particular transporter subtype and purinergic regulation.

Several experimental approaches have been used in this regard. NT transporter pharmacology is still poorly developed and no subtype-specific inhibitors are available for CNT proteins, although this is not the case for ENTs. Indeed, high-affinity inhibition of ENT1 by NMBPR has proven very helpful. In fact, the determination of NMBPR-specific binding sites has been used by different authors to quantify ENT1 expression at the plasma membrane, even long before ENT1 was identified at the molecular level (Pickard et al., 1973; Dahlig-Harley et al., 1981;

Marangos et al., 1982). Besides the pharmacological approach, functional genomics is also available for ENT1, since Choi colleagues reported the first NT-subtype knock out mouse model (Choi et al., 2004; Oliveros et al., 2017). Probably because of these circumstances, we can say that ENT1 is the most studied transporter among the two families (*SLC28* and *SLC29*), with plenty of literature showing a link between ENT1 function and purinergic regulation. Another experimental approach suitable for the analysis of adenosine transporters as players in the purinome, comes from the evidence that selected NT subtypes (including ENT1) are under purinergic control. This means that their function is regulated by P1 (but probably also by P2) type receptors. In the classical set up of purinome function one would envisage NT proteins being stimulated by adenosine acting on P1 receptors, thereby promoting extracellular adenosine removal and ending the purinergic signaling. Moreover, changes in the expression of particular NT subtypes in physiological and pathophysiological conditions known to be associated with increased adenosine levels, further support the role particular NT proteins might play in purinergic regulation.

ENT Proteins

ENT1 expression in the rat and human brain has been mapped by different means (i.e., NBMPR binding, mRNA *in situ* hybridization and others). ENT1 shows broad cellular and regional distribution and its role in adenosine signaling is relatively well-understood (Parkinson et al., 2011). Adenosine is known to be neuroprotective in various pathological conditions such as stroke (Cunha, 2016). This is the reason why physiological mechanisms governing adenosine extracellular levels have been comprehensively studied. A probable dual role of ENT proteins either as influx or efflux transporters has been reported in the CNS. Indeed, rat cortical neurons when cultured alone are able to release adenosine after *N*-methyl-D-aspartate (NMDA) stimulation, whereas the NMDA-triggered increase in extracellular adenosine concentration appears to be related to nucleotide degradation when neurons are co-cultured with astrocytes (Zamzow et al., 2008). In rat hippocampal slices it has been shown that ATP is able to promote adenosine release via ENT-type proteins, which in turn might activate A2A receptors (Almeida et al., 2003). Subsequently, A2A activation might promote adenosine uptake, as shown in hippocampal synaptosomes (Pinto-Duarte et al., 2005). In fact, adenosine uptake via ENT-type transporters appears to reduce extracellular adenosine levels in hypoxia which suggests that ENT proteins and probably ENT1 in particular might be suitable targets for the treatment of cerebral ischemia (Zhang et al., 2011). Interestingly, adenosine in the brain has also been related to addictive behaviors, among them alcohol addiction. It has been known for a long time that ethanol increases extracellular adenosine by inhibiting in a somehow selective manner ENT1 function (Nagy et al., 1990). Nevertheless the most conclusive evidence supporting this pharmacological effect comes from functional genomics. The ENT1 knock out mouse model shows reduced acute responses to ethanol intake and increased addiction to alcohol (Choi et al., 2004). This animal model has also been useful in the understanding of ENT1-related adenosine signaling in other organs. In fact, ENT1-null mice show increased adenosine plasma levels and are cardioprotected (Rose et al., 2010, 2011). Similarly, ENT1 appears to be implicated in adenosine-related protection in the liver during ischemia and reperfusion (Zimmerman et al., 2013).

Moreover, adenosine contributes to chronic kidney disease, particularly in diabetes. Increased adenosine signaling via A2B receptors has been reported to be involved in diabetic glomerulopathy (Cárdenas et al., 2013), and increased adenosine levels in insulin-deficient states have been associated with down-regulation of ENT2 transport function in podocytes (Alarcón et al., 2017). In a complementary manner, in proximal tubule cells, decreased ENT1 function has also been related to fibrosis in diabetic nephropathy (Kretschmar et al., 2016). In fact, ENT1 null mouse shows a spontaneous tendency to develop renal fibrosis whereas ENT1 silencing in human kidney epithelial (HK) cells results in the promotion of epithelial-to-mesenchymal transition (EMT) (Guillén-Gómez et al., 2012). Promotion of EMT in HK2 cells can be mimicked by TFG-β1, whereas adenosine itself mediates TFG-β1 release from glomeruli of diabetic rats via A2B receptor activation (Roa et al., 2009).

The involvement of ENT proteins in the regulation of adenosine tone in vascular endothelium has been comprehensively studied using Human Umbilical Vein Endothelial Cells (HUVECs) and Placenta Microvascular Endothelial Cells (PMECs) as experimental models (review in Sobrevia et al., 2011; Pardo et al., 2013). As in other cell types, it has been shown that control of extracellular adenosine levels via P1 receptors also involves hENT modulation, in particular the hENT1 and hENT2 subtypes (Escudero et al., 2008; Pardo et al., 2013). In some cases, opposite effects on each transporter protein have been reported, thereby suggesting either some sort of physiological compensation or an hENT-subtype specific effect impacting on the ability of removing from the extracellular milieu not only adenosine but also some of its catabolites. hENT2 is indeed a suitable hypoxanthine transporter. Interestingly, we have recently shown that hENT1 and hENT2 can form oligomers hENT1-hENT1, hENT2-hENT2, but also hENT1-hENT2, with multiple functional consequences (Grañé-Boladeras et al., 2002).

Overall, it is within this framework that the pharmacological use of ENT inhibitors such as dipyridamole and dilazep can be understood (Figueredo et al., 1999). Nevertheless, at least for cardioprotection, it has recently been argued that ENT4 could become a better target than ENT1, because of the more restricted tissue expression pattern of the former ENT subtype (Yang and Leung, 2015). As discussed above, ENT4 was shown to be a suitable cardiac adenosine transporter at acidic pH (Barnes et al., 2006). Then, the idea these authors discuss is that most cell types may rely upon ENT1 for nucleoside salvage purposes, thereby making any ENT1-targeting drug more likely to present adverse effects than newly developed molecules targeting ENT4.

CNT Proteins

As discussed above, hCNT2 and hCNT3 should be, by far, the best candidates for efficient removal of adenosine from the extracellular milieu. This statement is based upon their apparent high affinity for adenosine and for its concentrative capacity which is even 10 fold higher for hCNT3 than hCNT2. Nevertheless, hCNT pharmacology is very poor, even though some hCNT subtype specific inhibitors have been recently proposed (Kumar Deokar et al., 2017). In this regard the structural modeling of human CNT subtypes (Arimany-Nardi et al., 2017; Kumar Deokar et al., 2017; Latek, 2017; Mulinta et al., 2017) based upon the crystal structure of the *Vibrio cholerae* CNT ortholog (Johnson et al., 2012) might be particularly useful for future specific inhibitor design. This has been a major bottleneck to study the probable impact of acute CNT pharmacological inhibition on adenosine signaling. Nevertheless there is solid experimental evidence showing that CNT2 and CNT3 are under purinergic regulation, which suggests they contribute, as ENTs, to modulate extracellular adenosine levels and P1 signaling.

In liver parenchymal cells CNT2 is expressed at the basolateral (sinusoidal) and apical (canalicular) plasma membranes (Duflot et al., 2002; Govindarajan et al., 2008). In rat primary hepatocytes and hepatocarcinoma FAO cells the activity of this transporter protein is under purinergic regulation via A1 receptors (Duflot et al., 2004). This effect is relatively rapid (peaking between 5 and 10 min after agonist addition) and consistent with increased transport capacity (Vmax effect). Interestingly the magnitude of the effect (transport fold-induction) is dependent upon glucose concentration, being lower at high glucose (10 vs. 5 mM glucose). Indeed, CNT2 up-regulation could be blocked by inhibitors of KATP channels and mimicked by openers, which establishes a putative link between energy metabolism and purinergic regulation of CNT2. All the protein machinery likely to be implicated in this phenomenon, this is the KATP channel subunits Kir6.1, Kir6.2, SUR2A, SUR2B, as well as the transporter itself and A1 receptors were shown to co-localize in FAO cells. The physiological impact of the reduction of adenosine removal capacity triggered by high-glucose is not clear, although decreased hENT1 function and expression have been reported in HUVEC from diabetic patients and shown to be mimicked by high glucose in the culture medium (Sobrevia et al., 2011). It is interesting to keep in mind that extracellular adenosine has been reported to be able to modulate the AMP-dependent kinase AMPK, by a mechanism which depends on transporter function, also involving CNT2 in some cell types (Aymerich et al., 2006). Overall, CNT2 appears to be a suitable candidate to modulate purinergic signaling in hepatocytes, particularly considering that hCNT1 is not an adenosine transporter and hCNT3 expression in hepatocytes appears to be negligible. Interestingly, CNT2 function has recently been identified in primary rat bile duct epithelial cells where it is similarly found in both plasma membrane domains, apical and basolateral of cholangiocytes (Godoy et al., 2014). Luminal ATP, via P2Y receptors, down-regulates apical (lumen-facing) CNT2 activity by a Ca^{++}-dependent mechanism. Cholangiocytes also express CNT3 and its apical function is similarly down-regulated by nucleotides, such as ATP. However, A2A agonists (i.e., adenosine), acting from the luminal side, specifically activate apical CNT3, without modifying CNT2 function. CNT3 activation is consistent with transporter trafficking from intracellular vesicles to the plasma membrane. In practice this means that CNT2 and probably to more extent CNT3 are contributing to end up the purinergic regulation of bile flow by removing adenosine from the bile canaliculus. It makes sense that the adenosine precursor ATP reduces adenosine removal capacity by inhibiting both CNT2 and CNT3, whereas the differential regulation of both transporters by adenosine acting on A2A receptors may reflect basal (CNT2 and CNT3) and adenosine-induced (CNT3) capacity for its own removal.

CNT2, in parallel with ENT1, has also been mapped in the adult rat brain by *in situ* hybridization (Guillén-Gómez et al., 2004). Indeed, CNT2 is broadly distributed in the CNS with significant overlapping with ENT1. More recently, others have identified the CNT2 protein in plasma and vesicle membranes isolated from rat striatum (Melani et al., 2012). The possibility of CNT2 also playing a role in adenosine signaling in the brain is also supported by the evidence that its activity can be up-regulated by P1 receptor activation in differentiated neural PC12 cells (most probably A1 and A2A) (Medina-Pulido et al., 2013). CNT2 activation is relatively rapid, as in hepatocytes, peaking 15 min after P1 agonist addition. Interestingly, caffeine has been reported to inhibit CNT2 function with an apparent Ki value of 103 μM (Lang et al., 2004). Although this concentration might significantly exceed the one found in blood after coffee ingestion, it could still be relevant in heavy coffee drinkers (Nehlig and Debry, 1994). Taking together these observations suggest ENT1 may not be the only player regulating adenosine signaling in the brain, which in fact is consistent with the relatively mild phenotype of the ENT1 null mice.

Last, but not least, several physiological and pathophysiological observations also support a role for hCNT2 and hCNT3 as proteins relevant to purinergic signaling. The three hCNT genes are expressed in the nephron and accurate anatomic analysis of their distribution along it reveals a longitudinal pattern of expression consistent with nucleoside renal tubule reabsorption but also with adenosine-mediated tubulo-glomerular feedback regulation (Schnermann, 2015). Indeed, the three transporter proteins are expressed in the proximal convoluted tubule (PCT), where most nutrient reabsorption (glucose, amino acids) take place, but only the two adenosine transporters (CNT2 and CNT3), not CNT1, are also expressed in very specific distal segments of the nephron, the cortical collecting duct (CCD) (CNT3) and the outer medullary collecting duct (OMCD) (CNT2). This anatomical distribution is more consistent with adenosine signaling than with nucleoside reabsorption. Distribution of CNTs along the gastrointestinal tract (Pastor-Anglada et al., 2018) also points to this dual role of adenosine transporters. In fact, the CNT2 encoding gene (*SLC28A2*) is, by far, the one which is down-regulated the most (sevenfold) in inflamed ileon mucosa from Crohn's patients (Pérez-Torras et al., 2016). Even though the impact of inflammation is broad and down-regulates a broad cohort of genes, those associated with the purinome (transporters, receptors, and ectonucleotidases) are greatly affected.

In the rat brain, CNT2 is also down-regulated in situations known to be associated with increased adenosine concentrations. CNT2 mRNA levels are decreased in cortical samples from sleep-deprived rats, whereas ENT1 mRNA is not affected at all under the same circumstances (Guillén-Gómez et al., 2004).

CNT2-related mRNA tends to recover when animals are allowed to sleep. On the other hand, experimental ischemia *in vivo*, induced in rats by intraluminal middle cerebral arterial occlusion, also regulates nucleoside transporter encoding genes (Medina-Pulido et al., 2013). In this study, transcripts of both ENTs (ENT1 and ENT2) and the three CNT members were quantified in the ipsilateral cortex (infarcted) and compared to the contralateral cortex as its own control. Indeed, the mRNA levels of hENT1, hCNT2, but also hCNT3 (poorly studied in the brain), the three transporters more likely to modulate adenosine tone, were decreased in the infarcted tissue with no changes observed for hCNT1 and hENT2.

CONCLUDING REMARKS AND FUTURE PERSPECTIVES

Nucleoside transport by each particular nucleoside protein subtype cannot be measured directly, thereby resulting in some experimental variability likely to impact on the determination of adenosine affinity constants. Despite this limitation, we can conclude that adenosine transport mechanisms across the plasma membrane are well-understood with the only exception of ENT4, for which a clear role in the regulation of adenosine tone in some tissues (i.e., heart) still awaits clarification. Nevertheless, in general trends, who is who in adenosine transport is well-known.

Less clear is how each transporter subtype contributes to modulate adenosine levels, an issue of particular interest considering most cells show some apparent redundancy in the expression of adenosine transporters. ENT1 is by far the most studied adenosine transporter. This may be explained, as discussed above, not necessarily because of its ubiquitous expression, but because pharmacological tools and functional genomics have provided better chances to study it than for the other adenosine transporters. Nevertheless, the contribution of the other subtypes, particularly CNTs (CNT2 and CNT3) should not be ruled out and deserves further investigation.

Although CNT and ENT subtype expression appears to be polarized in (re)absorptive epithelia, thus allowing vectorial flux of substrates, in other epithelial cell types CNT and ENT proteins appear to be located in both poles (apical and basolateral), thereby anticipating other roles beyond absorption (Pastor-Anglada et al., 2018). Moreover, non-epithelial cells, such as adipocytes (Guallar et al., 2007) and immune system cells (Soler et al., 1998, 2001; Minuesa et al., 2009, 2011) also express ENT and CNT proteins. Whether particular subtypes are under purinergic regulation in these cells and tissues has not been properly addressed until now. Last, but not least, there is also the possibility of local regulation of selected adenosine transporters even at the single cell level, thereby providing some sort of compartmental regulation of biological functions. In this regard, ENT and CNT protein interactomics might help to unveil novel regulatory events likely to facilitate the fine tuning of purinergic regulation.

AUTHOR CONTRIBUTIONS

MP-A conceived the review and wrote the first draft of the manuscript. SP-T critiqued and revised the manuscript. SP-T and MP-A read the final version of the manuscript and approved it for submission.

FUNDING

This work was funded by SAF2011-23660 and SAF2014-52067-R (MINECO, Spain), Fundación Ramón Areces (Spain), and FEDER (European Union). MPET is a member of the Oncology Program of CIBER EHD. CIBER is an initiative of Instituto de Salud Carlos III (Spain).

ACKNOWLEDGMENTS

The authors would like to acknowledge past and present members of the MPET laboratory.

REFERENCES

Alarcón, S., Garrido, W., Cappelli, C., Suárez, R., Oyarzún, C., Quezada, C., et al. (2017). Deficient insulin-mediated upregulation of the equilibrative nucleoside transporter 2 contributes to chronically increased adenosine in diabetic glomerulopathy. *Sci. Rep.* 7:9439. doi: 10.1038/s41598-017-09783-0

Almeida, T., Rodrigues, R. J., de Mendonça, A., Ribeiro, J. A., and Cunha, R. A. (2003). Purinergic P2 receptors trigger adenosine release leading to adenosine A2A receptor activation and facilitation of long-term potentiation in rat hippocampal slices. *Neuroscience* 122, 111–121. doi: 10.1016/S0306-4522(03)00523-2

Arimany-Nardi, C., Claudio-Montero, A., Viel-Oliva, A., Schmidtke, P., Estarellas, C., Barril, X., et al. (2017). Identification and characterization of a secondary sodium-binding site and the main selectivity determinants in the human concentrative nucleoside transporter 3. *Mol. Pharm.* 14, 1980–1987. doi: 10.1021/acs.molpharmaceut.7b00085

Aymerich, I., Foufelle, F., Ferré, P., Casado, F. J., and Pastor-Anglada, M. (2006). Extracellular adenosine activates AMP-dependent protein kinase (AMPK). *J. Cell Sci.* 119(Pt 8), 1612–1621. doi: 10.1242/jcs.02865

Baldwin, S. A., Yao, S. Y., Hyde, R. J., Ng, A. M., Foppolo, S., Barnes, K., et al. (2005). Functional characterization of novel human and mouse equilibrative nucleoside transporters (hENT3 and mENT3) located in intracellular membranes. *J. Biol. Chem.* 280, 15880–15887. doi: 10.1074/jbc.M414337200

Barnes, K., Dobrzynski, H., Foppolo, S., Beal, P. R., Ismat, F., Scullion, E. R., et al. (2006). Distribution and functional characterization of equilibrative nucleoside transporter-4, a novel cardiac adenosine transporter activated at acidic pH. *Circ. Res.* 99, 510–519. doi: 10.1161/01.RES.0000238359.18495.42

Blay, J., White, T. D., and Hoskin, D. W. (1997). The extracellular fluid of solid carcinomas contains immunosuppressive concentrations of adenosine. *Cancer Res.* 57, 2602–2605.

Boleti, H., Coe, I. R., Baldwin, S. A., Young, J. D., and Cass, C. E. (1997). Molecular identification of the equilibrative NBMPR-sensitive (es) nucleoside transporter and demonstration of an equilibrative NBMPR-insensitive (ei) transport activity in human erythroleukemia (K562) cells. *Neuropharmacology* 36, 1167–1179. doi: 10.1016/S0028-3908(97)00136-6

Burnstock, G. (2017). Purinergic signalling: therapeutic developments. *Front. Pharmacol.* 8:661. doi: 10.3389/fphar.2017.00661

Cárdenas, A., Toledo, C., Oyarzún, C., Sepúlveda, A., Quezada, C., Guillén-Gómez, E., et al. (2013). Adenosine A(2B) receptor-mediated VEGF induction promotes diabetic glomerulopathy. *Lab. Invest.* 93, 135–144. doi: 10.1038/labinvest.2012.143

Casanello, P., Torres, A., Sanhueza, F., González, M., Farías, M., Gallardo, V., et al. (2005). Equilibrative nucleoside transporter 1 expression is downregulated by hypoxia in human umbilical vein endothelium. *Circ. Res.* 97, 16–24. doi: 10.1161/01.RES.0000172568.49367.f8

Celis, N., Araos, J., Sanhueza, C., Toledo, F., Beltrán, A. R., Pardo, F., et al. (2017). Intracellular acidification increases adenosine transport in human umbilical vein endothelial cells. *Placenta* 51, 10–17. doi: 10.1016/j.placenta.2017.01.120

Che, M., Ortiz, D. F., and Arias, I. M. (1995). Primary structure and functional expression of a cDNA encoding the bile canalicular, purine-specific Na(+)-nucleoside cotransporter. *J. Biol. Chem.* 270, 13596–13599. doi: 10.1074/jbc.270.23.13596

Choi, D. S., Cascini, M. G., Mailliard, W., Young, H., Paredes, P., and McMahon, T. (2004). The type 1 equilibrative nucleoside transporter regulates ethanol intoxication and preference. *Nat. Neurosci.* 7, 855–861. doi: 10.1038/nn1288

Cunha, R. A. (2016). How does adenosine control neuronal dysfunction and neurodegeneration? *J. Neurochem.* 139, 1019–1055. doi: 10.1111/jnc.13724

Dahlig-Harley, E., Eilam, Y., Paterson, A. R., and Cass, C. E. (1981). Binding of nitrobenzylthioinosine to high-affinity sites on the nucleoside-transport mechanism of HeLa cells. *Biochem. J.* 200, 295–305. doi: 10.1042/bj2000295

Damaraju, S., Zhang, J., Visser, F., Tackaberry, T., Dufour, J., Smith, K. M., et al. (2005). Identification and functional characterization of variants in human concentrative nucleoside transporter 3, hCNT3 (SLC28A3), arising from single nucleotide polymorphisms in coding regions of the hCNT3 gene. *Pharmacogenet. Genomics* 15, 173–182. doi: 10.1097/01213011-200503000-00006

de Andrade Mello, P., Coutinho-Silva, R., and Savio, L. E. B. (2017). Multifaceted effects of extracellular adenosine triphosphate and adenosine in the tumor-host interaction and therapeutic perspectives. *Front. Immunol.* 8:1526. doi: 10.3389/fimmu.2017.01526

Di Virgilio, F., and Adinolfi, E. (2017). Extracellular purines, purinergic receptors and tumor growth. *Oncogene* 36, 293–303. doi: 10.1038/onc.2016.206

Dos Santos-Rodrigues, A., Grane-Boladeras, N., Bicket, A., and Coe, I. R. (2014). Nucleoside transporters in the purinome. *Neurochem. Int.* 73, 229–237. doi: 10.1016/j.neuint.2014.03.014

Duflot, S., Calvo, M., Casado, F. J., Enrich, C., and Pastor-Anglada, M. (2002). Concentrative nucleoside transporter (rCNT1) is targeted to the apical membrane through the hepatic transcytotic pathway. *Exp. Cell Res.* 281, 77–85. doi: 10.1006/excr.2002.5641

Duflot, S., Riera, B., Fernández-Veledo, S., Casadó, V., Norman, R. I., Casado, F. J., et al. (2004). ATP-sensitive K(+) channels regulate the concentrative adenosine transporter CNT2 following activation by A(1) adenosine receptors. *Mol. Cell Biol.* 24, 2710–2719. doi: 10.1128/MCB.24.7.2710-2719.2004

Engel, K., Zhou, M., and Wang, J. (2004). Identification and characterization of a novel monoamine transporter in the human brain. *J. Biol. Chem.* 279, 50042–50049. doi: 10.1074/jbc.M407913200

Errasti-Murugarren, E., Cano-Soldado, P., Pastor-Anglada, M., and Casado, F. J. (2008). Functional characterization of a nucleoside-derived drug transporter variant (hCNT3C602R) showing altered sodium-binding capacity. *Mol. Pharmacol.* 73, 379–386. doi: 10.1124/mol.107.041848

Errasti-Murugarren, E., Molina-Arcas, M., Casado, F. J., and Pastor-Anglada, M. (2009). A splice variant of the SLC28A3 gene encodes a novel human concentrative nucleoside transporter-3 (hCNT3) protein localized in the endoplasmic reticulum. *FASEB J.* 23, 172–182. doi: 10.1096/fj.08-113902

Errasti-Murugarren, E., Molina-Arcas, M., Casado, F. J., and Pastor-Anglada, M. (2010). The human concentrative nucleoside transporter-3 C602R variant shows impaired sorting to lipid rafts and altered specificity for nucleoside-derived drugs. *Mol. Pharmacol.* 78, 157–165. doi: 10.1124/mol.110.063552

Escudero, C., Casanello, P., and Sobrevia, L. (2008). Human equilibrative nucleoside transporters 1 and 2 may be differentially modulated by A2B adenosine receptors in placenta microvascular endothelial cells from pre-eclampsia. *Placenta* 29, 816–825. doi: 10.1016/j.placenta.2008.06.014

Espinoza, J., Espinoza, A. F., and Power, G. G. (2011). High fetal plasma adenosine concentration: a role for the fetus in preeclampsia? *Am. J. Obstet. Gynecol.* 485, e424–e487. doi: 10.1016/j.ajog.2011.06.034

Fenton, R. A., and Dobson, J. G. Jr. (1992). Fluorometric quantitation of adenosine concentration in small samples of extracellular fluid. *Anal. Biochem.* 207, 134–141. doi: 10.1016/0003-2697(92)90514-8

Figueredo, V. M., Diamond, I., Zhou, H. Z., and Albert Camacho, S. (1999). Chronic dipyridamole therapy produces sustained protection against cardiac ischemia-reperfusion injury. *Am. J. Physiol.* 277(5 Pt 2), H2091–H2097. doi: 10.1152/ajpheart.1999.277.5.H2091

Fredholm, B. B., IJzerman, A. P., Jacobson, K. A., Linden, J., and Müller, C. E. (2011). International Union of Basic and Clinical Pharmacology. LXXXI. Nomenclature and classification of adenosine receptors–an update. *Pharmacol. Rev.* 63, 1–34. doi: 10.1124/pr.110.003285

Godoy, V., Banales, J. M., Medina, J. F., and Pastor-Anglada, M. (2014). Functional crosstalk between the adenosine transporter CNT3 and purinergic receptors in the biliary epithelia. *J. Hepatol.* 61, 1337–1343. doi: 10.1016/j.jhep.2014.06.036

Gorraitz, E., Pastor-Anglada, M., and Lostao, M. P. (2010). Effects of Na+ and H+ on steady-state and presteady-state currents of the human concentrative nucleoside transporter 3 (hCNT3). *Pflugers Arch.* 460, 617–632. doi: 10.1007/s00424-010-0846-9

Govindarajan, R., Endres, C. J., Whittington, D., LeCluyse, E., Pastor-Anglada, M., Tse, C. M., et al. (2008). Expression and hepatobiliary transport characteristics of the concentrative and equilibrative nucleoside transporters in sandwich-cultured human hepatocytes. *Am. J. Physiol. Gastrointest. Liver Physiol.* 295, G570–G580. doi: 10.1152/ajpgi.00542.2007

Grañé-Boladeras, N., Spring, C. M., Hanna, W. J., Pastor-Anglada, M., and Coe, I. R. (2016). Novel nuclear hENT2 isoforms regulate cell cycle progression via controlling nucleoside transport and nuclear reservoir. *Cell Mol. Life Sci.* 73, 4559–4575. doi: 10.1007/s00018-016-2288-9

Grañé-Boladeras, N., Williams, D., McKenzie, T., and Naydenova, Z. (2002). Oligomerisation of Equilibrative Nucleoside Transporters: a novel regulatory and functional mechanism involving PKC and PP1. *FASEB J.* 517, 201–205.

Guallar, J. P., Cano-Soldado, P., Aymerich, I., Domingo, J. C., Alegre, M., Domingo, P., et al. (2007). Altered expression of nucleoside transporter genes (SLC28 and SLC29) in adipose tissue from HIV-1-infected patients. *Antivir. Ther.* 12, 853–863.

Guillén-Gómez, E., Calbet, M., Casado, J., de Lecea, L., Soriano, E., Pastor-Anglada, M., et al. (2004). Distribution of CNT2 and ENT1 transcripts in rat brain: selective decrease of CNT2 mRNA in the cerebral cortex of sleep-deprived rats. *J. Neurochem.* 90, 883–893. doi: 10.1111/j.1471-4159.2004.02545.x

Guillén-Gómez, E., Pinilla-Macua, I., Pérez-Torras, S., Choi, D. S., Arce, Y., Ballarín, J. A., et al. (2012). New role of the human equilibrative nucleoside transporter 1 (hENT1) in epithelial-to-mesenchymal transition in renal tubular cells. *J. Cell Physiol.* 227, 1521–1528. doi: 10.1002/jcp.22869

Hsu, C. L., Lin, W., Seshasayee, D., Chen, Y. H., Ding, X., Lin, Z., et al. (2012). Equilibrative nucleoside transporter 3 deficiency perturbs lysosome function and macrophage homeostasis. *Science* 335, 89–92. doi: 10.1126/science.1213682

Huang, Q. Q., Yao, S. Y., Ritzel, M. W., Paterson, A. R., Cass, C. E., Young, J. D., et al. (1994). Cloning and functional expression of a complementary DNA encoding a mammalian nucleoside transport protein. *J. Biol. Chem.* 269, 17757–17760.

Johnson, Z. L., Cheong, C. G., and Lee, S. Y. (2012). Crystal structure of a concentrative nucleoside transporter from *Vibrio cholerae* at 2.4 A. *Nature* 483, 489–493. doi: 10.1038/nature10882

Kang, N., Jun, A. H., Bhutia, Y. D., Kannan, N., Unadkat, J. D., and Govindarajan, R. (2010). Human equilibrative nucleoside transporter-3 (hENT3) spectrum disorder mutations impair nucleoside transport, protein localization, and stability. *J. Biol. Chem.* 285, 28343–28352. doi: 10.1074/jbc.M110.109199

Kretschmar, C., Oyarzún, C., Villablanca, C., Jaramillo, C., Alarcón, S., Perez, G., et al. (2016). Reduced adenosine uptake and its contribution to signaling that mediates profibrotic activation in renal tubular epithelial cells: implication in diabetic nephropathy. *PLoS One* 11:e0147430. doi: 10.1371/journal.pone.0147430

Kumar Deokar, H., Barch, H. P., Barch, H. P., and Buolamwini, J. K. (2017). Homology modeling of human concentrative nucleoside transporters (hCNTs)

and validation by virtual screening and experimental testing to identify novel hCNT1 Inhibitors. *Drug Des.* 6:146. doi: 10.4172/2169-0138.1000146

Lang, T. T., Young, J. D., and Cass, C. E. (2004). Interactions of nucleoside analogs, caffeine, and nicotine with human concentrative nucleoside transporters 1 and 2 stably produced in a transport-defective human cell line. *Mol. Pharmacol.* 65, 925–933. doi: 10.1124/mol.65.4.925

Larráyoz, I. M., Casado, F. J., Pastor-Anglada, M., and Lostao, M. P. (2004). Electrophysiological characterization of the human Na(+)/nucleoside cotransporter 1 (hCNT1) and role of adenosine on hCNT1 function. *J. Biol. Chem.* 279, 8999–9007. doi: 10.1074/jbc.M311940200

Larráyoz, I. M., Fernández-Nistal, A., Garcés, A., Gorraitz, E., and Lostao, M. P. (2006). Characterization of the rat Na+/nucleoside cotransporter 2 and transport of nucleoside-derived drugs using electrophysiological methods. *Am. J. Physiol. Cell Physiol.* 291, C1395–C1404. doi: 10.1152/ajpcell.00110.2006

Latek, D. (2017). Rosetta Broker for membrane protein structure prediction: concentrative nucleoside transporter 3 and corticotropin-releasing factor receptor 1 test cases. *BMC Struct. Biol.* 17:8. doi: 10.1186/s12900-017-0078-8

Li, J. Y., Boado, R. J., and Pardridge, W. M. (2001). Differential kinetics of transport of 2′,3′-dideoxyinosine and adenosine via concentrative Na+ nucleoside transporter CNT2 cloned from rat blood-brain barrier. *J. Pharmacol. Exp. Ther.* 299, 735–740.

Lostao, M. P., Mata, J. F., Larrayoz, I. M., Inzillo, S. M., Casado, F. J., and Pastor-Anglada, M. (2000). Electrogenic uptake of nucleosides and nucleoside-derived drugs by the human nucleoside transporter 1 (hCNT1) expressed in Xenopus laevis oocytes. *FEBS Lett.* 481, 137–140. doi: 10.1016/S0014-5793(00)01983-9

Mackey, J. R., Mani, R. S., Selner, M., Mowles, D., Young, J. D., Belt, J. A., et al. (1998). Functional nucleoside transporters are required for gemcitabine influx and manifestation of toxicity in cancer cell lines. *Cancer Res.* 58, 4349–4357.

Marangos, P. J., Patel, J., Clark-Rosenberg, R., and Martino, A. M. (1982). [3H]nitrobenzylthioinosine binding as a probe for the study of adenosine uptake sites in brain. *J. Neurochem.* 39, 184–191. doi: 10.1111/j.1471-4159.1982.tb04717.x

Medina-Pulido, L., Molina-Arcas, M., Justicia, C., Soriano, E., Burgaya, F., Planas, A. M., et al. (2013). Hypoxia and P1 receptor activation regulate the high-affinity concentrative adenosine transporter CNT2 in differentiated neuronal PC12 cells. *Biochem. J.* 454, 437–445. doi: 10.1042/BJ20130231

Melani, A., Corti, F., Stephan, H., Müller, C. E., Donati, C., Bruni, P., et al. (2012). Ecto-ATPase inhibition: ATP and adenosine release under physiological and ischemic in vivo conditions in the rat striatum. *Exp. Neurol.* 233, 193–204. doi: 10.1016/j.expneurol.2011.09.036

Minuesa, G., Huber-Ruano, I., Pastor-Anglada, M., Koepsell, H., Clotet, B., and Martinez-Picado, J. (2011). Drug uptake transporters in antiretroviral therapy. *Pharmacol. Ther.* 132, 268–279. doi: 10.1016/j.pharmthera.2011.06.007

Minuesa, G., Volk, C., Molina-Arcas, M., Gorboulev, V., Erkizia, I., Arndt, P., et al. (2009). Transport of lamivudine [(-)-beta-L-2′,3′-dideoxy-3′-thiacytidine] and high-affinity interaction of nucleoside reverse transcriptase inhibitors with human organic cation transporters 1, 2, and 3. *J. Pharmacol. Exp. Ther.* 329, 252–261. doi: 10.1124/jpet.108.146225

Mulinta, R., Yao, S. Y. M., Ng, A. M. L., Cass, C. E., and Young, J. D. (2017). Substituted cysteine accessibility method (SCAM) analysis of the transport domain of human concentrative nucleoside transporter 3 (hCNT3) and other family members reveals features of structural and functional importance. *J. Biol. Chem.* 292, 9505–9522. doi: 10.1074/jbc.M116.743997

Muñoz, G., San Martín, R., Farías, M., Cea, L., Vecchiola, A., Casanello, P., et al. (2006). Insulin restores glucose inhibition of adenosine transport by increasing the expression and activity of the equilibrative nucleoside transporter 2 in human umbilical vein endothelium. *J. Cell Physiol.* 209, 826–835. doi: 10.1002/jcp.20769

Nagy, L. E., Diamond, I., Casso, D. J., Franklin, C., and Gordon, A. S. (1990). Ethanol increases extracellular adenosine by inhibiting adenosine uptake via the nucleoside transporter. *J. Biol. Chem.* 265, 1946–1951.

Nehlig, A., and Debry, G. (1994). Potential teratogenic and neurodevelopmental consequences of coffee and caffeine exposure: a review on human and animal data. *Neurotoxicol. Teratol.* 16, 531–543. doi: 10.1016/0892-0362(94)90032-9

Nguyen, M. D., Ross, A. E., Ryals, M., Lee, S. T., and Venton, B. J. (2015). Clearance of rapid adenosine release is regulated by nucleoside transporters and metabolism. *Pharmacol. Res. Perspect.* 3:e00189. doi: 10.1002/prp2.189

Oliveros, A., Starski, P., Lindberg, D., Choi, S., Heppelmann, C. J., Dasari, S., et al. (2017). Label-Free neuroproteomics of the hippocampal-accumbal circuit reveals deficits in neurotransmitter and neuropeptide signaling in mice lacking ethanol-sensitive adenosine transporter. *J. Proteome Res.* 16, 1445–1459. doi: 10.1021/acs.jproteome.6b00830

Pardo, F., Arroyo, P., Salomón, C., Westermeier, F., Salsoso, R., Sáez, T., et al. (2013). Role of equilibrative adenosine transporters and adenosine receptors as modulators of the human placental endothelium in gestational diabetes mellitus. *Placenta* 34, 1121–1127. doi: 10.1016/j.placenta.2013.09.007

Parkinson, F. E., Damaraju, V. L., Graham, K., Yao, S. Y., Baldwin, S. A., Cass, C. E., et al. (2011). Molecular biology of nucleoside transporters and their distributions and functions in the brain. *Curr. Top. Med. Chem.* 11, 948–972. doi: 10.2174/156802611795347582

Pastor-Anglada, M., Urtasun, N., and Pérez-Torras, S. (2018). Intestinal nucleoside transporters: function, expression and regulation. *Comp. Physiol.* (in press).

Pérez-Torras, S., Iglesias, I., Llopis, M., Lozano, J. J., Antolín, M., Guarner, F., et al. (2016). Transportome profiling identifies profound alterations in crohn's disease partially restored by commensal bacteria. *J. Crohns Colitis* 10, 850–859. doi: 10.1093/ecco-jcc/jjw042

Pickard, M. A., Brown, R. R., Paul, B., and Paterson, A. R. (1973). Binding of the nucleoside transport inhibitor 4-nitrobenzylthioinosine to erythrocyte membranes. *Can. J. Biochem.* 51, 666–672. doi: 10.1139/o73-083

Pinto-Duarte, A., Coelho, J. E., Cunha, R. A., Ribeiro, J. A., and Sebastião, A. M. (2005). Adenosine A2A receptors control the extracellular levels of adenosine through modulation of nucleoside transporters activity in the rat hippocampus. *J. Neurochem.* 93, 595–604. doi: 10.1111/j.1471-4159.2005.03071.x

Rahman, M. F., Askwith, C., and Govindarajan, R. (2017). Molecular determinants of acidic pH-dependent transport of human equilibrative nucleoside transporter 3. *J. Biol. Chem.* 292, 14775–14785. doi: 10.1074/jbc.M117.787952

Ritzel, M. W., Ng, A. M., Yao, S. Y., Graham, K., Loewen, S. K., Smith, K. M., et al. (2001). Molecular identification and characterization of novel human and mouse concentrative Na+-nucleoside cotransporter proteins (hCNT3 and mCNT3) broadly selective for purine and pyrimidine nucleosides (system cib). *J. Biol. Chem.* 276, 2914–2927. doi: 10.1074/jbc.M007746200

Roa, H., Gajardo, C., Troncoso, E., Fuentealba, V., Escudero, C., Yáñez, A., et al. (2009). Adenosine mediates transforming growth factor-beta 1 release in kidney glomeruli of diabetic rats. *FEBS Lett.* 583, 3192–3198. doi: 10.1016/j.febslet.2009.09.003

Rose, J. B., Naydenova, Z., Bang, A., Eguchi, M., Sweeney, G., Choi, D. S., et al. (2010). Equilibrative nucleoside transporter 1 plays an essential role in cardioprotection. *Am. J. Physiol. Heart Circ. Physiol.* 298, H771–H777. doi: 10.1152/ajpheart.00711.2009

Rose, J. B., Naydenova, Z., Bang, A., Ramadan, A., Klawitter, J., Schram, K., et al. (2011). Absence of equilibrative nucleoside transporter 1 in ENT1 knockout mice leads to altered nucleoside levels following hypoxic challenge. *Life Sci.* 89, 621–630. doi: 10.1016/j.lfs.2011.08.007

Salomón, C., Westermeier, F., Puebla, C., Arroyo, P., Guzmán-Gutiérrez, E., Pardo, F., et al. (2012). Gestational diabetes reduces adenosine transport in human placental microvascular endothelium, an effect reversed by insulin. *PLoS One* 7:e40578. doi: 10.1371/journal.pone.0040578

Schnermann, J. (2015). Concurrent activation of multiple vasoactive signaling pathways in vasoconstriction caused by tubuloglomerular feedback: a quantitative assessment. *Annu. Rev. Physiol.* 77, 301–322. doi: 10.1146/annurev-physiol-021014-071829

Slugoski, M. D., Smith, K. M., Mulinta, R., Ng, A. M., Yao, S. Y., Morrison, E. L., et al. (2008). A conformationally mobile cysteine residue (Cys-561) modulates Na+ and H+ activation of human CNT3. *J. Biol. Chem.* 283, 24922–24934. doi: 10.1074/jbc.M801793200

Smith, K. M., Ng, A. M., Yao, S. Y., Labedz, K. A., Knaus, E. E., Wiebe, L. I., et al. (2004). Electrophysiological characterization of a recombinant human Na+-coupled nucleoside transporter (hCNT1) produced in Xenopus oocytes. *J. Physiol.* 558(Pt 3), 807–823.

Sobrevia, L., Abarzúa, F., Nien, J. K., Salomón, C., Westermeier, F., Puebla, C., et al. (2011). Review: differential placental macrovascular and microvascular endothelial dysfunction in gestational diabetes. *Placenta* 32(Suppl. 2), S159–S164. doi: 10.1016/j.placenta.2010.12.011

Soler, C., Felipe, A., Mata, J. F., Casado, F. J., Celada, A., Pastor-Anglada, M., et al. (1998). Regulation of nucleoside transport by lipopolysaccharide, phorbol esters, and tumor necrosis factor-alpha in human B-lymphocytes. *J. Biol. Chem.* 273, 26939–26945. doi: 10.1074/jbc.273.41.26939

Soler, C., Valdés, R., Garcia-Manteiga, J., Xaus, J., Comalada, M., Casado, F. J., et al. (2001). Lipopolysaccharide-induced apoptosis of macrophages determines the up-regulation of concentrative nucleoside transporters Cnt1 and Cnt2 through tumor necrosis factor-alpha-dependent and -independent mechanisms. *J. Biol. Chem.* 276, 30043–30049. doi: 10.1074/jbc.M101807200

Ward, J. L., Sherali, A., Mo, Z. P., and Tse, C. M. (2000). Kinetic and pharmacological properties of cloned human equilibrative nucleoside transporters, ENT1 and ENT2, stably expressed in nucleoside transporter-deficient PK15 cells. Ent2 exhibits a low affinity for guanosine and cytidine but a high affinity for inosine. *J. Biol. Chem.* 275, 8375–8381. doi: 10.1074/jbc.275.12.8375

Westermeier, F., Salomón, C., González, M., Puebla, C., Guzmán-Gutiérrez, E., Cifuentes, F., et al. (2011). Insulin restores gestational diabetes mellitus-reduced adenosine transport involving differential expression of insulin receptor isoforms in human umbilical vein endothelium. *Diabetes* 60, 1677–1687. doi: 10.2337/db11-0155

Yang, C., and Leung, G. P. (2015). Equilibrative nucleoside transporters 1 and 4: which one is a better target for cardioprotection against ischemia-reperfusion injury? *J. Cardiovasc. Pharmacol.* 65, 517–521. doi: 10.1097/FJC.0000000000000194

Yao, S. Y., Ng, A. M., Ritzel, M. W., Gati, W. P., Cass, C. E., and Young, J. D. (1996). Transport of adenosine by recombinant purine- and pyrimidine-selective sodium/nucleoside cotransporters from rat jejunum expressed in Xenopus laevis oocytes. *Mol. Pharmacol.* 50, 1529–1535.

Young, J. D. (2016). The SLC28 (CNT) and SLC29 (ENT) nucleoside transporter families: a 30-year collaborative odyssey. *Biochem. Soc. Trans.* 44, 869–876. doi: 10.1042/BST20160038

Young, J. D., Yao, S. Y., Baldwin, J. M., Cass, C. E., and Baldwin, S. A. (2013). The human concentrative and equilibrative nucleoside transporter families, SLC28 and SLC29. *Mol. Aspects Med.* 34, 529–547. doi: 10.1016/j.mam.2012.05.007

Zamzow, C. R., Xiong, W., and Parkinson, F. E. (2008). Adenosine produced by neurons is metabolized to hypoxanthine by astrocytes. *J. Neurosci. Res.* 86, 3447–3455. doi: 10.1002/jnr.21789

Zhang, D., Xiong, W., Albensi, B. C., and Parkinson, F. E. (2011). Expression of human equilibrative nucleoside transporter 1 in mouse neurons regulates adenosine levels in physiological and hypoxic-ischemic conditions. *J. Neurochem.* 118, 4–11. doi: 10.1111/j.1471-4159.2011.07242.x

Zimmerman, M. A., Tak, E., Ehrentraut, S. F., Kaplan, M., Giebler, A., Weng, T., et al. (2013). Equilibrative nucleoside transporter (ENT)-1-dependent elevation of extracellular adenosine protects the liver during ischemia and reperfusion. *Hepatology* 58, 1766–1778. doi: 10.1002/hep.26505

2

Microglia $P2Y_{13}$ Receptors Prevent Astrocyte Proliferation Mediated by $P2Y_1$ Receptors

*Clara Quintas[1,2], Nuno Vale[1,3], Jorge Gonçalves[1,4] and Glória Queiroz[1,4]**

[1] *Laboratory of Pharmacology, Department of Drug Sciences, Faculty of Pharmacy, University of Porto, Porto, Portugal,*
[2] *REQUIMTE/LAQV, University of Porto, Porto, Portugal,* [3] *REQUIMTE/UCIBIO, University of Porto, Porto, Portugal,*
[4] *MedInUP, University of Porto, Porto, Portugal*

***Correspondence:**
Glória Queiroz
gloria@ff.up.pt

Cerebral inflammation is a common feature of several neurodegenerative diseases that requires a fine interplay between astrocytes and microglia to acquire appropriate phenotypes for an efficient response to neuronal damage. During brain inflammation, ATP is massively released into the extracellular medium and converted into ADP. Both nucleotides acting on P2 receptors, modulate astrogliosis through mechanisms involving microglia-astrocytes communication. In previous studies, primary cultures of astrocytes and co-cultures of astrocytes and microglia were used to investigate the influence of microglia on astroglial proliferation induced by ADPβS, a stable ADP analog. In astrocyte cultures, ADPβS increased cell proliferation through activation of $P2Y_1$ and $P2Y_{12}$ receptors, an effect abolished in co-cultures (of astrocytes with ~12.5% microglia). The possibility that the loss of the ADPβS-mediated effect could have been caused by a microglia-induced degradation of ADPβS or by a preferential microglial localization of $P2Y_1$ or $P2Y_{12}$ receptors was excluded. Since ADPβS also activates $P2Y_{13}$ receptors, the contribution of microglial $P2Y_{13}$ receptors to prevent the proliferative effect of ADPβS in co-cultures was investigated. The results obtained indicate that $P2Y_{13}$ receptors are low expressed in astrocytes and mainly expressed in microglia. Furthermore, in co-cultures, ADPβS induced astroglial proliferation in the presence of the selective $P2Y_{13}$ antagonist MRS 2211 (3 μM) and of the selective $P2Y_{12}$ antagonist AR-C66096 (0.1 μM), suggesting that activation of microglial $P2Y_{12}$ and $P2Y_{13}$ receptors may induce the release of messengers that inhibit astroglial proliferation mediated by $P2Y_{1,12}$ receptors. In this microglia-astrocyte paracrine communication, $P2Y_{12}$ receptors exert opposite effects in astroglial proliferation as a result of its cellular localization: cooperating in astrocytes with $P2Y_1$ receptors to directly stimulate proliferation and in microglia with $P2Y_{13}$ receptors to prevent proliferation. IL-1β also attenuated the proliferative effect of ADPβS in astrocyte cultures. However, in co-cultures, the anti-IL-1β antibody was unable to recover the ADPβS-proliferative effect, an effect that was achieved by the anti-IL-1α and anti-TNF-α antibodies. It is concluded that microglia control the $P2Y_{1,12}$ receptor-mediated astroglial proliferation through a $P2Y_{12,13}$ receptor-mediated mechanism alternative to the IL-1β suppressive pathway that may involve the contribution of the cytokines IL-1α and TNF-α.

Keywords: $P2Y_{13}$ receptors, $P2Y_1$ receptors, microglia, cell proliferation, astrocyte-microglia communication, IL-1β, anti-IL-1α, anti-TNF-α

INTRODUCTION

Astrocytes and microglia respond to all types of central nervous system (CNS) insults, undergoing through several morphological and functional changes to adapt to the requirements of the surrounding inflammatory response. Microglia initiate a response that starts with their activation and with a rapid mobilization to the site of injury, to phagocyte death cells and to remove cell debris (Hanisch and Kettenmann, 2007). Astrocytes also become reactive, coursing with glial fibrillary acidic protein up-regulation, hypertrophy and, in some cases, proliferation, to form a glial scar that limits the damaged area and prevents widespread inflammation (Sofroniew, 2014).

Pro-inflammatory cytokines attain high extracellular concentrations at the early stages of the inflammatory response and trigger, or modulate, the course of astrogliosis (Buffo et al., 2010). Since microglia are the main source of inflammatory mediators, these cells are regarded as active players in orchestrating the progression of astrogliosis. Microglia activation, and an increase in microglia-derived mediators, are primary events that occur in the inflammatory response, even before the astrocytes response (Zhang et al., 2010), supporting the relevance of a continuous communication between microglia and astrocytes during inflammatory insults, to control astrogliosis.

Purinergic signaling plays a central role in the microglia-astrocyte communication during the CNS inflammatory response. Nucleotides, leaked from dying or damaged cells, act as damage-associated molecular patterns, signaling the damage and triggering different actions through activation of ionotropic P2X or metabotropic P2Y receptors, expressed in astrocytes and microglia (Di Virgilio et al., 2009). For example, ATP and its metabolite ADP, activate microglia $P2Y_1$, $P2Y_{12}$ and $P2X_4$ receptors (Ohsawa et al., 2007; De Simone et al., 2010) that act as sensors to guide microglia to the site where the inflammatory response is occurring (Davalos et al., 2005). In astrocytes, activation of $P2Y_1$ and $P2Y_{12}$ receptors causes hypertrophy and stimulates proliferation, to create the glial scar that confines the lesion site, restraining the secondary neuronal damage (Franke et al., 2004; Quintas et al., 2011a).

It is also known that inflammatory mediators, released by microglia, modulate the expression and function of G protein-coupled receptors that induce an increase in $[Ca^{2+}]_i$ in astrocytes (Hamby et al., 2012). $P2Y_1$ receptors are metabotropic receptors which, in astrocytes, mediate an increase in $[Ca^{2+}]_i$ (Fischer et al., 2009) and trigger astroglial proliferation, an hallmark of astrogliosis (Franke et al., 2004). Therefore, it is expectable that microglia inflammatory mediators may modulate $P2Y_1$ receptors activity and consequently, influence astrogliosis progression.

We have previously confirmed that astroglial proliferation may be induced not only by activation of astrocyte $P2Y_1$ receptors, but also by $P2Y_{12}$ receptors (Quintas et al., 2011a). It was further demonstrated that $P2Y_{1,12}$ receptor-mediated astroglial proliferation is inhibited in co-cultures of astrocytes and microglia, when microglia P2Y receptors are also activated (Quintas et al., 2011b). In those studies, it was excluded the possibility that the loss of the ADPβS-mediated effect could have been caused by a microglia-induced metabolisation of the compound or by a preferential microglial localization of $P2Y_1$ or $P2Y_{12}$ receptors, but it was evident that microglial P2Y receptors induced the release of diffusible paracrine mediator(s) to prevent ADPβS-mediated astroglial proliferation. Since ADPβS also activates $P2Y_{13}$ receptors, this subtype arise as a promising candidate to mediate this microglia-astrocytes communication.

Expression of $P2Y_{13}$ receptors was previously detected in microglia from the whole brain of mice (Crain et al., 2009), but also in astrocytes of several brain regions (Fumagalli et al., 2004; Carrasquero et al., 2005; Fischer et al., 2009), and functional studies support the relevance of these receptor subtypes in both types of cells. $P2Y_{13}$ receptors activation was shown to elicit $[Ca^{2+}]_i$ increase in microglia (Zeng et al., 2014) and astrocytes (Carrasquero et al., 2009; Fischer et al., 2009) and to mediate the release of several pro-inflammatory cytokines by microglia, such as IL-1β, IL-6 and TNF-α (Liu et al., 2017).

In the previous studies, P2Y receptor-mediated astrocyte proliferation was induced by ADPβS, a stable ADP analog selective for $P2Y_1$, $P2Y_{12}$ and $P2Y_{13}$ receptors (Quintas et al., 2011a). However, the mechanisms behind this P2Y receptor-mediated communication between microglia and astrocytes are still largely unknown, namely the subtype of receptors involved and the identity of such mediator(s). Therefore, the aim of the present study was to clarify the role of each of these P2Y receptor subtypes in the microglia modulation of astroglial proliferation.

It is concluded that microglial $P2Y_{12}$ and $P2Y_{13}$ are the receptor subtypes involved in preventing astroglial proliferation mediated by ADPβS in co-cultures of astrocytes and microglia. As far as putative mediator(s) are concerned, the present study further shows that, in spite of all indications that microglia-derived IL-1β could be a strong candidate to prevent ADPβS-induced astroglial proliferation, the microglial P2Y receptor inhibition of astrocyte proliferation occurs through a IL-1β independent mechanism, which involves the release of IL-1α and TNF-α.

MATERIALS AND METHODS

Drugs and Antibodies

The following antibodies and drugs were used: goat anti-mouse IgG conjugated to Alexa Fluor 488 from Invitrogen (Barcelona, Spain); rabbit polyclonal anti-$P2Y_{13}$ from Alomone Laboratories (Jerusalem, Israel); mouse monoclonal anti-CD11b, and goat anti-rabbit IgG conjugated to horseradish peroxidase from Santa Cruz Biotechnology (Santa Cruz, CA, United States); 5-bromo-20-deoxyuridine (BrdU), rabbit polyclonal anti-BrdU, rabbit polyclonal anti-α tubulin, goat anti-rabbit IgG conjugated to Alexa Fluor 594 from Abcam (Cambridge, United Kingdom); rabbit and mouse anti-glial fibrillary acidic protein (anti-GFAP), recombinant rat interleukin-1β, rabbit polyclonal anti-interleukin-1β antibody, adenosine 5'-*O*-(3-thio)-diphosphate tetralithium (ADPβS), 2′-(4-hydroxyphenyl)-5-(4-methyl-1-piperazinyl)-2,5′-bi-1H-benzimidazole trihydrochloride hydrate (Hoechst 33258), penicillin and streptomycin from Sigma-Aldrich (Sintra, Portugal); 2-(propylthio)adenosine-5′-*O*-(β,γ-difluoromethylene)triphosphate tetrasodium (AR-C66096),

2-[(2-chloro-5-nitrophenyl) azo]-5-hydroxy-6-methyl-3-[(phosphonooxy)methyl]-4-pyridinecarboxaldehyde disodium (MRS 2211) and (1R*,2S*)-4-[2-Iodo-6-(methylamino)-9H-purin-9-yl]-2-(phosphonooxy)bicyclo[3.1.0]hexane-1-methanol dihydrogen phosphate ester tetraammonium (MRS 2500) from Tocris (Bristol, United Kingdom); *methyl*-[^{3}H]-thymidine (specific activity 80–86 Ci.mmol^{-1}) and enhanced chemiluminescence (ECL) Western blotting system from Amersham Biosciences (Lisbon, Portugal); goat polyclonal IL-1α antibody, mouse polyclonal TNF-α antibody from ThermoFisher Scientific (Lisbon, Portugal). Stock solutions of drugs were prepared with distilled water and kept at −20°C. Solutions of drugs were prepared from stock solutions diluted in culture medium immediately before use.

Cell Cultures

Animal handling and experiments were conducted according to the guidelines of the Directive 2010/63/EU of the European Parliament and the Council of the European Union and the Organismo Responsável pelo Bem-Estar Animal (ORBEA) from ICBAS-UP. Primary cortical astroglial cultures were prepared from offspring of Wistar rats (Charles River, Barcelona, Spain) as previously described (McCarthy and de Vellis, 1980). Briefly, the brains were placed in ice-cold Dulbecco's phosphate buffered calcium-free saline solution (DPBS) containing 0.2% glucose. The meninges and blood vessels were removed from hemispheres and after washing twice with ice-cold DPBS, they were cut into small pieces in culture medium, i.e., Dulbecco's modified Eagle medium containing 3.7 g/L $NaHCO_3$, 1.0 g/L D-glucose and stable glutamine, supplemented with 50 U/ml penicillin, 50 μg/ml streptomycin. Tissue from two hemispheres was dissociated by triturating in 10 ml culture medium. The cell suspension obtained was passed through a 40-μm pore nylon mesh and then centrifuged at 200 × *g* for 5 min and the supernatant discharged. Centrifugation followed by cell suspension was repeated twice and the pellet obtained was suspended in culture medium supplemented with 10% foetal bovine serum (FBS), and seeded at a density of 2 × 10^5cells/ml. Cultures were incubated at 37°C in a humidified atmosphere of 95% air, 5% CO_2 and the medium was replaced 1 day after preparation and subsequently twice a week. Confluent co-cultures of astrocytes and microglia were obtained at DIV14-18.

To prepare highly enriched astroglial cultures, that were named astrocytes cultures, confluent co-cultures were shaken overnight at 200 rpm to detach microglia sitting on the top of the astroglial monolayer and then trypsinized and subcultured to remove microglia trapped within the astroglial monolayer (Saura, 2007).

The suppernant obtained from confluent co-cultures after shaken overnight, which was enriched in microglia, was not discharged being used to prepared microglia cultures as previously described (Ni and Aschner, 2010; Deierborg, 2013). Briefly, the suppernant of shaken co-cultures was collect in 50 ml tubes previously cooled to 4°C and centrifuged at 1000 rpm for 10 min at 4°C. The supernant was discarded, the pellet obtained was resuspended in complete medium and cells were seeded at a density of 10^6 cells/ml. The surface of the supports used for culturing micoglia were previously coated with poly-L-lysine for better cell adhesion. To promote selective adhesion of microglia, culture medium was changed 1 h after seeding and replaced by complete medium containing 5 ng/ml M-CSF to promote microglial growth.

Co-cultures were used in experiments at DIV23. Highly enriched astrocyte cultures and microglia cultures were used at DIV6 after purification. All types of cultures were synchronized to a quiescent phase of the cell cycle, by shifting serum concentration to 0.1% FBS for 48 h before performing the experiments.

DNA Synthesis

At DIV23, cultures grown in 24-well plates, were incubated with ADPβS, IL-1β, or solvent for 48 h and methyl-[^{3}H]-thymidine was added to the medium in the last 24 h, at a concentration of 1 μCi/ml. When present, antagonists were added to the medium 1 h before ADPβS. IL-1β and the anti-ILs antibodies tested were added at the same time as ADPβS. At the end of the 48 h period of incubation, cells were rinsed with PBS, fixed with 10% of trichloroacetic acid for 30 min at 4°C, washed with ice-cold 5% trichloroacetic acid and rinsed again with PBS. Protein content and methyl-[^{3}H]-thymidine incorporation were evaluated after cell lysis with 0.2 M NaOH. The effect of drugs in cell proliferation was determined by *methyl*-[^{3}H]-thymidine incorporation, quantified by liquid scintillation spectrometry (Beckman LS 6500, Beckman Instruments, Fullerton, CA, United States) and normalized by the protein content determined by the Bradford method.

Immunocytochemistry

Cell cultures grown on 13 mm round coverslips were fixed in 4% paraformaldehyde and 4% sucrose in phosphate buffered saline (PBS; 100 mM NaH_2PO_4, 50 mM NaCl, pH adjusted to 7.3) and then incubated with 10% FBS, 1% bovine serum albumin, 0.1% Triton X, 0.05% NaN3 in PBS for 1 h. For double labeling astrocytes and microglia, and for $P2Y_{13}$ receptors localization, cultures were incubated overnight at 4°C with the following primary antibodies, diluted in 5% FBS, 1% bovine serum albumin, 0.1% Triton X, 0.05% NaN3 in PBS: rabbit or mouse anti-glial fibrillary acidic protein (anti-GFAP, 1:600), mouse anti-CD11b (1:50) and rabbit anti-$P2Y_{13}$ (1:200). Visualization of GFAP, CD11b and $P2Y_{13}$ receptors positive cells was accomplished upon 1 h incubation, at room temperature, with the secondary antibodies anti-rabbit IgG conjugated to Alexa Fluor 594 and anti-mouse IgG conjugated to Alexa Fluor 488 (both at 1:400). In negative controls, the primary antibody was omitted. Cell nuclei were labeled with Hoechst 33258 (5 μg/ml) for 1 min at room temperature. To evaluate the percentage of microglia, the two types of cultures were processed in parallel and about 200 cells were counted in each culture. The number of CD11b positive cells was expressed as percentage of the total number of cells counted. Images were captured with Lionheart^{TM} FX Automated Microscope (Biotek, United Kingdom).

BrdU Staining

In astrocyte cultures, proliferation of astrocytes or contaminating microglia was identified through double labeling of GFAP or CD11b and 5-bromo-20-deoxyuridine (BrdU) positive cells. Astrocytes cultures grown on 13 mm round coverslips were incubated with ADPβS 300 μM for 48 h. BrdU (100 μM) was added to the medium for the last 24 h, after which time the cells were incubated with mouse anti-CD11b (1:50) for 30 min at 37°C and then fixed with in 4% paraformaldehyde and 4% sucrose in PBS for 15 min at room temperature. Coverslips were washed with PBS and then incubated for 20 min with methanol to permeabilize the membranes. The BrdU epitope was exposed by incubating the cells in 2 M hydrochloric acid for 1 h at 37°C followed by neutralization with 0.1 M sodium borate, pH 8.5 for 20 min. Cell cultures were blocked with 3% FBS and then incubated with mouse anti-GFAP (1:600) and rabbit anti-BrdU (1:300) for 1 h, at room temperature. Visualization of GFAP or CD11b and BrdU positive cells was accomplished upon 1 h incubation, at room temperature, with the secondary antibodies anti-rabbit IgG conjugated to Alexa Fluor 594 and anti-mouse IgG conjugated to Alexa Fluor 488 (both at 1:400). In negative controls, the primary antibody was omitted. Images were captured with Lionheart^{TM} FX Automated Microscope (Biotek, United Kingdom).

Real Time RT-qPCR Analysis

RNA was extracted from astrocyte and microglia cultures with the RNeasy Mini Kit (QIAGEN), according to manufacturer's instructions. RNA purity and concentration was confirmed using a Synergy HT spectrophotometer (Biotek, United Kingdom). Nine hundred ng of RNA (astrocytes) or 70 ng of RNA (microglia) were used as a template for reverse-transcriptase reactions using the NZY First-Strand cDNA Synthesis kit (NZYTech). The primer sequences, listed in **Table 1**, were designed and evaluated with Beacon Designer^{TM} Software 7 (PREMIER Biosoft). Primer specificity was assessed through NCBI BLAST analysis prior to use and, for each sample following PCR, it was verified that the dissociation curve had a single peak with an observed Tm consistent with the amplicon length. Standard dilutions of the cDNA were used to check the relative efficiency and quality of primers. Negative controls (no template cDNA) were included in all qPCR.

qPCR amplifications were performed in duplicate, using 0.125 μM of each primer,10 μl of 2X iTaqTM Universal SYBR Green Supermix (Bio-Rad) and 1 μl of template cDNA. qPCRs were carried out on a CFX96 Touch^{TM} Real-Time PCR Detection System (Bio-Rad) and conditions were as follows: 95°C for 3 min followed by 40 cycles of denaturation at 95°C for 10 s, 60°C annealing temperature for 30 s. Melting curves of the PCR amplicons were then generated with temperatures ranging from 55°C to 95°C, with increments of 0.5°C at a rate of 10 s/step. The melting curve data were analyzed with the CFX Manager^{TM} (ver. 2.0, Bio-Rad). The data obtained were analyzed using the method described by Pfaffl (2001). Ct values from duplicate measurements were averaged, and relative expression levels were determined by the $2^{-\Delta C_T}$ method. While PCRs were run to 40 cycles, all detected genes had Ct values below 31 in all of the samples examined. For each analysis GAPDH and β-actin were used for normalization.

Western Blot Analysis

Cell cultures were rinsed with ice-cold PBS and total cell protein extracted in lysis buffer with protease inhibitors (1 mM Na_3VO_4, 1 mM NaF, 1 mM PMSF, 2 μg/ml aprotinin and 2 μg/ml leupeptin). Ceramic beads with 1.4 mm were added to the samples, which were disrupted with two cycles of 15 s at 5800 rpm in the Precellys Evolution homogenizer (Bertin Instruments, France). The lysate was incubated on ice for 1 h and then centrifuged at 20,000 × *g* for 45 min at 4°C. The protein concentration was determined in the supernatant and equal amounts of protein (50 μg) were boiled at 70°C for 10 min in 6x sample buffer (0.35 M Tris–HCl at pH 6.8, 10% SDS, 30% glycerol, 9.3% dithiothreitol, 0.01% bromphenol blue, 5% mercaptoethanol) and subjected to 12% SDS-PAGE (SDS-polyacrylamide gel electrophoresis). Proteins were electrotransferred onto nitrocellulose membranes overnight at 40 V in transfer buffer. Membranes were blocked at room temperature for 2 h with 5% of bovine serum albumin in PBS, and then probed for 2 h at room temperature with primary polyclonal antibody rabbit anti-$P2Y_{13}$ (1:200) followed by the secondary antibody goat anti-rabbit IgG conjugated to horseradish peroxidase (1:10,000). Immunoblots were then stripped by incubation in stripping buffer (62.5 mM Tris-HCl, 100 mM 2-mercaptoethanol and 2% SDS, pH adjusted to 6.8) for 15 min at 50°C and blocked overnight with 5% of bovine serum albumin in PBS. Subsequently, membranes were re-probed with the primary polyclonal antibody rabbit anti-atubulin (1:1000) for 1 h at room temperature, followed by the secondary antibody. Immunocomplexes were detected using Novex ECL Chemiluminescent kit (Life Technologies) and ChemiDoc MP Imaging System (Bio-Rad, Portugal).

TABLE 1 | Primer sequence table.

Gene	Forward primer	Reverse primer
$P2Y_1$	5′-CTGATCTTGGGCTGTTATGG-3′	5′-GCTGTTGAGACTTGCTAGAC-3′
$P2Y_{12}$	5′-TGTTCCTGCTGTCACTGCCTAA-3′	5′-CTCGTGCCAGACCAGACCAA-3′
$P2Y_{13}$	5′-TGCACTTTCTCATCCGTGGT-3′	5′-GGCAGGGAGATGAGGAACAT-3′
β-actin	5′-CTGTGCTATGTTGCCCTA-3′	5′-CCGATAGTGATGACCTGAC-3′
GAPDH	5′-TTCAACGGCACAGTCAAG-3′	5′-TACTCAGCACCAGCATCA-3′

Statistical Analysis

Data are expressed as means ± standard errors of the mean (S.E.M.) from n independent cell cultures tested in triplicated, or duplicated in qRT-PCR experiments. Statistical analysis was carried out using the unpaired Student's *t*-test or one-way analysis of variance (ANOVA) followed by Dunnett's multiple comparison test. Statistical analysis performed on $2^{-\Delta C_T}$ data was carried out using one-way ANOVA followed by Bonferroni's *post hoc* comparisons tests. *P*-values lower than 0.05 were considered to indicate significant differences.

RESULTS

Characterization of Glial Cultures

Two types of cell cultures were prepared, astrocytes being the predominant cell type. When no treatment was applied, cultures could be described as a monolayer of astrocytes containing a significant percentage of microglia 12.5 ± 0.2% ($n = 4$). Cultures obtained under these conditions were named astrocyte-microglia co-cultures or, more briefly, co-cultures. Confluent astrocyte-microglia co-cultures were treated to eliminate microglia (see section "Materials and Methods"), resulting in cell cultures of astrocytes with much less microglia (1.6 ± 0.1%; $n = 4$). Cultures obtained under these conditions were named astrocyte cultures. Both types of cultures, co-cultures and astrocyte cultures, were used in the experiments to identify microglia P2Y receptor subtype(s) and to explore potential paracrine mechanisms involved in the control of the ADPβS-induced astroglial proliferation.

Glial P2Y Receptor Subtype(s) Involved in the Modulation of ADPβS-Induced Astroglial Proliferation

The proliferative effect of ADPβS was compared in astrocyte cultures and in co-cultures to clarify the influence of microglia in the astrocyte proliferation elicited by this more stable ADP analog, selective for $P2Y_1$, $P2Y_{12}$ and $P2Y_{13}$ receptors.

In astrocyte cultures, ADPβS (1–300 μM), increased astroglial proliferation in a concentration-dependent manner, up to 201 ± 10% ($n = 4$; **Figure 1**). Although astroglial cultures had about 2% of contaminating microglia (see above), proliferation of astrocytes and microglia was differentiated through a double labeling of GFAP or CD11b with 5-bromo-20-deoxyuridine (BrdU), to identify the type of BrdU positive cells. The results indicate that the main proliferating cells, the BrdU positive cells, were astrocytes (**Figure 2**).

The proliferative effect caused by ADPβS (300 μM) was antagonized by MRS 2500 (1 μM), a selective antagonist of $P2Y_1$ receptor, by AR-C66096 (0.1 μM), a selective antagonist of $P2Y_{12}$ receptor, but not by MRS 2211 (3 μM), a selective antagonist of $P2Y_{13}$ receptor (**Figure 2A**). No additive antagonism was observed when both MRS 2500 (1 μM) and AR-C66096 (0.1 μM) were tested simultaneously (**Figure 3A**).

In co-cultures, ADPβS failed to cause astroglial proliferation. However, the ADPβS-induced astroglial proliferation was almost restored in the presence of MRS 2211 (3 μM), reaching proliferation levels similar to those observed in astrocyte cultures, and only partially restored by AR-C66096 (0.1 μM). When $P2Y_{12}$ and $P2Y_{13}$ receptors were blocked simultaneously, ADPβS proliferative effect was similar to that observed in the presence of the $P2Y_{13}$ antagonist alone (**Figure 3B**).

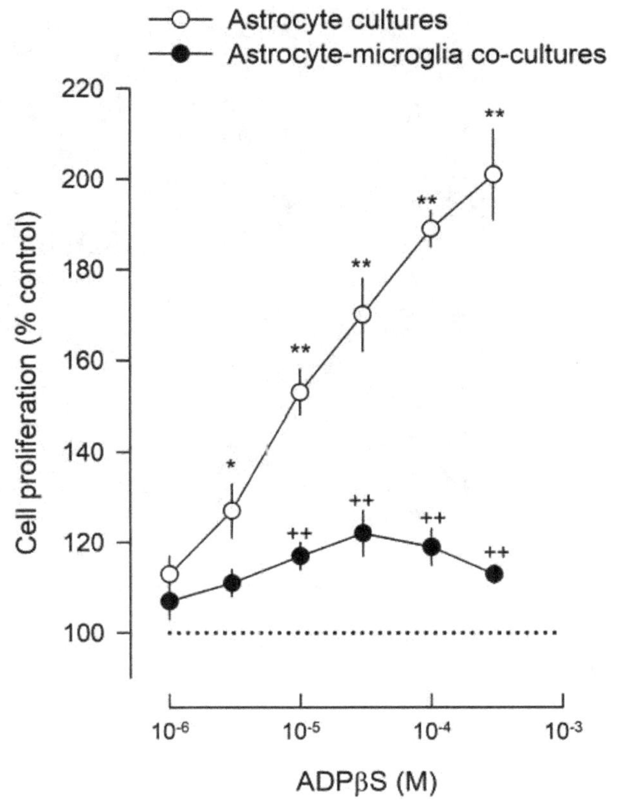

FIGURE 1 | Astroglial proliferation in astrocyte cultures and astrocyte-microglia co-cultures induced by ADPβS. Cultures were incubated with ADPβS or solvent for 48 h and *methyl*-[^{3}H]-thymidine (1 μCi/ml) was added in the last 24 h. Cell proliferation was estimated by *methyl*-[^{3}H]-thymidine incorporation and expressed in percentage of control. Values are means ± SEM from 4 different cultures. $^*P < 0.05$ and $^{**}P < 0.01$, significant differences from control (solvent). $^{++}P < 0.01$, significant differences from the ADPβS in astrocyte cultures.

Expression and Cellular Localization of $P2Y_{13}$ in Glial Cultures

$P2Y_1$ and $P2Y_{12}$ receptor subtypes are known to be expressed both in astrocytes (Fumagalli et al., 2003; Franke et al., 2004; Amadio et al., 2010) and microglia (Bianco et al., 2005; Ohsawa et al., 2007; De Simone et al., 2010) and expression levels of these receptor subtypes was found to be similar in both types of cultures, without any predominant cell-type localization (Quintas et al., 2011b). Therefore, considering these observations, and the results from the pharmacological approach, it remains to be explored a putative role for $P2Y_{13}$ receptor as candidate to mediate the loss of ADPβS-induced astroglial proliferation in co-cultures. Therefore, the expression of $P2Y_{13}$ receptors was

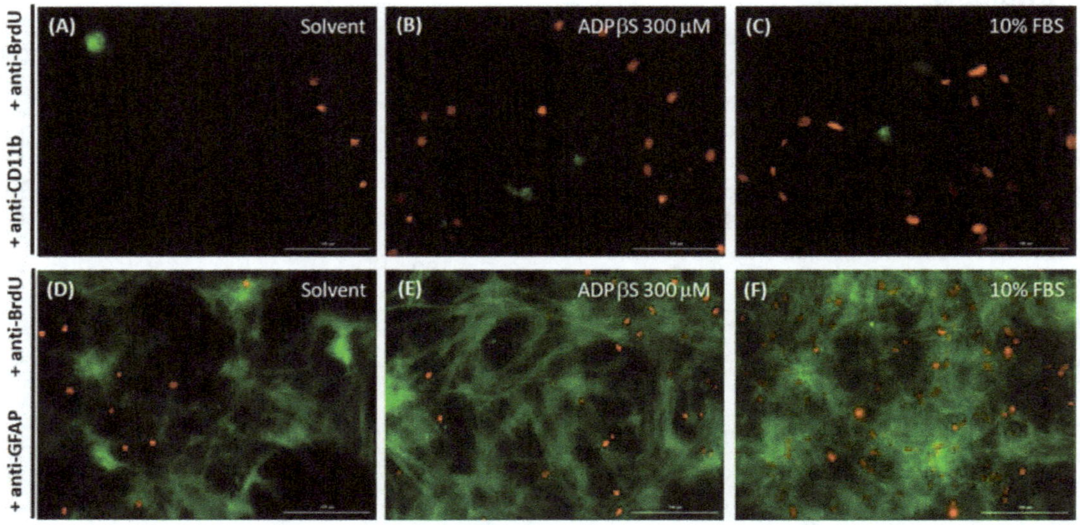

FIGURE 2 | BrdU staining and its cellular localization in astrocyte cultures. Astrocyte cultures were incubated with solvent **(A,D)**, ADPβS **(B,E)** or 10% FBS, a positive control for cell proliferation **(C,F)**, for 48 h. BrdU (100 μM) was added to the medium for the last 24 h and then stained with rabbit anti-BrdU (Alexa Fluor 594, red) to visualize BrdU incorporation. Microglia were then co-labeled with mouse anti-Cd11b (**A–C**; Alexa Fluor 488, green) and astrocytes, with mouse anti-GFAP (**D–F**; Alexa Fluor 488, green). BrdU positive nuclei co-localize mainly with astrocytes, showing they are the main proliferating cells within the astrocyte cultures. Representative images from 3 different cultures. Scale bar: 100 μm.

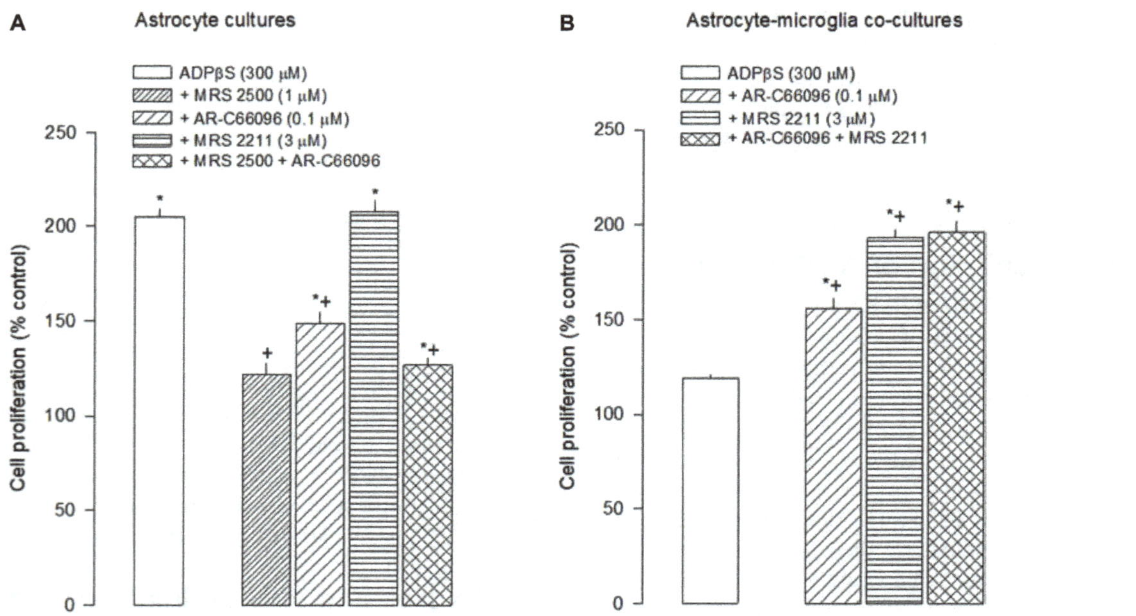

FIGURE 3 | Pharmacological characterization of P2Y receptors involved in the modulation of ADPβS-mediated astroglial proliferation. **(A)** Astrocyte cultures and **(B)** astrocyte-microglia co-cultures were incubated with ADPβS or solvent for 48 h and *methyl*-[^{3}H]-thymidine (1 μCi/mL) was added in the last 24 h. The P2Y antagonists: MRS 2500 (anti-P2Y$_1$R), AR-C66096 (anti-P2Y$_{12}$R) and MRS 2211 (anti-P2Y$_{13}$R) were added to the medium 1 h before ADPβS. Cell proliferation was estimated by *methyl*-[^{3}H]-thymidine incorporation and expressed in percentage of control. Values are means ± SEM from 6 to 10 different cultures. *$P < 0.05$, significant differences from control (solvent). $^+P < 0.05$, significant differences from ADPβS alone.

further analyzed in both types of cultures and their cellular localization was characterized in co-cultures.

In western blot assays, P2Y$_{13}$ receptors expression was evidenced by two immunoreactive bands of 32 and 52 kDa that reacted with the anti-P2Y$_{13}$ antibody. These bands were absent in the presence of the P2Y$_{13}$ neutralizing peptide, indicating they represent specific epitopes for the anti-P2Y$_{13}$ receptor antibody (**Figure 4A**, see also Supplementary Material). qRT-PCR experiments confirm the expression of the three receptor subtypes in astrocyte cultures, despite the significant lower

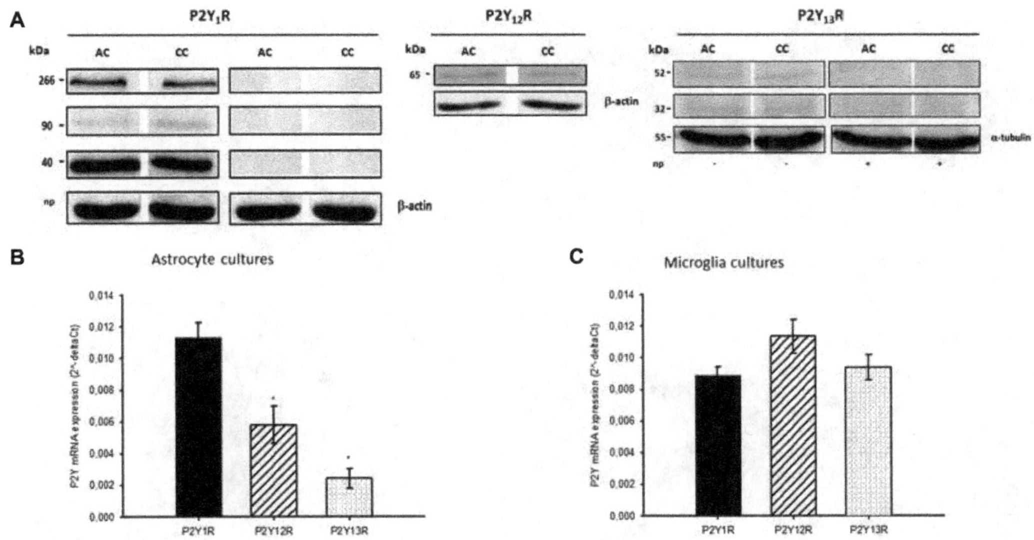

FIGURE 4 | Expression of $P2Y_1$, $P2Y_{12}$ and $P2Y_{13}$ receptors. **(A)** Representative Western blots of $P2Y_1$, $P2Y_{12}$ and $P2Y_{13}$ receptors ($P2Y_1R$, $P2Y_{12}R$ and $P2Y_{13}R$) expression in astrocyte-microglia co-cultures (CC) and astrocyte cultures (AC). $P2Y_1R$, $P2Y_{12}R$ and β-actin (43 kDa) expression data previously published by Quintas et al. (2011a,b). $P2Y_{13}$ receptors ($P2Y_{13}R$) and α-tubulin (55 kDa) expression were obtained from whole cell lysates. Two immunoreactive bands of 32 and 52 kDa specifically reacted with rabbit anti-$P2Y_{13}$ antibody. These bands were absent in the presence of the respective neutralising peptide (np). mRNA expression of P2YR in **(B)** astrocyte cultures and **(C)** microglia cultures. mRNA P2YR expression were determined using qRT-PCR and normalized to GAPDH (astrocytes cultures) or β-actin (microglial). Values are means ± SEM from 3 different cultures. $^*P < 0.05$, significant differences from $P2Y_1R$ expression.

expression of $P2Y_{12}$ and $P2Y_{13}$ receptors, when compared to that of $P2Y_1$ receptors (**Figure 4B**). In contrast, the expression of these receptor subtypes was similar in microglia cultures (**Figure 4C**). The results obtained indicate that, even though at low expression levels, $P2Y_{13}$ receptors are present in co-cultures and astrocyte cultures and that both cell types, astrocytes and microglia, express the receptor.

Immunocytochemistry analysis of co-cultures, revealed low immunoreactivity for $P2Y_{13}$ receptors in astrocytes (**Figures 5A–C**), and a preferentially localization in microglial cells ($P2Y_{13}$ receptor subtype in red and the CD11b integrin in green; **Figures 5D–F**). Although astrocytes express $P2Y_{13}$ receptors, it is clear that $P2Y_{13}$ receptors are mostly localized in microglia, and thus, may have a more relevant role in controlling the ADPβS-induced astroglial proliferation through $P2Y_{1,12}$ receptors.

On the Microglia Paracrine Mediator That Prevents the ADPβS-Induced Astroglial Proliferation

Previous studies have shown that, in co-cultures, ADPβS activates microglia P2Y receptors, inducing release of non-identified diffusible messenger(s) that attenuated its proliferative effect in astrocytes (Quintas et al., 2011b). Interleukins are potential candidates, since recently it was demonstrated that activation of microglia $P2Y_{12,13}$ receptors induces the release of IL-1β, TNF-α and IL-6 (Liu et al., 2017). Furthermore, IL-1β has been shown to decrease the activity of $P2Y_1$ receptors (Scemes, 2008). In preliminary experiments, the presence of IL-1β was detected by ELISA in the supernatant of co-cultures treated with ADPβS (not shown). Therefore, it was hypothesized that activation of microglial $P2Y_{12,13}$ receptors by ADPβS may induce release of IL-1β from microglia, which in turn interacts with $P2Y_1$ receptors expressed in astrocytes, to prevent the ADPβS-induced astroglial proliferation.

In agreement with this hypothesis, in astrocyte cultures, IL-1β attenuated ADPβS-induced astroglial proliferation, and this effect was prevented by the anti-IL-1β antibody (**Figure 6A**), supporting the view that IL-1β has conditions to exert such role. Additionally, when tested alone, the anti-IL-1β antibody had no effect, suggesting that there is no significant tonic release of IL-1β by astrocytes or by the small percentage of contaminating microglia.

Considering the hypothesis that IL-1β could be the soluble messenger produced by microglia, responsible for preventing ADPβS-induced astroglial proliferation, the anti-IL-1β antibody was tested in co-cultures to investigate whether, after IL-1β neutralization, ADPβS was able to induce astroglial proliferation. In co-cultures, when tested alone, the anti-IL-1β antibody induced cell proliferation up to 142 ± 4 ($n = 5$; $P < 0.05$), suggesting the occurrence of a basal release of IL-1β by microglia exerting a tonic inhibition of astroglial proliferation. However, the anti-IL-1β antibody was unable to restore the ADPβS proliferative effect (**Figure 6B**), indicating that there is no additional significant release of IL-1β, when ADPβS activates microglial P2Y receptors (not shown).

Following the same hypothesis, and considering the contribution of activated microglia to the release of other interleukins, such as IL-1α and TNF-α (Liu et al., 2017; Liddelow et al., 2017), that have been shown to change de reactivity of astrocytes (Liddelow et al., 2017), the interaction between

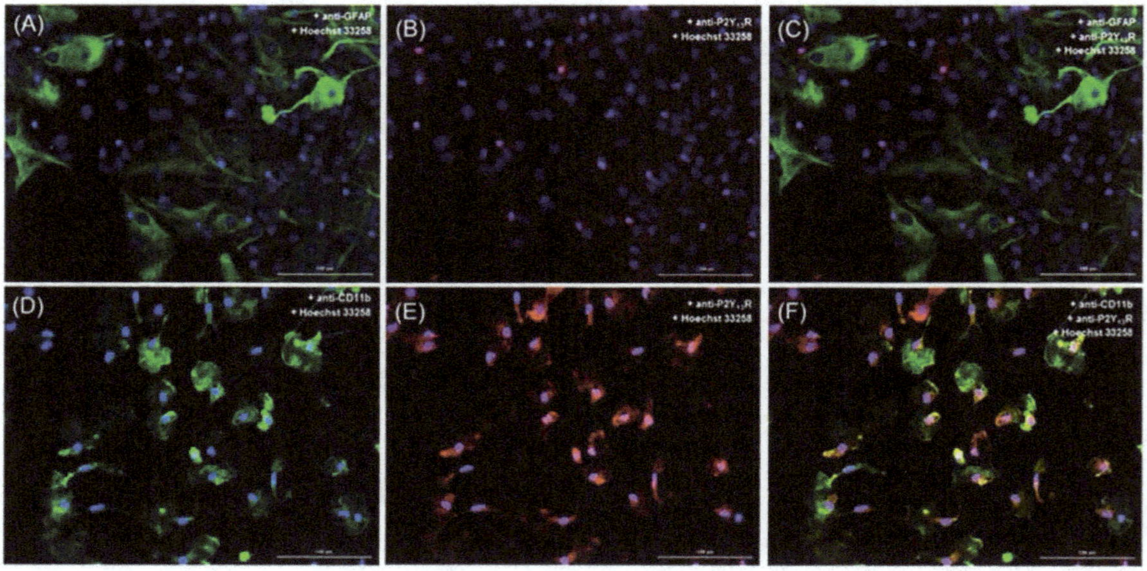

FIGURE 5 | Cellular distribution and localization of $P2Y_{13}$ receptors in astrocyte-microglia co-cultures. Astrocytes were double labeled with **(A)** mouse anti-GFAP (Alexa Fluor 488, green) and with **(B)** rabbit anti-$P2Y_{13}$ receptor (Alexa Fluor 594, red). Microglia were double labeled with **(D)** mouse anti-CD11b (Alexa Fluor 488, green) and with **(E)** rabbit anti-$P2Y_{13}$ receptor (Alexa Fluor 594, red). Nuclei were labeled with Hoechst 33258 (blue). $P2Y_{13}$ receptors (red) co-localize with astrocytes **(C)** but mainly with microglia **(F)**. Scale bar: 100 μm.

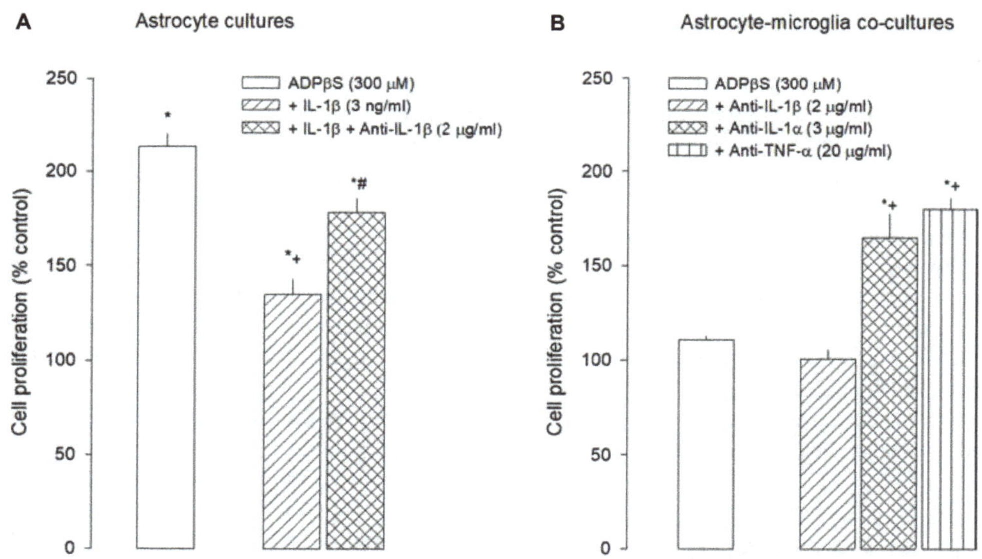

FIGURE 6 | Effect of IL-1β and anti-IL-1β antibody on proliferation induced by ADPβS in astrocyte cultures **(A)** and effect of antibodies anti-IL-1β, anti-IL-1α, and anti-TNF-α in proliferation induced by ADPβS on astrocyte-microglia co-cultures **(B)**. **(A)** Astrocyte cultures were incubated with ADPβS alone or in combination with IL-1β or IL-1β plus anti-IL-1β antibody for 48 h. **(B)** Astrocyte-microglia co-cultures were incubated with ADPβS or with anti-ILs antibodies alone or with ADPβS plus anti-ILs antibodies for 48 h. Anti-ILs antibodies, when present were added at the same time as ADPβS or solvent. *Methyl*-[^{3}H]-thymidine (1 μCi/mL) was added in the last 24 h and cell proliferation was estimated by *methyl*-[^{3}H]-thymidine incorporation and expressed in percentage of control. Values are means ± SEM from 4 to 5 different cultures. $^*P < 0.05$, significant differences from the respective control; $^+P < 0.05$, significant differences from ADPβS alone and $^\#P < 0.05$, significant differences from ADPβS plus the anti-IL-l1β antibody.

ADPβS and the antibodies anti-IL-1α and anti-TNF-α was tested in co-cultures. Unlike the anti-IL-1β antibody, both the anti-IL-1α and the anti-TNF-α antibodies had no effect when tested alone, but restored the ADPβS-proliferative effect to levels close to those observed in astrocyte cultures (**Figure 6B**). These results suggest that activation of microglia $P2Y_{12,13}$ receptors by ADPβS may induce the release of IL-1α and TNF-α that control astroglial proliferation.

DISCUSSION

Nucleotides, such as ATP and ADP are massively present in the extracellular medium during brain lesion, and were shown to activate P2Y receptors, modulating astroglial proliferation through mechanisms that involve communication between microglia and astrocytes (Quintas et al., 2011b). ADPβS is a stable ADP analog, selective for $P2Y_1$, $P2Y_{12}$, and $P2Y_{13}$ receptor subtypes, and was shown to cause cell proliferation in astrocyte cultures, an effect mediated by $P2Y_1$ and $P2Y_{12}$ receptors (Quintas et al., 2011a). The ADPβS-induced astroglial proliferation was abolished when the percentage of microglia cells increased to about 10–13% microglia (Quintas et al., 2011b). In these previous studies, it was excluded the possibility that a lower expression of $P2Y_1$ and/or $P2Y_{12}$ receptors, or a preferential microglial localization of these P2Y receptor subtypes could explain the absence of ADPβS-induced proliferative effect observed in co-cultures. It was also demonstrated that the presence of microglia did not influence metabolic degradation of ADPβS. Therefore, an activation of microglia P2Y receptors by ADPβS, was seen as the more solid explanation for the lack of ADPβS proliferative effect observed in co-cultures. However, the microglial P2Y receptor subtype(s) involved in the modulation of astroglial proliferation remained to be identified.

In the present study, it was confirmed that, in astrocyte cultures, ADPβS induces cell proliferation. Despite the minor contamination of astrocyte cultures with microglia, we have demonstrated, by BrdU incorporation, that astrocytes are the main proliferating cells. ADPβS proliferative effect in these cultures is triggered through activation of $P2Y_1$ and $P2Y_{12}$ receptor subtypes. The ADPβS proliferative effect was attenuated by the selective $P2Y_1$ receptor antagonist, MRS 2500 (1 μM; Houston et al., 2006) and by the selective $P2Y_{12}$ receptor antagonist, AR-C66096 (0.1 μM; Humphries et al., 1994). Interestingly, no additive effect was observed when both antagonists were tested simultaneously. A possible explanation is that, although they are coupled to different transduction mechanisms, they may convey in a common pathway. In fact, $P2Y_1$ receptors, are coupled to G(q) proteins and mediate astroglial proliferation through activation of phospholipase (PLC)-protein kinase C (PKC)-extracellular signal-regulated kinase 1/2 (ERK1/2) pathway (Neary et al., 2003; Quintas et al., 2011a), whereas $P2Y_{12}$ receptor activation may lead to G(i) βγ-dependent PLC-PKC-ERK1/2 pathway, as seen in 1321N1 human astrocytoma cells (Mamedova et al., 2006) or to a PLC-independent activation of PKC, as seems to occur in glioma C6 cells (Grobben et al., 2001; Van Kolen and Slegers, 2006). Therefore, $P2Y_1$ and $P2Y_{12}$ receptors subtypes, despite being coupled to different G proteins, may activate converging pathways, leading to ERK1/2 activation and cell proliferation. The results obtained in astrocyte cultures further demonstrate that $P2Y_{13}$ receptors are not involved in astroglial proliferation, because the antagonist of $P2Y_{13}$ receptor MRS 2211 (3 μM; Kim et al., 2005) did not change the ADPβS-induced astroglial proliferation.

In co-cultures, the results obtained with ADPβS on proliferation contrast with those observed in astrocyte cultures. In co-cultures, ADPβS failed to induce astroglial proliferation. However, the proliferative effect of ADPβS was restored, to levels similar to those observed in astrocyte cultures, when $P2Y_{13}$ receptors were blocked with MRS 2211, and partially recovered when $P2Y_{12}$ receptors were blocked with AR-C66096.

$P2Y_{12}$ receptors have been shown to be expressed either by microglia (Haynes et al., 2006; Ohsawa et al., 2007; De Simone et al., 2010) or by astrocytes (Fumagalli et al., 2003, 2004; Carrasquero et al., 2005; Amadio et al., 2010). Additionally, our previous studies demonstrated, by western blot and by immunocytochemical assays, that $P2Y_{12}$ receptors are expressed in both astrocytes cultures and co-cultures, by astrocytes and by microglial cells, with no preferential cellular localization (Quintas et al., 2011b). In this study, $P2Y_{12}$ receptors expression in astrocytes and microglia was further supported by quantification of $P2Y_{12}$ transcripts.

Concerning to the $P2Y_{13}$ receptors, they were expressed at low levels either in astrocyte cultures or co-cultures, which is in agreement with its lower mRNA expression in astrocytes. $P2Y_{13}$ receptors have been shown to be expressed in astrocytes of several brain regions, inducing $[Ca^{2+}]_i$ increase (Fumagalli et al., 2004; Carrasquero et al., 2009; Fischer et al., 2009), which suggest a possible role for this receptor subtype in the modulation of astrogliosis. In the present work, $P2Y_{13}$ receptors were shown to be residually expressed by astrocytes, but do not directly modulate of astroglial proliferation. Results obtained by immunocytochemistry showed that they were preferentially expressed by microglia, an observation in line with previous studies that demonstrated the expression of $P2Y_{13}$ receptors in microglia from the whole brain (Crain et al., 2009) and spinal cord, where they elicit $[Ca^{2+}]_i$ increase (Zeng et al., 2014) and the release of several pro-inflammatory cytokines, such as IL-1β, IL-6 and TNF-α (Liu et al., 2017).

From the pharmacological and molecular biology results, it may be concluded that astrocyte $P2Y_{13}$ receptors do not directly mediate astroglial proliferation, but rather act indirectly, through microglia, to regulate P2Y-mediated astroglial proliferation. The $P2Y_{12}$ receptors seem to cooperate with $P2Y_{13}$ receptors to restrain astroglial proliferation in co-cultures.

In co-cultures, $P2Y_{12}$ and $P2Y_{13}$ receptors also do not cause additive effects in preventing the ADPβS-induced astroglial proliferation. Likely, because $P2Y_{12}$ and $P2Y_{13}$ share the same transduction pathways. Both receptor subtypes are coupled to G(i) proteins (Marteau et al., 2003) and/or to an increase in $[Ca^{2+}]_i$, as described in microglial cells (Bianco et al., 2005).

We have previously shown that conditioned medium of microglia treated with ADPβS prevented the proliferative effect mediated by $P2Y_{1,12}$ receptors in astrocyte cultures, supporting the view that, in co-cultures, activation of microglia P2Y receptors induced the release of diffusible paracrine mediator(s) responsible for the inhibitory influence in the ADPβS-induced astroglial proliferation (Quintas et al., 2011b).

A recent report has shown that microglial cytokines, such as IL-1β, TNF-α and IL-6, transform astrocytes into a neuroprotective phenotype, involving downregulation of $P2Y_1$ receptors (Shinozaki et al., 2017). We have also shown that, the presence of microglia was associated with a loss of $P2Y_1$ receptor function, but without changing the expression levels (Quintas et al., 2011b). In line with our observations, it was seen a correlation between the presence of the pro-inflammatory IL-1β and the loss of $P2Y_1$ receptors function in astrocytes, without modifying its expression levels, possibly due to protein-protein interactions (Scemes, 2008). Thus, it was considered the hypothesis that microglial $P2Y_{12,13}$ receptors could induce the release of IL-1β which, acting on astrocytes, would prevent the $P2Y_{1,12}$-mediated proliferation. According to this hypothesis, IL-1β inhibited ADPβS-induced proliferation in astrocytes cultures, an effect prevented by the anti-IL-1β antibody. In co-cultures, but not in astrocyte cultures, the anti-IL-1β antibody, induced astroglial proliferation, suggesting that there is a microglial basal release of IL-1β that tonically inhibits astroglial proliferation. However, ADPβS was still unable to induce astroglial proliferation in the presence of anti-IL-1β antibody, excluding any significant contribution of IL-1β to the microglial $P2Y_{12,13}$ receptor-mediated inhibition of astroglial proliferation.

Another recent study, indicated that activated microglia release IL-1α, TNF-α and the complement factor Cq1, which are involved in phenotypical changes in astrocytes that may lead to a less proliferative and more aggressive profile to neurons (Liddelow et al., 2017). In line with this study it was hypothesized that in co-cultures, ADPβS-activated microglia could release IL-1α, TNF-α, and that these interleukins could be paracrine mediators involved in the inhibition of ADPβS-mediated astroglial proliferation. In co-cultures, both anti-IL-1α and anti-TNF-α antibodies restored, almost completely, the ADPβS proliferative effect, without causing significant effects on basal proliferation, supporting the conclusion that activation of microglia $P2Y_{12,13}$ receptors by ADPβS may induce the release of IL-1α and TNF-α that control $P2Y_{1,12}$ astroglial proliferation.

Taken together, the present results evidence the existence of two distinct pair of receptors controlling astroglial proliferation induced by extracellular purine nucleotides: $P2Y_1$ and $P2Y_{12}$ receptors, present in astrocytes and causing proliferation, and $P2Y_{12}$ and $P2Y_{13}$ receptors, present in microglia, causing a suppression of astroglial proliferation due to the release of soluble messenger(s), on a paracrine mode of communication that is independent of IL-1β, but seems to involve the release of IL-1α and TNF-α.

This purinergic interaction between microglia and astrocytes may be relevant under physiopathological conditions, during the initial phase of the inflammatory response, when there is cell death and inflammation, recruitment of microglia and other inflammatory and immune cells to remove cell debris (Burda and Sofroniew, 2014). Nucleotides are released to the lesion core at these early stages of CNS insult and may coordinate multicellular responses, activating purinergic receptors in astrocytes, microglia and surrounding cells (Buffo et al., 2010). Adenine nucleotides have been shown to induce astroglial proliferation mediated by $P2Y_{1,12}$ receptors (Franke et al., 2004; Quintas et al., 2011a) and would also act as chemotactic signals through activation of $P2Y_{12}$ receptors, causing microglia mobilization to reach the damaged site and to modulate the inflammatory response (Davalos et al., 2005). Here, we demonstrate that activation of microglial $P2Y_{12,13}$ receptors control $P2Y_{1,12}$ receptor-mediated astroglial proliferation. With the arrival of microglia to the lesion core, microglial $P2Y_{12,13}$ receptors would silence $P2Y_{1,12}$ receptor-mediated astroglial proliferation, by the release of paracrine mediators, delaying the formation of the astrocytic scar and, therefore, keeping open the path for more immune cells infiltration. As inflammation is resolved, microglia will change their phenotype, releasing astrocytes from the $P2Y_{12,13}$ proliferative brake, and pave the way for a full remodeling and repair.

ETHICS STATEMENT

Animal handling and experiments were conducted according to the guidelines of the Directive 2010/63/EU of the European Parliament and the Council of the European Union. Ethical commission of the animal house, called Organismo Responsável pelo Bem-Estar Animal (ORBEA), which in English corresponds to "Commission responsible for Animal Welfare," approved this study. Additionally, a qualified veterinary supervised the most critical part, which consisted in the euthanasia of newborn rats.

AUTHOR CONTRIBUTIONS

GQ supervised the entire work, prepared the cell cultures, and performed the experiments of DNA synthesis. CQ prepared the cell cultures and performed the experiments of immunofluorescence and molecular biology. GQ and CQ conceived and designed the experiments and analyzed the data. JG and NV analyzed the data and critically revised the manuscript. All authors discussed the results and contributed to manuscript writing.

ACKNOWLEDGMENTS

We would like to thank Maria do Céu Pereira, Mónica Caldas (Faculty of Pharmacy, University of Porto), and Paula Magalhães (i3S, University of Porto) for their technical assistance. We also thank the University of Porto, Faculty of Pharmacy for the financial support.

REFERENCES

Amadio, S., Montilli, C., Magliozzi, R., Bernardi, G., Reynolds, R., and Volonté, C. (2010). P2Y12 receptor protein in cortical gray matter lesions in multiple sclerosis. *Cereb. Cortex* 20, 1263–1273. doi: 10.1093/cercor/bhp193

Bianco, F., Fumagalli, M., Pravettoni, E., D'Ambrosi, N., Volonte, C., and Matteoli, M. (2005). Pathophysiological roles of extracellular nucleotides in glial cells: differential expression of purinergic receptors in resting and activated microglia. *Brain Res. Brain Res. Rev.* 48, 144–156. doi: 10.1016/j.brainresrev.2004.12.004

Buffo, A., Rolando, C., and Ceruti, S. (2010). Astrocytes in the damaged brain: molecular and cellular insights into their reactive response and healing potential. *Biochem. Pharmacol.* 79, 77–89. doi: 10.1016/j.bcp.2009.09.014

Burda, J. E., and Sofroniew, M. V. (2014). Reactive gliosis and the multicellular response to CNS damage and disease. *Neuron* 81, 229–248. doi: 10.1016/j.neuron.2013.12.034

Carrasquero, L. M., Delicado, E. G., Bustillo, D., Gutiérrez-Martín, Y., Artalejo, A. R., and Miras-Portugal, M. T. (2009). P2X7 and P2Y13 purinergic receptors mediate intracellular calcium responses to BzATP in rat cerebellar astrocytes. *J. Neurochem.* 110, 879–889. doi: 10.1111/j.1471-4159.2009.06179.x

Carrasquero, L. M., Delicado, E. G., Jiménez, A. I., Pérez-Sem, R., and Miras-Portugal, M. T. (2005). Cerebellar astrocytes co-express several ADP receptors. Presence of functional P2Y(13)-like receptors. *Purinergic Signal.* 1, 153–159. doi: 10.1007/s11302-005-6211-3

Crain, J. M., Nikodemova, M., and Watters, J. J. (2009). Expression of P2 nucleotide receptors varies with age and sex in murine brain microglia. *J. Neuroinflammation* 6:24. doi: 10.1186/1742-2094-6-24

Davalos, D., Grutzendler, J., Yang, G., Kim, J. V., Zuo, Y., and Jung, S. (2005). ATP mediates rapid microglial response to local brain injury *in vivo*. *Nat. Neurosci.* 8, 752–758. doi: 10.1038/nn1472

De Simone, R., Niturad, C. E., De Nuccio, C., Ajmone-Cat, M. A., Visentin, S., and Minghetti, L. (2010). TGF-β and LPS modulate ADP-induced migration of microglial cells through P2Y1 and P2Y12 receptor expression. *J. Neurochem.* 115, 450–459. doi: 10.1111/j.1471-4159.2010.06937.x

Deierborg, T. (2013). Preparation of primary microglia cultures from postnatal mouse and rat brains. *Methods Mol. Biol.* 1041, 25–31. doi: 10.1007/978-1-62703-520-0_4

Di Virgilio, F., Ceruti, S., Bramanti, P., and Abbracchio, M. P. (2009). Purinergic signalling in inflammation of the central nervous system. *Trends Neurosci.* 32, 79–87. doi: 10.1016/j.tins.2008.11.003

Fischer, W., Appelt, K., Grohmann, M., Franke, H., Norenberg, W., and Illes, P. (2009). Increase of intracellular Ca2+ by P2X and P2Y receptor-subtypes in cultured cortical astroglia of the rat. *Neuroscience* 160, 767–783. doi: 10.1016/j.neuroscience.2009.02.026

Franke, H., Krugel, U., Grosche, J., Heine, C., Hartig, W., and Allgaier, C. (2004). P2Y receptor expression on astrocytes in the nucleus accumbens of rats. *Neuroscience* 127, 431–441. doi: 10.1016/j.neuroscience.2004.05.003

Fumagalli, M., Brambilla, R., D'Ambrosi, N., Volonté, C., Matteoli, M., and Verderio, C. (2003). Nucleotide-mediated calcium signaling in rat cortical astrocytes: role of P2X and P2Y receptors. *Glia* 43, 218–303. doi: 10.1002/glia.10248

Fumagalli, M., Trincavelli, L., Lecca, D., Martini, C., Ciana, P., and Abbracchio, M. P. (2004). Cloning, pharmacological characterisation and distribution of the rat G-protein-coupled P2Y(13) receptor. *Biochem. Pharmacol.* 68, 113–124. doi: 10.1016/j.bcp.2004.02.038

Grobben, B., Claes, P., Van Kolen, K., Roymans, D., Fransen, P., and Sys, S. U. (2001). Agonists of the P2Y(AC)-receptor activate MAP kinase by a ras-independent pathway in rat C6 glioma. *J. Neurochem.* 78, 1325–1338. doi: 10.1046/j.1471-4159.2001.00524.x

Hamby, M. E., Coppola, G., Ao, Y., Geschwind, D. H., Khakh, B. S., and Sofroniew, M. V. (2012). Inflammatory mediators alter the astrocyte transcriptome and calcium signaling elicited by multiple G-protein-coupled receptors. *J. Neurosci.* 32, 14489–14510. doi: 10.1523/JNEUROSCI.1256-12.2012

Hanisch, U. K., and Kettenmann, H. (2007). Microglia: active sensor and versatile effector cells in the normal and pathologic brain. *Nat. Neurosci.* 10, 1387–1394. doi: 10.1038/nn1997

Haynes, S. E., Hollopeter, G., Yang, G., Kurpius, D., Dailey, M. E., and Gan, W. B. (2006). The P2Y12 receptor regulates microglial activation by extracellular nucleotides. *Nat. Neurosci.* 9, 1512–1519. doi: 10.1038/nn1805

Houston, D., Ohno, M., Nicholas, R. A., Jacobson, K. A., and Harden, T. K. (2006). [^{32}P]2-iodo-N^6-methyl-(N)-methanocarba-2′-deoxyadenosine-3′,5′-bisphosphate ([^{32}P]MRS2500), a novel radioligand for quantification of native P2Y$_1$ receptors. *Br. J. Pharmacol.* 147, 459–467. doi: 10.1038/sj.bjp.0706453

Humphries, R. G., Tomlinson, W., Ingall, A. H., Cage, P. A., and Leff, P. (1994). FPL 66096: a novel, highly potent and selective antagonist at human platelet P$_{2T}$-purinoceptors. *Br. J. Pharmacol.* 113, 1057–1063. doi: 10.1111/j.1476-5381.1994.tb17100.x

Kim, Y.-C., Lee, J.-S., Sak, K., Marteau, F., Mamedova, L., Boeynaems, J. M., et al. (2005). Synthesis of pyridoxal phosphate derivatives with antagonist activity at the P2Y$_{13}$ receptor. *Biochem. Pharmacol.* 70, 266–274. doi: 10.1016/j.bcp.2005.04.021

Liddelow, S. A., Guttenplan, K. A., Clarke, L. E., Bennett, F. C., Bohlen, C. J., Schirmer, L., et al. (2017). Neurotoxic reactive astrocytes are induced by activated microglia. *Nature* 541, 481–487. doi: 10.1038/nature21029

Liu, P. W., Yue, M. X., Zhou, R., Niu, J., Huang, D. J., and Xu, T. (2017). P2Y$_{12}$ and P2Y$_{13}$ receptors involved in ADPβs induced the release of IL-1β, IL-6 and TNF-α from cultured dorsal horn microglia. *J. Pain Res.* 10, 1755–1767. doi: 10.2147/JPR.S137131

Mamedova, L. K., Gao, Z. G., and Jacobson, K. A. (2006). Regulation of death and survival in astrocytes by ADP activating P2Y1 and P2Y12 receptors. *Biochem. Pharmacol.* 72, 1031–1041. doi: 10.1016/j.bcp.2006.07.017

Marteau, F., Le Poul, E., Communi, D., Communi, D., Labouret, C., and Savi, P. (2003). Pharmacological characterization of the human P2Y13 receptor. *Mol. Pharmacol.* 64, 104–112. doi: 10.1124/mol.64.1.104

McCarthy, K. D., and de Vellis, J. (1980). Preparation of separate astroglial and oligodendroglial cell cultures from rat cerebral tissue. *J. Cell Biol.* 85, 890–902. doi: 10.1083/jcb.85.3.890

Neary, J. T., Kang, Y., Willoughby, K. A., and Ellis, E. F. (2003). Activation of extracellular signal-regulated kinase by stretch-induced injury in astrocytes involves extracellular ATP and P2 purinergic receptors. *J. Neurosci.* 23, 2348–2356. doi: 10.1523/JNEUROSCI.23-06-02348.2003

Ni, M., and Aschner, M. (2010). Neonatal rat primary microglia: isolation, culturing, and selected applications. *Curr. Protoc. Toxicol.* 43, 12.17.1–12.17.16. doi: 10.1002/0471140856.tx1217s43

Ohsawa, K., Irino, Y., Nakamura, Y., Akazawa, C., Inoue, K., and Kohsaka, S. (2007). Involvement of P2X4 and P2Y12 receptors in ATP-induced microglial chemotaxis. *Glia* 55, 604–616. doi: 10.1002/glia.20489

Pfaffl, M. W. (2001). A new mathematical model for relative quantification in real-time RT-PCR. *Nucleic Acids Res.* 29:e45. doi: 10.1093/nar/29.9.e45

Quintas, C., Fraga, S., Goncalves, J., and Queiroz, G. (2011a). Opposite modulation of astroglial proliferation by adenosine 5′-O-(2-thio)-diphosphate and 2-methylthioadenosine-5′-diphosphate: mechanisms involved. *Neuroscience* 182, 32–42. doi: 10.1016/j.neuroscience.2011.03.009

Quintas, C., Fraga, S., Goncalves, J., and Queiroz, G. (2011b). P2Y receptors on astrocytes and microglia mediate opposite effects in astroglial proliferation. *Purinergic Signal.* 7, 251–263. doi: 10.1007/s11302-011-9235-x

Saura, J. (2007). Microglial cells in astroglial cultures: a cautionary note. *J. Neuroinflammation* 4:26. doi: 10.1186/1742-2094-4-26

Scemes, E. (2008). Modulation of astrocyte P2Y1 receptors by the carboxyl terminal domain of the gap junction protein Cx43. *Glia* 56, 145–153. doi: 10.1002/glia.20598

Shinozaki, Y., Shibata, K., Yoshida, K., Shigetomi, E., Gachet, C., and Ikenaka, K. (2017). Transformation of astrocytes to a neuroprotective phenotype by microglia via P2Y1 receptor downregulation. *Cell Rep.* 19, 1151–1164. doi: 10.1016/j.celrep.2017.04.047

Sofroniew, M. V. (2014). Astrogliosis. *Cold Spring Harb. Perspect. Biol.* 7:a020420. doi: 10.1101/cshperspect.a020420

Van Kolen, K., and Slegers, H. (2006). Atypical PKCzeta is involved in RhoA-dependent mitogenic signaling by the P2Y(12) receptor in C6 cells. *FEBS J.* 273, 1843–1854. doi: 10.1111/j.1742-4658.2006.05205.x

Zeng, J., Wang, G., Liu, X., Wang, C., Tian, H., and Liu, A. (2014). P2Y13 receptor-mediated rapid increase in intracellular calcium induced by ADP in cultured dorsal spinal cord microglia. *Neurochem. Res.* 39, 2240–2250. doi: 10.1007/s11064-014-1426-8

Zhang, D., Hu, X., Qian, L., O'Callaghan, J. P., and Hong, J. S. (2010). Astrogliosis in CNS pathologies: is there a role for microglia? *Mol. Neurobiol.* 41, 232–241. doi: 10.1007/s12035-010-8098-4

3

The Selective Antagonism of Adenosine A_{2B} Receptors Reduces the Synaptic Failure and Neuronal Death Induced by Oxygen and Glucose Deprivation in Rat CA1 Hippocampus *in Vitro*

Irene Fusco[1†], Filippo Ugolini[2†], Daniele Lana[2], Elisabetta Coppi[1], Ilaria Dettori[1], Lisa Gaviano[1], Daniele Nosi[3], Federica Cherchi[1], Felicita Pedata[1], Maria G. Giovannini[2] and Anna M. Pugliese[1*]

[1] Department of Neuroscience, Psychology, Drug Research and Child Health, NEUROFARBA, Section of Pharmacology and Toxicology, University of Florence, Florence, Italy, [2] Department of Health Sciences, Section of Clinical Pharmacology and Oncology, University of Florence, Florence, Italy, [3] Department of Experimental and Clinical Medicine, University of Florence, Florence, Italy

***Correspondence:**
Anna M. Pugliese
annamaria.pugliese@unifi.it

† These authors have contributed equally to this work.

Ischemia is a multifactorial pathology characterized by different events evolving in time. Immediately after the ischemic insult, primary brain damage is due to the massive increase of extracellular glutamate. Adenosine in the brain increases dramatically during ischemia in concentrations able to stimulate all its receptors, A_1, A_{2A}, A_{2B}, and A_3. Although adenosine exerts clear neuroprotective effects through A_1 receptors during ischemia, the use of selective A_1 receptor agonists is hampered by their undesirable peripheral side effects. So far, no evidence is available on the involvement of adenosine A_{2B} receptors in cerebral ischemia. This study explored the role of adenosine A_{2B} receptors on synaptic and cellular responses during oxygen and glucose deprivation (OGD) in the CA1 region of rat hippocampus *in vitro*. We conducted extracellular recordings of CA1 field excitatory post-synaptic potentials (fEPSPs); the extent of damage on neurons and glia was assessed by immunohistochemistry. Seven min OGD induced anoxic depolarization (AD) in all hippocampal slices tested and completely abolished fEPSPs that did not recover after return to normoxic condition. Seven minutes OGD was applied in the presence of the selective adenosine A_{2B} receptor antagonists MRS1754 (500 nM) or PSB603 (50 nM), separately administered 15 min before, during and 5 min after OGD. Both antagonists were able to prevent or delay the appearance of AD and to modify synaptic responses after OGD, allowing significant recovery of neurotransmission. Adenosine A_{2B} receptor antagonism also counteracted the reduction of neuronal density in CA1 stratum pyramidale, decreased apoptosis at least up to 3 h after the end of OGD, and maintained activated mTOR levels similar to those of controls, thus sparing neurons from the degenerative effects caused by the simil-ischemic conditions. Astrocytes significantly proliferated in CA1 stratum radiatum already 3 h after the end of OGD, possibly due to increased glutamate release.

A_{2B}receptor antagonism significantly prevented astrocyte modifications. Both A_{2B} receptor antagonists did not protect CA1 neurons from the neurodegeneration induced by glutamate application, indicating that the antagonistic effect is upstream of glutamate release. The selective antagonists of the adenosine A_{2B} receptor subtype may thus represent a new class of neuroprotective drugs in ischemia.

Keywords: apoptosis, MRS1754, PSB603, OGD, anoxic depolarization, mTOR, confocal microscopy, neurodegeneration

INTRODUCTION

Cerebral ischemic stroke represents a life threatening neurological disorder that leads to mortality and long-term disability in surviving patients. Ischemic stroke remains one of the main causes of death and disability in the western countries with only very limited therapeutic options (Dirnagl, 2012).

Acute brain injury after stroke is caused primarily by the lack of oxygen and glucose. In such conditions, mammalian neurons rapidly depolarize, and excessive release of glutamate occurs, causing excitotoxic cell death, largely due to over-activation of glutamatergic *N*-methyl-D-aspartate (NMDA) receptors. NMDA receptors are highly permeable to Ca^{2+} and are responsible for intracellular Ca^{2+} increase that reaches neurotoxic levels which, by activating cell lipases, endonucleases, proteases, and phosphatases, ultimately bring to acute excitotoxic cell death (Choi, 1992). Also, one of the early events occurring by an ischemic episode *in vivo* and during oxygen and glucose deprivation (OGD) *in vitro*, is the release of substantial amounts of adenosine (Latini et al., 1998; Melani et al., 1999; Frenguelli et al., 2007).

Adenosine exerts its biological functions via four receptors subtypes, A_1, A_{2A}, A_{2B}, and A_3 (Latini and Pedata, 2001). Many studies indicate that A_1 receptors play a prominent inhibitory tone on synaptic transmission and that adenosine selective antagonists, acting on this receptor subtype, has a protective role under ischemia (Pedata et al., 2016). Unfortunately, the development of A_1 receptor selective agonists as possible anti-ischemic drugs has been stalled by their sedative and cardiovascular side effects, including bradycardia and hypotension. Therefore, in order to identify putative targets for therapeutic intervention, the research on possible anti-ischemic drugs has focussed on the contribution of the other adenosine receptors. The role of the adenosine A_{2A} receptor under ischemia has been largely investigated (Chen et al., 2007; Pedata et al., 2014). Among adenosine receptors, the A_{2B} receptor subtype is the least studied and still remains the most enigmatic, because of the relatively low potency of adenosine for this receptor (Fredholm et al., 2011) and the very few selective ligands that have been described so far. Most of the present knowledge on A_{2B} receptors originates from their peripheral role on the control of cardiac myocyte contractility, intestinal tone, asthma, inflammation, cancer and diabetes (Feoktistov et al., 1998; Kolachala et al., 2008; Chandrasekera et al., 2010; Merighi et al., 2015; Allard et al., 2017). A_{2B} receptors play proinflammatory roles in human asthma, in chronic obstructive pulmonary disease and murine colitis (Feoktistov et al., 1998; Csóka et al., 2007; Kolachala et al., 2008). In the central nervous system (CNS), adenosine A_{2B} receptors, although scarcely, are uniformly expressed (Dixon et al., 1996) including in the hippocampus (Perez-Buira et al., 2007), but their role or function and in particular under ischemic/hypoxic conditions is still to be clarified. Understanding the processes by which the applications of these compounds confer neuroprotection should shed light on mechanisms to delay or mitigate the pathophysiological effects of ischemic injury.

In this paper we investigated the role of adenosine A_{2B} receptors during OGD in the CA1 region of rat hippocampus, the most susceptible hippocampal area to an ischemic insult. For this purpose two selective adenosine A_{2B} receptor antagonists were used. In order to characterize the OGD-induced cell injury and putative pharmacological protection, we conducted extracellular recordings of CA1 field excitatory post-synaptic potentials (fEPSPs) after a severe (7 min or 30 min) simil-ischemic insult. The response to ischemia consists of complex, concerted actions of the CNS and the peripheral immune system, that is very difficult to reproduce in *in vitro* model. However, these OGD episodes bring about irreversible depression of neurotransmission and the appearance of anoxic depolarization (AD) (Frenguelli et al., 2007; Pugliese et al., 2007). AD is a severe neuronal depolarization, which is an early and critical event that has been demonstrated both *in vivo* (Somjen, 2001) and *in vitro* (Tanaka et al., 1997; Pugliese et al., 2006). AD triggers a variety of molecular events, contributes to cell death and represents an unequivocal sign of neuronal injury (Somjen, 2001). The amount of time spent by neurons in AD is an important determinant of neuron fate. Propagation of AD from the ischemic core is one major factor contributing to neuronal death in the area surrounding the ischemic core (the penumbra) (Koroleva and Bures, 1996). The penumbra constitutes potentially salvageable tissue and hence a pharmacological treatment that delays the onset of AD would help to protect brain tissue from ischemia (Jarvis et al., 2001; Somjen, 2001).

Cell viability, extent of neuronal damage, astrocytes immunoreactivity and activation of apoptosis markers were also assessed by immunohistochemical analysis. Preliminary data were presented at the Society for Neuroscience Meeting (Ugolini et al., 2017).

MATERIALS AND METHODS

All animal experiments were performed according to the Italian Law on Animal Welfare (DL 26/2014), approved by the

Institutional Animal Care and Use Committee of the University of Florence and by the Italian Ministry of Health. All efforts were made to minimize animal sufferings and to use only the number of animals necessary to produce reliable scientific data. Male Wistar rats (Envigo, Italy, 150–200 g body weight) were used. Experiments were carried out on acute rat hippocampal slices, prepared as previously described (Pugliese et al., 2006, 2009).

Preparation of Slices

Animals were killed with a guillotine under anesthesia with isoflurane (Baxter, Rome, Italy) and hippocampi were rapidly removed and placed in ice-cold oxygenated (95% O_2–5% CO_2) artificial cerebrospinal fluid (aCSF) of the following composition (mM): NaCl 124, KCl 3.33, KH_2PO_4 1.25, $MgSO_4$ 1.4, $CaCl_2$ 2.5, $NaHCO_3$ 25, and D-glucose 10. Slices (400 μm nominal thickness) were cut using a McIlwain Tissue Chopper (Mickle Laboratory Engineering Co. Ltd., Gomshall, United Kingdom) and kept in oxygenated aCSF for at least 1 h at room temperature. A single slice was then placed on a nylon mesh, completely submerged in a small chamber (0.8 ml) and superfused with oxygenated aCSF (31–32°C) at a constant flow rate of 1.5 ml/min. The treated solutions reached the preparation in 60 s and this delay was taken into account in our calculations.

Extracellular Recordings

Test pulses (80 μs, 0.066 Hz) were delivered through a bipolar nichrome electrode positioned in the stratum radiatum of the CA1 region of the hippocampus to stimulate the Schaffer collateral-commissural pathway (**Figure 1A**). Evoked potentials were extracellularly recorded with glass microelectrodes (2–10 MΩ, Harvard Apparatus LTD, United Kingdom) filled with 150 mM NaCl. The recording electrode was placed at the dendritic level of the CA1 region to record field excitatory postsynaptic potentials (fEPSPs) (**Figure 1A**). Responses were amplified (200×, BM 622, Mangoni, Pisa, Italy), digitized (sample rate, 33.33 kHz), and stored for later analysis with LTP (version 2.30D) program (Anderson and Collingridge, 2001). The amplitude of fEPSP was measured as the difference between the negative peak following the afferent fiber volley and the baseline value preceding the stimulus artifact. In some experiments both the amplitude and the initial slope of fEPSP were quantified, but since no appreciable difference between these two parameters was observed under control conditions, in the presence of drugs or during *in vitro* ischemia, only the measure of the amplitude was expressed in the figures. When a stable baseline of evoked responses was reached, fEPSP amplitudes were routinely measured and expressed as the percentage of the mean value recorded 5 min before the application of any treatment (in particular pre-OGD). Stimulus-response curves were obtained by gradual increase in stimulus strength at the beginning of each experiment. The test stimulus strength was then adjusted to produce a response whose amplitude was 40% of the maximum and was kept constant throughout the experiment. Simultaneously, with fEPSP amplitude, AD was recorded as negative extracellular direct current (d.c.) shifts induced by OGD. The d.c. potential is an extracellular recording considered to provide an index of the polarization of cells surrounding the

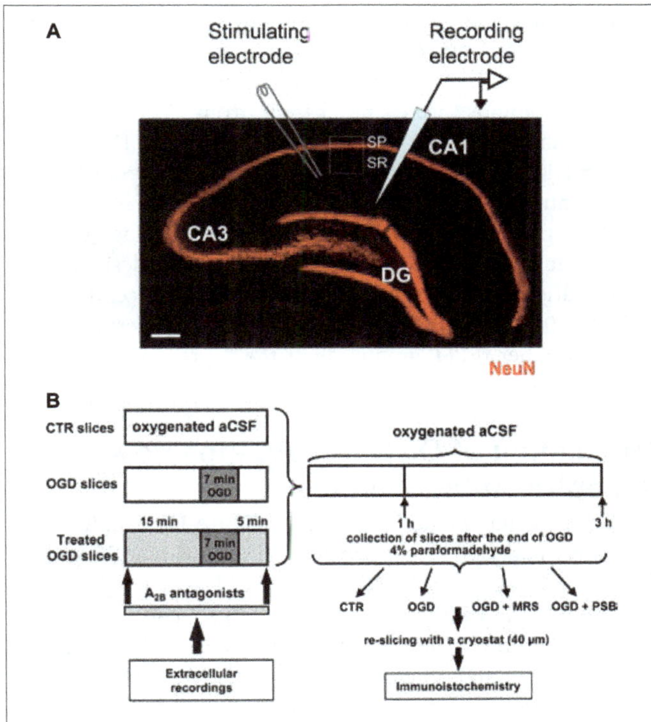

FIGURE 1 | Experimental methods. **(A)** Microphotography of an hippocampal slice showing the three subregions, the localization of the stimulating and recording electrodes and the region of interest (ROI, framed area) for the immunohistochemical analyses. SP, stratum pyramidale; SR, stratum radiatum. Scale bar: 200 μm. **(B)** Schematic representation of the experimental method.

tip of the glass electrode (Farkas et al., 2008). AD latency, expressed in min, was calculated from the beginning of OGD; AD amplitude, expressed in mV, was calculated at the maximal negativity peak. In the text and bar graphs, AD amplitude values were expressed as positive values. The terms "irreversible synaptic failure" or "irreversible loss of synaptic transmission" used in the present work refer to the maximal time window of cell viability in our experimental model (acutely isolated hippocampal slice preparation) which, according to our previous results is 24 h (Pugliese et al., 2009).

Paired-Pulse Facilitation

To elicit paired-pulse facilitation (PPF) of fEPSP, we stimulated the Schaffer collateral-commissural fibers twice with a 40-ms interpulse interval. Double stimulation was evoked once every 15 s. The synaptic facilitation was quantified as the ratio (P2/P1) between the slope of the fEPSP elicited by the second (P2) and the first (P1) stimuli. PPF was monitored in control conditions for at least 5 min before the application of BAY606583. The effect of BAY606583 on PPF was evaluated by measuring the P2/P1 ratio during at least 5 min after 15 min of agonist application.

Drugs

Two selective adenosine A_{2B} receptors antagonists, N-(4-Cyanophenyl)-2-[4-(2,3,6,7-tetrahydro-2,6-dioxo-1,3-dip-ropyl-1H-purin-8-yl)phenoxy]-acetamide) (MRS1754) and 8-[4-[4-

(4-Chlorophenzyl) piperazide-1-sulfonyl) phenyl]]-1-propyl xanthine (PSB603) were used. D-2-amino-5-phosphonovalerate, a selective NMDA receptor antagonist was used. All these compounds were purchased from Tocris (Bristol, United Kingdom). The A_1 receptor antagonist DPCPX (8-cyclopentyl-1,3-dipropylxanthine) was purchased from SIGMA Aldrich (https://www.sigmaaldrich.com).

All drugs were dissolved in dimethyl sulphoxide (DMSO). Stock solutions, of 1000–10,000 times the desired final concentration, were stored at −20°C. The final concentration of DMSO (0.05% and 0.1% in aCSF) used in our experiments did not affect either fEPSP amplitude or the depression of synaptic potentials induced by OGD (data not shown).

Application of OGD and Adenosine A_{2B} Receptor Antagonists

The experimental method is shown in **Figure 1B**. Conditions of OGD were obtained by superfusing the slice with aCSF without glucose and gassed with nitrogen (95% N_2–5% CO_2) (Pedata et al., 1993). This causes a drop in pO_2 in the recording chamber from ~500 mmHg (normoxia) to a range of 35–75 mmHg (after 7 min OGD) (Pugliese et al., 2003). At the end of the ischemic period, the slice was again superfused with normal, glucose-containing, oxygenated aCSF. The terms 'OGD slices' or 'treated OGD slices' refer to hippocampal slices in which OGD was applied in the absence or in the presence of A_{2B} receptor antagonists, respectively. Control slices were not subjected to OGD or treatment with A_{2B} receptor antagonists but were incubated in oxygenated aCSF for identical time intervals. All the selective adenosine A_{2B} receptors antagonists were applied 15 min before, during and 5 min after OGD. In a typical experimental day, first a control slice was subjected to 7 min of OGD. If the recovery of fEPSP amplitude after 60 min of reperfusion with glucose containing and normally oxygenated aCSF was ≤15% of the pre-OGD value, and AD developed into 7 min OGD, a second slice from the same rat was subjected to an OGD insult in the presence of the A_{2B} receptor antagonist under investigation. To confirm the result obtained in the treated group, a third slice was taken from the same rat and another 7 min OGD was performed under control conditions to verify that no difference between slices was caused by the time gap between the experiments. In some slices the OGD period was prolonged to 30 min and the A_{2B} receptor antagonists were applied 15 min before and during OGD application. After the extracellular recordings, slices were maintained in separate chambers for 1 or 3 h from the end of OGD in oxygenated aCSF at room temperature (RT). At the end, slices were harvested and fixed overnight at 4°C in 4% paraformaldehyde in PBS, cryopreserved in 18% sucrose for 48 h, and resliced as written below.

Treatment of Hippocampal Slices With Glutamate *in Vitro*

Experiments were carried out on acute hippocampal slices, prepared from male Wistar rats as described above. The A_{2B} receptor antagonists were dissolved in DMSO to obtain a stock solution suitable for a 1:2000 dilution. Slices, maintained oxygenated throughout the procedure, were incubated according to the following scheme:

- Control slices were incubated for 1 h in aCSF and then for 25 min in aCSF with DMSO (1:2000; 0.05%);
- Glutamate (GLU) treated slices were incubated 1 h in aCSF and then for 10 min with 100 μM glutamate in aCSF;
- MRS+GLU treated slices were incubated for 1 h in aCSF, then for 15 min with 500 nM MRS1754 and for further 10 min with 500 nM MRS1754 plus 100 μM glutamate, in aCSF;
- PSB+GLU treated slices were incubated for 1 h in aCSF, then for 15 min with 50 nM PSB603, and for further 15 min with 50 nM PSB603 plus 100 μM glutamate in aCSF;

After the incubation with glutamate and A_{2B} receptor antagonists, slices were further incubated for 3 h in aCSF, and then harvested and fixed overnight at 4°C in 4% paraformaldehyde in PBS, cryopreserved in 18% sucrose for 48 h, and resliced as written below.

Immunohistochemistry

One hour or 3 h after OGD, or after the incubation with glutamate and A_{2B} receptor antagonists, the 400 μm thick slices fixed in paraformaldehyde were placed on an agar support (6% agar in normal saline), included in an embedding matrix and re-sliced with a cryostat to obtain 40 μm thick slices. The more superficial sections were eliminated, while those obtained from the inner part of the slice were collected and stored in vials with 1 ml of antifreeze solution at −20°C until immunohistochemical analyses. From the 400 μm thick slices on average only a maximum of 2–3 complete 40 μm thick slices were obtained, which were then randomly allocated to the fluorescent immunohistochemical staining groups.

Antibodies Used – Primary Antibodies

Neurons were immunostained with a mouse monoclonal anti-NeuN antibody (1:200, MilliporeSigma, Carlsbad, CA, United States), astrocytes were detected by means of a polyclonal rabbit antibody anti-Glial Fibrillary Acidic Protein (GFAP, 1:500, DakoCytomation, Glostrup, Denmark), Cytochrome C with a mouse monoclonal antibody (1:200, Abcam, Cambridge, United Kingdom). Activated mTOR was detected using a polyclonal rabbit primary antibody raised against phospho-(Ser2448)-mTOR (1:100, Abcam, Cambridge, United Kingdom). Fluorescent secondary antibodies: Alexa Fluor 488 donkey anti rabbit (fluorescence in green, 1:400), Alexa Fluor 555 donkey anti mouse (fluorescence in red, 1:400), Alexa Fluor 635 goat anti-rabbit (fluorescence in far red, 1:400) (all from Life Technologies, Carlsbad, CA, United States). All primary and secondary antibodies were dissolved in Blocking Buffer (BB, 10% Normal Goat Serum, 0.05% NaN_3 in PBS-TX). All procedures were carried out with the free-floating method in wells of a 24-well plate (Cerbai et al., 2012; Lana et al., 2013).

Day 1

The sections were washed (3 times, 5 min each) in PBS-0.3% Triton X-100 (PBS-TX), blocked with 500 μl BB for 1 h, at RT under slight agitation and then incubated overnight at 4°C with the primary antibody under slight agitation.

Day 2

After washing in PBS-TX (3 times, 5 min each), sections were incubated for 2 h at room temperature in the dark with a solution containing one or two (for double immunostaining) fluorescent secondary antibodies, as appropriate. Sections were washed (3 times, 5 min each) with BB and then with 1 ml of distilled H_2O at RT in the dark, mounted on gelatinized microscopy slides, dried and coverslipped with a mounting medium containing DAPI to counterstain nuclei (Vectashield, Hard set mounting medium with DAPI, Vector Laboratories, Burlingame, CA, United States). Sections were kept refrigerated in the dark until microscopy analyses.

Day 3

Qualitative and quantitative analyses of NeuN positive neurons, CytC and phospho-mTOR positive cell bodies were performed in CA1 stratum pyramidale (SP), while astrocytes, phospho-mTOR positive dendrites and microglia were performed in CA1 stratum radiatum (SR) as shown in **Figure 1A**. Epifluorescence microscopy: sections were observed under an Olympus BX63 microscope equipped with an Olympus DP 50 digital camera (Olympus, Milan, Italy). For quantitative analysis images were acquired at 20× magnification with the digital camera.

Confocal Microscopy

Scans were taken at 0.3 μm z-step, keeping constant all the parameters (pinhole, contrast, and brightness), using a LEICA TCS SP5 confocal laser scanning microscope (Leica Microsystems CMS GmbH, Mannheim, Germany). Images were converted to green, or red using ImageJ (freeware provided by National Institute of Health[1]). The region of interest (ROI) in CA1, containing stratum pyramidalis and stratum radiatum was consistently analyzed in all slices, as shown in **Figure 1A** (Lana et al., 2014). Quantitative analyses of $NeuN^+$ neurons, HDN neurons, LDN neurons, $GFAP^+$ astrocytes, $CytC^+$ apoptotic neurons and phospho-mTOR positive cell bodies and dendrites were performed blind by two experimenters and results were averaged. Areas were expresses as mm^2. Digitized images were transformed into TIFF files and thresholded using ImageJ. Care was taken to maintain the same threshold in all sections within the same experiment. In CA1 pyramidal layer, the area labeled above the set threshold with NeuN or phospho-mTOR was calculated in pixels and expressed as $NeuN^+$ pixels/mm^2 or phospho-$mTOR^+$ pixels/mm^2. HDN neurons, LDN neurons, Cytochrome C-positive ($CytC^-$) apoptotic neurons in CA1 stratum pyramidale and $GFAP^+$ astrocytes in CA1 stratum radiatum were counted and were expressed as number of cells/mm^2. In order to evaluate mTOR activation in basal dendrites the length of phospho-$mTOR^+$ dendrites was measured at three fixed locations, equal in all slices and evenly distributed throughout the CA1 stratum radiatum ROI, and results were averaged.

[1]http://rsb.info.nih.gov/ij

Statistical Analysis

Statistical significance was evaluated by Student's paired or unpaired *t*-tests. Analysis of variance (one-way ANOVA), followed by Newman–Keuls multiple comparison *post hoc* test was used, as appropriate. *P*-values from both Student's paired and unpaired *t*-tests are two-tailed. Data were analyzed using software package GraphPad Prism (version 7.0; GraphPad Software, San Diego, CA, United States). All numerical data are expressed as the mean ± standard error of the mean (SEM). A value of $P < 0.05$ was considered significant.

RESULTS

Electrophysiological Experiments

It has been established that 7 min OGD episodes bring about irreversible depression of neurotransmission and the appearance of a severe neuronal depolarization or AD (Pugliese et al., 2006, 2007, 2009), a critical event that has been demonstrated both *in vivo* (Somjen, 2001) and *in vitro* (Fowler, 1992; Pearson et al., 2006; Pugliese et al., 2006, 2007, 2009; Frenguelli et al., 2007). Therefore, we studied the effects of two selective adenosine A_{2B} receptor antagonists, MRS1754 and PSB603, on AD development in the CA1 region of acute rat hippocampal slices under severe OGD episodes by extracellular recording of fEPSPs on 133 hippocampal slices taken from 42 rats.

The Selective Adenosine A_{2B} Receptor Antagonism Prevents or Delays AD Development and Protects From Synaptic Failure Induced by Severe OGD in CA1 Hippocampus

In agreement with our previous results (Pugliese et al., 2006, 2007, 2009), in untreated OGD slices the d.c. shift presented a mean latency of 6.04 ± 0.2 min (calculated from the beginning of OGD) and a mean peak amplitude of −6.7 ± 0.4 mV (n = 24) (**Figure 2A**). Seven min OGD exposure induced a rapid and irreversible depression of fEPSPs amplitude evoked by Schaffer-collateral stimulation, since synaptic potentials did not recover their amplitude after return to oxygenated aCSF (**Figure 2D**, n = 24, 2.5 ± 2.7% of pre-OGD level, calculated 50 min from the end of OGD). Control slices, followed for up to 3 h in oxygenated aCSF, maintained stable fEPSPs for the entire experimental time recording and never developed the d.c. shift (data not shown).

Oxygen and glucose deprivation was then applied in the presence of the selective adenosine A_{2B} receptor antagonists MRS1754 or PSB603, administered 15 min before, during and 5 min after OGD.

The two A_{2B} receptor antagonists did not modify basal synaptic transmission measured before OGD. Indeed, MRS1754 (500 nM, n = 17) did not modify fEPSPs amplitude under

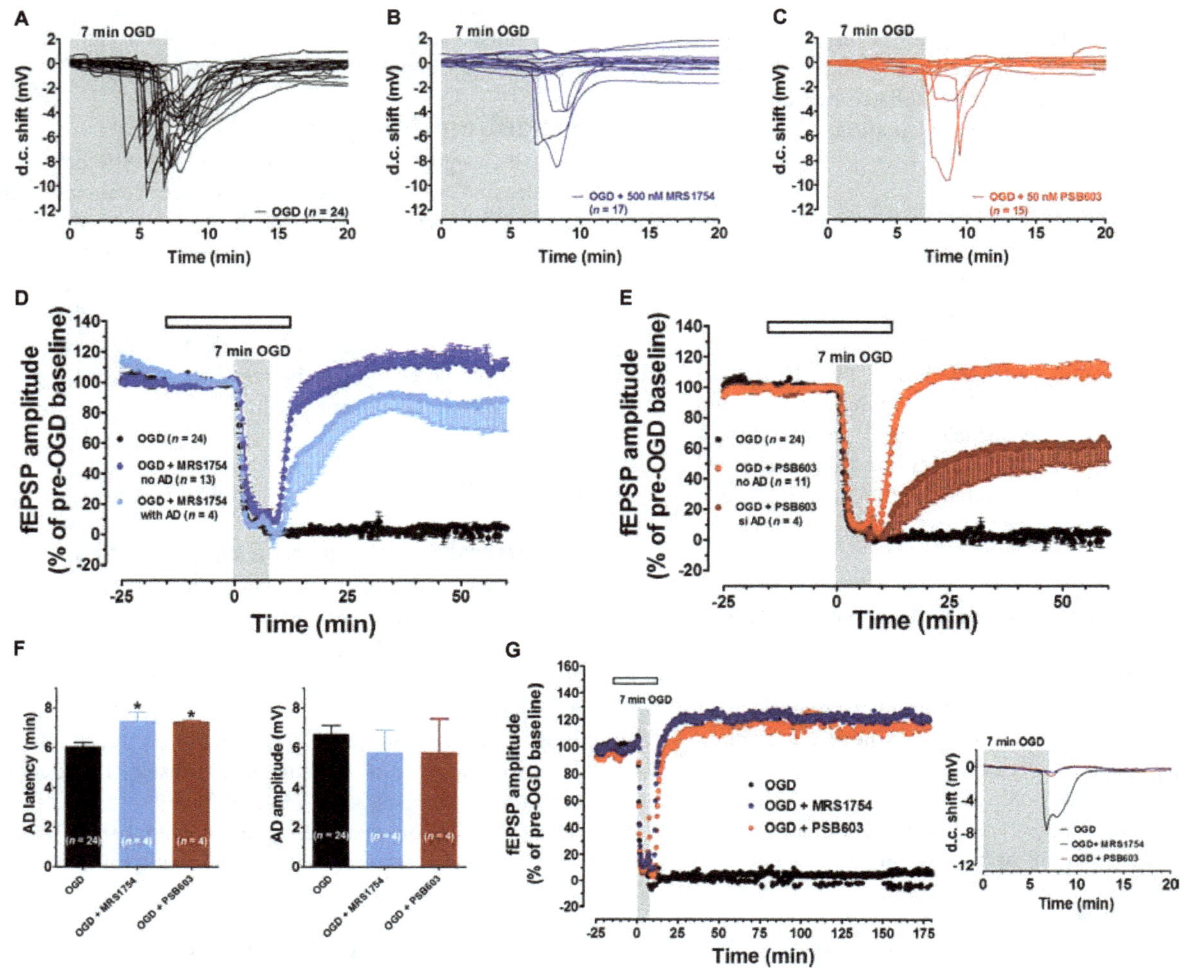

FIGURE 2 | The selective adenosine A_{2B} receptor antagonists MRS1754 or PSB603 significantly reduced the synaptic failure induced by 7 min oxygen and glucose deprivation (OGD) in the CA1 region of rat hippocampal slices. **(A–C)** anoxic depolarization (AD) was recorded as a negative direct current (d.c.) shift in response to 7 min OGD in untreated OGD slices **(A)**, in 500 nM MRS1754-treated slices **(B)**, or 50 nM PSB603-treated slices **(C)**. Note that MRS1754 prevented the appearance of AD in 13 out of 17 slices, while PSB603 in 11 out of 15 slices. **(D)** The graph shows the time-course of the effect of 7 min OGD on field excitatory post-synaptic potential (fEPSP) amplitude, expressed as percentage of pre-OGD baseline in the CA1 hippocampal region in the absence (n = 24) or in the presence of 500 nM MRS1754 (n = 17). Note that, in untreated slices, the ischemic-like insult caused gradual reduction, up to disappearance, of fEPSPs amplitude that did not recover after washing in oxygenated artificial cerebrospinal fluid (aCSF). On the contrary, after reperfusion in oxygenated standard solution, a recovery of fEPSP in all MRS1754 treated OGD slices was found, even in those in which AD developed. **(E)** The graph shows the time course of the effect of 7 min OGD on fEPSP amplitude in 50 nM PSB603 treated OGD slices. Note that, after reperfusion in normal oxygenated standard solution, a recovery of fEPSP was found in all OGD-treated PSB603 slices, even those in which AD occurred. **(F, Left)** each column represents the mean ± SEM of AD latency recorded in the CA1 region during 7 min OGD in the absence or in the presence of MRS1754 (500 nM) or PSB603 (50 nM). AD latency was measured from the beginning of OGD insult. Note that when OGD was applied in the presence of MRS1754 or PSB603 the appearance of AD was significantly delayed in comparison to OGD untreated slices. *$P < 0.05$ vs. OGD, One-way ANOVA followed by Newman–Keuls Multiple comparison test. **(Right)** each column represents the mean ± SEM of AD amplitude recorded in the CA1 during 7 min OGD. The number of slices is reported in the columns. **(G)** The graph shows the time course of the effect of 7 min OGD on fEPSP amplitude in OGD-untreated slices and in 500 nM MRS1754- or 50 nM PSB603-treated slices. The selective antagonism of adenosine A_{2B} receptors counteracted the CA1 synaptic damage induced by severe OGD up to 3 h from the end of the insult. Inset: 7 min OGD induced AD was recorded untreated OGD slices, but not in the presence of 500 nM MRS1754 or 50 nM PSB603. Gray bar: OGD time duration. Open bar: time of drug application. Amplitude of fEPSPs (mean ± SEM) is expressed as percentage of pre-OGD baseline.

normoxic conditions (from 1.05 ± 0.06 mV immediately before to 1.01 ± 0.08 mV after 15 min drug application, n = 17). Also, PSB603 did not change the amplitude of synaptic potentials under normoxic conditions (from 1.32 ± 0.12 mV before to 1.35 ± 0.14 mV after 15 min drug application, n = 15). These data indicate that the blockade of A_{2B} receptors does not modify low-frequency-induced CA1 synaptic transmission under normoxic conditions, in agreement with results reported in mouse hippocampal slices (Gonçalves et al., 2015).

Nevertheless, the two A_{2B} receptor antagonists were able to prevent or delay the appearance of AD and to modify synaptic responses after OGD.

During 7 min OGD, MRS1754 prevented the appearance of AD in 13 out of 17 slices tested (**Figure 2B**). In these 13 slices a complete recovery of fEPSPs was recorded (111.9 ± 7.4%, calculated 50 min from the end of OGD, **Figure 2D**). In the remaining 4 slices, AD developed, although at later times (**Figure 2F**, mean AD latency: 7.37 ± 0.41 min; mean peak amplitude: −5.8 ± 1.1 mV, n = 4), and, unexpectedly, was followed by a consistent fEPSP recovery (85.2 ± 15.3%, n = 4, **Figure 2D**).

During 7 min OGD, PSB603 prevented the appearance of AD in 11 out of 15 slices tested (**Figure 2C**). In these 11 slices a complete recovery of fEPSPs was found (110.4 ± 10.2%, n = 11, **Figure 2E**). In the remaining four slices in which AD appeared, a delay in AD latency was recorded (**Figure 2F**, mean AD latency: 7.33 ± 0.08 min; mean peak amplitude: −6.8 ± 1.9 mV, n = 4). Moreover, in these four PSB603-treated slices, a significant recovery of fEPSP (36.2 ± 19.7%, n = 4, **Figure 2E**) was found.

In the slices in which AD appeared in the presence of MRS1754 or PSB603, we compared the time of AD appearance in the absence and in the presence of drugs. As illustrated in **Figure 2F**, during 7 min OGD, AD appeared in OGD slices with a mean latency of 6.04 ± 0.2 min (Left panel) and a mean peak amplitude of 6.7 ± 0.4 mV (n = 24, Right panel). When 7 min OGD was applied in the presence of 500 nM MRS1754 or 50 nM PSB603 the d.c. shifts were always delayed (**Figure 2F**, Left panel), while AD amplitude values were not significantly modified in comparison to OGD slices (**Figure 2F**, Right panel).

In an experimental group of slices which never developed AD in the presence of PSB603 (50 nM) (n = 6) and MRS1754 (500 nM) (n = 6), we followed the evolution of the synaptic response for 3 h after the end of the 7 min ischemic like insult in comparison to untreated OGD slices (n = 6). As reported in the representative electrophysiological traces shown in **Figure 2G**, PSB603 (50 nM) and MRS1754 (500 nM) allowed the recovery of synaptic potentials for at least 3 h after 7 min OGD.

Furthermore, in order to confirm that both the recovery of fEPSP and the irreversible loss of neurotransmission after 7 min OGD observed in the different experimental groups were not transient, we tested slice viability 24 h after the OGD insult in control, untreated, slices and slices treated with A_{2B}-receptor antagonists. In agreement with our previously published results (Pugliese et al., 2009), we showed that untreated OGD slices, which did not recover any synaptic activity within 1 h after the insult, maintained synaptic impairment when tested 24 h later (Supplementary Figure 1A shows a representative experiment out of a total of six slices). On the contrary, MRS1754- or PSB603-treated OGD slices, which recovered initial fEPSP amplitude 1 h after OGD, preserved neurotransmission for at least 24 h after the insult (Supplementary Figure 1B shows a representative experiment out of a total of four slices, and Supplementary Figure 1C shows a representative experiment out of a total of five slices for MRS1754 and PSB603, respectively).

In order to characterize the role of adenosine A_{2B} receptors on AD development, in a next series of experiments we prolonged the OGD duration up to 30 min, in order to allow AD to unavoidably appear in all experimental groups. This longer duration of OGD is invariably associated with tissue damage (Pearson et al., 2006). We compared the latency and the magnitude of depolarizing d.c. shifts recorded in the absence or presence of PSB603 or MRS1754. As illustrated in **Figure 3A**, 30 min OGD elicited the appearance of AD in all slices, with a mean peak amplitude of −7.5 ± 0.7 mV (n = 8) and a mean latency of 5.8 ± 0.3 min, as shown in **Figures 3D,E**. When OGD was applied in the presence of 500 nM MRS1754, the d.c. shift was significantly delayed to 9.2 ± 0.7 min (**Figures 3B, D**; n = 5), although the AD amplitude (−5.7 ± 0.7 mV) was not significantly changed (**Figure 3E**). Similarly, when OGD was applied in the presence of 50 nM PSB603, the d.c. shift was significantly delayed to 7.7 ± 0.3 min (**Figures 3C,D**; n = 7) whereas AD amplitude (−7.7 ± 0.7 mV) was unchanged (**Figure 3E**).

Data in the literature demonstrate that adenosine A_{2B} receptors exert their effects through a control of A_1 receptor function in the hippocampus under simil-physiological, normoxic, conditions (Gonçalves et al., 2015). In order to test this possibility, we studied whether A_{2B} receptor antagonists were still effective in inhibiting OGD-induced alterations of synaptic transmission in the presence of the A_1 receptor antagonist DPCPX. As shown in Supplementary Figures 2A–C, we applied DPCPX before, during and after a 7 min OGD and, unexpectedly, we found that 2 out of 6 slices tested did not undergo AD and completely recovered their synaptic activity. This unexpected result was possibly due to the unselective block of A_{2A} receptors by DPCPX, as already described in hippocampal slices during OGD (Sperlágh et al., 2007). Therefore, we reduced DPCPX concentration to 100 nM and we prolonged the OGD period up to 30 min (Supplementary Figure 2D). Under these experimental conditions, DPCPX-exposed slices presented a delayed AD appearance (mean AD peak time = 8.4 ± 0.5 min) in comparison to control, untreated, OGD slices (mean AD peak time = 6.8 ± 0.2 min) thus confirming that DPCPX protects hippocampal slices from OGD insults (Supplementary Figure 2E). The time window of A_{2B} or A_1 receptor-mediated effects found in the present studies overlaps with the delay found treating the slices with glutamate receptor antagonists (Tanaka et al., 1997; Yamamoto et al., 1997), or blocking NMDA receptors that are involved both in initiation and propagation of AD (Herreras and Somjen, 1993; Somjen, 2001). In a further series of experiments, we demonstrated that D-AP5 (50 μM) significantly delayed AD appearance (from 6.8 ± 0.2 min in untreated OGD slices to 9.8 ± 1.0 min in D-AP5-treated OGD slices, Supplementary Figure 2E).

For this reason, in order to assess the involvement of A_1 receptors in A_{2B} receptor-mediated effects, we choose a different protocol. It has been shown that short-term plasticity, measured by PPF, is modified by A_{2B} receptor activation in mouse hippocampal slices in a DPCPX-sensitive manner (Gonçalves et al., 2015). We confirmed that the A_{2B} receptor agonist BAY606583, at 200 nM concentration, significantly decreased PPF in rat CA1 hippocampus (**Figure 4**), thus indicating an increase of presynaptic glutamate release upon A_{2B} receptor activation. This effect was blocked not only by the A_{2B} receptor antagonists PSB603 and MRS1754, but also by the A_1 receptor antagonist DPCPX (**Figure 4B**), thus confirming that A_{2B} receptor effects are mediated by the inhibition of the A_1 subtype, as already stated by Gonçalves et al. (2015).

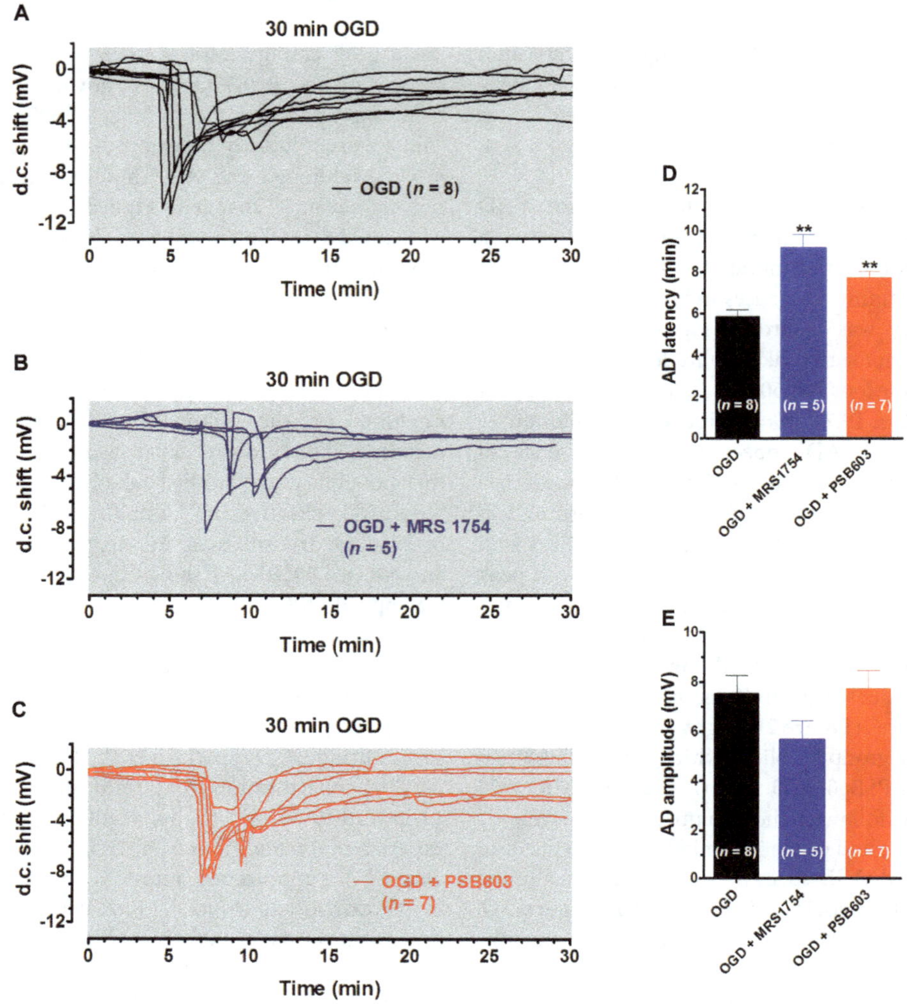

FIGURE 3 | MRS1754 and PSB603 delayed the appearance of AD induced by 30 min OGD in rat hippocampal slices. **(A–C)** The graphs show the d.c. shift traces during 30 min OGD in untreated OGD slices (**A**, $n = 8$), in the presence of 500 nM MRS1754 (**B**, $n = 5$), or 50 nM PSB603 (**C**, $n = 7$). **(D)** Each column represents the mean ± SEM of AD latency recorded in hippocampal slices during 30 min OGD in different experimental groups. AD was measured from the beginning of OGD insult. Note that both adenosine A_{2B} receptor antagonists significantly delayed AD development. $^{**}P < 0.01$ vs. OGD, One-way ANOVA followed by Newman–Keuls Multiple comparison test. **(E)** Each column represents the mean ± SEM of AD amplitude recorded in the CA1 during 30 min OGD. The number of slices is reported in the columns.

Analysis of Neuronal Damage in CA1 Stratum Pyramidale 1 and 3 h After the End of 7 min OGD

The extent of neuronal damage caused by 7 min OGD in stratum pyramidale of hippocampal CA1 was assessed by immunohistochemistry using the anti-NeuN antibody in control slices, in slices after 7 min OGD alone, and after 7 min OGD in the presence of 500 nM MRS1754 or 50 nM PSB603, both at 1 and 3 h after the end of OGD. Representative images of NeuN immunostaining in CA1 of slices collected 1 h after the end of OGD are shown in **Figures 5A–D**.

Figures 5E,F show the quantitative analyses of the area of NeuN$^+$ immunofluorescence in CA1, which represents an index of the number of pyramidal neurons, 1 and 3 h after the end of OGD, respectively. The data demonstrate that NeuN$^+$ CA1 pyramidal neurons significantly decreased both 1 h (**Figure 5E**) and 3 h (**Figure 5F**) after the end of 7 min OGD. Statistical analysis showed that 7 min OGD caused a statistically significant reduction of NeuN$^+$ area at 1 h (−29.6%, $^*P < 0.05$ vs. control slices) and at 3 h (−41%, $^*P < 0.05$ vs. control slices). The time-course of the effect, indicating that the decrease of NeuN$^+$ area was more pronounced at 3 h than at 1 h after the end of OGD, demonstrates that neuronal degeneration is an ongoing process at least at these time points.

The decrease of NeuN$^+$ area in CA1 stratum pyramidale was completely antagonized by treatment with 50 nM PSB603 (−1% at 1 h and −14% at 3 h, ns vs. control slices). This effect was statistically significant vs. 7 min OGD slices both at 1 and 3 h after the end of OGD ($^{\$}P < 0.05$ vs. respective OGD). Treatment with 500 nM MRS1754 completely blocked the decrease of NeuN$^+$

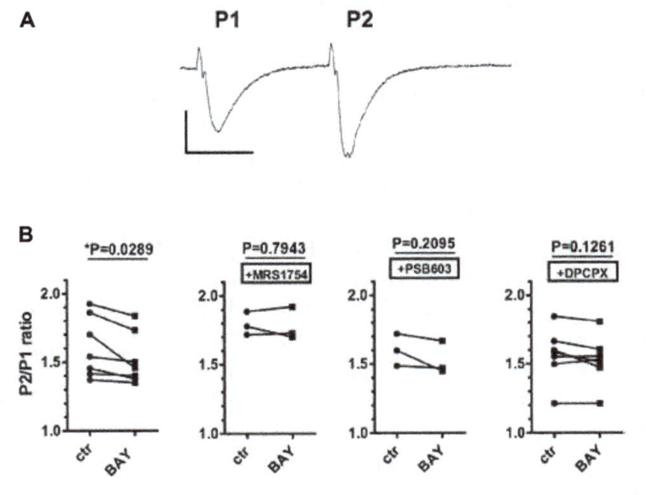

FIGURE 4 | The selective stimulation of adenosine A_{2B} receptors reduced paired-pulse facilitation (PPF) in rat hippocampal slices. **(A)** Trace of fEPSP responses to PPF protocol (40-ms interval), taken from a typical experiment. Calibration: 0.5 mV, 20 ms. **(B)** Each graph shows PPF quantified as the ratio (P2/P1) between the slope of the second fEPSP (P2) and the slope first fEPSP (P1). The effect of BAY606583 (BAY, 200 nM) on PPF was investigated in the absence ($n = 7$) or in the presence of MRS1754 (500 nM, $n = 3$), PSB603 (50 nM, $n = 3$), or DPCPX (100 nM, $n = 7$). $*P < 0.05$ vs. ctr, paired Student's *t*-test.

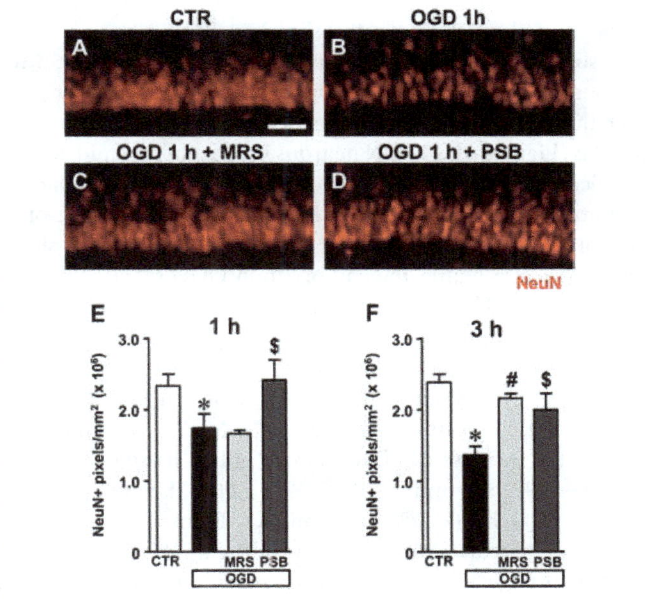

FIGURE 5 | Analysis of NeuN$^+$ immunofluorescence in CA1 stratum pyramidale after the simil-ischemic insult. **(A–D)** Representative images of NeuN$^+$ immunofluorescence in the ROI of CA1 of a control slice (CTR, **A**), a slice collected 1 h after 7 min OGD (OGD, **B**), a slice treated with 500 nM MRS1754 (OGD+MRS, **C**), and a slice treated with 50 nM PSB603 (OGD+PSB, **D**), all harvested 1 h after the end of 7 min OGD. Scale bar: 75 μm. **(E,F)** Quantitative analyses of NeuN$^+$ immunofluorescence in the four experimental groups 1 h **(E)** and 3 h **(F)** after the end of 7 min OGD. Each column represents the area, expressed in pixels ($\times 10^6$) above a threshold, maintained constant for all slices investigated. **(E)** Statistical analysis: One-way ANOVA: $F_{(3;13)} = 6.296$, $P < 0.01$, Newman–Keuls multiple comparison test: $*P < 0.05$, OGD vs. CTR; $^{\$}P < 0.05$, OGD+PSB vs. OGD. CTR, $n = 6$; OGD, $n = 5$; OGD+PSB, $n = 3$; OGD+MRS, $n = 3$. **(F)** Statistical analysis: One-way ANOVA: $F_{(3,16)} = 4.924$, $P < 0.02$; Newman–Keuls multiple comparison test: $*P < 0.05$ OGD vs. CTR, $^{\#}P < 0.05$ OGD+MRS vs. OGD, $^{\$}P < 0.05$ OGD+PSB vs. OGD. CTR, $n = 6$; OGD, $n = 3$; OGD+PSB, $n = 4$; OGD+MRS $n = 4$. All data in the graphs are expressed as mean ± SEM.

area in CA1 stratum pyramidale 3 h after the end of OGD (−7% vs. control slices, ns; $^{\#}P < 0.05$ vs. OGD). MRS1754 had no effect 1 h after the end of OGD (−31.5% vs. control slices; ns vs. OGD). Therefore, antagonism of A_{2B} receptors blocked the neuronal damage induced by 7 min OGD up to 3 h after the end of the simil-ischemic insult. In the OGD slices treated either with MRS1754 or PSB603 that developed AD we found a partial reduction of neuronal damage at 1 h after the end of OGD (data not shown).

Closer examination of CA1 stratum pyramidale with confocal microscopy indicated the presence of many damaged neurons both 1 and 3 h after the end of 7 min OGD. The representative confocal z stacks in **Figures 5B**, **6B**, each obtained stacking 37 consecutive confocal z-scans (0.3 μm each, total thickness 11.1 μm) through the thickness of CA1, show that 3 h after the end of OGD the layout and morphology of CA1 pyramidal neurons was significantly different from that of the control slice (**Figure 6A**). **Figures 6A1,B1** are magnification of the framed areas in **Figures 6A,B**, and show stacks of two consecutive z-scans, 0.3 μm each, total thickness 0.6 μm, taken at 2.1 μm depth inside the neurons. It appears evident from panel **Figure 6B1** the altered morphology of pyramidal neurons after OGD, in comparison to those of the control slice shown in **Figure 6A1**. Indeed, in CA1 stratum pyramidale of OGD slices, both at 1 and 3 h after the end of OGD, we observed the presence of many neurons with nuclei that exhibit a highly condensed NeuN-positive nucleus and very faint NeuN cytoplasmic labeling (**Figures 6B,B1**, open arrows). We defined these neurons as High Density Nucleus neurons, "HDN neurons." Furthermore, we observed many NeuN$^+$ neurons that have lost the NeuN$^+$ nuclear immunofluorescence, an index of damaged nuclei, while NeuN$^+$ immunofluorescence persists in the cytoplasm (**Figures 6B,B1**, white arrows). We defined these neurons as Low Density Nucleus neurons, "LDN neurons."

In order to better characterize this phenomenon, we performed the quantitative analysis of HDN and LDN neurons in control, 7 min OGD, 7 min OGD plus MRS1754 and 7 min OGD plus PSB603 slices at 1 and 3 h after the end of OGD. The results, presented in **Figures 6C,D**, show that HDN neurons increased significantly in 7 min OGD slices both at 1 h (+603% vs. control slices, $^{**}P < 0.01$) and 3 h (+794% vs. control slices, $^{***}P < 0.001$) after the end of OGD. The increase of damaged, HDN neurons in the CA1 area caused by the simil-ischemic insult was significantly blocked by treatment with 50 nM PSB603 at 1 and 3 h after the end of OGD (−97% at 1 h, and −77% at 3 h vs. 7 min OGD slices, both $^{\$\$\$}P < 0.001$; ns vs. controls). Conversely, treatment with 500 nM MRS1754 significantly blocked the increase of HDN neurons only 3 h after the end of OGD (−70% vs. 7 min OGD slices, $^{\#\#\#}P < 0.001$; ns vs.

control slices), but not 1 h after the end of OGD (+12% vs. OGD slices, ns; $^{\#\#}P < 0.01$ vs. control slices).

Also, as shown by the representative images in **Figures 6B,B1**, we found many LDN neurons in stratum pyramidale 1 and 3 h after the end of 7 min OGD. As demonstrated by quantitative analysis (**Figures 6E,F**) LDN neurons in stratum pyramidale were significantly increased both 1 and 3 h after OGD, in comparison to control slices. The increase of LDN neurons, in comparison to control slices, was 1489% at 1 h ($^{***}P < 0.01$ vs. control slices) and 1033% at 3 h after the end of 7 min OGD ($^{***}P < 0.01$ vs. control slices). The increase of damaged, LDN neurons brought about by the simil-ischemic insult was significantly blocked by treatment with 50 nM PSB603 both at 1 and 3 h after the end of OGD (−98% at 1 h, and −62% at 3 h vs. OGD, both $^{\$\$\$}P < 0.001$). Treatment with 500 nM MRS1754 significantly blocked the increase of LDN neurons only 3 h after the end of OGD (−52% vs. 7 min OGD,$^{\#\#\#}P < 0.001$), but not 1 h after the end of OGD (−17% vs. 7 min OGD, ns; $^{\#\#}P < 0.01$ vs. controls). These data further confirm the efficacy of the two A_{2B} receptor antagonists, and particularly of PSB603, in reducing not only the electrophysiological effects but also the morphological modifications that OGD caused on CA1 pyramidal neurons, up to 3 h after the end of the ischemic-like insult.

Analysis of Apoptotic Neurons in Stratum Pyramidale of CA1 1 and 3 h After 7 min OGD

These data demonstrate that 7 min OGD can induce neuronal damage in CA1 stratum pyramidale, as evidenced by immunohistochemical analyses that highlight conformational modifications of pyramidal neurons that may subtend cell death. Therefore, we studied whether all the above-described effects and the decrease of neurons in CA1 stratum pyramidale might be caused by apoptosis. To this end, as an apoptosis marker we used CytC, a protein which, in physiological conditions, is found in mitochondria but in the most advanced stages of apoptosis is intensely and diffusely released in the cytoplasm, where it activates caspases (Kluck et al., 1997; Yang et al., 1997; Jiang and Wang, 2004; Suen et al., 2008) and can be used as a marker of apoptosis using immunohistochemical analysis (Martínez-Fábregas et al., 2014). Using a selective antibody, CytC can be visualized in apoptotic cells as an intense and diffuse cytoplasmic immunostaining, as shown by the white arrows in the representative confocal images of an OGD slice 1 h after the end of OGD (**Figures 7A–A2**). As shown in the confocal subslice of the framed area of **Figure 7A2**, obtained stacking 17 consecutive confocal z-scans through the $CytC^+$ neuron (0.3 μm each, total thickness 5.1 μm), it is evident that the $CytC^+$ positive neuron is a LDN neuron (**Figures 7B–B2**, open arrow), thus demonstrating that LDN neurons are apoptotic.

From the quantitative analysis of $CytC^+$ neurons in CA1 stratum pyramidale, we demonstrated that both 1 and 3 h after the end of 7 min OGD many CA1 pyramidal neurons were apoptotic (**Figures 7C,D**). The increase was statistically significant in comparison to control slices both at 1 h (+277% vs. control slices, $^{***}P < 0.001$) and at 3 h (+107% vs. control slices, $^{**}P < 0.01$) after OGD. These data indicate that in CA1 area, already after 1 h from the end of OGD, neurons had clear signs of apoptotic processes. In the presence of MRS1754 or PSB603, there was a significant reduction of CytC immunostaining, both at 1 and 3 h after the end of OGD, showing that antagonism of A_{2B} receptors significantly reduced neuronal death by apoptosis at both times investigated. Indeed, treatment with MRS1754 decreased apoptotic neurons by 61% at 1 h ($^{\#\#\#}P < 0.001$ vs. 7 min OGD; ns vs. control slices) and by 33% at 3 h ($^{\#}P < 0.05$ vs. 7 min OGD; ns vs. control slices), in comparison to OGD slices. Treatment with PSB603 decreased apoptotic neurons by 63% ($^{\$\$\$}P < 0.001$ vs. 7 min OGD; ns vs. control slices) and by 46% ($^{\$\$}P < 0.001$ vs. 7 min OGD; ns vs. control slices) in comparison to OGD slices. In the OGD slices treated either with MRS1754 or PSB603 that developed AD the number of HDN and LDN neurons were partially decreased in comparison to OGD slices (data not shown).

These data indicate that in the CA1 area already 1 h after the end of OGD, when there was still no recovery of neurotransmission, neurons showed obvious signs of apoptosis. These data demonstrate that antagonism of A_{2B} receptors brought about significant protection against neuron degeneration.

Analysis of Phospho-mTOR in Area CA1 of the Hippocampus 1 and 3 h After 7 min OGD

We used a selective antibody for phospho-(Ser244)-mTOR, the activated form of mTOR, to investigate whether mTOR activation might be modified in our experimental conditions (**Figures 8A–D1**). Representative qualitative images of mTOR activation in cell bodies and dendrites of CA1 pyramidal neurons in a control slice are shown in **Figure 8A1** (green). Neurons were also immunolabelled with anti-NeuN antibody (red). The merge of the immunofluorescence (yellow-orange) in a control slice is shown in **Figure 8A**. It is evident from the images that activated mTOR is present in CA1 pyramidal neurons in basal, control conditions where it is localized both in the cell body and in neuronal apical dendritic tree spanning throughout the stratum radiatum. The simil-ischemic condition caused a significant decrease of mTOR activation 3 h after the end of OGD, as shown in the representative image of **Figures 8B,B1**. This effect is more evident in **Figures 8E,F**, that represent digital subslices obtained stacking nine consecutive confocal z-scans throughout the neuronal cell bodies (0.3 μm each, total thickness 2.7 μm) of control and OGD slices. The images clearly show that in control conditions phospho-mTOR was present both in the cell body (**Figure 8E**, open arrow) and in the dendrites (**Figure 8E**, white arrows), while 3 h after 7 min OGD activation of mTOR decreased both in cell body and dendrites (**Figure 8F**). Quantitative analysis showed that in slices harvested 1 h after the end of 7 min OGD, no significant modification of activated mTOR immunostaining was present in the neuronal cell body (**Figure 8G**) or in the apical dendrites of CA1 pyramidal neurons in any of the groups investigated (**Figure 8I**). On the contrary, in slices harvested 3 h after the

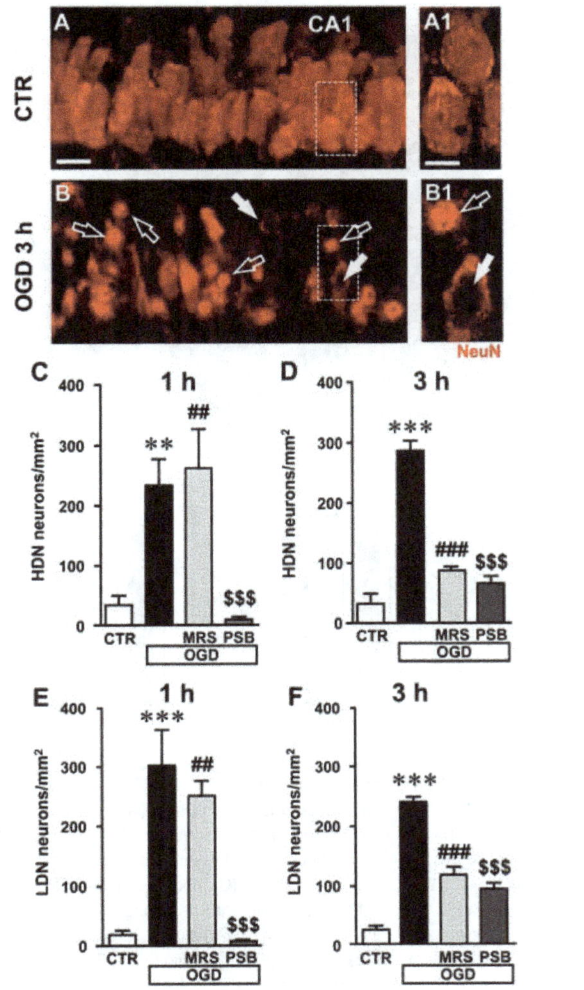

FIGURE 6 | Analysis of damaged neurons in CA1 stratum pyramidale after the simil-ischemic insult. **(A–B1)** Representative images of NeuN$^+$ immunofluorescence in the CA1 area of a control slice (CTR, **A,A1**), and of a slice harvested 3 h after the end of 7 min OGD (OGD, **B,B1**). **(A1–B1)** magnification of digital subslices of the framed areas in **A,B** (stacks of two consecutive z-scans taken at 2.1 μm depth inside the neurons, total thickness 0.6 μm). Note the presence of many HDN neurons (open arrows) and LDN neurons (white arrows) in CA1 stratum pyramidale after OGD **(B,B1)**. Scale bars: **A,B**: 25 μm; **A1,B1**: 10 μm. **(C,D)** Quantitative analyses of NeuN$^+$ HDN neurons in CA1 stratum pyramidale 1 h **(C)** and 3 h **(D)** after the end of OGD. **(C)** One-way ANOVA: $F_{(3;12)} = 11.32$, $P < 0.001$. Newman–Keuls multiple comparison test: $^{**}P < 0.01$, OGD vs. CTR; $^{\#\#}P < 0.01$, OGD+MRS vs. CTR;$^{\$\$\$}P < 0.001$ OGD+PSB vs. OGD. CTR, $n = 5$; OGD, $n = 5$; OGD+PSB, $n = 3$; OGD+MRS, $n = 3$. **(D)** One-way ANOVA: $F_{(3;12)} = 64.33$, $P < 0.001$. Newman–Keuls multiple comparison test: $^{***}P < 0.001$, OGD vs. CTR; $^{\#\#\#}P < 0.001$, OGD+MRS vs. OGD;$^{\$\$\$}P < 0.001$ OGD+PSB vs. OGD. CTR, $n = 5$; OGD, $n = 3$; OGD+PSB, $n = 4$; OGD+MRS, $n = 4$. **(E–F)**: Quantitative analysis of NeuN$^+$ LDN neurons in CA1 stratum pyramidale 1 h **(E)** and 3 h **(F)** after the end of OGD. **(E)** One-way ANOVA: $F_{(3;14)} = 13.80$, $P < 0.001$. Newman–Keuls multiple comparison test: $^{***}P < 0.01$, OGD vs. CTR; $^{\#\#}P < 0.01$, OGD+MRS vs. CTR;$^{\$\$\$}P < 0.001$ OGD+PSB vs. OGD. CTR, $n = 6$; OGD, $n = 6$; OGD+PSB, $n = 3$; OGD+MRS, $n = 3$. **(F)** One-way ANOVA: $F_{(3;12)} = 69.77$, $P < 0.001$. Newman–Keuls multiple comparison test: $^{***}P < 0.001$, OGD vs. CTR; $^{\#\#\#}P < 0.001$, OGD+MRS vs. OGD;$^{\$\$\$}P < 0.001$ OGD+PSB vs. OGD. CTR, $n = 5$; OGD, $n = 3$; OGD+PSB, $n = 4$; OGD+MRS, $n = 4$. All data in the graphs are expressed as mean ± SEM.

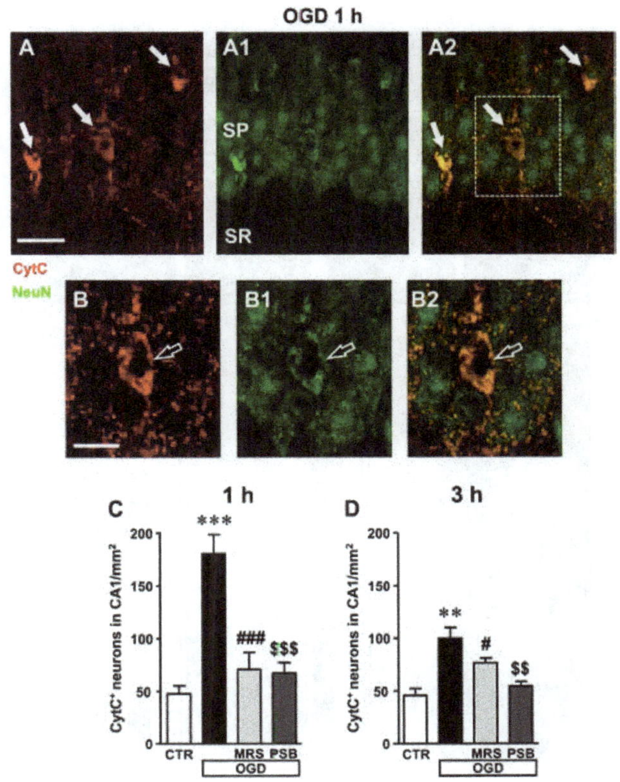

FIGURE 7 | Analysis of CytocromeC$^+$ (CytC$^+$) neurons in CA1 stratum pyramidale after the simil-ischemic insult. **(A–A2)** Representative microphotographs, taken at the laser scanning confocal microscope, of apoptotic neurons labeled with anti-CytC antibody (**A**, red), of pyramidal neurons labeled with anti-NeuN antibody (**A1**, green) and the merge of the two previous images **(A2)**. NeuN$^+$ and CytC$^+$ apoptotic neurons in CA1 stratum pyramidale are indicated by the arrows (yellow-orange color in **A2**). Scale bar: 25 μm. **(B–B2)** Subslice of the framed area in **A2**, obtained stacking 17 consecutive confocal z-scans (5.1 μm total thickness), shown at higher magnification (2×). The open arrow shows an LDN apoptotic pyramidal neuron. Scale bar: 10 μm. **(C,D)** Quantitative analysis of NeuN$^+$ and CytC$^+$ neurons in CA1 stratum pyramidale at 1 h **(C)** and 3 h **(D)** after the end of 7 min OGD. Note the significant increase of CytC$^+$ neurons both 1 and 3 h after the end of OGD. **(C)** Statistical analysis: One-way ANOVA: $F_{(3;11)} = 18.40$, $P < 0.001$, Newman–Keuls multiple comparison test: $^{***}P < 0.001$, OGD vs. CTR; $^{\#\#\#}P < 0.001$, OGD+MRS vs. OGD; $^{\$\$\$}P < 0.001$, OGD+PSB vs. OGD. CTR, $n = 4$; OGD, $n = 3$; OGD+PSB, $n = 4$; OGD+MRS, $n = 4$. **(D)** Statistical analysis: One-way ANOVA: $F_{(3;11)} = 11.41$, $P < 0.02$, Newman–Keuls multiple comparison test: $^{**}P < 0.01$, OGD vs. CTR; $^{\#}P < 0.05$, OGD+MRS vs. OGD; $^{\$\$}P < 0.01$, OGD+PSB vs. OGD. CTR, $n = 4$; OGD, $n = 3$; OGD+PSB, $n = 4$; OGD+MRS, $n = 4$. All data in the graphs are expressed as mean ± SEM.

end of 7 min OGD, we found highly significant decrease of activated mTOR immunostaining in the cytoplasm and dendrites of CA1 pyramidal neurons (**Figures 8H,J**). Indeed, statistical analysis, shown in **Figure 8H**, demonstrates that 3 h after the end of 7 min OGD there was a statistically significant reduction of activated mTOR immunostaining in the cytoplasm of CA1 pyramidal neurons (−74.8%, $^{***}P < 0.001$ vs. control slices, **Figure 8H**) in comparison to control slices. As shown in **Figure 8H**, treatment with 50 nM PSB603 blocked this effect

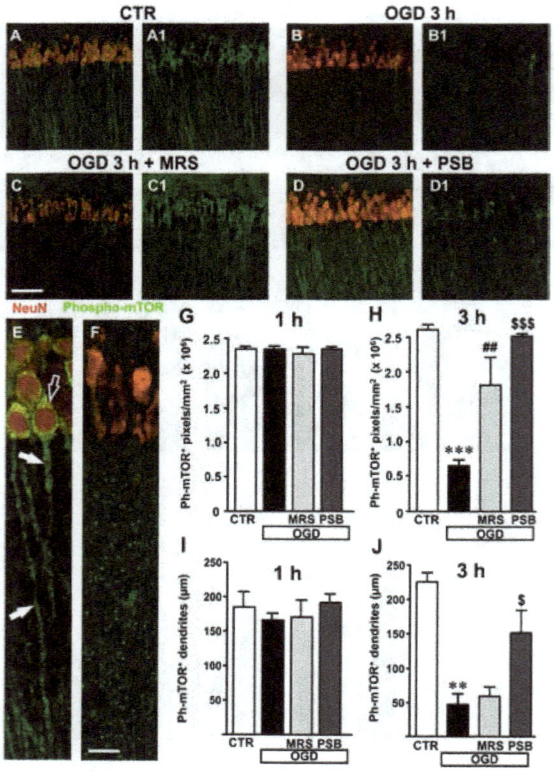

FIGURE 8 | mTOR activation in CA1 stratum pyramidale and stratum radiatum after the simil-ischemic insult. Representative microphotographs, taken at the laser scanning confocal microscope, showing immunolabelling with anti-NeuN antibody (red) and anti-phospho-mTOR antibody (green) of a control slice **(A,A1)**, a slice harvested 3 h after 7 min OGD **(B,B1)**, a slice treated with MRS1754 and harvested 3 h after 7 min OGD **(C,C1)**, and a slice treated with PSB603 and harvested 3 h after 7 min OGD **(D,D1)**. Scale bar: 75 μm. **(E,F)** Digital subslices of a control slice **(E)** and a slice collected 3 h after 7 min OGD **(F)** immunostained for phospho-mTOR (green) and NeuN (red). The open arrow shows the presence of activated mTOR in the cell body and arrows in the dendrites of pyramidal neurons in the control slice **(E)**. **(G,H)** Quantitative analysis of activated mTOR in CA1 stratum pyramidale in the different experimental conditions. Each column represents the mTOR$^+$ immunofluorescent area calculated using the ImageJ program (number of pixels above a reference, fixed threshold). **(G)** No difference among the four experimental groups, was found 1 h after the end of 7 min OGD. Statistical analysis: One-way ANOVA: $F_{(3;11)} = 0.4563$, $P > 0.05$, ns. **(H)** Slices harvested 3 h after the end of 7 min OGD. Note the significant decrease of activated mTOR in CA1 pyramidal neurons 3 h after the end of OGD. Both MRS1754 and PSB603 significantly blocked this effect. Statistical analysis: One-way ANOVA: $F_{(3;10)} = 26.99$, $P < 0.001$, Newman–Keuls multiple comparison test: $^{***}P < 0.001$, OGD vs. CTR; $^{\#\#}P < 0.01$, OGD+MRS vs. OGD; $^{\$\$\$}P < 0.001$, OGD +PSB vs. OGD. CTR, $n = 4$; OGD, $n = 3$; OGD+PSB, $n = 3$; OGD+MRS, $n = 4$. All data are expressed as mean ± SEM. **(I,J)** Quantitative analysis of phospho-mTOR$^+$ dendrites in CA1 stratum radiatum in the different experimental conditions. **(I)** Length of phospho-mTOR$^+$ dendrites in CA1 stratum radiatum 1 h after the end of 7 min OGD. No difference among the four experimental groups was observed. Statistical analysis: One-way ANOVA: $F_{(3;11)} = 0.7143$, $P > 0.05$, ns. **(J)** Length of mTOR$^+$ dendrites in CA1 stratum radiatum 3 h after the end of 7 min OGD. Note the significant decrease of activated mTOR in dendrites 3 h after the end of OGD. PSB603 significantly blocked this effect. Statistical analysis: One-way ANOVA: $F_{(3;9)} = 12.38$, $P < 0.02$, Newman–Keuls multiple comparison test: $^{**}P < 0.01$, OGD vs. CTR; $^{\$}P < 0.05$, OGD+PSB vs. OGD. CTR, $n = 3$; OGD, $n = 3$; OGD+PSB, $n = 3$; OGD+MRS, $n = 4$. All data in the graphs are expressed as mean ± SEM.

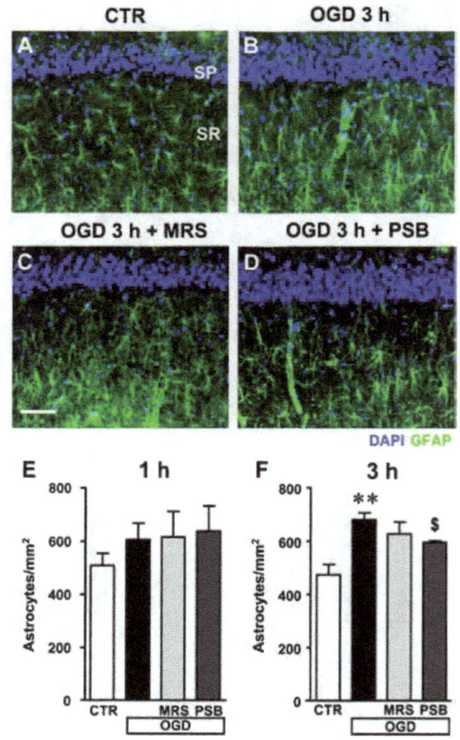

FIGURE 9 | Quantitative analysis of astrocytes in the CA1 area in the different experimental conditions after the simil-ischemic insult. **(A–D)** Representative microphotographs, taken at the epifluorescence microscope, of astrocytes immunolabelled with anti-GFAP antibodies in the stratum radiatum (green) of a control **(A)**, OGD **(B)**, OGD plus MRS1754 **(C)**, and OGD plus PSB603 **(D)** slice. Scale bar: 50 μm. **(E,F)** Quantitative analysis of astrocytes in the stratum radiatum of CA1 in control, OGD, OGD plus MRS1754, and OGD plus PSB603 slices at 1 h **(E)** and 3 h **(F)** after 7 min OGD. **(E)** No significant differences among the four experimental groups analyzed was found. Statistical analysis: One-way ANOVA: $F_{(3;18)} = 0.877$, $P > 0.05$, ns. CTR, $n = 8$; OGD, $n = 7$; OGD+PSB, $n = 3$; OGD+MRS, $n = 4$. **(F)** Statistical analysis: One-way ANOVA: $F_{(3;15)} = 6.734$, $P < 0.01$, Newman–Keuls multiple comparison test: $^{**}P < 0.01$, OGD vs. CTR; $^{\$}P < 0.05$, OGD+PSB vs. OGD. CTR, $n = 7$; OGD, $n = 4$; OGD+PSB, $n = 4$; OGD+MRS, $n = 4$. All data in the graphs are expressed as mean ± SEM.

(−4% vs. control slices, ns, $^{\$\$\$}P < 0.001$ vs. 7 min OGD), while treatment with 500 nM MRS1754 partially, but still significantly attenuated this effect (−31% vs. controls, ns, $^{\#\#}P < 0.01$ vs. 7 min OGD).

We used, as a determinant of mTOR activation in the dendrites, the analysis of the length of phospho-mTOR positive dendrites, as reported in the methods. The results shown in **Figure 8I** reveal that mTOR activation was not statistically significant among the four experimental groups 1 h after the end of 7 min OGD. However, in the slices collected 3 h after the end of 7 min OGD we found a significant decrease of mTOR positive dendrites in the stratum radiatum of the CA1 area (**Figure 8J**). From the statistical analysis we demonstrated a significant decrease of mTOR immunopositive dendrites in CA1 stratum radiatum of 7 min OGD slices 3 h after the end of OGD (−80% vs. controls, $^{**}P < 0.01$, **Figure 8J**). The selective antagonist MRS1754, did not significantly modify this effect, while treatment with PSB603 partially, but significantly, reversed this effect (+226% vs. 7 min OGD,$^{\$}P < 0.05$). These data demonstrate that OGD significantly decreased mTOR activation and that the selective antagonism selective antagonism of A_{2B} receptors significantly reduced this impairment, a further indication of prevention of neuronal degeneration by blockade of this receptor.

Analysis of Astrocytes in CA1 Stratum Radiatum After 7 min OGD

Astrocytes were labeled with the anti-GFAP antibody and quantified in the stratum radiatum of CA1 hippocampus in the four experimental conditions: in control slices, in slices after 7 min OGD alone, and after 7 min OGD in the presence of 500 nM MRS1754 or 50 nM PSB603, both at 1 and 3 h after the end of OGD, as shown in the representative microphotographs in **Figures 9A–D**, taken at 3 h after the end of OGD.

In the stratum radiatum of slices harvested 1 h after the end of 7 min OGD we found a slight, not significant increase of astrocytes (**Figure 9E**, +19%, ns vs. controls), which became significant at 3 h after the end of 7 min OGD (**Figure 9F**, +43% vs. control slices, $^{**}P < 0.01$). Both A_{2B} receptor antagonists, partially but significantly, reduced the increase of astrocytes caused by the simil-ischemic conditions. MRS1754 decreased the number of astrocytes by 10% (ns vs. OGD), while PSB603 by 13% ($^{\$}P < 0.05$ vs. OGD).

Quantitative analysis of total microglia did not reveal statistically significant modifications in the different experimental conditions both at 1 and 3 h after the end of 7 min OGD (data not shown).

Neurodegeneration of CA1 Pyramidal Neurons Induced by Glutamate Was Not Prevented by Adenosine A_{2B} Receptor Antagonists

In order to have an insight into the mechanism of A_{2B} receptor antagonism-induced neuroprotection, we verified whether MRS1754 and PSB603 might protect CA1 pyramidal neurons from the well-known neurodegenerative effects caused by glutamate exposure. We incubated the hippocampal slices *in vitro* with 100 μM glutamate for 10 min and verified the effect of MRS1754 and PSB603 on glutamate-induced cell death (**Figures 10A–D**).

Administration of 100 μM glutamate for 10 min caused significant damage to pyramidal neurons at 3 h after the end of incubation, evidenced by the significant increase of HDN neurons in hippocampal CA1, as shown in the representative image presented in **Figure 10B**. Quantitative analysis (**Figure 10D**) demonstrated that the increase of HDN neurons was statistically significant in comparison to control slices, and that neither MRS1754 nor PSB603 protected CA1 pyramidal neurons from the excitotoxic effect of glutamate ($^{*}P < 0.05$ vs. all other groups).

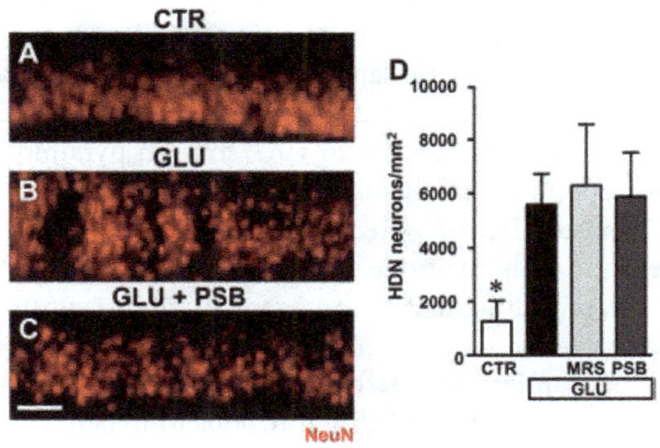

FIGURE 10 | Evaluation of glutamate induced neurotoxicity in CA1 stratum pyramidale in the different experimental conditions. **(A–C)** Representative microphotographs, taken at the epifluorescence microscope, of CA1 pyramidal neurons immunolabelled with anti-NeuN antibodies in a control slice **(A)**, a slice treated with glutamate (GLU, **B**), a slice treated with glutamate plus PSB603 (GLU+ PSB, **C**) slice. Scale bar: 50 μm. **(D)** Quantitative analyses of $NeuN^+$ HDN neurons in the four experimental groups 3 h after the end of drug incubation. Statistical analysis: One-way ANOVA: $F_{(3;15)} = 3.313$, $P < 0.05$, Newman–Keuls multiple comparison test: $^{*}P < 0.05$, vs. all other groups. CTR, $n = 6$; GLU, $n = 6$; GLU+PSB, $n = 3$; GLU+MRS, $n = 4$.

DISCUSSION

The putative protective role of adenosine A_{2B} receptors in cerebral ischemia was studied in the CA1 region of hippocampal slices under oxygen-glucose deprivation, an experimental condition that mimics, albeit with the limits of *in vitro* methodology, the most common causes of cerebral ischemia, such as vessel occlusion. *In vitro* slices give a partial view of the physiology of the brain because of the absence of an intact vascular system and the altered tridimensional microenvironment. These alterations involve not only neurons but also glia, and more generally the physiology of the neurovascular unit formed by astrocytes, pericytes, microglia, neurons, and the extracellular matrix (Holloway and Gavins, 2016). Nevertheless, the *in vitro* systems have many benefits such as the opportunity to obtain highly valuable information in terms of the time-course of the electrophysiological events, changes in membrane potential (AD), changes in synaptic transmission and morphological and biochemical changes in neurons and glia. Our results confirm that in the CA1 region of rat hippocampus, the application of a 7 min OGD episode induced the appearance of AD which was followed by irreversible synaptic damage and neurodegeneration of CA1 pyramidal neurons (Pugliese et al., 2003, 2006, 2009; Coppi et al., 2007; Traini et al., 2011). We now demonstrate that these events are accompanied by neurodegeneration of CA1 pyramidal neurons, with reduction of neuronal density and significant increase of apoptotic neurons. For the first time we demonstrated here that antagonism of A_{2B} receptors using the selective ligands MRS1754 or PSB603, applied before, during and after OGD, prevented or delayed the appearance of AD, and prevented the irreversible loss of neurotransmission induced by 7 min OGD. Furthermore, we demonstrated that the selective blockade of A_{2B} receptors during a prolonged (30 min) OGD insult delays the appearance of AD indicating an extension of the time window between the start of the insult and the appearance of excitotoxic damage. Adenosine A_{2B} receptor antagonism also counteracted the reduction of neuronal density in CA1 stratum pyramidale and decreased apoptosis mechanisms at least up to 3 h after the end of the insult. Both A_{2B} receptor antagonists did not protect CA1 neurons from neurodegeneration induced by glutamate application, indicating that the antagonistic effect is upstream of glutamate release.

The hippocampus, and particularly CA1 stratum pyramidale, is one of the most vulnerable brain regions to ischemic damage. We used the acute rat hippocampal slice preparation which allows measurements of synaptic transmission with good spatial and temporal resolution. In the early phases, hypoxia/ischemia is known to induce a massive increase of extracellular glutamate levels which trigger hyperactivation of glutamate receptors, production of reactive oxygen species, pathological increase of intracellular Ca^{2+}, rapid decrease in ATP reserves and activation of various proteolytic enzymes (Káradóttir et al., 2005; Al-Majed et al., 2006; Kovacs et al., 2006). In hippocampal slices, a severe OGD insult as that applied in the present experiments (7 min) elicits the appearance of AD within the OGD period and is invariably followed by irreversible loss of neurotransmission (Frenguelli et al., 2007; Pugliese et al., 2007, 2009), an index of cell suffering, damage to neurons and to the surrounding tissue (Somjen, 2001). AD is caused by the sudden increase of extracellular K^{+} and by the contemporary explosive rise in glutamate extracellular concentration (Somjen, 2001). Contemporarily to the extracellular increase of glutamate, the extracellular concentration of adenosine significantly increases, as demonstrated both in *in vivo* and *in vitro* experiments (Latini and Pedata, 2001). After 5 min OGD, adenosine reaches an extracellular concentration of 30 μM in hippocampal slices (Latini et al., 1999; Pearson et al., 2006). At such high concentration adenosine can stimulate all receptor subtypes, including the A_{2B} receptor, which exhibits affinity for adenosine with an EC_{50} in the range of 5–20 μM, lower than all other subtypes (Fredholm et al., 2011). For this reason, it is possible that activation of A_{2B} receptors occurs mainly during pathological conditions, such as inflammation, hypoxia, trauma, and ischemia (Fredholm et al., 2001).

Our data show that A_{2B} receptor antagonists, by preventing or delaying the onset of AD, prevent the irreversible loss of neurotransmission induced by 7 min OGD allowing complete recovery of synaptic potentials. We showed for the first time a partial recovery of neurotransmission was also observed in a group of hippocampal slices, treated with A_{2B} receptor antagonists, that developed AD immediately after reoxygenation. This delay of AD appearance might account for the partial recovery of neurotransmission observed in these slices. The occurrence of AD after the end of OGD period is a peculiar characteristic that we observed in our hippocampal preparation. We envisage that when the AD appears during the reoxygenation period, similarly to the phenomenon of spreading depression (Somjen, 2001), neurons are less damaged, and they can partially recover their electrical activity. Thus, even in those slices treated with the A_{2B} receptor antagonists in which AD takes place, this event is less harmful to neuronal viability. This is a substantial difference from A_{2A} receptor antagonist-mediated neuroprotection during a 7 min OGD insult. Indeed, fEPSP recovery was never observed in those few slices undergoing AD in the presence of the A_{2A} receptor blocker ZM241385, as previously published (Pugliese et al., 2009).

As to the mechanism by which A_{2B} receptor antagonists protect from hypoxia/ischemia, recent studies by Gonçalves et al. (2015) have demonstrated that in mouse hippocampus A_{2B} receptors are expressed on glutamatergic terminals anatomically comparable to those from which our recordings were performed. Their selective stimulation counteracts the predominant A_1 receptor-mediated inhibition of synaptic transmission. We confirmed this assumption by performing PPF experiments in rat hippocampal slices in which the A_{2B} receptor agonist BAY606583 was able to reduce PPF ratio, which is known to be caused by increased glutamate release at presynaptic level. This effect is counteracted not only by the A_{2B} receptor antagonists MRS1754 and PSB603 but also by the A_1 receptor antagonist DPCPX. As already hypothesized (Moriyama and Sitkovsky, 2010; Gonçalves et al., 2015), this result may be related to the existence of an A_1/A_{2B} receptor heterodimer in the CA1 hippocampal region. On these bases, our purpose was to study the possible involvement of A_1 receptors in the neuroprotective effects elicited by the two A_{2B} receptor antagonists during OGD. In accordance to data reported by Canals et al. (2008) in a model of chemical penumbra produced by a mitochondrial gliotoxin in the hippocampus *in vitro*, we would have expected conservation of synaptic transmission during the first min of OGD and acceleration of AD appearance. In our conditions, a similar response was observed only in a limited number of slices during 7 min OGD. Instead, in most of the slices we demonstrated that DPCPX induced neuroprotection during OGD, delaying AD appearance. This unexpected result may be due to a different response of A_1 receptors during OGD in our experimental conditions. Our data could also be explained considering the results obtained by Sperlágh et al. (2007) who demonstrated that DPCPX decreases glutamate release from hippocampal slices subjected to OGD and that this effect is mimicked and occluded by the A_{2A} receptor antagonist ZM241385. The same Authors hypothesize that DPCPX, even at low nanomolar concentrations, would directly bind to A_{2A} receptors during severe ischemia (in accordance with our previously published results, Pugliese et al., 2009). The rational for this assumption is that the A_{2A} receptor agonist CGS21680 displays two distinct binding sites in the hippocampus: a "typical" (striatal-like) binding site which is displayed by DPCPX only at high (submicromolar) concentrations, and an "atypical" binding site, which shows high affinity for DPCPX (Johansson and Fredholm, 1995; Cunha et al., 1996). On these bases, we can hypothesize that, in our OGD experiments, DPCPX binds to this "atypical" binding site (i.e., an A_1–A_{2A} receptor heterodimer) thus decreasing glutamate outflow and protecting hippocampal slices from OGD insults. Furthermore, when overstimulated such as during ischemia, A_1 receptors undergo desensitization (Siniscalchi et al., 1999).

This phenomenon can be further increased by A_{2B} receptors activation, triggering a vicious circle in which the beneficial effect of A_1 receptor stimulation is overcome by the noxious effect of A_{2B} receptors activation (Gonçalves et al., 2015) as already suggested for A_{2A} adenosine receptors (Pugliese et al., 2009). Further mechanistic studies suggest that the A_{2A} receptor, when stimulated, facilitates A_{2B} receptor externalization from the endoplasmic reticulum to the plasma membrane, possibly increasing the formation of the A_{2A}–A_{2B} dimer (Moriyama and Sitkovsky, 2010). All these results taken together may explain the deleterious activity of adenosine A_{2B} receptor stimulation during an ischemic insult, and the protective effect of A_{2B} receptor antagonists in this condition. Finally, observation that the A_{2B} receptor antagonists did not protect CA1 neurons from neurodegeneration induced by direct glutamate application, confirms that the mechanism underlying their protection against ischemia-induced neurodegeneration is exerted at adenosine receptors that, by the abovementioned mechanisms, regulate extracellular glutamate release. Alternatively, since OGD is above all a problem of efficient energy recovery, the demonstration that A_{2B} receptors control astrocytic and neuronal glycogen metabolism (Magistretti et al., 1986; Allaman et al., 2003) and glucose utilization by hippocampal slices (Lemos et al., 2015) may suggest an additional effect of these receptors on metabolic activity during OGD.

Severe OGD increased apoptosis and damaged CA1 pyramidal neurons at 1 and 3 h after the end of the ischemic insult. Immunohistochemistry showed that CA1 pyramidal neurons had significant morphological changes, with increased density of nuclei (HDN neurons), karyorrhexis (LDN neurons) and possibly nuclear fragmentation, as evidenced by the significantly higher number of LDN neurons and cell death after OGD. These results are in agreement with those found by Ünal-Çevik et al. (2004) in the cerebral cortex of the rat after mild ischemia. Pyknosis is typical of apoptotic cells (Elmore, 2007) and may precede karyorrhexis. We demonstrated that LDN neurons, being highly positive for CytC, were undergoing apoptosis. It has been demonstrated that CytC released into the cytosol binds to apoptotic protease activating factor-1, which leads to activation of caspase-9 which is important in neuronal cell death following ischemia (Kluck et al., 1997; Yang et al., 1997; Love, 2003; Jiang and Wang, 2004; Suen et al., 2008; Lana et al., 2014, 2016, 2017a,b; Martínez-Fábregas et al., 2014). In turn, caspase-9 is activated by high glutamate levels, as occurs during ischemia (Li et al., 2009). As reported in the literature, activation of mTOR, which has multiple roles in cells among which local protein synthesis at the dendritic and spine level (Frey and Morris, 1997; Tsokas et al., 2007; Thoreen et al., 2012), can be modified in ischemic conditions (Dennis et al., 2001; Laplante and Sabatini, 2012). As already reported (Gegelashvili et al., 2001; Maragakis and Rothstein, 2004), the decrease of mTOR activation may be secondary to the excitotoxic mechanisms evoked by massive increase of glutamate during OGD, which is known to be an important component of neuronal injury *in vitro* (Newell et al., 1995). The participation of decreased mTOR activation in OGD-induced neuronal damage is supported by our results showing decreased activation of mTOR both in the cell body and dendrites of CA1 neurons 3 h after the end of OGD.

Within the limits of the *in vitro* model and the alteration of the neurovascular unit and of neuro glia interplay, we found interesting effects on astrocytic responses. Indeed, astrocytes proliferation, possibly caused, among other stimuli, by increased release of glutamate, is one of the early events that takes place after acute focal CNS damage (Burda and Sofroniew, 2014). In accordance to our previous results (Pugliese et al., 2009), we found evidence of significant, although limited, astrocytic proliferation in CA1 stratum radiatum already 3 h after the end of OGD, possibly caused by increased glutamate release. A_{2B} receptor antagonism significantly prevented all the above neuronal and astrocytic modifications, sparing neurons from the degenerative effects caused by the simil-ischemic conditions, and reducing astrocytes proliferation. CA1 pyramidal neurons treated with the A_{2B} receptor antagonists had a similar morphology to those of control slices, had neither increased nor decreased nuclear density, did not undergo apoptosis, and had activated mTOR levels similar to those of controls.

The similar effects obtained using two different A_{2B} receptor antagonists strengthen the hypothesis that the A_{2B} receptor is involved in the mechanisms of cerebral ischemia. Nevertheless, MRS1754 seems to have lower efficiency than PSB603 on some of the parameters investigated. It is possible that the two drugs act with a different time-course or that PSB603 is more efficacious than MRS1754 in this model.

In summary, our data demonstrate that antagonists of adenosine A_{2B} receptors protect the CA1 area of the hippocampus from an acute damage induced by severe hypoxic/ischemic conditions. The mechanism likely resides in protection from the acute increase of glutamate extracellular concentrations and consequent excitotoxicity. It is worth noticing that since A_{2B} receptors have low affinity for the endogenous ligand adenosine, they are activated only at high extracellular adenosine concentrations that can be reached under pathological conditions such as ischemia, thus representing a selective target (Popoli and Pepponi, 2012).

AUTHOR CONTRIBUTIONS

MG and AP designed the research. FU, DL, DN, IF, LG, ID, and FC performed the experiments. FU, DL, EC, MG and AP analyzed the data. DL, MG, EC, AP and FP interpreted the results and the experiments. DL, MG, FU, AP and IF prepared the figures. MG and AP drafted the manuscript. DL, MG, FU, FP, AP and EC edited and revised the manuscript. All authors read and approved the final version of the manuscript.

FUNDING

DL was partly funded by Ente Cassa di Risparmio di Firenze (ECRF_2014_0663_Giovannini) and by

University of Florence Dean's Postdoctoral Fellowship. This research was funded in part by University of Florence (Fondi Ateneo Ricerca: AP, FP, and MG), and in part by MIUR-PRIN (2015E8EMCM_006, MG) and (2015E8EMCM_002, AP). The funding sources had no involvement in the conduct of the research, in preparation of the article, in study design; in the collection, analysis and interpretation of data; in the writing of the report; and in the decision to submit the article for publication.

ACKNOWLEDGMENTS

We thank Dr. F. Trombetta for the helpful technical assistance.

REFERENCES

Allaman, I., Lengacher, S., Magistretti, P. J., and Pellerin, L. (2003). A2B receptor activation promotes glycogen synthesis in astrocytes through modulation of gene expression. *Am. J. Physiol. Cell Physiol.* 284, C696–C704. doi: 10.1152/ajpcell.00202.2002

Allard, D., Turcotte, M., and Stagg, J. (2017). Targeting A2 adenosine receptors in cancer. *Immunol. Cell Biol.* 95, 333–339. doi: 10.1038/icb.2017.8

Al-Majed, A. A., Sayed-Ahmed, M. M., Al-Omar, F. A., Al-Yahya, A. A., Aleisa, A. M., and Al-Shabanah, O. A. (2006). Carnitine esters prevent oxidative stress damage and energy depletion following transient forebrain ischaemia in the rat hippocampus. *Clin. Exp. Pharmacol. Physiol.* 33, 725–733. doi: 10.1111/j.1440-1681.2006.04425.x

Anderson, W. W., and Collingridge, G. L. (2001). The LTP Program: a data acquisition program for on-line analysis of long-term potentiation and other synaptic events. *J. Neurosci. Methods* 108, 71–83. doi: 10.1016/S0165-0270(01)00374-0

Burda, J. E., and Sofroniew, M. V. (2014). Reactive gliosis and the multicellular response to CNS damage and disease. *Neuron* 81, 229–248. doi: 10.1016/j.neuron.2013.12.034

Canals, S., Larrosa, B., Pintor, J., Mena, M. A., and Herreras, O. (2008). Metabolic challenge to glia activates an adenosine-mediated safety mechanism that promotes neuronal survival by delaying the onset of spreading depression waves. *J. Cereb. Blood Flow Metab.* 28, 1835–1844. doi: 10.1038/jcbfm.2008.71

Cerbai, F., Lana, D., Nosi, D., Petkova-Kirova, P., Zecchi, S., Brothers, H. M., et al. (2012). The neuron-astrocyte-microglia triad in normal brain ageing and in a model of neuroinflammation in the rat hippocampus. *PLoS One* 7:e45250. doi: 10.1371/journal.pone.0045250

Chandrasekera, P. C., McIntosh, V. J., Cao, F. X., and Lasley, R. D. (2010). Differential effects of adenosine A2a and A2b receptors on cardiac contractility. *Am. J. Physiol. Heart Circ. Physiol.* 299, H2082–H2089. doi: 10.1152/ajpheart.00511.2010

Chen, J. F., Sonsalla, P., Pedata, F., Melani, A., Domenici, M. R., Popoli, P., et al. (2007). Adenosine A2A receptors and brain injury: broad spectrum of neuroprotection, multi-faced actions and "fine tuning" modulation. *Prog. Neurobiol.* 83, 310–331. doi: 10.1016/j.pneurobio.2007.09.002

Choi, D. W. (1992). Excitotoxic cell death. *J. Neurobiol.* 23, 1261–1276. doi: 10.1002/neu.480230915

Coppi, E., Pugliese, A. M., Stephan, H., Müller, C. E., and Pedata, F. (2007). Role of P2 purinergic receptors in synaptic transmission under normoxic and ischaemic conditions in the CA1 region of rat hippocampal slices. *Purinergic Signal.* 3, 203–219. doi: 10.1007/s11302-006-9049-4

Csóka, B., Németh, Z. H., Selmeczy, Z., Koscsó, B., Pacher, P., Vizi, E. S., et al. (2007). Role of A(2A) adenosine receptors in regulation of opsonized *E. coli*-induced macrophage function. *Purinergic Signal.* 3, 447–452. doi: 10.1007/s11302-007-9075-x

Cunha, R. A., Johansson, B., Constantino, M. D., Sebastião, A. M., and Fredholm, B. B. (1996). Evidence for high-affinity binding sites for the adenosine A2A receptor agonist [3H] CGS 21680 in the rat hippocampus and cerebral cortex that are different from striatal A2A receptors. *Naunyn Schmiedebergs Arch. Pharmacol.* 353, 261–271. doi: 10.1007/BF00168627

Dennis, P. B., Jaeschke, A., Saitoh, M., Fowler, B., Kozma, S. C., and Thomas, G. (2001). Mammalian TOR: a homeostatic ATP sensor. *Science* 294, 1102–1105. doi: 10.1126/science.1063518

Dirnagl, U. (2012). Pathobiology of injury after stroke: the neurovascular unit and beyond. *Ann. N. Y. Acad. Sci.* 1268, 21–25. doi: 10.1111/j.1749-6632.2012.06691.x

Dixon, A. K., Gubitz, A. K., Sirinathsinghji, D. J., Richardson, P. J., and Freeman, T. C. (1996). Tissue distribution of adenosine receptor mRNAs in the rat. *Br. J. Pharmacol.* 118, 1461–1468. doi: 10.1111/j.1476-5381.1996.tb15561.x

Elmore, S. (2007). Apoptosis: a review of programmed cell death. *Toxicol. Pathol.* 35, 495–516. doi: 10.1080/01926230701320337

Farkas, E., Pratt, R., Sengpiel, F., and Obrenovitch, T. P. (2008). Direct, live imaging of cortical spreading depression and anoxic depolarisation using a fluorescent, voltage-sensitive dye. *J. Cereb. Blood Flow Metab.* 28, 251–262. doi: 10.1038/sj.jcbfm.9600569

Feoktistov, I., Polosa, R., Holgate, S. T., and Biaggioni, I. (1998). Adenosine A2B receptors: a novel therapeutic target in asthma? *Trends Pharmacol. Sci.* 19, 148–153.

Fowler, J. C. (1992). Escape from inhibition of synaptic transmission during in vitro hypoxia and hypoglycemia in the hippocampus. *Brain Res.* 573, 169–173. doi: 10.1016/0006-8993(92)90128-V

Fredholm, B. B., IJzerman, A. P., Jacobson, K. A., Linden, J., and Müller, C. E. (2011). International union of basic and clinical pharmacology. LXXXI. Nomenclature and classification of adenosine receptors–an update. *Pharmacol. Rev.* 63, 1–34. doi: 10.1124/pr.110.003285

Fredholm, B. B., Irenius, E., Kull, B., and Schulte, G. (2001). Comparison of the potency of adenosine as an agonist at human adenosine receptors expressed in Chinese hamster ovary cells. *Biochem. Pharmacol.* 61, 443–448. doi: 10.1016/S0006-2952(00)00570-0

Frenguelli, B. G., Wigmore, G., Llaudet, E., and Dale, N. (2007). Temporal and mechanistic dissociation of ATP and adenosine release during ischaemia in the mammalian hippocampus. *J. Neurochem.* 101, 1400–1413. doi: 10.1111/j.1471-4159.2007.04425.x

Frey, U., and Morris, R. G. (1997). Synaptic tagging and long-term potentiation. *Nature* 385, 533–536. doi: 10.1038/385533a0

Gegelashvili, G., Robinson, M. B., Trotti, D., and Rauen, T. (2001). Regulation of glutamate transporters in health and disease. *Prog. Brain Res.* 132, 267–286. doi: 10.1016/S0079-6123(01)32082-4

Gonçalves, F. Q., Pires, J., Pliassova, A., Beleza, R., Lemos, C., Marques, J. M., et al. (2015). Adenosine A2b receptors control A1 receptor-mediated inhibition of synaptic transmission in the mouse hippocampus. *Eur. J. Neurosci.* 41, 878–888. doi: 10.1111/ejn.12851

Herreras, O., and Somjen, G. G. (1993). Propagation of spreading depression among dendrites and somata of the same cell population. *Brain Res.* 610, 276–282. doi: 10.1016/0006-8993(93)91411-K

Holloway, P. M., and Gavins, F. N. (2016). Modeling ischemic stroke in vitro: status quo and future perspectives. *Stroke* 47, 561–569. doi: 10.1161/STROKEAHA.115.011932

Jarvis, C. R., Anderson, T. R., and Andrew, R. D. (2001). Anoxic depolarization mediates acute damage independent of glutamate in neocortical brain slices. *Cereb. Cortex* 11, 249–259. doi: 10.1093/cercor/11.3.249

Jiang, X., and Wang, X. (2004). Cytochrome C-mediated apoptosis. *Annu. Rev. Biochem.* 73, 87–106. doi: 10.1146/annurev.biochem.73.011303.073706

Johansson, B., and Fredholm, B. B. (1995). Further characterization of the binding of the adenosine receptor agonist [3H]CGS 21680 to rat brain using autoradiography. *Neuropharmacology* 34, 393–403. doi: 10.1016/0028-3908(95)00009-U

Káradóttir, R., Cavelier, P., Bergersen, L. H., and Attwell, D. (2005). NMDA receptors are expressed in oligodendrocytes and activated in ischaemia. *Nature* 438, 1162–1166. doi: 10.1038/nature04302

Kluck, R. M., Bossy-Wetzel, E., Green, D. R., and Newmeyer, D. D. (1997). The release of cytochrome c from mitochondria: a primary site for Bcl-2 regulation of apoptosis. *Science* 275, 1132–1136. doi: 10.1126/science.275.5303.1132

Kolachala, V., Ruble, B., Vijay-Kumar, M., Wang, L., Mwangi, S., Figler, H., et al. (2008). Blockade of adenosine A2B receptors ameliorates murine colitis. *Br. J. Pharmacol.* 155, 127–137. doi: 10.1038/bjp.2008.227

Koroleva, V. I., and Bures, J. (1996). The use of spreading depression waves for acute and long-term monitoring of the penumbra zone of focal ischemic damage in rats. *Proc. Natl. Acad. Sci. U.S.A.* 93, 3710–3714. doi: 10.1073/pnas.93.8.3710

Kovacs, K., Toth, A., Deres, P., Kalai, T., Hideg, K., Gallyas, F. Jr., et al. (2006). Critical role of PI3-kinase/Akt activation in the PARP inhibitor induced heart function recovery during ischemia-reperfusion. *Biochem. Pharmacol.* 71, 441–452. doi: 10.1016/j.bcp.2005.05.036

Lana, D., Cerbai, F., Di Russo, J., Boscaro, F., Giannetti, A., Petkova-Kirova, P., et al. (2013). Hippocampal long term memory: effect of the cholinergic system on local protein synthesis. *Neurobiol. Learn. Mem.* 106, 246–257. doi: 10.1016/j.nlm.2013.09.013

Lana, D., Iovino, L., Nosi, D., Wenk, G. L., and Giovannini, M. G. (2016). The neuron-astrocyte-microglia triad involvement in neuroinflammaging mechanisms in the CA3 hippocampus of memory-impaired aged rats. *Exp. Gerontol.* 83, 71–88. doi: 10.1016/j.exger.2016.07.011

Lana, D., Melani, A., Pugliese, A. M., Cipriani, S., Nosi, D., Pedata, F., et al. (2014). The neuron-astrocyte-microglia triad in a rat model of chronic cerebral hypoperfusion: protective effect of dipyridamole. *Front. Aging Neurosci.* 6:322. doi: 10.3389/fnagi.2014.00322

Lana, D., Ugolini, F., Melani, A., Nosi, D., Pedata, F., and Giovannini, M. G. (2017a). The neuron-astrocyte-microglia triad in CA3 after chronic cerebral hypoperfusion in the rat: protective effect of dipyridamole. *Exp. Gerontol.* 96, 46–62. doi: 10.1016/j.exger.2017.06.006

Lana, D., Ugolini, F., Nosi, D., Wenk, G. L., and Giovannini, M. G. (2017b). Alterations in the interplay between neurons, astrocytes and microglia in the rat dentate gyrus in experimental models of neurodegeneration. *Front. Aging Neurosci.* 9:296. doi: 10.3389/fnagi.2017.00296

Laplante, M., and Sabatini, D. M. (2012). mTOR signaling in growth control and disease. *Cell* 149, 274–293. doi: 10.1016/j.cell.2012.03.017

Latini, S., Bordoni, F., Corradetti, R., Pepeu, G., and Pedata, F. (1998). Temporal correlation between adenosine outflow and synaptic potential inhibition in rat hippocampal slices during ischemia-like conditions. *Brain Res.* 794, 325–328. doi: 10.1016/S0006-8993(98)00304-7

Latini, S., Bordoni, F., Corradetti, R., Pepeu, G., and Pedata, F. (1999). Effect of A2A adenosine receptor stimulation and antagonism on synaptic depression induced by in vitro ischaemia in rat hippocampal slices. *Br. J. Pharmacol.* 128, 1035–1044. doi: 10.1038/sj.bjp.0702888

Latini, S., and Pedata, F. (2001). Adenosine in the central nervous system: release mechanisms and extracellular concentrations. *J. Neurochem.* 79, 463–484. doi: 10.1046/j.1471-4159.2001.00607.x

Lemos, C., Pinheiro, B. S., Beleza, R. O., Marques, J. M., Rodrigues, R. J., Cunha, R. A., et al. (2015). Adenosine A2B receptor activation stimulates glucose uptake in the mouse forebrain. *Purinergic Signal.* 1, 561–569. doi: 10.1007/s11302-015-9474-3

Li, S. Q., Zhang, Y., and Tang, D. B. (2009). Possible mechanisms of Cyclosporin A ameliorated the ischemic microenvironment and inhibited mitochondria stress in tree shrews' hippocampus. *Pathophysiology* 16, 279–284. doi: 10.1016/j.pathophys.2009.02.014

Love, S. (2003). Apoptosis and brain ischaemia. *Prog. Neuropsychopharmacol. Biol. Psychiatry* 27, 267–282.

Magistretti, P. J., Hof, P. R., and Martin, J. L. (1986). Adenosine stimulates glycogenolysis in mouse cerebral cortex: a possible coupling mechanism between neuronal activity and energy metabolism. *J. Neurosci.* 6, 2558–2562. doi: 10.1523/JNEUROSCI.06-09-02558.1986

Maragakis, N. J., and Rothstein, J. D. (2004). Glutamate transporters: animal models to neurologic diseases. *Neurobiol. Dis.* 15, 461–473. doi: 10.1016/j.nbd.2003.12.007

Martínez-Fábregas, J., Díaz-Moreno, I., González-Arzola, K., Janocha, S., Navarro, J. A., Hervás, M., et al. (2014). Structural and functional analysis of novel human cytochrome C targets in apoptosis. *Mol. Cell. Proteomics* 13, 1439–1456. doi: 10.1074/mcp.M113.034322

Melani, A., Pantoni, L., Corsi, C., Bianchi, L., Monopoli, A., Bertorelli, R., et al. (1999). Striatal outflow of adenosine, excitatory amino acids, gamma-aminobutyric acid, and taurine in awake freely moving rats after middle cerebral artery occlusion: correlations with neurological deficit and histopathological damage. *Stroke* 30, 2448–2454. doi: 10.1161/01.STR.30.11.2448

Merighi, S., Borea, P. A., and Gessi, S. (2015). Adenosine receptors and diabetes: Focus on the A(2B) adenosine receptor subtype. *Pharmacol. Res.* 99, 229–236. doi: 10.1016/j.phrs.2015.06.015

Moriyama, K., and Sitkovsky, M. V. (2010). Adenosine A2A receptor is involved in cell surface expression of A2B receptor. *J. Biol. Chem.* 285, 39271–39288. doi: 10.1074/jbc.M109.098293

Newell, D. W., Barth, A., Papermaster, V., and Malouf, A. T. (1995). Glutamate and non-glutamate receptor mediated toxicity caused by oxygen, and glucose deprivation in organotypic hippocampal cultures. *J. Neurosci.* 15, 7702–7711. doi: 10.1523/JNEUROSCI.15-11-07702.1995

Pearson, T., Damian, K., Lynas, R. E., and Frenguelli, B. G. (2006). Sustained elevation of extracellular adenosine and activation of A1 receptors underlie the post-ischaemic inhibition of neuronal function in rat hippocampus in vitro. *J. Neurochem.* 97, 1357–1368. doi: 10.1111/j.1471-4159.2006.03823.x

Pedata, F., Dettori, I., Coppi, E., Melani, A., Fusco, I., Corradetti, R., et al. (2016). Purinergic signalling in brain ischemia. *Neuropharmacology* 104, 105–130. doi: 10.1016/j.neuropharm.2015.11.007

Pedata, F., Latini, S., Pugliese, A. M., and Pepeu, G. (1993). Investigations into the adenosine outflow from hippocampal slices evoked by ischemia-like conditions. *J. Neurochem.* 61, 284–289. doi: 10.1111/j.1471-4159.1993.tb03566.x

Pedata, F., Pugliese, A. M., Coppi, E., Dettori, I., Maraula, G., Cellai, L., et al. (2014). Adenosine A2A receptors modulate acute injury and neuroinflammation in brain ischemia. *Mediators Inflamm.* 2014:805198. doi: 10.1155/2014/805198

Perez-Buira, S., Barrachina, M., Rodriguez, A., Albasanz, J. L., Martín, M., Ferrer, I., et al. (2007). Expression levels of adenosine receptors in hippocampus and frontal cortex in argyrophilic grain disease. *Neurosci. Lett.* 423, 194–199. doi: 10.1016/j.neulet.2007.06.049

Popoli, P., and Pepponi, R. (2012). Potential therapeutic relevance of adenosine A2B and A2A receptors in the central nervous system. *CNS Neurol. Disord. Drug Targets* 11, 664–674. doi: 10.2174/187152712803581100

Pugliese, A. M., Coppi, E., Spalluto, G., Corradetti, R., and Pedata, F. (2006). A3 adenosine receptor antagonists delay irreversible synaptic failure caused by oxygen and glucose deprivation in the rat CA1 hippocampus in vitro. *Br. J. Pharmacol.* 147, 524–532. doi: 10.1038/sj.bjp.0706646

Pugliese, A. M., Coppi, E., Volpini, R., Cristalli, G., Corradetti, R., Jeong, L. S., et al. (2007). Role of adenosine A3 receptors on CA1 hippocampal neurotransmission during oxygen-glucose deprivation episodes of different duration. *Biochem. Pharmacol.* 74, 768–779. doi: 10.1016/j.bcp.2007.06.003

Pugliese, A. M., Latini, S., Corradetti, R., and Pedata, F. (2003). Brief, repeated, oxygen-glucose deprivation episodes protect neurotransmission from a longer ischemic episode in the in vitro hippocampus: role of adenosine receptors. *Br. J. Pharmacol.* 140, 305–314. doi: 10.1038/sj.bjp.0705442

Pugliese, A. M., Traini, C., Cipriani, S., Gianfriddo, M., Mello, T., Giovannini, M. G., et al. (2009). The adenosine A2A receptor antagonist ZM241385 enhances neuronal survival after oxygen-glucose deprivation in rat CA1 hippocampal slices. *Br. J. Pharmacol.* 157, 818–830. doi: 10.1111/j.1476-5381.2009.00218.x

Siniscalchi, A., Rodi, D., Gessi, S., Campi, F., and Borea, P. A. (1999). Early changes in adenosine A1 receptors in cerebral cortex slices submitted to in vitro ischemia. *Neurochem. Int.* 34, 517–522. doi: 10.1016/S0197-0186(99)00028-5

Somjen, G. G. (2001). Mechanisms of spreading depression and hypoxic spreading depression-like depolarization. *Physiol. Rev.* 81, 1065–1096. doi: 10.1152/physrev.2001.81.3.1065

Sperlágh, B., Zsilla, G., Baranyi, M., Illes, P., and Vizi, E. S. (2007). Purinergic modulation of glutamate release under ischemic-like conditions in the hippocampus. *Neuroscience* 149, 99–111. doi: 10.1016/j.neuroscience.2007.07.035

Suen, D. F., Norris, K. L., and Youle, R. J. (2008). Mitochondrial dynamics and apoptosis. *Genes Dev.* 22, 1577–1590. doi: 10.1101/gad.1658508

Tanaka, E., Yamamoto, S., Kudo, Y., Mihara, S., and Higashi, H. (1997). Mechanisms underlying the rapid depolarization produced by deprivation of oxygen and glucose in rat hippocampal CA1 neurons in vitro. *J. Neurophysiol.* 78, 891–902. doi: 10.1152/jn.1997.78.2.891

Thoreen, C. C., Chantranupong, L., Keys, H. R., Wang, T., Gray, N. S., and Sabatini, D. M. (2012). A unifying model for mTORC1-mediated regulation of mRNA translation. *Nature* 485, 109–113. doi: 10.1038/nature11083

Traini, C., Pedata, F., Cipriani, S., Mello, T., Galli, A., Giovannini, M. G., et al. (2011). P2 receptor antagonists prevent synaptic failure and extracellular signal-regulated kinase 1/2 activation induced by oxygen and glucose deprivation in rat CA1 hippocampus in vitro. *Eur. J. Neurosci.* 33, 2203–2215. doi: 10.1111/j.1460-9568.2011.07667.x

Tsokas, P., Ma, T., Iyengar, R., Landau, E. M., and Blitzer, R. D. (2007). Mitogen-activated protein kinase upregulates the dendritic translation machinery in long-term potentiation by controlling the mammalian target of rapamycin pathway. *J. Neurosci.* 27, 5885–5894. doi: 10.1523/JNEUROSCI.4548-06.2007

Ugolini, F., Lana, D., Fusco, I., Coppi, E., Dettori, I., Gaviano, L., et al. (2017). "The selective antagonism of adenosine A2B receptors prevents synaptic and neuronal damage induced by oxygen and glucose deprivation in CA1 rat hippocampus," in *Proceedings of the Neuroscience 47th Annual Meeting*, Washington, DC.

Ünal-Çevik, I., Kilinç, M., Gürsoy-Ozdemir, Y., Gurer, G., and Dalkara, T. (2004). Loss of NeuN immunoreactivity after cerebral ischemia does not indicate neuronal cell loss: a cautionary note. *Brain Res.* 1015, 169–174. doi: 10.1016/j.brainres.2004.04.032

Yamamoto, S., Tanaka, E., Shoji, Y., Kudo, Y., Inokuchi, H., and Higashi, H. (1997). Factors that reverse the persistent depolarization produced by deprivation of oxygen and glucose in rat hippocampal CA1 neurons in vitro. *J. Neurophysiol.* 78, 903–911. doi: 10.1152/jn.1997.78.2.903

Yang, J., Liu, X., Bhalla, K., Kim, C. N., Ibrado, A. M., Cai, J., et al. (1997). Prevention of apoptosis by Bcl-2: release of cytochrome c from mitochondria blocked. *Science* 275, 1129–1132. doi: 10.1126/science.275.5303.1129

4

Extracellular Guanosine 5′-Triphosphate Induces Human Muscle Satellite Cells to Release Exosomes Stuffed with Guanosine

Tiziana Pietrangelo[1†], Ester S. Di Filippo[1†], Marcello Locatelli[2], Francesco Piacenza[3], Marco Farina[4], Eleonora Pavoni[4], Andrea Di Donato[5], Denise Innosa[6], Mauro Provinciali[3] and Stefania Fulle[1]*

[1] Dipartimento Neuroscienze Imaging and Scienze Cliniche, Università degli Studi "G. d'Annunzio" Chieti-Pescara, Chieti, Italy, [2] Dipartimento di Farmacia, Università degli Studi "G. d'Annunzio" Chieti-Pescara, Chieti, Italy, [3] IRCCS-Istituto Nazionale di Riposo e Cura per Anziani, Polo Scientifico e Tecnologico, Centro di Tecnologie Avanzate nell'Invecchiamento Ancona, Italy, [4] Dipartimento di Ingegneria dell'Informazione, Università Politecnica delle Marche, Ancona, Italy, [5] Harvard John A. Paulson School of Engineering and Applied Sciences, Harvard University, Cambridge, MA, United States, [6] Facoltà di Bioscienze e Tecnologie Agro-Alimentari e Ambientali, Università di Teramo, Teramo, Italy

***Correspondence:**
Tiziana Pietrangelo
tiziana.pietrangelo@unich.it

† These authors have contributed equally to this work.

The extracellular guanosine 5′-triphosphate, GTP, has been demonstrated to be an enhancer of myogenic cell differentiation in a murine cell line, not yet in human muscle cells. Our hypothesis was that GTP could influence also human skeletal muscle regeneration, specifically in the first phases. We tested GTP stimulus on human muscle precursor cells established in culture by human satellite cells derived from Vastus Lateralis of three young male. Our data show that extracellular GTP (a) up-regulated miRNA (specifically miR133a and miR133b) and myogenic regulator factor and (b) induces human myogenic precursor cells to release exosomes stuffed with guanosine based molecules (mainly guanosine) in the extracellular milieu. We think that probably these exosomes could be addressed to influence by means of their content (mainly guanosine) in paracrine or autocrine manner the surrounding cells and/or at distance other muscles or tissues.

Keywords: satellite cells, guanosine, guanosine 5′-triphosphate, myomiRNA, exosomes, skeletal muscle regeneration

INTRODUCTION

It has been extensively demonstrated that extracellular nucleotides are important intercellular messengers that mediate their signals through activation of P2 purinoceptors on the cell membrane (Burnstock, 2017). However, to date no indication exists about other ways of nucleotide signaling. In the last years, the communication by extracellular vesicles in muscle has received a great attention due to their importance as intercellular mediators bearing proteins, lipids, RNAs, and miRNAs through the entire body (Murphy et al., 2017). Exosomes are secreted by cells and released in the extracellular *melieu* where they could keep in contact with the surrounding cells or could be captured into the flowing blood or the lymph and addressed to the entire body. In this manner, the exosomes, and specifically their content, keep in contact different tissues influencing them as physiologycal mediators and/or pathological inductors. The adult skeletal muscle stem cells, satellite cells, provide a high degree of plasticity to muscles. During youth, the activated satellite cells form new myofiber and make hypertrophic the existing ones; during adulthood they compensate for muscle turnover due to daily wear (Yin et al., 2013). Recently, it has been demonstrated that satellite cells are involved in the cellular turnover in response to the ingestion of protein dense foods and exercise (Burd and De Lisio, 2017). Moreover, the skeletal muscle regeneration greatly relies on the dynamic interplay between satellite cells and their cellular niche. The 3D culture model of fibers has been demonstrated to be physiologically relevant to study *in vitro* this niche and the signals present in it (Said et al., 2017; Kasper et al., 2018). The interest on studying skeletal muscle regeneration is exponentially increasing due to also its implication in nutritional aspects, exercise and healthy life. Many papers and reviews outline the role of satellite cells in muscle homeostasis during exercise stimulus or in pathological conditions, when the relative roles of intrinsic vs. extrinsic factors contribute to satellite cell dysfunction (Pietrangelo et al., 2015; Cornelison, 2018).

The pools of satellite cells are activated to proliferate under myogenic regulator factors that control both an initial boost of proliferation and differentiation. These phases influence and in turn are influenced both by myogenic regulator factors as Myogenin and by myo-microRNA, specifically miR-1, miR133a/b, and miR-206 (Drummond et al., 2011; Di Filippo et al., 2017). To date, the study of the role of nucleotide signaling in skeletal muscle regeneration is underestimated. We previously demonstrated that extracellular GTP is able to bind specific sites on plasma membrane and it participates in the early phases of myogenic differentiation process of murine C2C12 cells, modifying the plasma membrane potential toward hyperpolarized state and accelerating the proliferative boost (Pietrangelo et al., 2002, 2006a; Mancinelli et al., 2012). To date it is not known whether extracellular GTP also affects the human satellite cells in the phases of differentiation process. We therefore, hypothesize that extracellular GTP could influence the satellite stem cells via both typical signal transduction (binding on receptors) and/or by release of exosomes stuffed with guanosine based molecules.

MATERIALS AND METHODS

Cell Cultures

The Vastus Lateralis skeletal muscle biopsies were obtained by means of tiny percutaneous needle-biopsy (Pietrangelo et al., 2011).

The subjects who volunteered to have Vastus lateralis needle-biopsy to collect satellite cells provided written informed consent. The study was conducted according to the Helsinki Declaration (as amended in 2000) and approved by the Ethics Committee of the Università degli Studi "G. d'Annunzio" Chieti-Pescara, Italy (protocol no. 773 COET).

To obtain satellite sells, the skeletal muscle was processed according to the method described in Mancinelli et al. (2016). Human satellite cells were isolated from three young male volunteers (22.7 $\pm$ 2.1 years; $n = 3$), were grown as human myogenic precursor cells (MPCs) at 37°C in 5% CO_2 humidity, in Growth Medium (GM): HAM's Nutrient Mixture F10 medium (Euroclone, Milan, Italy, product #ECB7503SL) supplemented with 20% fetal bovine serum (FBS; Hyclone, Euroclone, product #SH30070.03), 100 U/ml penicillin, 100 μg/ml streptomycin, 50 μg/ml gentamycin (Euroclone, product #ECM0011B) and 1% glutamax. The MPCs were plated at a confluence of 15,000 cells/cm^2 and maintained for 2 days in Growth Medium. After 2 days in GM, the cells were cultivated with fresh GM for additional 24 h (CTR-undiff) or stimulated by addition of 500 μM GTP for the following 24 h (GTP-undiff). Differentiation was induced by replacing the GM with the Differentiation Medium (DM) on cells plated on growth condition 3 days before. The differentiating cells were regularly cultivated for 24 h (CTR-diff) or stimulated by addition of 500 μM GTP for 24 h (GTP-diff). DM is composed of DMEM high Glucose (Euroclone, product #ECB7501L) supplemented with 5% heat-inactivated Horse Serum (HS) (56°C, 30 min) (HS; Euroclone, product #ECS0091L), 50 μg/ml gentamycin (Euroclone, product #ECM0011B), 10 μg/ml insulin (Sigma-Aldrich, Milan, Italy, product #I-0516) and 100 μg/ml of apo-transferrin (Sigma-Aldrich, product #T2036).

Immunocytochemistry and Flow Cytometric Analysis

To estimate the myogenic purity of our cultures, we performed immunocytochemistry assays using Desmin as a marker. Desmin is a cytoskeletal intermediate filament protein early expressed in myogenic cell populations and not in fibroblasts. The myogenic purity of each MPC culture was estimated using Desmin antibody D33 as marker (DAKO, product #M0760). Specific antibody binding was revealed using the streptavidin biotinylated peroxidase visualization reagent (StreptABComplex DAKO). The percentage of desmin positive myoblasts was estimated as the number of positive cells vs. the total number of cells. Furthermore, human cell cultures were analyzed by flow cytometric analysis for surface myogenic markers using CD56 Mouse monoclonal antibody (Abcam, Cambridge, United Kingdom) and 5.1H11 policlonal antibody [Developmental Studies Hybridoma Bank (DSHB), Iowa City, IA, United States] (Di Filippo et al., 2016).

Gene Expression Profile

The RNA was extracted from the human MPCs in undifferentiated cells (CTR-undiff) and with GTP stimulation for 24 h (GTP-undiff), and also in differentiation medium for 24 h (CTR-diff) and with GTP stimulation 24 h (GTP-diff)

TABLE 1 | Gradient elution profile used for the four analytes.

Time (min)	Flow rate (mL/min)	%A	%B
0	1 mL/min	100	0
5		80	20
7		80	20
7.10		100	0
18		100	0

TABLE 2 | Calibration parameters for the four analytes.

Analytes	Retention times (min)	Wavelengths (nm)	LOQ (LOD) (μg/mL)	Linearity (μg/mL)	r^2
GTP	3.34 ± 0.03	256	0.1 (0.03)	0.1–5	0.9987
GDP	3.64 ± 0.05	256	0.1 (0.03)	0.1–5	0.9996
GMP	4.46 ± 0.08	256	0.1 (0.03)	0.1–5	0.9997
Guanosine	6.03 ± 0.06	259	0.1 (0.03)	0.1–5	0.9980

LOD, limit of detection; LOQ, limit of quantification.

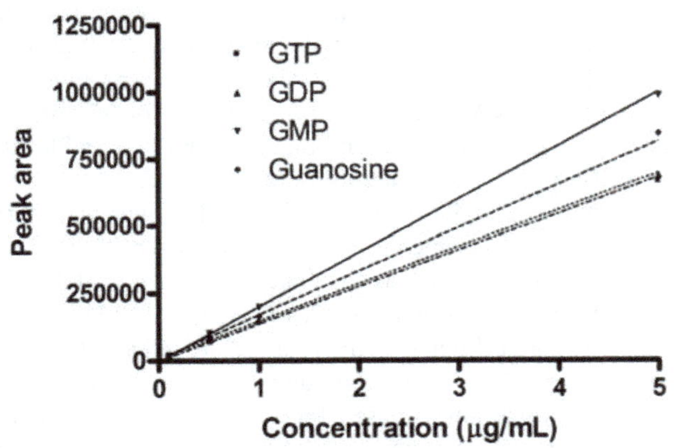

FIGURE 1 | Calibration curves. Calibration curves obtained for the four guanosine-based analytes. The graph shows the concentrations of guanosine-based molecules and the relative peak area measured on the developed HPLC procedure.

using PureLink RNA mini kit (Life Technologies). After RNA quantification using a NanoDrop^{TM} spectrophotometer, 500 ng was processed to obtain cDNA by High Capacity cDNA Reverse Transcription (#4368814; Applied Biosystems). We evaluated by quantitative real-time PCR the following genes: paired box (Pax) 7 (#4331182, Hs00242962_m1); myogenic differentiation (MyoD) 1 (#4331182, Hs00159528_m1), myogenin (#4331182, Hs 01072232GEXper-design_m1). Glyceraldehyde-3-phosphate dehydrogenase (GAPDH; #4331182, Hs99999905_m1) was used as the internal control, and the data are shown as difference in cycle threshold (ΔCt). An Applied Biosystems Prism 7900HT Sequence Detection System was used, with the Sequence Detector Software (SDS version 2.0; Applied Biosystems) (Di Filippo et al., 2017).

GTP-Dependent microRNA Expression Profile

To perform the microRNA analysis, small RNA extractions from the human MPCs in undifferentiated cells (CTR-undiff) and with GTP stimulation for 24 h (GTP-undiff), and also in differentiation medium for 24 h (CTR-diff) and with GTP stimulation 24 h (GTP-diff) was isolated using PureLink miRNA Isolation kits (Invitrogen, Life Technologies) following the manufacturer instructions and according to the procedure of Mancinelli et al. (2016). We also evaluated the following microRNA, called myomiRs: has-miR-1 (#0 02222); has-miR-206 (#00 0510); has-miR-133b (#00 2247); has-miR-16-5p (#00 0391). miR-16 was used as an internal control. The relative quantification of the miRNA targets was carried out using the ΔCt formula ($Ct_{miRNAofinterest}$ e Ct_{miR-16}), according to the Ct method.

Exosome Isolation and Purification From Cellular Media

Exosomes have been purified from both GM and DM and from media conditioned with cell culture as CTR-undiff and -diff and GTP-undiff and -diff samples following the method published by Thery et al. (2006). In detail, after a first centrifugation

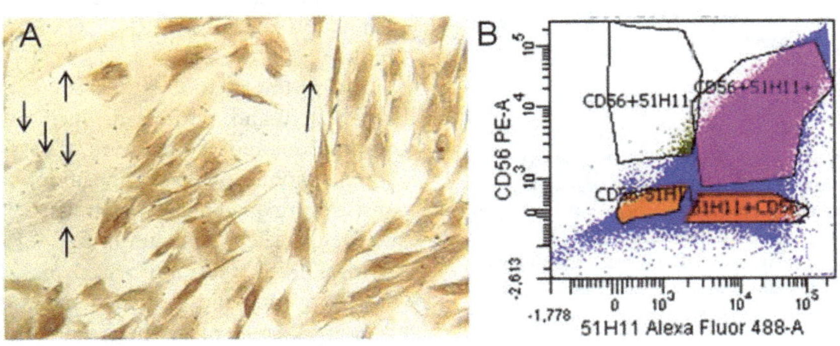

FIGURE 2 | Human myogenic precursor cells (MPCs). Human MPCs characterization. **(A)** Representative example of Desmin-positive (brown) and Desmin-negative (arrows) cells revealed by biotin-streptavidin complex method. **(B)** Representative example of flow cytometric analysis for two surface myogenic markers (CD56 and 5.1H11). In the example the percentage of CD56+/5.1H11+ cells was 75.1% and CD56–/5.1H11– cell was 11.2%.

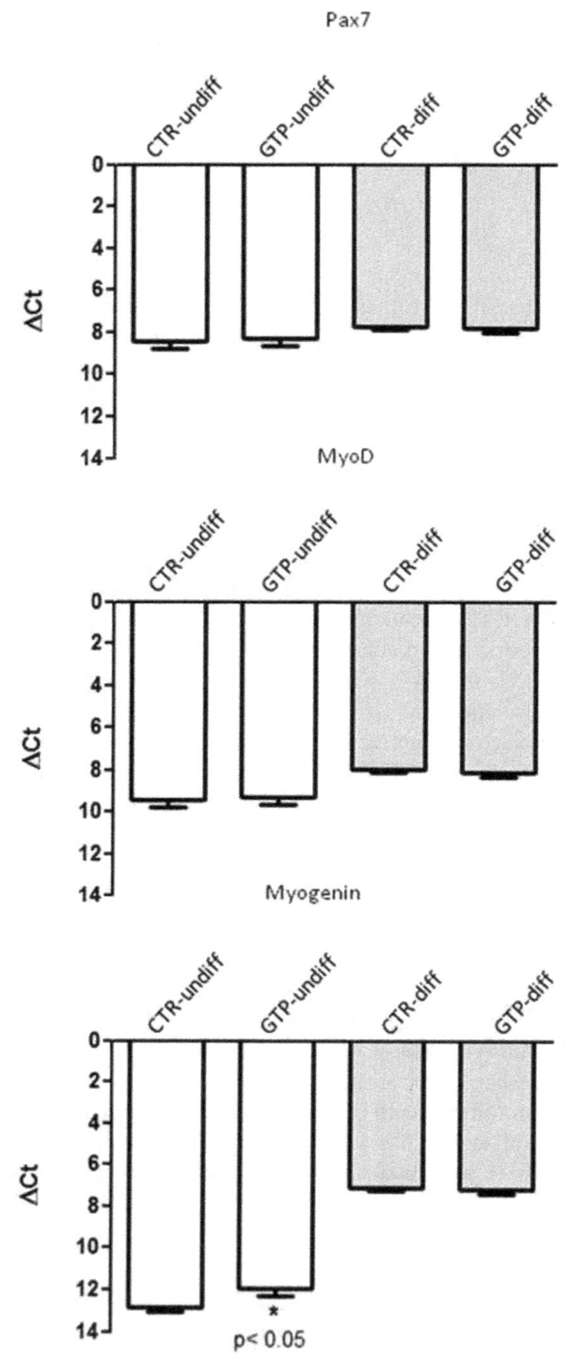

FIGURE 3 | GTP-dependent Myogenic regulator factors in human MPCs. The graphs show the relative expression of Pax7, MyoD, and Myogenin genes in undifferentiated MPCs (CTR-undiff) and with GTP stimulation (GTP-undiff) and in MPCs after 24 h of differentiation medium (CTR-diff) and with GTP stimulation (GTP-diff). The data are as mean and SD for $n = 3$ independent experiments, each performed in triplicate.

10 min at 300 *g*, 4°C to pellet cells, the conditioned-cell culture media was centrifuged 20 min at 2,000 *g*, 4°C in order to remove dead cells. The supernatant was then centrifuged 30 min at 10,000 *g*, 4°C to remove cell debris. The resulting supernatant was centrifuged 70 min at 1,00,000 *g*, 4°C to collect the pellet containing exosomes. A final step at the same speed was performed to obtain purified exosomes. The resulting pellet was resuspended in 150 μL of PBS. All the centrifugation steps were performed with the Sorvall Discovery 90SE Centrifuge.

Western Blotting for Exosome Identification

Exosomes were lysed with Exosome Resuspension Buffer (Thermo Fisher Scientific, Cat # 4478545), and denatured for 5 min at 75°C, loaded onto Bolt™ 4–12% Bis-Tris Plus Gels (invitrogen REF NW04120BOX), run at 150 V for 35 min and transferred to nitrocellulose membrane with iBlot 2 Dry Blotting System (Thermo Fisher Scientific, Cat # IB21001). Membrane was blocked 1 h at RT with 5% Skim-milk (Sigma-Aldrich) in TBS buffer supplemented with 0.1% Tween-20 (Sigma-Aldrich), the membrane was incubated overnight at 4°C with primary antibodies, as follows: CD63 (MX-49.129.5, sc-5275, Santa Cruz Biotechnology, Inc.) at 1:200, CD81 (1.3.3.22, sc-7637, Santa Cruz Biotechnology, Inc.) at 1:200. After incubation with anti-mouse IgG, HRP-linked Antibody (Cell Signaling Technology) at 1:5000 for 1 h at RT. Immunodetection was performed with the LiteAblot PLUS enhanced chemiluminiscent substrate (EuroClone). Images were taken at UVITEC machine (Cambridge).

Guanosine-Based Molecules Determination by HPLC-PDA

For the guanosine based-molecules separation was used a mobile phase composed by phosphate buffer (pH 7, concentration 40 mM) as solvent A and acetonitrile as solvent B at a flow rate of 1 mL/min. The column used for analytes resolution is the XTIMATE C18 (4.6 mm × 250 mm, 5 μm, Welch, Shanghai, China) and the system was thermostated at 25°C (±1°C). The gradient profile used to resolve the four compounds was reported in **Table 1**. The samples (20 μL) were directly injected into the HPLC-PDA system after a preliminary centrifuged at 12,000 rpm and without further pre-treatment. All the analytes were detected and quantified at their corresponding maximum wavelengths, such as 256 nm for GTP, GDP, GMP, and 259 nm for guanosine (**Table 2**).

During the method development, several parameters have been tested and optimized, such as column, mobile phase composition and temperature. The first parameter evaluated was the mobile phase composition, which was optimal when consisting of phosphate buffer (pH 7, concentration 40 mM) and acetonitrile. The column used for analytes resolution is the XTIMATE C18 (4.6 mm × 250 mm, 5 μm, Welch, Shanghai, China). Among the evaluated parameters, however, it is also necessary to remember the type of elution chosen. Firstly, was tested isocratic elution with PBS and AcN in ratio 97:3 in order to retain the more hydrophobic compounds and to reduce the total run-time. Isocratic conditions were tested in order to avoid transferability drawbacks. Unfortunately, these conditions do not

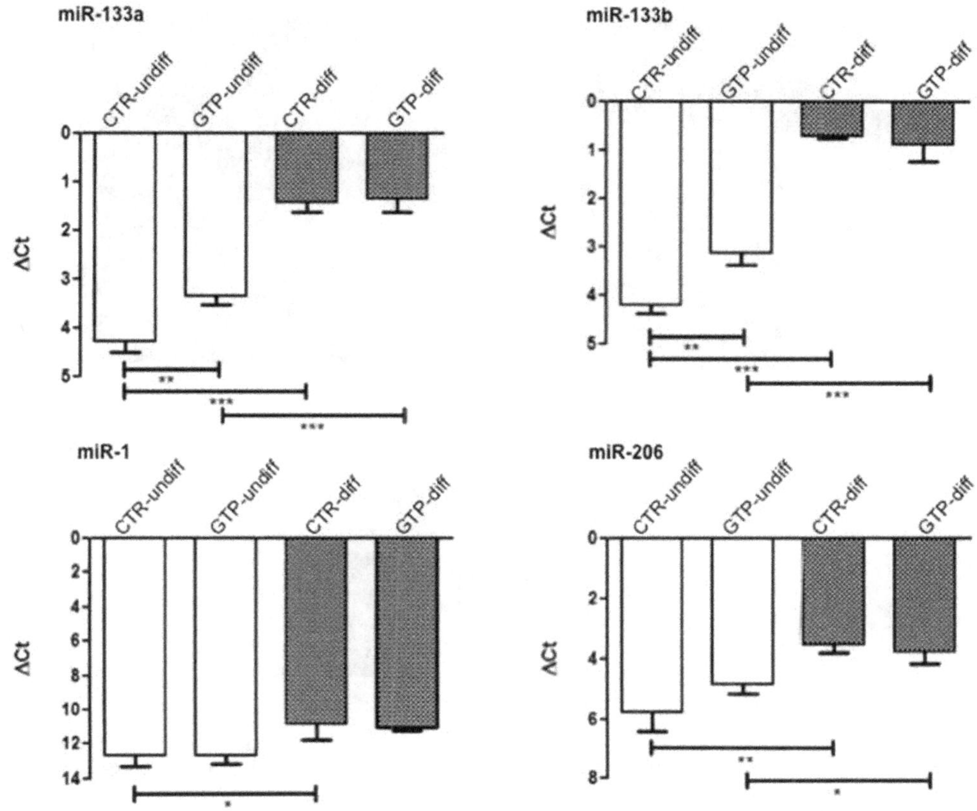

FIGURE 4 | microRNA expression profile in human MPC cells after GTP stimulation. The graphs show the relative expression of miR-133a, miR-133b, miR-1, and miR-206 both in myoblasts (CTR-undiff), in cells differentiated for 24 h in DM (CTR-diff) and in 500 μM GTP-stimulated myoblasts and differentiating cells (GTP-undiff and GTP-diff, respectively). Mean ± SD, $n = 3$ independent experiments, each performed in triplicate. $^*p < 0.05$, $^{**}p < 0.005$, $^{***}p < 0.0001$.

allow to fully resolving the analyte peaks and it was therefore necessary to proceed using gradient elution. Some gradient elution profiles were tested and the best conditions in terms of total run-time and peaks resolution were observed using the gradient reported in **Table 1** at 25°C.

In this range of linearity (**Figure 1**), the HPLC procedure fulfills the validation parameters as requested by International Guidelines (CDER and CVM Guidance for Industry, 2001; Taverniers et al., 2004; ICH, 2005).

Preliminary analysis of exosomes deriving from fresh media GM and DM, revealed the only presence of GDP as 0.10–$0.12 \pm 0.01\ \mu g\ mL^{-1}$.

Nanometric Scanning of Exosomes by Atomic Force Microscopy

The exosomes derived from media conditioned by MPCs in presence or not of extracellular GTP were scanned to analyze their physical properties. Experimental data were obtained using the NT-MDT Solver Pro P-47 AF. The measurements were collected in semi-contact mode by using a probe with a resonant frequency of 130 kHz and a spring constant of 4.4 N/m (HA_NC ETALON, NT-MDT). The images were obtained by plotting the error signal (mag) over 256 × 256 (x,y) positions; the mag signal is related to the oscillation amplitude of the cantilever and corresponds to the error signal of the feedback loop when working in semi-contact mode; the error signal is used for a more detailed information on the surface topography. Particle size distribution was performed with Nova Software in 1 μm × 1 μm scan area and by using a threshold of 10 nm. A statistical t-test has been used to evaluate the significance between the diameter distribution ($p < 0.05$).

Statistical Analysis

Data were expressed as means ± standard deviations. Statistical significance was set at $p < 0.05$ and was calculated using the unpaired Student's t-test. Prism5 GraphPad software (Abacus Concepts GraphPad Software, San Diego, CA, United States).

RESULTS

Human Myogenic Precursor Cells

We obtained three different human MPC culture named #1 (85.31% desmin positivity), #2 (61.6% desmin positivity), and #3 (77.8% desmin positivity). The MPC cultures were analyzed by flow cytometric analysis for surface myogenic markers using the mouse monoclonal antibody CD56 (Abcam,

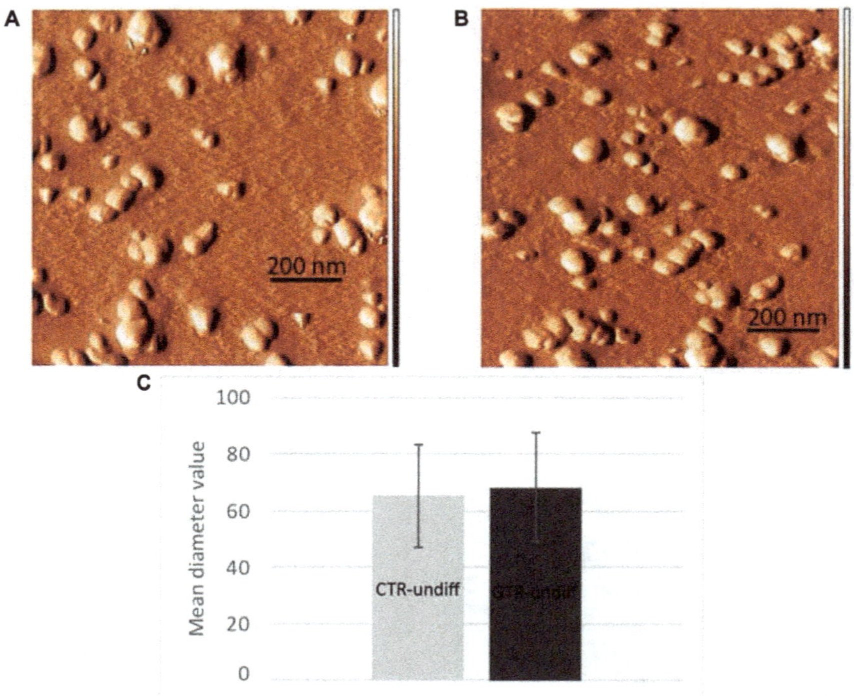

FIGURE 5 | Nanometric scanning of exosomes by atomic force microscopy. The exosomes are rounded shaped structures showing dimensions of about 60–70 nm as mean diameter. Images represent an example of exosome topography acquired in semicontact scanning. AFM error signal images obtained in semi-contact mode [scan area 1 μm × 1 μm (x,y)] of undifferentiated control (**A**, CTR-undiff) and GTP-treated (**B**, GTP-undiff) exosomes. Mean diameter particle size distribution **(C)** evaluated in 1 μm × 1 μm scan area by using a threshold of 10 nm.

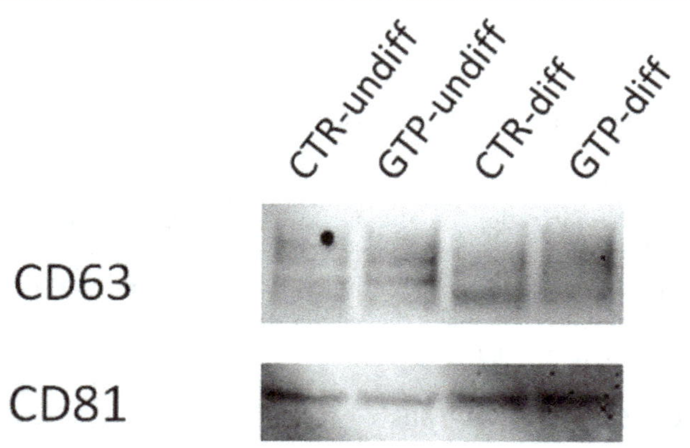

FIGURE 6 | Western blotting for exosome identification. Representative image of Western blotting analysis of CD63 and CD81 expression on exosomes obtained by cell culture media named CTR-undiff and CTR–diff and GTP-undiff and GTP-diff samples. The image showed the presence of these proteins in the exosome samples we isolated by ultracentrifugation (see section "Materials and Methods").

Cambridge, United Kingdom) and policlonal antibody 5.1H11 [Developmental Studies Hybridoma Bank (DSHB), Iowa City, IA, United States] to confirm the percentage of myogenicity. The percentage of $CD56^{+}/5.1H11^{+}$ cells was 75.1% and those $CD56^{-}/5.1H11^{-}$ was 11.2% (**Figure 2**).

Quantitative Gene Expression RT-PCR on Myogenic Regulatory Factors

The most important myogenic regulatory factors such as Pax7, MyoD, and Myogenin were assessed in our samples in order to investigate their involvement with GTP stimulation. Pax7 and MyoD1 did not change their expression in our samples, neither with respect to undifferentiated and 24-h differentiation (**Figure 3**). Myogenin was up-regulated after 24 h of differentiation stimulation both in CTR-diff and GTP-diff compared to CTR-undiff and GTP-undiff. Strikingly, we found Myogenin up-regulated after 24 h of 500 μM GTP stimulation in growth medium (GTP-undiff compared to CTR-undiff), but no differences were found in 24-h differentiated samples between CTR-diff and GTP-diff (**Figure 3**).

GTP-Induced microRNA Modulation

miR-133a and miR-133b were significantly up-regulated after 24 h of 500 μM GTP stimulation of myoblasts (GTP-undiff) compared to control (CTR-undiff). Furthermore, these microRNAs were found highly up-regulated in differentiation media both in CTR-diff and in GTP-diff. Also miR-1, that in myoblasts (CTR-undiff; GTP-undiff) does not change its expression, in differentiative condition, was slightly up-regulated both on CTR-diff and GTP-diff both at the same extent. Similarly, miR-206 was significant up-regulated after 24 h of differentiation stimulation both CTR-diff and

GTP-diff compared to CTR-undiff and GTP-undiff, but no differences were found between CTR-diff and GTP-diff (**Figure 4**).

Nanometric Scanning of Exosomes by Atomic Force Microscopy

The images obtained by AFM (**Figures 5A,B**) show the typical round-shaped structure of exosomes with diameter values ranging between 30 and 100 nm. Specifically, the diameter values were 65 ± 18 and 68 ± 19 nm for CTR-undiff and GTP-undiff exosomes, respectively (**Figure 5C**). Both samples, control and GTP-treated exosomes, were analyzed in terms of diameter distribution and as can be seen from the images, the exosomes were not found to be significantly different ($p < 0.05$).

Western Blotting for Exosome Identification

The western blot analysis using antibodies CD63 and CD81 (specifically expressed on exosomes), revealed the presence of these proteins on our isolated nanovesicles (**Figure 6**).

HPLC-PDA Guanosine-Based Molecules Determination Into Exosomes

The exosomes obtained by both simple and cell-conditioned media with and without GTP were analyzed to detect guanosine-based molecules. The herein reported HPLC-PDA method allows quantify simultaneously the four guanosine-based molecules in exosomes extracted from culture media. The gradient elution allows separate and analyze these compounds better than isocratic condition, within an overall runtime of 18 min. The quantitative data are reported in **Table 3**.

DISCUSSION AND CONCLUSION

We previously demonstrated that extracellular GTP binds its specific binding site on C2C12 myoblasts and triggers specific signal transduction that lead the myoblasts to increase the intracellular calcium and to hyperpolarize the plasma membrane (Pietrangelo et al., 2006a). However, GTP works also as intracellular signal, it triggers molecules for the G-coupled receptor signaling or its de-phosphorylation is instrumental for effector enzyme activation. In addition, GTP shows inhibitory effect at uncoupling proteins of the mitochondrial anion carrier protein family (Woyda-Ploszczyca and Jarmuszkiewicz, 2017). Low mitochondrial potential increases the inhibitory effect of GTP. In particular, GTP–GDP inhibits the proton leak mediated by these carriers across the inner mitochondrial membrane in lizard skeletal muscle mitochondria (Rey et al., 2008). In the cytoplasm GTP is present at mM level but also externally its effective concentration is in the order of 100s of micromolar (Azzu and Brand, 2010). Moreover, the cells are able to phosphorylate guanosine molecule to obtain GMP, GDP, and GTP and in turn they could be released. However, in the extracellular space, the ectonucleotidase binds and hydrolyze the GTP to GDP, GMP, and guanosine (Kovács et al., 2011). In this scenario, it is difficult to understand how guanosine-based molecules and particularly GTP could be secreted in the extracellular space and directed toward cell target, escaping the ectonucleotide degradation. The exosomes are small vesicles that protect and carry molecules to specific target. Our hypothesis that the GTP-incubated cells could produce some categories of exosomes stuffed with guanosine-based purines has been verified because we found mainly guanosine in the exosomes, but also GTP, GDP, and GMP even if in few samples. Specifically, the human MPCs that we stimulated with 500 μM extracellular GTP for 24 h, both in proliferative and differentiative conditions,

TABLE 3 | Concentration of guanosine-based molecules contained into exosome samples deriving from three different MPC culture of young subjects.

Samples	Concentration ($\mu g\ mL^{-1}$)			
	GTP	GDP	GMP	Guanosine
#1 Exosomes from CTR-undiff	nd	nd	nd	nd
#1 Exosomes from CTR-diff	nd	nd	nd	nd
#1 Exosomes from GTP-undiff	nd	0.10 ± 0.01	nd	1.70 ± 0.18
#1 Exosomes from GTP-diff	nd	0.36 ± 0.04	nd	2.52 ± 0.25
#2 Exosomes from CTR-undiff	nd	nd	nd	nd
#2 Exosomes from CTR-diff	nd	nd	nd	nd
#2 Exosomes from GTP-undiff	nd	nd	0.15 ± 0.02	4.17 ± 0.35
#2 Exosomes from GTP-diff	0.33 ± 0.03	0.19 ± 0.01	nd	0.20 ± 0.02
#3 Exosomes from CTR-undiff	nd	nd	nd	nd
#3 Exosomes from CTR-diff	nd	nd	nd	nd
#3 Exosomes from GTP-undiff	nd	nd	nd	1.51 ± 0.12
#3 Exosomes from GTP-diff	0.16 ± 0.02	0.17 ± 0.02	nd	0.70 ± 0.05

nd, not detected. #1, #2, #3 three different young volunteers from whom we obtained myogenic precursor cells. CTR-undiff = the exosomes obtained from the medium conditioned with the human MPC cells in proliferative state for3 days in GM. CTR-diff = the exosomes obtained from the medium conditioned with the human MPC cells in differentiative state for 24 h. GTP-undiff = the exosomes obtained from the medium conditioned with the human MPC cells in proliferative state for additional 24 h after 2 days of regular cultivation in GM. GTP-diff = the exosomes obtained from the medium conditioned with the human MPC cells in differentiative state in presence of 500 μM extracellular GTP for 24 h.

secreted exosomes stuffed with guanosine in the range of 1.51–4.17 and 0.2–2.5 $\mu g\,mL^{-1}$, respectively. This result suggests that extracellular GTP influences skeletal muscle exosome release in order to direct guanosine molecules via exosomes as both paracrine and endocrine transmission in the body. We think that these exosomes containing guanosine could influence surrounding cells in the niche of regenerating skeletal muscle and in addition could spread out in all other muscles of the body and other tissue via blood and/or lymphatic fluxes. The scenario we envisioned if that the extracellular free GTP could derive from a damaged skeletal fiber after injury or after vigorous muscle contractions following specific training and/or could be released physiologically during muscle growth. The extracellular free GTP stimulus in a specific fiber, could influence the entire skeletal tissue on the same muscle (Vastus Lateralis, for instance) or other skeletal muscles in the body via exosomes stuffed with guanosine, probably in a different manner with respect to the typical binding of ligand on a receptor. In our previous paper (Pietrangelo et al., 2006a) we demonstrated a specific free GTP effect in the first stage (the proliferative phase of myogenesis) of murine skeletal muscle regeneration. Here, we confirm that free GTP stimulates human MPCs in the proliferative boost phase of differentiation. In fact, extracellular GTP up-regulated the miR-133a and miR133b expression. These myo-miRNA are specifically linked to myogenic proliferation (La Rovere et al., 2014). The enhancer toward the differentiation process mediated by free extracellular GTP is confirmed by Myogenin gene upregulation during proliferation state. These results are in concordance with the fact that the pool of satellite cells is activated to proliferate under myogenic regulator factors that control both an initial boost of proliferation and a push of differentiation (Ceafalan et al., 2014). In conclusion, we think that free extracellular GTP elicited two effects: miRNA-myogenic regulator factor modulation and exosome stuffed with guanosine and guanosine-based molecules secretion. We think that these effects are sequential, in the sense that free GTP immediately influence MPC proliferation-differentiation step and in turn after 24 h induces secretion of exosomes contained-guanosine both in proliferative and differentiative conditions.

At the current state of the study, we do not have evidence for saying that exosome contained-guanosine based molecules could influence regeneration or differentiation. What we can hypothesize for future study is that these exosome stuffed with guanosine and guanosine based molecules (GMP, GDP, GTP) could be transferred into other tissues as neuronal and glial ones where exert specific effects (Gysbers et al., 2000; Pietrangelo et al., 2006b; Guarnieri et al., 2009; Giuliani et al., 2012, 2015; Mancinelli et al., 2014).

AUTHOR CONTRIBUTIONS

All authors listed have made a substantial, direct and intellectual contribution to the work, and approved it for publication.

FUNDING

This study was funded by Università degli Studi "G. d'Annunzio" Chieti-Pescara (2012N8YJC3_003 PRIN) to TP.

ACKNOWLEDGMENTS

The authors would like to thank Dr. Elisa De Luca for her kindly collaboration during the first steps of this project. They also thank Dr. Tereza Jandova for English language revision.

REFERENCES

Azzu, V., and Brand, M. D. (2010). The on-off switches of the mitochondrial uncoupling proteins. *Trends Biochem. Sci.* 35, 298–307. doi: 10.1016/j.tibs.2009.11.001

Burd, N. A., and De Lisio, M. (2017). Skeletal muscle remodeling: interconnections between stem cells and protein turnover. *Exerc. Sport Sci. Rev.* 45, 187–191. doi: 10.1249/JES.0000000000000117

Burnstock, G. (2017). Purinergic signalling: therapeutic developments. *Front. Pharmacol.* 8:661. doi: 10.3389/fphar.2017.00661

CDER and CVM Guidance for Industry (2001). *Bioanalytical Method Validation.* Silver Spring, MD: Food and Drug Administration.

Ceafalan, C. L., Popescu, B. O., and Hinescu, M. E. (2014). Cellular players in skeletal muscle regeneration. *Biomed Res. Int.* 2014:957014. doi: 10.1155/2014/957014

Cornelison, D. (2018). "Known unknowns": current questions in muscle satellite cell biology. *Curr. Top. Dev. Biol.* 126, 205–233. doi: 10.1016/bs.ctdb.2017.08.006

Di Filippo, E. S., Mancinelli, R., Marrone, M., Doria, C., Verratti, V., Toniolo, L., et al. (2017). Neuromuscular electrical stimulation improves skeletal muscle regeneration through satellite cell fusion with myofibers in healthy elderly subjects. *J. Appl. Physiol.* 123, 501–512. doi: 10.1152/japplphysiol.00855.201

Di Filippo, E. S., Mancinelli, R., Pietrangelo, T., La Rovere, R. M., Quattrocelli, M., Sampaolesi, M., et al. (2016). Myomir dysregulation and reactive oxygen species in aged human satellite cells. *Biochem. Biophys. Res. Commun.* 473, 462–470. doi: 10.1016/j.bbrc.2016.03.030

Drummond, M. J., McCarthy, J. J., Sinha, M., Spratt, H. M., Volpi, E., Esser, K. A., et al. (2011). Aging and microRNA expression in human skeletal muscle: a microarray and bioinformatics analysis. *Physiol. Genomics* 43, 595–603. doi: 10.1152/physiolgenomics.00148.2010

Giuliani, P., Ballerini, P., Buccella, S., Ciccarelli, R., Rathbone, M. P., Romano, S., et al. (2015). Guanosine protects glial cells against 6-hydroxydopamine toxicuity. *Adv. Exp. Med. Biol.* 837, 23–33. doi: 10.1007/5584_2014_73

Giuliani, P., Romano, S., Ballerini, P., Ciccarelli, R., Petragnani, N., Cicchitti, S., et al. (2012). Protective activity of guanosine in an in vitro model of parkinson's disease. *Panminerva Med.* 54(1 Suppl. 4), 43–51.

Guarnieri, S., Pilla, R., Morabito, C., Sacchetti, S., Mancinelli, R., Fanò, G., et al. (2009). Extracellular guanosine and GTP promote expression of differentiation markers and induce S-phase cell-cycle arrest in human SH-SY5Y neuroblastoma cells. *Int. J. Dev. Neurosci.* 27, 135–147. doi: 10.1016/j.ijdevneu.2008.11.007

Gysbers, J. W., Guarnieri, S., Mariggiol̀, M. A., Pietrangelo, T., Fanol̀, G., and Rathbone, M. P. (2000). Extracellular guanosine 5′-triphosphate enhances nerve-growth-factor-induced neurite outgrowth via increases in intracellular calcium. *Neuroscience* 96, 817–824. doi: 10.1016/S0306-4522(99)00588-6

ICH (2005). *International Conference on Harmonisation of Technical Requirements for Registration of Pharmaceuticals for Human Use.* Geneva: ICH.

Kasper, A. M., Turner, D. C., Martin, N. R. W., and Sharples, A. P. (2018). Mimicking exercise in three-dimensional bioengineered skeletal muscle to investigate cellular and molecular mechanisms of physiological adaptation. *J. Cell. Physiol.* 233, 1985–1998. doi: 10.1002/jcp.25840

Kovács, Z., Juhász, G., Palkovits, M., Dobolyi, A., and Kékesi, K. A. (2011). Area, age and gender dependence of the nucleoside system in the brain: a review of current literature. *Curr. Top. Med. Chem.* 11, 1012–1033. doi: 10.2174/156802611795347636

La Rovere, R. M., Quattrocelli, M., Pietrangelo, T., Di Filippo, E. S., Maccatrozzo, L., Cassano, M., et al. (2014). Myogenic potential of canine craniofacial satellite cells. *Front. Aging Neurosci.* 6:90. doi: 10.3389/fnagi.2014.00090

Mancinelli, R., Di Filippo, E. S., Verratti, V., Fulle, S., Toniolo, L., Reggiani, C., et al. (2016). The regenerative potential of female skeletal muscle upon hypobaric hypoxic exposure. *Front. Physiol.* 7:303. doi: 10.3389/fphys.2016.00303

Mancinelli, R., La Rovere, R. M., Fulle, S., Miscia, S., Marchisio, M., Pierdomenico, L., et al. (2014). Extracellular GTP is a potent water-transport regulator via aquaporin 5 plasma-membrane insertion in M1-CCD epithelial cortical collecting duct cells. *Cell Physiol. Biochem.* 33, 731–746. doi: 10.1159/000358648

Mancinelli, R., Pietrangelo, T., Burnstock, G., Fanò, G., and Fulle, S. (2012). Transcriptional profile of GTP-mediated differentiation of C2C12 skeletal muscle cells. *Purinergic Signal.* 8, 207–221. doi: 10.1007/s11302-011-9266-3

Murphy, C., Withrow, J., Hunter, M., Liu, Y., Tang, Y. L., Fulzele, S., et al. (2017). Emerging role of extracellular vesicles in musculoskeletal diseases. *Mol. Aspects Med.* doi: 10.1016/j.mam.2017.09.006 [Epub ahead of print].

Pietrangelo, T., D'Amelio, L., Doria, C., Mancinelli, R., Fulle, S., and Fano, G. (2011). Tiny percutaneous needle biopsy: an efficient method for studying cellular and molecular aspects of skeletal muscle in humans. *Int. J. Mol. Med.* 27, 361–367. doi: 10.3892/ijmm.2010.582

Pietrangelo, T., Di Filippo, E. S., Mancinelli, R., Doria, C., Rotini, A., Fanò-Illic, G., et al. (2015). Low intensity exercise training improves skeletal muscle regeneration potential. *Front. Physiol.* 6:399. doi: 10.3389/fphys.2015.00399

Pietrangelo, T., Fioretti, B., Mancinelli, R., Catacuzzeno, L., Franciolini, F., Fanoì, G., et al. (2006a). Extracellular guanosine 5′-triphosphate modulates myogenesis via intermediate Ca2+-activated K+ currents in C2C12 mouse cells. *J Physiol.* 572, 721–733.

Pietrangelo, T., Guarnieri, S., Fulle, S., Fanò, G., and Mariggiò, M. A. (2006b). Signal transduction events induced by extracellular guanosine 5′ triphosphate in excitable cells. *Purinergic Signal.* 2, 633–636. doi: 10.1007/s11302-006-9021-3

Pietrangelo, T., Mariggioì, M. A., Lorenzon, P., Fulle, S., Protasi, F., Rathbone, M., et al. (2002). Characterization of specific GTP binding sites in C2C12 mouse skeletal muscle cells. *J. Muscle Res. Cell Motil.* 23, 107–118. doi: 10.1023/A:1020288117082

Rey, B., Sibille, B., Romestaing, C., Belouze, M., Letexier, D., Servais, S., et al. (2008). Reptilian uncoupling protein: functionality and expression in sub-zero temperatures. *J. Exp. Biol.* 211(Pt 9), 1456–1462. doi: 10.1242/jeb.012328

Said, S. R., Mustafa, A. G., Asfour, H. A., and Shaqoura, E. I. (2017). Myogenic satellite cells: biological milieu and possible clinical applications. *Pak. J. Biol. Sci.* 20, 1–11. doi: 10.3923/pjbs.2017.1.11

Taverniers, E., Van Bockstaele, M., and De Loose, M. (2004). Trends in quality in the analytical laboratory. II. Analytical method validation and quality assurance. *Trend Anal. Chem.* 23, 535–552. doi: 10.1016/j.trac.2004.04.001

Thery, C., Clayton, A., Amigorena, S., and Raposo, G. (2006). Isolation and characterization of exosomes from cell culture supernatants and biological fluids. *Curr. Protoc. Cell Biol.* 30, 3.22.1–3.22.29. doi: 10.1002/0471143030.cb0322s30

Woyda-Ploszczyca, A. M., and Jarmuszkiewicz, W. (2017). The conserved regulation of mitochondrial uncoupling proteins: from unicellular eukaryotes to mammals. *Biochim. Biophys. Acta* 1858, 21–33.

Yin, H., Price, F., and Rudnicki, M. A. (2013). Satellite cells and the muscle stem cell niche. *Physiol. Rev.* 93, 23–67. doi: 10.1152/physrev.00043.2011

5

Cytokine-Induced Killer Cells Express CD39, CD38, CD203a, CD73 Ectoenzymes and P1 Adenosinergic Receptors

Alberto L. Horenstein[1], Antonella Chillemi[1], Roberta Zini[2], Valeria Quarona[1], Nicoletta Bianchi[3], Rossella Manfredini[2], Roberto Gambari[3], Fabio Malavasi[1†] and Davide Ferrari[3†]*

[1] Laboratory of Immunogenetics and CeRMS, Department of Medical Sciences, University of Torino, Torino, Italy, [2] Centre for Regenerative Medicine "Stefano Ferrari," Department of Life Sciences, University of Modena and Reggio Emilia, Modena, Italy, [3] Department of Life Science and Biotechnology, Section of Microbiology and Applied Pathology, University of Ferrara, Ferrara, Italy

***Correspondence:**
Davide Ferrari
dfr@unife.it

† Same authorship.

Cytokine-induced killer (CIK) cells, a heterogeneous T cell population obtained by *in vitro* differentiation of peripheral blood mononuclear cells (PBMC), represent a promising immunological approach in cancer. Numerous studies have explored the role of CD38, CD39, CD203a/PC-1, and CD73 in generating extracellular adenosine (ADO) and thus in shaping the tumor niche in favor of proliferation. The findings shown here reveal that CIK cells are able to produce extracellular ADO via traditional (CD39/CD73) and/or alternative (CD38/CD203a/CD73 or CD203a/CD73) pathways. Transcriptome analysis showed the mRNA expression of these molecules and their modulation during PBMC to CIK differentiation. When PBMC from normal subjects or cancer bearing patients were differentiated into CIK cells under normoxic conditions, CD38 and CD39 were greatly up-regulated while the number of CD203a, and CD73 positive cells underwent minor changes. Since hypoxic conditions are often found in tumors, we asked whether CD39, CD38, CD203a, and CD73 expressed by CIK cells were modulated by hypoxia. PBMC isolated from cancer patients and differentiated into CIK cells in hypoxic conditions did not show relevant changes in CD38, CD39, CD73, CD203a, and CD26. CIK cells also expressed A_1, A_{2A}, and A_{2B} ADO receptors and they only underwent minor changes as a consequence of hypoxia. The present study sheds light on a previously unknown functional aspect of CIK cells, opening the possibility of pharmacologically modulated ADO-generating ectoezymes to improve CIK cells performance.

Keywords: CIK, adenosine, CD38, CD39, CD73, CD203a/PC-1, hypoxia, P1 receptors

INTRODUCTION

CIK cells are polyclonal T effector cells sharing immunological properties and receptors with NK cells. They are attracting increasing interest for their ability to perform non-MHC-restricted cytolytic activities toward susceptible autologous and allogeneic cancer cells (Schmidt-Wolf et al., 1991; Lu and Negrin, 1994). This capacity, along with their safety and easy *in vitro* generation has opened the door to multiple applications of CIK adoptive immunotherapy against different types of cancer. Hence, CIK can be employed against solid and hematological tumors, either alone or together with chemotherapy. An experimental CIK based approach has been undertaken for the following neoplasms: chronic and acute lymphocytic leukemias, lymphomas, kidney carcinoma, renal, liver and stomach cancer, melanomas and bone sarcomas (Linn and Hui, 2010; Gammaitoni et al., 2013; Jiang et al., 2013; Sangiolo et al., 2014). CIK cells are generated by *ex vivo* cultivation of human PBMC in the presence of the cytokine interferon gamma (IFN-γ), the anti-CD3 monoclonal antibody OKT3, and then adding recombinant human IL-2 (rhIL-2) (Introna et al., 2007; Jiang et al., 2013; Giraudo et al., 2015). The addition of IFN-γ has the main goal of activating monocytes present in the mixed PBMC population to secrete IL-12, which favors CD58/LFA-3-mediated activation, while the binding of anti-CD3 antibody to CD3 membrane antigen expressed by T lymphocytes and the addition of IL-2 provides cells with the mitogenic stimuli they need for proliferation (Franceschetti et al., 2009). CIK cells are a heterogeneous population comprising $CD3^+CD8^+$ T cells, $CD3^+CD56^-$ T cells (from 20 to 60% of total CIK), and $CD3^+CD56^+$ double positive cells (from 40 to 80% of total CIK), as well as of a small number of $CD3^-CD56^+$ NK cells (from 1 to 10%) (Franceschetti et al., 2009; Pievani et al., 2011; Introna et al., 2013; Valgardsdottir et al., 2014).

Immune cells interact with cancer cells in the so called "tumor niche," i.e., in a localized neoplastic tissue context; therefore they are heavily influenced by the superimposed tumor conditions. Some of the most influential extracellular mediators in the niche are the nucleotides and nucleosides. Adenosine (ADO), the main nucleoside mediator generated both intracellularly and extracellularly, suppresses the anti-tumoral immune response, thus favoring metastasis to the detriment of the host organism. Once present in the extracellular *milieu*, nucleotides and nucleosides bind purinergic receptors, i.e., specific plasma membrane receptors necessary for cell-to-cell communication and named P2 (activated by ATP, UTP, ADP, UDP, UDP-glucose, and NAD^+) and P1 receptors (G protein-coupled, activated by ADO). P1 are further divided into four subtypes (A_1R, $A_{2A}R$, $A_{2B}R$, A_3R) (Burnstock, 2007; Surprenant and North, 2009; Harden et al., 2010; Plattner and Verkhratsky, 2016).

Extracellular nucleotides and nucleosides are subjected to continuous transformation. The main canonical actors of this function are four ectonucleotidases: ectonucleoside triphosphate diphosphohydrolase (NTPDase, CD39), ectonucleotide pyrophosphatase/phosphodiesterase (NPP, CD203a) or PC-1, ecto-5′nucleotidase (CD73), and alkaline phosphatases (Yegutkin, 2008; Zimmermann et al., 2012) which degrade ATP and its metabolites, eventually leading to ADO production and the subsequent activation of P1 receptors (Fredholm et al., 2001). Transformation of extracellular ATP into its metabolites requires the sequential participation of the CD39 ectoenzyme (stepwise forming extracellular AMP) subsequently metabolized by CD73 into ADO (Yegutkin, 2008; Zimmermann et al., 2012).

Another pathway generating extracellular AMP, which can then be transformed into ADO, involves participation of extracellular NAD^+ and CD38 an ADP-ribosyl cyclase/cyclic ADP-ribose (cADPR) hydrolase. Expression of CD203a (ectonucleotide pyrophosphatase/phosphodiesterase-1) accompanied by the extracellular presence of its substrate ADPR (product of the deconstruction of NAD^+ by CD38) favors the generation of additional AMP (Horenstein et al., 2013).

ADO plays multiple roles as an extracellular mediator both in physiological and pathological conditions. It is released in different tissue contexts, including neurons, kidney cells, cardiomyocytes, vascular endothelium and immune cells (Shryock and Belardinelli, 1997; Latini and Pedata, 2001; Dale and Frenguelli, 2009; Praetorius and Leipziger, 2010; Morandi et al., 2015; Silva, 2016). However, the interest in ADO and ectoenzymes involved in ADO formation (CD38, CD39, CD73 and CD203a) was prompted by growing evidence of their role in cancer biology. Indeed, ADO suppresses immune responses against tumor cells, and cancer-derived ADO is recognized as a crucial extracellular immune checkpoint target for re-establishing immune-surveillance mechanisms (Young et al., 2014; Hatfield and Sitkovsky, 2016; Allard et al., 2017).

A role in favoring cancer growth and dissemination has been described for each of the extracellular enzymes involved in nucleotide/nucleoside and NAD^+ metabolism (i.e., CD39, CD38, CD203a and CD73) and for the complexing ADO deaminase (ADA)/CD26 molecules, a controller of ADO in the extracellular space. CD39 is involved in colorectal cancer dissemination (Stagg and Smyth, 2010) as well as in the metastatic competence of non-small-cell lung cancer (NSCLC) (Schmid et al., 2015; Ferrari et al., 2017). CD73 is involved in the spread of cancer and in reducing immune-surveillance (Wang et al., 2008; Antonioli et al., 2016a,b; Ferrari et al., 2017). This is achieved by using antibodies to CD73 and CD39 (Young et al., 2014; Allard et al., 2017; Kazemi et al., 2017) to block ADO, a normal immune regulator, which is hijacked by tumors to evade immune attack. Likewise, human CD38 (Malavasi et al., 2008) is implicated in multiple myeloma, where it is main target of therapeutic treatments (Horenstein et al., 2015; Sanchez et al., 2016; Costa et al., 2017; Shallis et al., 2017). Concerning P1, $A_{2A}R$ and $A_{2B}R$ have been indicated as the main candidate receptors in cancer therapy (Beavis et al., 2013; Desmet et al., 2013; Hatfield and Sitkovsky, 2016; Allard et al., 2017; Garber, 2017; Mittal et al., 2017).

However, so far, there is no information on P1, CD39, CD38, CD203a, CD73, and CD26 expression in CIK cells. In view of the important immunosuppressive role played by ADO and the promising use of CIK cells in adoptive cancer therapy, we investigated the metabolic processes of ADO generated during the differentiation of human T cells present into the PBMC fraction into CIK cells under normoxic and hypoxic conditions.

Abbreviations: ADO, adenosine; ADA, adenosine deaminase; AR, adenosine receptor; ADPR, ADP-ribose; CD38, ADP-ribosyl cyclase/cyclic ADPR-hydrolase; CD39, ecto-nucleoside triphosphate diphosphohydrolase (NTPDase); CD73, ecto-5′-nucleotidase (5′-NT); CD203a/PC-1, ectonucleotide pyrophosphatase/phosphodiesterase-1 (NPP-1); CIK, cytokine-induced killer; EHNA, erytro-9 (2-hydroxy-3-nonyl) adenine; GIST, Gastrointestinal Stromal Tumor; PBMC, peripheral blood mononuclear cells; OS, osteosarcoma.

MATERIALS AND METHODS

CIK Cell Production and Characterization

PBMC cells from 11 donors, five healthy donors, five patients with histologic confirmed Gastrointestinal Stromal Tumors (GIST) and 1 patient with osteosarcoma (OS). Blood samples were obtained through an ongoing collaboration with Dr D. Sangiolo at the Candiolo Cancer Institute FPO-IRCCS Fondazione del Piemonte per l'Oncologia. Patients provided written informed consent for blood donation according to a protocol approved by the internal review board and ethic committee (Ethic Committee, IRCCS Candiolo Cancer Institute, Turin, Italy. Prot. CE IRCCS 244/2015).

Cryopreserved PBMC were seeded at a concentration of $2x10^6$ cells/ml according to the standard protocols (Gammaitoni et al., 2013; Sangiolo et al., 2014), including 21 days of culture in RPMI-1640 medium (Gibco BRL Life Technologies Italia, Monza, Italy) supplemented with 10% fetal bovine serum (Sigma Aldrich, MI, Italy) 100 U/ml penicillin, and 100 U/ml streptomycin (Gibco BRL Life Technologies Italia, Italy) at 37°C and 5% CO_2, with the timed addition of IFN-γ (1,000 U/ml on day 0), Ab anti-CD3 OKT3 (50 ng/ml on day 1) and IL-2 (300 U/ml on day 1 up to the end, refreshing the medium every 2-3 days) (all factors are from Miltenyi Biotec S.r.l., Calderara di Reno, BO, Italy). In parallel with the standard *ex vivo* cultures, at day 0 an aliquot (7×10^6) of PBMC was seeded (2×10^6 cells/ml) in RPMI-1640 medium with 10% fetal bovine serum, 100 U/ml penicillin and streptomycin at 37°C and 5% CO_2) but without the addition of INF-γ to perform mRNA analysis. At day 1 of culture, 3×10^6 of these cells were collected for RNA extraction. Cells were lysed in Invitrogen™ TRIzol™ (Thermo Fisher Scientific S.p.a., MI, Italy) and stored at−80°C. RNA extraction was repeated with the same procedure for each CIK cells cultures at day 14 and 21.

Phenotype of CIK cells was weekly analyzed starting from day 0 by standard flow cytometric assays. The following monoclonal antibodies (mAb) were used: CD3-FITC, CD4-PE, CD56-APC, CD8-PE, and CD314-APC (anti-NKG2D) (all mAb are from Miltenyi Biotec S.r.l., BO, Italy). Labeled cells were read on FACS Cyan (Cyan ADP, Beckman Coulter s.r.l., Cassina De' Pecchi, MI, Italy) and analyzed using Summit Software.

Evaluation of Ectoenzyme Expression on CIK Cells by Flow Cytometry

FACS analysis of $CD56^+CD3^+$ CIK cells was performed using FITC-labeled anti-CD56 (Beckman Coulter Inc., Brea CA, USA) and PE-Cy7-labeled anti-CD3 antibodies (BioLegend, Milan, Italy). Expression of ectoezymes was detected by using the following mAbs generated and purified in-house by two-step HPLC chromatography (Horenstein et al., 2003) and APC-conjugated by Aczon (BO, Italy): anti-CD38 (clone IB4), anti-CD73 (clone CB73), anti-CD203a (clone 3E8, kindly provided by J. Goding) and anti-CD26 (clone BT5.9). CD39 expression was analyzed using anti-CD39 APC mAb (clone eBioA1, eBiosciences, San Diego, CA, USA). Tests were performed on cells washed in phosphate buffered saline (PBS) containing 1% bovine serum albumin (BSA) + NaN_3 and incubated with APC-conjugated mAb for 1 h at 4°C. The samples were then washed, resuspended in PBS and acquired on a FACSort flow cytometer (Becton-Dickinson, USA) using CellQuest Software (Becton-Dickinson). Data were analyzed using FlowJo Software (TreeStar).

Expression of ADO receptors was evaluated on CIK cells gated for $CD3^+$ $CD56^+$ and assayed in PBMC and in the corresponding CIK cells using the following antibodies: purified rabbit polyclonal anti-A_1R (LifeSpan BioSciences, Inc., USA), rabbit polyclonal anti-$A_{2A}R$ and rabbit polyclonal anti-$A_{2B}R$ (Thermo Scientific, USA). PE-conjugated goat anti-rabbit Ig (Beckman Coulter, USA) was used as secondary reagent. Data were expressed as mean relative of fluorescence intensity (MRFI), obtained as follows: mean fluorescence obtained with specific mAb/mean fluorescence obtained with irrelevant isotype-matched mAb.

For FACS analysis under hypoxic culture conditions, total cryopreserved PBMC were seeded at a concentration of 2×10^6 cells/ml in a humidified CO_2 incubator (Thermo Scientific Water Jacketed 3010) and differentiated into CIK cells by using the standard procedure. Culture conditions were 21% (normoxia) or 1% (hypoxia) O_2, 5% CO_2 at 37°C. The phenotype was weekly analyzed starting from day 0 by standard flow cytometric assays.

Quantification of ADO Production by CIK Cells

CIK (1×10^6/ml) were incubated in 500 µl HBSS at 37°C and 5% CO_2 in 24 well plates (Costar Corning) and pre-treated with 50 µL of stop solution [EHNA (5 µM) + Dipyridamole (20 µM) + Levamisole (30 µM) + Deoxycoformicin (50 µM)], in the presence (or absence) of NAD^+, ADPR, ATP or AMP (100 µM). At the end of the incubation time (30 min), supernatants were collected and acetonitrile (ACN, Sigma Aldrich) was immediately added (1:2 ratio) to stabilize ADO. Samples were then centrifuged at 13,700 × g, collected and stored at −80°C until use. The presence of NAD^+, ATP, ADPR, AMP, and ADO was investigated by high-pressure liquid chromatography (HPLC, Beckman Gold 126/166NM, Beckman Coulter) equipped with a reversed-phase column (Synergi Polar C18, 5 µm; 150 × 4.5 mm, Phenomenex). The metabolites were separated using a pH 5.1 mobile-phase buffer (0.125 M citric acid and 0.025 M KH_2PO_4 containing 8% ACN) over ten min with a flow rate of 0.8 mL/min and UV detection set at 254 nm. Peak identities were confirmed by using standard compounds. The presence of ADO was also confirmed by spiking standard (50 µM ADO), followed by chromatography. The retention times (Rt, in min) of standards were: ATP, 2.00; AMP, 2.35; NAD^+, 2.8; ADPR, 3.44, and ADO; 5.56. All concentrations measured on CIK-derived supernatants were normalized to cell number and volume.

Expression Profile of Adenosinergic Ectoenzymes and P1 Purinergic Receptors in CIK Cells

The mRNA expression data of PBMC and CIK cells originate from Mesiano et al. (2017) and were deposited in the Gene Expression Omnibus repository (https://www.ncbi.nlm.nih.gov/geo/query/acc.cgi?acc=GSE97581).

Briefly, we performed the gene expression profile (GEP) of PBMC (day 1, absence of INF- γ) and CIK cells (day 14) obtained from 3 GIST patients by means of HG-U219 Array Strip (Affymetrix; Santa Clara, CA, USA) (Mesiano et al., 2017). Microarray data were analyzed by using the Partek GS 6.6 Software Package and normalized using the robust multiarray average (RMA) procedure (Irizarry et al., 2003).

Differentially expressed genes (DEGs) were then selected using a supervised approach with the ANOVA module included in Partek GS package. In particular, we considered differentially expressed genes (DEGs) all the probe sets with a fold change contrast $\geq$ 1.4 in the pairwise comparison of CIK cells with PBMCs, and a false discovery rate (FDR) (q-value) < 0.5.

Statistical Analysis

p-value was calculated using an unpaired nonparametric test, two-tailed Mann-Whitney for GraphPad Prism 6. Reported data are expressed as mean values ± SD.

RESULTS

Transcriptome Analysis on Adenosinergic Ectoenzymes

In vitro differentiation of CIK cells starts with cultivation of PBMC according to standard protocols (Gammaitoni et al., 2013; Sangiolo et al., 2014). To shed light on extracellular enzymes involved in nucleotide/nucleoside and NAD^+ metabolism we checked the expression levels of CD39, CD38, CD203a and CD73 during CIK cell differentiation. As shown in **Figure 1**, CD38 and CD39 were up-regulated in CIK cells form 3 GIST subjects (day 14) vs. PBMC (day 1, absence of INF-γ), whereas CD73 and CD203a resulted down-regulated.

Expression of Nucleotide-Hydrolyzing Ectoenzymes in PBMC and CIK Cells

Firstly, cell cultures were gated for $CD3^+CD56^+$ expression and CD38, CD39, CD203a, and CD73 were assayed both in PBMC and in the corresponding CIK cells. A representative gating of the CIK population at the third week of culture is shown in **Figure 2A**. Expression of the assayed markers is represented by white peaks (**Figure 2B**). Cytofluorometric analysis revealed that the NAD^+-consuming CD38 ectoenzyme was present in 45.7% of the PBMC while it was expressed by the vast majority (98.9 ± 1%) of CIK cells, with minor variations in mean fluorescence intensity (MFI; mean ± SD, 148 ± 25). The expression of CD39 increased during PBMC to CIK differentiation (PBMC 35.7 ± 1.89; CIK 97.9 ± 2.34). CD203a and CD73 were also monitored (**Figure 2B**). In contrast to CD38 and CD39, CD203a was barely expressed by PBMC and increased in CIK cells (PBMC 7.7 ± 0.29; CIK 14.9 ± 0.34); while expression of CD73 was almost unchanged during differentiation (28.8 ± 3.65 vs. 23.8 ± 12.1).

While day 0 corresponds to withdrawal of PBMC, day 21 is usually chosen as end of *in vitro* differentiation period to start procedures for CIK cell infusion into cancer patients. **Figure 2C** shows that $CD3^+$ $CD56^+$ CIK cells from 6 subjects 5 GIST and 1 OS) maintained the initial high levels of CD38 with a mean value of 62.5% (min 53.2%, max 75.0%) vs. 92.5% (min 81.5%, max 98.8%); CD39 had a mean value of 13.2% (min 2.3%, max 23.5%) vs. 53.3% (min 32.2%, max 75.2%) associated to a significant increase at day 21 of the expression of CD26 as compared to resting PBMC with a mean value of 20.5% (min 6.8%, max 23.1%) vs. 91.2% (min 76.5%, max 96.5%), along with minimal CD203a up-regulation with a mean value of 15.1% (min 2.5%, max 24.1%) vs. 23.5% (min. 13.6%, max 35.1%), and stable expression of CD73 with a mean value of 75.2% (min 63.5%, max 80.30%) vs. 93.6% (min 77.5%, max 97.6%). These results indicate that CIK cells are provided with a complete ectoenzymatic machinery able to produce ADO through the traditional (CD39/CD73) as well as alternative (CD38/CD203a/CD73 or CD203a/CD73) pathways.

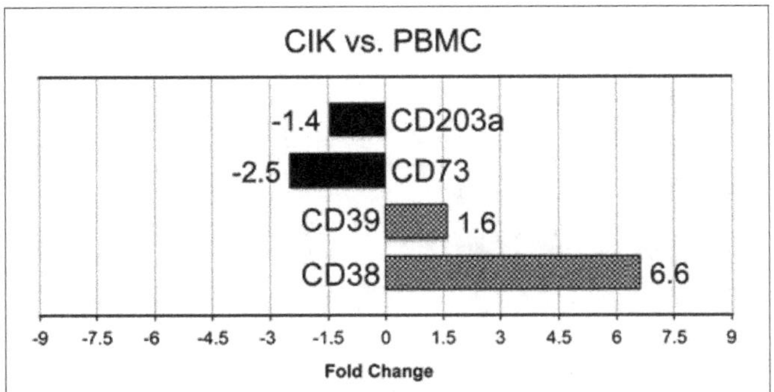

FIGURE 1 | Transcriptome analysis of CIK ectoenzymes. mRNA expression was analyzed in PBMC (day 1, absence of INF-γ) and CIK cells (day 14) obtained from 3 GIST patients. The black blocks display the transcripts that are down-regulated during CIK differentiation; whereas, the chess pattern displays the mRNAs that are up-regulated during CIK differentiation.

Extracellular ADO Production by CIK Cells

The role of ADO as potent suppressor of immune-surveillance has been well ascertained and has adopted by many cancer types as a mechanism of escape from the deleterious activity of macrophages, dendritic cells, T lymphocytes and NK (Morandi et al., 2015; Antonioli et al., 2016a,b). For adoptive immunotherapy CIK cells are usually infused as bulk into tumor bearing patients. Therefore, we checked whether the adenosinergic ectoenzymes expressed by bulk CIK cells deriving from PBMC of cancer patients were functional. To address this issue, we evaluated ADO produced by CIK cells obtained from 6 subjects (5 GIST and 1 OS). ADO release was investigated in supernatants from CIK cells incubated with NAD^+ (CD38 substrate), ADPR (CD203a substrate) and AMP (CD73 substrate) in the presence of EHNA (adenosine deaminase inhibitor).

Metabolism of Extracellular NAD^+

HPLC-assisted analysis of the supernatants of bulk CIK cells revealed the presence of non-consumed NAD^+ together with the enzymatic products ADPR and nicotinamide (NIC) ($n = 5$) (**Figure 3**). Besides the non-consumed NAD^+, which could be identified in the HPLC assay by its unique retention time (R_t) of 2.80 min, the metabolic products of CIK cells were ADPR,

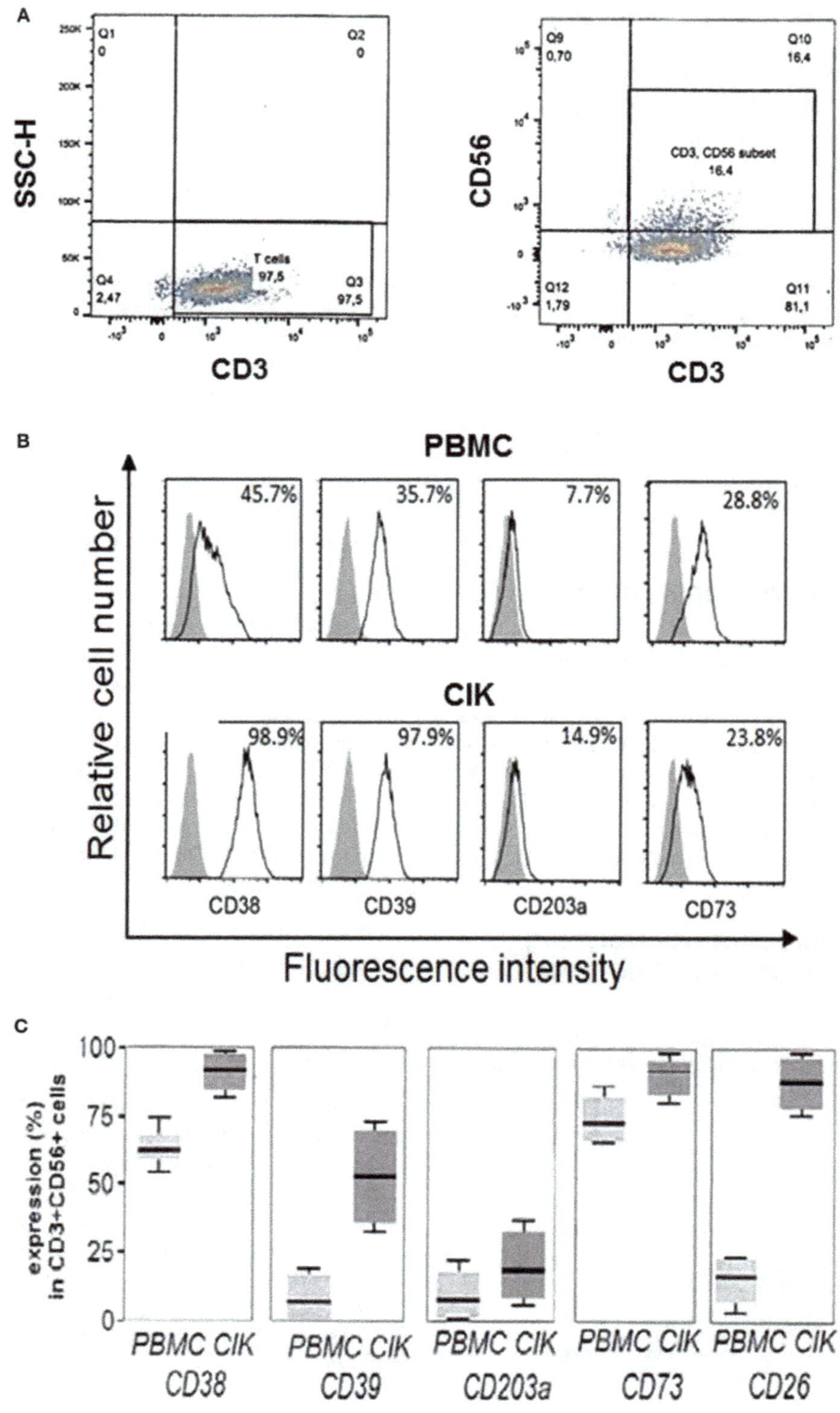

FIGURE 2 | Expression of CD38, CD39, CD203a, and CD73 in CD3$^+$CD56$^+$ human PBMC and in the corresponding CIK cells. **(A)** Representative gating of CD3$^+$ and CD3$^+$CD56$^+$ populations present in CIK cells at the third week of culture. Analysis was performed by using the fluorophores PE-Cy7 or FITC for CD3 and CD56 antigens, respectively. **(B)** Cytofluorometric expression analysis of ectoenzymes (white peaks) in PBMC at day 0 (upper panel) and CIK cells at day 21 (lower panel). CD38, CD39, CD73, and CD203a were detected by APC conjugated antibodies. Gray peaks demarcate isotype control staining. Percentage of positive cells is indicated. **(C)** Percentage of expression of the different markers in PBMC (day 0) and CIK cells (day 21). Cells were from 6 subjects (5 gastrointestinal stromal tumors and 1 osteosarcoma). In **C**, data are expressed as mean, minimum and maximum values.

NIC and AMP, exhibiting corresponding R_t of 3.44, 6.87, and 2.35 min, respectively.

The NAD^+ hydrolytic profile of CIK cells, converting extracellular NAD^+ into AMP, can be attributed to the ADP-ribosyl cyclase/cyclic ADPR-hydrolase activity of CD38 and CD203a, which exhibits nucleotide pyrophosphatase/phosphodiesterase activity. ADPR produced by CD38 upon the partial breakdown of NAD^+ can subsequently be degraded to AMP by CD203a, confirming the observations reported in other cell systems (Horenstein et al., 2015, 2016).

Since ADPR was the principal product of exogenously applied NAD^+, we wondered whether it would be source of the AMP generated by CIK cells. Thus, we tested the functional activity of CD203a by directly applying ADPR, a known substrate for this ectoenzyme (**Figure 3**). CIK cells displayed an ADPR-hydrolyzing activity leading to AMP, supporting our hypothesis that the NAD^+ converting pathway leading to AMP is operative in CIK cells concomitantly expressing CD38 and CD203a.

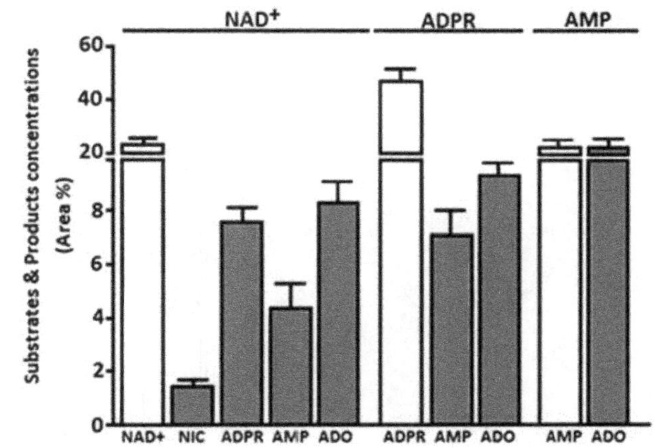

FIGURE 3 | Extracellular products of CIK enzymatic reactions using NAD^+, ADPR, and AMP as substrates. Products (NIC, ADPR, AMP, or ADO) obtained from bulk CIK cell cultures ($n = 5$) using (i) NAD^+, (ii) ADPR or (iii) AMP as substrates, were evaluated by HPLC assays in the presence of the adenosine deaminase inhibitor (EHNA) as described in Materials and Methods. Products (gray bars) are expressed as area percentage (Area %) for each enzymatic product as compared to the total components present in the ACN-treated CIK cell supernatant (100%). Substrates are represented as Area % of consumed substrate (white bars). Results indicate that bulk CIK cells efficiently hydrolyze NAD^+, ADPR and AMP to generate ADO. Of note, CIK cells produce low or undetectable amounts of ADO when incubated with NAD^+, ADPR, or AMP substrates in the absence of EHNA (not shown). The identity of peaks was confirmed by the co-migration of reference standards.

Metabolism of Extracellular ATP

The canonical adenosinergic pathway in CIK cells was investigated using ATP, a known substrate for CD39 or alternatively for CD203a (**Figures 4A,B**). Therefore, analysis ($n = 5$) of ATP consumption by CIK cells allowed a comparison of both nucleotide transformation pathways. The incubation of CIK cells with ATP led to a predominant accumulation of AMP, with low levels of ADP due to the catabolism of ATP by CD39 ectoenzyme (**Figure 4A**). However, at variance with reports pointing to the exclusive CD39-mediated ATP hydrolysis to ADP and AMP by lymphoid cells, CIK cells converted part of the ATP substrate directly to AMP, confirming the simultaneous presence of functional CD203a. This finding was confirmed by the attenuation (~50%) of the metabolic conversion of ATP into AMP in the presence of the CD39 inhibitor POM-1 (**Figures 4A,B**). These experiments support the view that the enzymatic activity of CD203a produced AMP also by a secondary conversion of ADPR (arising from the breakdown of NAD^+ by CD38), in a CD39-independent manner.

Metabolism of Extracellular AMP

The 5′-NT CD73 is expressed on the surface of select lymphoid cells. Thus, the heterogeneous T cell population composing CIK cells, ought to display AMP-degrading activity toward ADO generation. Indeed, these cells provided the proper phenotypic background with the capacity to degrade extracellular AMP to ADO (see the complete cellular phenotype of CIK cells in **Figure 1**).

HPLC experiments confirmed that CIK cells dephosphorylate extracellular AMP (**Figure 3**). HPLC analysis showed that AMP was dephosphorylated to ADO: AMP (R_t = 2.35 min) was metabolized (~80% within 30 min) by CIK cells resulting in a production of ADO (R_t = 5.56 min). Low level of inosine (INO, R_t = 3.26 min) was detected in the absence of EHNA (CD26 inhibitor) (not shown). Inhibition experiments further evinced the role of CD73 in the conversion of AMP. When CIK cells were incubated with AMP in the presence of α,β-methylene-ADP (APCP, a CD73 inhibitor), the catabolism of AMP and the formation of ADO were strongly decreased (~80%). These results indicate that the CD73 was the predominant ectoenzyme participating in ADO generation by CIK cells.

Metabolism of Extracellular ADO

Extracellular ADO may partially accumulate in the culture medium (or tumor extracellular *milieu*) where it binds specific P1 receptors or be internalized through nucleoside transporters. Alternatively, surface adenosine deaminase (ADA), complexed to CD26, converts ADO to INO (**Figure 4B**). PBMC expressed CD26 (6.8%) and during the cytokine-dependent differentiation to CIK cells the molecule raised to 89.4%. We confirmed such feature of CIK cells by measuring the increment of ADO production upon the incubation of these cells with AMP in the presence of EHNA (an inhibitor of ADA). Consequently, ADA on the surface of CIK cells, anchored to the CD26 receptor, offer to a combination of ectoenzymes [CD38 (cyclase/hydrolase), CD203a (NPP) or CD39 (NTDase) along with CD73 (5′-NT)] a machinery for ADO generation (**Figure 4B**). Indeed, results obtained indicated that consumption of 50% of the added ATP produced AMP (20%) and ADO (23%) after 30 min of incubation (**Figure 4A**). The presence of ADO indicated that the ectoenzyme clustering on the surface of CIK cells leaded to the production of the nucleoside. The consumption of NAD^+ by CIK cell in 30 min was, however, kinetically slower. As shown in **Figure 3**, consumed NAD^+ (22%) leaded to the production of 8% of ADPR, 5% of AMP and only 8% of ADO. Taking into consideration that low metabolization of

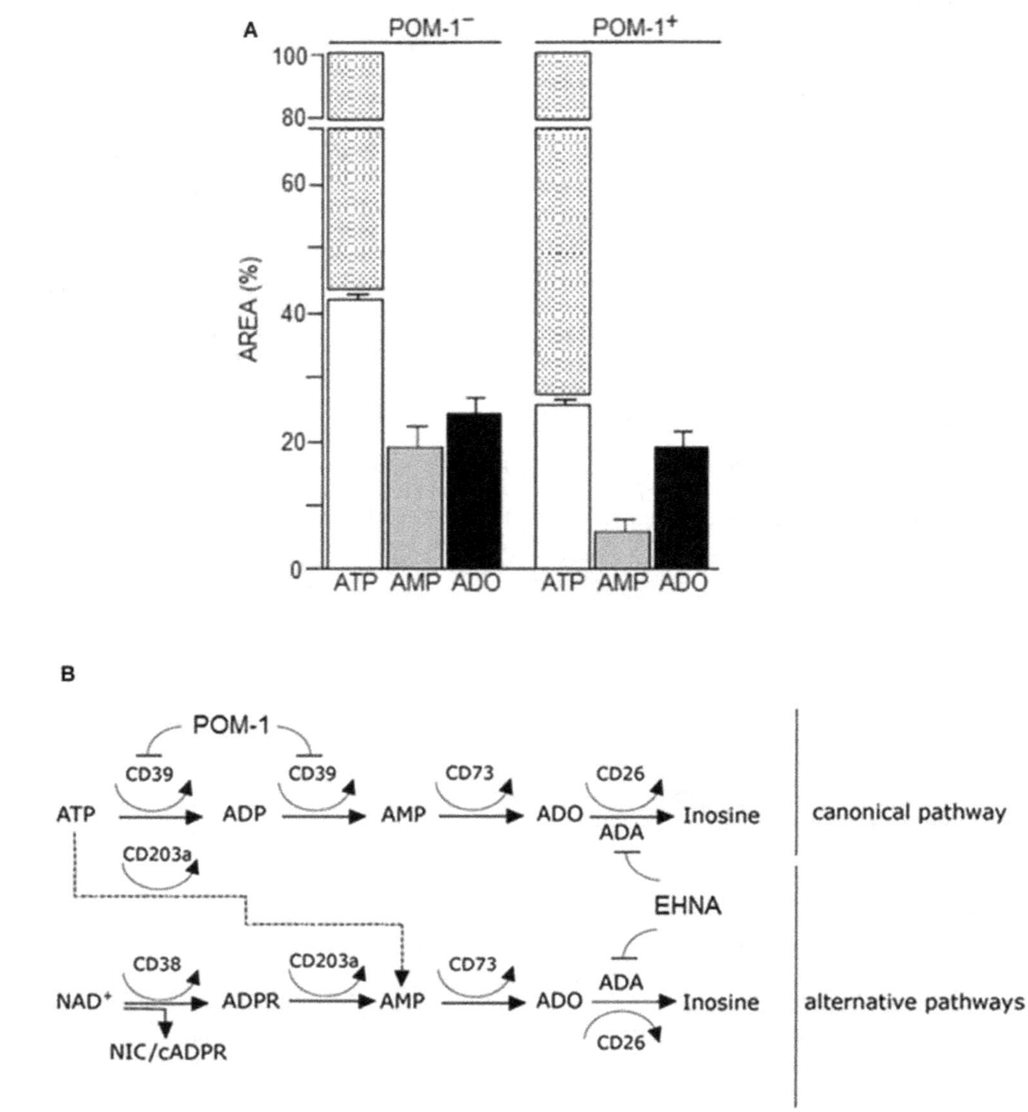

FIGURE 4 | Canonical adenosinergic pathway in CIK cells. **(A)** To prove the existence of ATP adenosinergic pathway in CIK cells, production of ADO was investigated in CIK supernatants collected 30 min after 100 μM ATP addition. White columns indicate the concentration of consumed ATP in the presence or absence of POM-1 (inhibitor of CD39). White/dotted columns indicate the total area of the substrate ATP (100%). Generated products (AMP and ADO) are indicated by grey and black columns, respectively. Data are expressed as area percentage (AREA %) of AMP and ADO. **(B)** Canonical and alternative scheme pathways of ADO production showing the enzymatic targets of POM-1 (inhibitor of CD39) and EHNA (inhibitor of adenosine deaminase, ADA).

AMP as substrate (20%) was paralleled by a high efficiency of ADO production (20%) confirmed the observation of a reduced expression of CD203a. Alternatively, a plausible explanation is a low enzymatic efficiency of CD203a to catalyze the conversion of ADPR into AMP. Accordingly, ADO production by CIK cells using NAD^+ was lower than using ATP either by CD39 or CD203a. In conclusion, CIK cells are equipped with a functional ectoenzymatic machinery leading to ADO production in the extracellular *milieu* (~25 μmol/min/10^6 cells). However, CIK cells produced low amounts of ADO when incubated with NAD^+, ADPR, AMP, or ATP as substrates in the absence of EHNA (CD26/ADA tandem inhibitor), confirming the presence of ADA (evaluated by measuring the expression of the surrogate CD26 molecule) as shown in **Figure 3**.

Expression of P1 Receptors During CIK Cell Differentiation

Cellular responses to ADO are induced through activation of four subtypes of specific G protein-coupled receptors (A_1R, $A_{2A}R$, $A_{2B}R$, and A_3R) (Chen et al., 2013). Extracellular ADO generated by canonical (CD39/CD73) or alternative (CD38/CD203a/CD73 and CD203a/CD73) pathways, can be captured by the cells, thereby explaining its local signaling. Therefore, next step was to detect at mRNA and protein levels, the expression of these receptors during CIK cell differentiation. As shown in **Figure 5**, mRNA expression level of $A_{2A}R$, $A_{2B}R$, and A_3R were decreased in CIK cells compared to PBMC, while A_1R expression was not changed ($n = 3$).

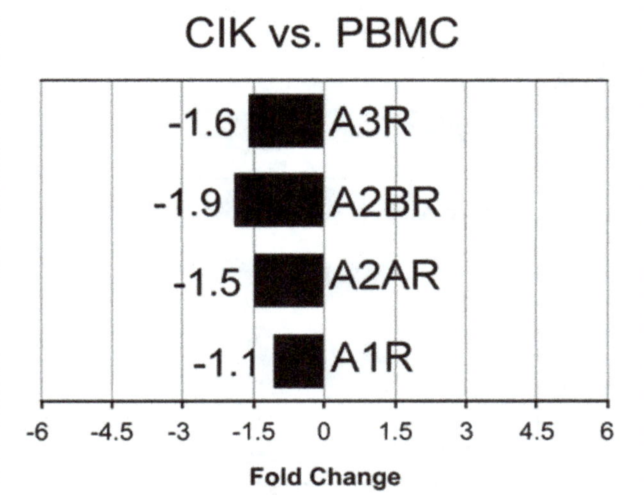

FIGURE 5 | Transcriptome analysis of P1 receptors in CIK cells. mRNA expression of A_1R, $A_{2A}R$, $A_{2B}R$, A_3R was analyzed in PBMC (day 1, absence of INF-γ) and CIK cells (day 14) obtained from 3 GIST patients as described in Materials and Methods.

To further investigate CIK immune regulation mechanisms, we analyzed the expression of ADO receptors at the protein level. Results obtained in additional patients confirmed that CIK cells of further expressed A_1R, $A_{2A}R$, and $A_{2B}R$ (see below), a feature that can be exploited by CIK cells to modulate intracellular cyclic AMP (cAMP). $A_{2A}R$ plays a role in lymphocyte deactivation by ADO and accumulation of high extracellular ADO in the absence of ADA is lymphotoxic (Huang et al., 1997; Burnstock and Boeynaems, 2014). Hence, to support cytotoxic CIK properties, the final product of the adenosinergic reaction might be devoid of an autocrine cAMP-dependent signaling. To comply with this condition, we hypothesized that a CIK active ADA/CD26 complex might scavenge pericellular ADO from the extracellular environment to facilitate their own survival and to protect its cytotoxic activities. In fact, we were unable to detect physiological levels of ADO when HPLC assays were carried in the absence of EHNA, an inhibitor of adenosine deaminase (**Figure 3**).

CIK Cell Ectoenzymes and Purinergic Receptors in Hypoxic Conditions

Hypoxic microenvironment has been shown to be one of the main drivers for the accumulation of ADO in different cancers and in some cases it increases the expression of CD39 and CD73 (Sitkovsky et al., 2014; Allard et al., 2016). CIK cells have a mixed

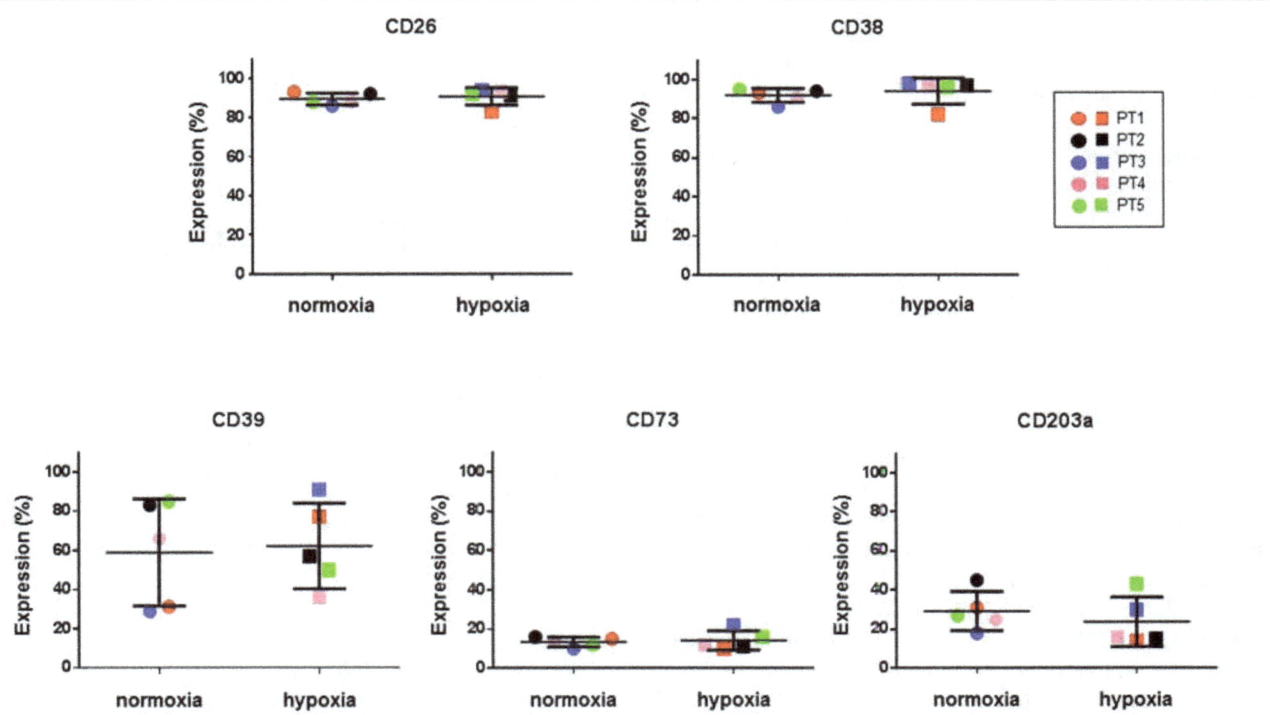

FIGURE 6 | Expression of ectoenzymes in CIK cells under normoxic and hypoxic conditions. Comparative cytofluorimetric analysis of CIK cells stained with primary antibodies to various ectonucleotidases as reported in Materials and Methods. To compare hypoxia and normoxia we used unpaired nonparametric test, two-tailed Mann-Whitney for GraphPad Prism 6. Circles, normoxia; squares, hypoxia. Patients are as following: PT1, red; PT2, black; PT3, blue; PT4, pink; PT5, green. Reported data are expressed as mean values ± SD.

T- and NK cell-like phenotype and ADO has been shown to hamper anti-tumor functions of these cells. For these reasons, the expression of CD39, CD38, CD203a and CD73 was monitored during CIK differentiation of cells from 5 patients, both in normoxic and hypoxic culture conditions. **Figure 6** shows that no significant ($p > 0.05$) differences were evidenced between values obtained in normoxia and hypoxia. ADO receptors are known to suppress immune responses against tumors. Expression analysis of A_1R, $A_{2A}R$, and $A_{2B}R$ was also performed, showing that ADO receptors only underwent minor, non-significant ($p > 0.05$) changes as a consequence of hypoxia (**Figure 7**).

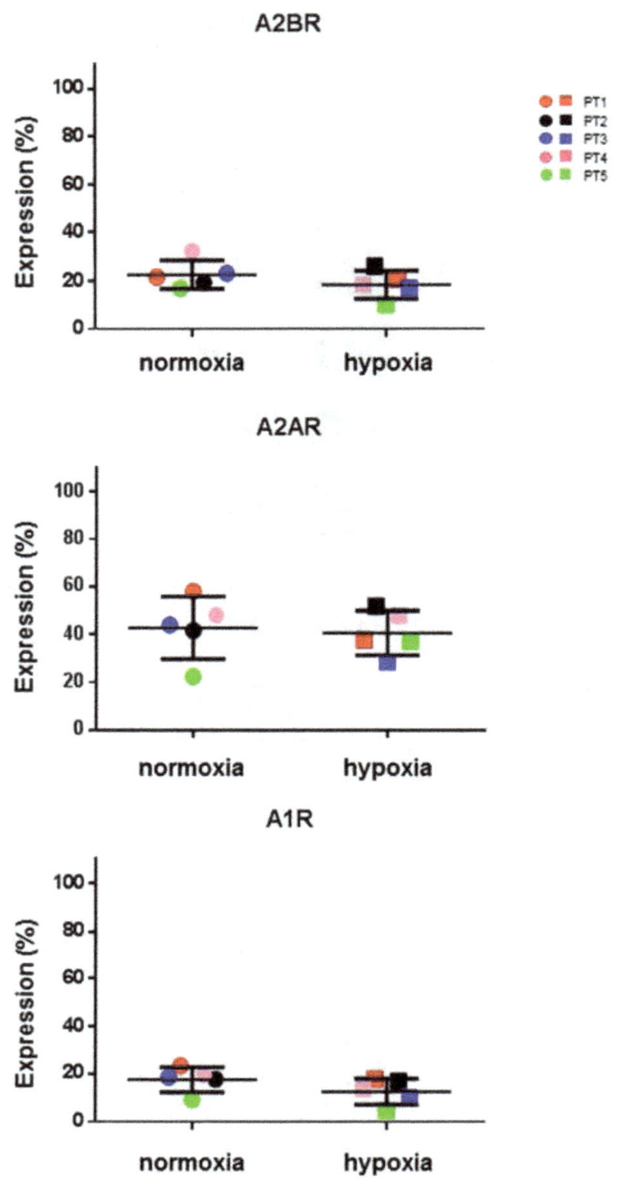

FIGURE 7 | Expression of P1 receptors in normal and hypoxic conditions. Comparative cytofluorometric analysis of A_1R, $A_{2A}R$ and $A_{2B}R$ expression in CIK cells stained with primary antibodies to various P1 receptors and detected with fluorescein (FITC)-conjugated secondary antibodies as reported in Materials and Methods. To compare data obtained in hypoxia and normoxia we used unpaired nonparametric test, two-tailed Mann-Whitney for GraphPad Prism 6. Circles, normoxia; squares, hypoxia. Patients are as following: PT1, red; PT2, black; PT3, blue; PT4, pink; PT5, green. Reported data are expressed as mean values ± SD.

DISCUSSION

Adoptive immunotherapy consists in potentiating the anticancer effects of selected immune populations. CIK cells represent a fundamental advancement in immunotherapy because of their ability to eradicate transformed cells, while sparing normal tissues (Vesely et al., 2011; Gajewski et al., 2013). However, in some cases tumors evade the killing activities of these cells. Numerous attempts are being made to enhance the potency and specificity of CIK cells (Wong et al., 2013).

Purine nucleoside adenosine (ADO) is attributed important roles in physiology and pathology. In immunity, ADO has immunosuppressive functions through activation of P1 purinergic receptors expressed by immune cells. ADO is produced from the dismantling of mono- and dinucleotides (ATP and NAD^+) and their byproducts (ADP, ADPR, AMP) by a set of ectoenzymes (CD39, CD38, CD203a, and CD73), of interest to both basic and clinical research because of their involvement in tumor biology and immune response.

The canonical pathway of ADO production originates from CD39, which metabolizes ATP. However, it was recently demonstrated that CD38 leads to an alternative pathway, whose substrate is NAD^+ (Horenstein et al., 2013). Both pathways converge into AMP, produced either from ATP/ADP (by means of CD39) or from ADPR (by means of CD203a/PC-1). AMP is then converted to ADO by CD73, the bottleneck enzyme for both adenosinergic pathways. These ectoenzymes are expressed by different normal cells (such as immune effectors) and by tumor cells. In the latter instance, these ectoenzymes grant immunosuppressive properties to the tumor cells by means of ligation of adenosine receptors (A_1R, $A_{2A}R$, $A_{2B}R$, and A_3R).

The aim of this study was to investigate expression and function of plasma membrane molecules involved in the adenosinergic pathways in PBMC and CIK cells. Here we showed that CIK cells are characterized by a combination of functional CD38, CD39, CD203a/PC-1, and CD73 ectonucleotidases. Consequently, these cells are potentially able to exploit *ex vivo* the coexistence of the canonical (CD39/CD73) and the alternative (CD38/CD203a/CD73 or CD203a/CD73) pathways. As a result they are able to generate the immunosuppressive purine nucleoside ADO, which either arises from the degradation of ATP or NAD^+ substrates. Accordingly, the substrates (ATP, NAD^+) were added to cell cultures, and their products (ADPR, NIC, AMP, ADO and INO) were quantified in the supernatants by means of a dedicated HPLC assay.

At the head of the alternative network converting extracellular NAD^+ is CD38, a molecule with multiple functions. As an ectoenzyme, CD38 acts as a primary regulator of extracellular NAD^+ levels (Malavasi et al., 2008). The next component in the ectonucleotidase cascade is CD203a, an ectoenzyme initially

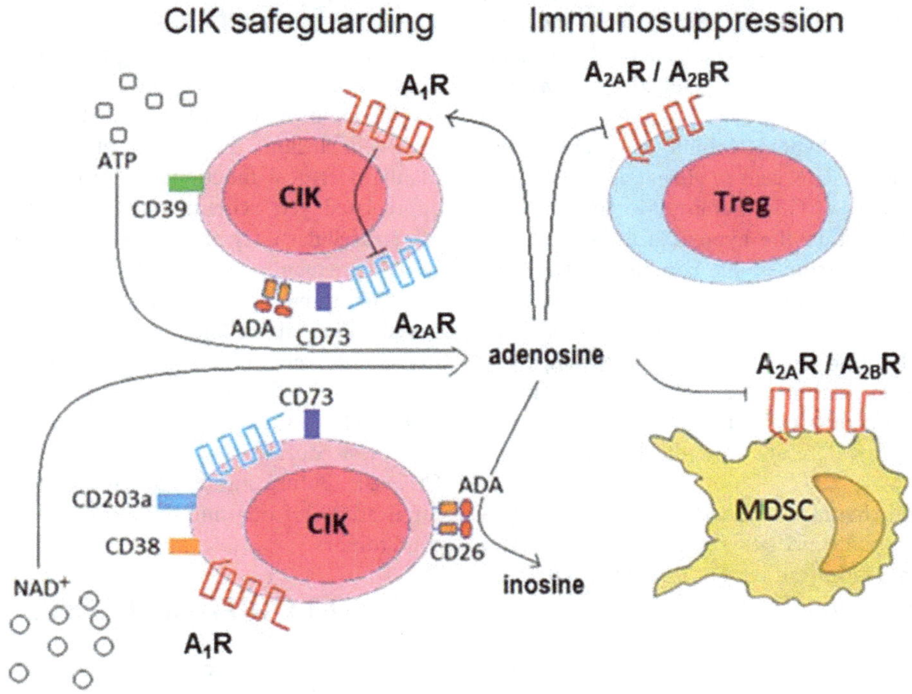

FIGURE 8 | Conceptual model of the role of ADO production, metabolism and receptor ligation in the cytotoxic activity of CIK cells. CIK cells prevent the induction of an autocrine immunosuppression by abrogating $A_{2A}R$-mediated signaling (by A_1R activation) and deamination of ADO catalyzed by the CD26/ADA complex. In turn, ADO produced by CIK cells can reduce pro-cancer immune responses through paracrine cell inhibition (e.g., Treg, MDSC functions).

known as Plasma Cell-1 (PC-1) (Goding et al., 1998). The interactions between extracellular NAD^+ and the CD38/CD203a enzymatic tandem can be exploited by CIK to generate AMP. Indeed, the addition of NAD^+ to CIK cells causes production of ADPR and NIC (products of the enzymatic activity of CD38) and AMP, in the culture supernatants. These results indicate that the outer plasma membrane of CIK cells is equipped with molecules endowed with hydrolytic activities that determine the fate of extracellular NAD^+. Lastly, we demonstrate that ADPR or AMP added exogenously to CIK cell cultures are further metabolized to produce ADO.

Extracellular ADO homeostasis is influenced by the presence of ADA, which irreversibly deaminates ADO, converting it to the related nucleoside inosine. This means that generated ADO is *in vivo* partially transformed by the cells of the surrounding environment, consequently locking the immunosuppressive effects of the nucleoside. Indeed, the low production of ADO in the absence of EHNA (a CD26/ADA inhibitor) is not ascribable to the high expression of ectonucleotidases by CIK cells. There are at least two possible explanations for this lowered production: either up-regulation of the ADA (as inferred by proxy from the increase in its surrogate, CD26) or low expression of CD203a, both of which are observed in differentiated CIK cells. Under such conditions, CIK cells would protect their ability to generate toxic effects against neoplastic cells. The remnant ADO generated by CIK cells in the extracellular medium is however available for binding to P1 purinergic receptors. Alternatively, it can be internalized by nucleoside transporters. This internalization step through the nucleoside transport was not observed in the system analyzed. Indeed, the addition of dipyridamole, an inhibitor of nucleoside transporters, was not followed by an increase in ADO. Things become even more complex considering the finding that CIK cells express high affinity A_1R and $A_{2A}R$. The presence of the two receptors would support the hypothesis that CIK cells take advantage of the P1 receptors to achieve autocrine signaling and thus self-regulation. Indeed, it is known that many cells express more than one purinergic receptor along with nucleotides degrading ectoenzymes, establishing a regulatory membrane network (Volonté et al., 2006). Therefore, trace amount of pericellular ADO may be sufficient to bind and activate (high affinity) $A_{2A}R$ on the surface of CIK cells (inducing a reduction in their immune activity). Nonetheless, $A_{2A}R$ activation is reported as being self-inhibited through the action of A_1R. This effect allow us to postulate that ADO binding to A_1R expressed by CIK cells can induce an autocrine inhibition of the nucleoside immunosuppressive effect, as depicted in **Figure 8**. Extracellular nucleoside concentrations can potentially favor (or suppress) the local immune responses, depending on its concentration as well as the relative abundance of P1 receptor subtypes expressed by CIK cells. These P1 receptor subtypes are coupled to different combinations of G-protein family members, namely A_1 receptors to G_i/G_o, A_{2a} receptors to G_s/G_{olf}, and A_{2b} receptors to G_s/G_q. Accordingly, engagement of A_{2a} and A_{2b} activates adenyl cyclase, leading to elevated levels of cellular cyclic AMP (cAMP). Instead,

A_1 stimulation inhibits adenyl cyclase, resulting in decreased cellular levels of cAMP. Accordingly, the observed biphasic effect of extracellular ADO could be explained by the peculiar functionality of A_1 and A_{2a} receptors (Cunha, 2005; Milne and Palmer, 2011).

It has been reported that hypoxia inhibit the proliferation, cytotoxicity and migration of CIK cells *in vitro* (Shi et al., 2013), hampering the effectiveness of CIK therapy. Moreover, the *ex vivo* infiltration of CIK cells in the hypoxic area is hindered, suggesting that a high expression of the complex CD26/ADA might be a condition *sine-qua-non* to warrant cytotoxicity to infused CIK cells. On this premise, we elaborate a model for CD26/ADA action at the CIK cell surface, where human ADA fine-tune ADO concentrations protecting CIK cells from an ADO mediated inhibition of proliferation. Consequently, this versatile strategy would provide a safety lock of CIK cell cytotoxic activities (**Figure 8**).

Treg cells and mesenchymal derived stromal cells (MDSC) are widely considered immune mediators of peripheral tolerance, playing a pivotal role in limiting anti-tumor immunity (Quarona et al., 2015; Chillemi et al., 2017). Therefore, pathways leading to ADO synthesis on CIK cells may contribute to the induction of paracrine suppression of the Tregs and MDSC immune activities (**Figure 8**).

A *bona fide* conclusion of the present study is that CIK cells are equipped with a surface machinery leading to ADO production. Moreover, CIK cells are characterized by the expression of ADO receptors with high affinity (A_1R and A_{2A}R): the activation occurs when ADO reaches 1-3 nM concentrations (Burnstock, 2007). CIK cells may produce microenvironmental ADO concentrations above the affinity constant (Ka) of adenosinergic A_1 and A_{2A} receptors present on the same cells and on immune effectors (e.g., Treg, MDSC). This sequence of events may occur *in situ* in the microenvironment or at a distance. The final outcome is an implementation by CIK cells of an autocrine/paracrine network required for optimal physiological activities. Support for this hypothesis comes from a recent study that showed T helper (Th) 17 cells ($CD26^+$) are also equipped with an adenosinergic machinery, which induces a negative regulation of the immune response of Tregs through the production of ADO (Bailey et al., 2014).

In conclusion, the results of this work consented us to highlight critical functional features of human CIK cells, not appreciated yet. Schematically, CIK cells express (i) a panel of extracellular enzymes involved in nucleotide/nucleoside and NAD^+ metabolism i.e., CD39, CD38, CD203a, and CD73. (ii) The same cells exploit the chain CD26/ADA/ADO to govern the extracellular concentration of ADO. The same effects are likely to be extended at distance, providing negative signals to T lymphocyte populations (De Meester et al., 1999). The results of this work pave the way to verify this hypothesis during the discrete steps of the induction of the CIK cells. Future studies are required to explore the functional implications of our findings within the challenging setting of solid tumors.

AUTHOR CONTRIBUTIONS

AH, FM, and DF: Conceived and designed the experiments; AH, AC, and RZ: Performed the experiments; AH, AC, FM, VQ, NB, and DF: Analyzed the data; FM, RM, and RG: Contributed reagents; AH, FM, and DF: Wrote the paper.

ACKNOWLEDGMENTS

We are thankful to Dr. Sangiolo D., Mesiano G., Grignani G., and Aglietta M for providing biological CIK samples. RZ and RM were financiated by Associazione Italiana per la Ricerca sul Cancro (AIRC), project number #10005 Special Program Molecular Clinical Oncology 5x1000 to AGIMM (AIRC-Gruppo Italiano Malattie Mieloproliferative, http://www.progettoagimm.it); AIRC project number #19818.

REFERENCES

Allard, B., Beavis, P. A., Darcy, P. K., and Stagg, J. (2016). Immunosuppressive activities of adenosine in cancer. *Curr. Opin. Pharmacol.* 29, 7–16. doi: 10.1016/j.coph.2016.04.001

Allard, D., Turcotte, M., and Stagg, J. (2017). Targeting A2 adenosine receptors in cancer. *Immunol. Cell Biol.* 95, 333–339. doi: 10.1038/icb.2017.8

Antonioli, L., Blandizzi, C., Malavasi, F., Ferrari, D., and Haskó, G. (2016a). Anti-CD73 immunotherapy: a viable way to reprogram the tumor microenvironment. *Oncoimmunology* 5:e1216292. doi: 10.1080/2162402X.2016.1216292

Antonioli, L., Yegutkin, G. G., Pacher, P., Blandizzi, C., and Haskó, G. (2016b). Anti-CD73 in cancer immunotherapy: awakening new opportunities. *Trends Cancer.* 2, 95–109. doi: 10.1016/j.trecan.2016.01.003

Bailey, S. R., Nelson, M. H., Himes, R. A., Li, Z., Mehrotra, S., and Paulos, C. M. (2014). Th17 cells in cancer: the ultimate identity crisis. *Front. Immunol.* 5:276. doi: 10.3389/fimmu.2014.00276

Beavis, P. A., Milenkovski, N., Stagg, J., Smyth, M. J., and Darcy, P. K. (2013). A2A blockade enhances anti-metastatic immune responses. *Oncoimmunology* 2:e26705. doi: 10.4161/onci.26705

Burnstock, G. (2007). Purine and pyrimidine receptors. *Cell. Mol. Life. Sci.* 64, 1471–1483. doi: 10.1007/s00018-007-6497-0

Burnstock, G., and Boeynaems, J. M. (2014). Purinergic signalling and immune cells. *Purinergic Signal.* 10, 529–564. doi: 10.1007/s11302-014-9427-2

Chen, J. F., Eltzschig, H. K., and Fredholm, B. B. (2013). Adenosine receptors as drug targets–what are the challenges? *Nat. Rev. Drug Discov.* 12, 265–286. doi: 10.1038/nrd3955

Chillemi, A., Quarona, V., Antonioli, L., Ferrari, D., Horenstein, A. L., and Malavasi, F. (2017). Roles and modalities of ectonucleotidases in remodeling the multiple myeloma niche. *Front. Immunol.* 8:305. doi: 10.3389/fimmu.2017.00305

Costa, F., Toscani, D., Chillemi, A., Quarona, V., Bolzoni, M., Marchica, V., et al. (2017). Expression of CD38 in myeloma bone niche: A rational basis for the use of anti-CD38 immunotherapy to inhibit osteoclast formation. *Oncotarget* 8, 56598–56611. doi: 10.18632/oncotarget.17896

Cunha, R. A. (2005). Neuroprotection by adenosine in the brain: From A1 receptor activation to A2A receptor blockade. *Purinergic Signal.* 1, 111–134. doi: 10.1007/s11302-005-0649-1

Dale, N., and Frenguelli, B. G. (2009). Release of adenosine and ATP during ischemia and epilepsy. *Curr. Neuropharmacol.* 7, 160–179. doi: 10.2174/157015909789152146

De Meester, I., Korom, S., Van Damme, J., and Scharpé, S. (1999). CD26, let it cut or cut it down. *Immunol Today.* 20, 367–375. doi: 10.1016/S0167-5699(99)01486-3

Desmet, C. J., Gallenne, T., Prieur, A., Reyal, F., Visser, N. L., Wittner, B. S., et al. (2013). Identification of a pharmacologically tractable Fra-1/ADORA2B axis promoting breast cancer metastasis. *Proc. Natl. Acad. Sci. U.S.A.* 110, 5139–5144. doi: 10.1073/pnas.1222085110

Ferrari, D., Malavasi, F., and Antonioli, L. (2017). A Purinergic trail for metastases. *Trends Pharmacol. Sci.* 38, 277–290. doi: 10.1016/j.tips.2016.11.010

Franceschetti, M., Pievani, A., Borleri, G., Vago, L., Fleischhauer, K., Golay, J., et al. (2009). Cytokine-induced killer cells are terminally differentiated activated CD8 cytotoxic T-EMRA lymphocytes. *Exp. Hematol.* 37, 616–628.e2. doi: 10.1016/j.exphem.2009.01.010

Fredholm, B. B., IJzerman, A. P., Jacobson, K. A., Klotz, K. N., and Linden, J. (2001). International Union of Pharmacology. XXV. Nomenclature and classification of adenosine receptors. *Pharmacol. Rev.* 53, 527–552.

Gajewski, T. F., Schreiber, H., and Fu, Y. X. (2013). Innate and adaptive immune cells in the tumor microenvironment. *Nat. Immunol.* 14, 1014–1022. doi: 10.1038/ni.2703

Gammaitoni, L., Giraudo, L., Leuci, V., Todorovic, M., Mesiano, G., Picciotto, F., et al. (2013). Effective activity of cytokine-induced killer cells against autologous metastatic melanoma including cells with stemness features. *Clin Cancer Res.* 19, 4347–4358. doi: 10.1158/1078-0432.CCR-13-0061

Garber, K. (2017). Industry 'road tests' new wave of immune checkpoints. *Nat. Biotechnol.* 35, 487–488. doi: 10.1038/nbt0617-487

Giraudo, L., Gammaitoni, L., Cangemi, M., Rotolo, R., Aglietta, M., and Sangiolo, D. (2015). Cytokine-induced killer cells as immunotherapy for solid tumors: current evidences and perspectives. *Immunotherapy* 7, 999–1010. doi: 10.2217/imt.15.61

Goding, J. W., Terkeltaub, R., Maurice, M., Deterre, P., Sali, A., and Belli, S. I. (1998). Ecto-phosphodiesterase/pyrophosphatase of lymphocytes and non-lymphoid cells: structure and function of the PC-1 family. *Immunol Rev.*161, 11–26. doi: 10.1111/j.1600-065X.1998.tb01568.x

Harden, T. K., Sesma, J. I., Fricks, I. P., and Lazarowski, E. R. (2010). Signalling and pharmacological properties of the P2Y receptor. *Acta Physiol.* 199, 149–160. doi: 10.1111/j.1748-1716.2010.02116.x

Hatfield, S. M., and Sitkovsky, M. (2016). A2A adenosine receptor antagonists to weaken the hypoxia-HIF-1α driven immunosuppression and improve immunotherapies of cancer. *Curr. Opin. Pharmacol.* 29, 90–96. doi: 10.1016/j.coph.2016.06.009

Horenstein, A. L., Chillemi, A., Quarona, V., Zito, A., Roato, I., Morandi, F., et al. (2015). NAD^+-Metabolizing ectoenzymes in remodeling tumor-host interactions: the human myeloma model. *Cells* 4, 520–537. doi: 10.3390/cells4030520

Horenstein, A. L., Chillemi, A., Zaccarello, G., Bruzzone, S., Quarona, V., Zito, A., et al. (2013). A CD38/CD203a/CD73 ectoenzymatic pathway independent of CD39 drives a novel adenosinergic loop in human T lymphocytes. *Oncoimmunology* 2:e26246. doi: 10.4161/onci.26246

Horenstein, A. L., Crivellin, F., Funaro, A., Said, M., and Malavasi, F. (2003). Design and scaleup of downstream processing of monoclonal antibodies for cancer therapy: from research to clinical proof of principle. *J. Immunol. Methods.* 275, 99–112. doi: 10.1016/S0022-1759(03)00006-1

Horenstein, A. L., Quarona, V., Toscani, D., Costa, F., Chillemi, A., Pistoia, V., et al. (2016). Adenosine generated in the bone marrow niche through a cd38-mediated pathway correlates with progression of human myeloma. *Mol. Med.* 22, 694–704. doi: 10.2119/molmed.2016.00198

Huang, S., Apasov, S., Koshiba, M., and Sitkovsky, M. (1997). Role of A2a extracellular adenosine receptor-mediated signaling in adenosine-mediated inhibition of T-cell activation and expansion. *Blood.* 90, 1600–1610.

Introna, M., Borleri, G., Conti, E., Franceschetti, M., Barbui, A. M., Broady, R., et al. (2007). Repeated infusions of donor-derived cytokine-induced killer cells in patients relapsing after allogeneic stem cell transplantation: a phase I study. *Haematologica* 92, 952–959. doi: 10.3324/haematol.11132

Introna, M., Golay, J., and Rambaldi, A. (2013). Cytokine Induced Killer (CIK) cells for the treatment of haematological neoplasms. *Immunol. Lett.* 155, 27–30. doi: 10.1016/j.imlet.2013.09.017

Irizarry, R. A., Hobbs, B., Collin, F., Beazer-Barclay, Y. D., Antonellis, K. J., Scherf, U., et al. (2003). Exploration, normalization, and summaries of high density oligonucleotide array prove level data. *Biostatistics* 4, 249–264. doi: 10.1093/biostatistics/4.2.249

Jiang, J., Wu, C., and Lu, B. (2013). Cytokine-induced killer cells promote antitumor immunity. *J. Transl. Med.* 11:83. doi: 10.1186/1479-5876-11-83

Kazemi, M. H., Raoofi Mohseni, S., Hojjat-Farsangi, M., Anvari, E., Ghalamfarsa, G., Mohammadi, H., et al. (2017). Adenosine and adenosine receptors in the immunopathogenesis and treatment of cancer. *J. Cell Physiol.* 233, 2032–2057. doi: 10.1002/jcp.25873

Latini, S., and Pedata, F. (2001). Adenosine in the central nervous system: release mechanisms and extracellular concentrations. *J. Neurochem.* 79, 463–484. doi: 10.1046/j.1471-4159.2001.00607.x

Linn, Y. C., and Hui, K. M. (2010). Cytokine-induced NK-like T cells: from bench to bedside. *J. Biomed. Biotechnol.* 2010:435745. doi: 10.1155/2010/435745

Lu, P. H., and Negrin, R. S. (1994). A novel population of expanded human CD3+CD56+ cells derived from T cells with potent in vivo antitumor activity in mice with severe combined immunodeficiency. *J. Immunol.* 153, 1687–1696.

Malavasi, F., Deaglio, S., Funaro, A., Ferrero, E., Horenstein, A. L., Ortolan, E., et al. (2008). Evolution and function of the ADP ribosyl cyclase/CD38 gene family in physiology and pathology. *Physiol. Rev.* 88, 841–886. doi: 10.1152/physrev.00035.2007

Mesiano, G., Zini, R., Montagner, G., Bianchi, N., Manfredini, R., Chillemi, A., et al. (2017). Analytic and dynamic secretory profile of patient-derived cytokine-induced killer cells. *Mol. Med.* doi: 10.2119/molmed.2017.00084. [Epub ahead of print].

Milne, G. R., and Palmer, T. M. (2011). Anti-inflammatory and immunosuppressive effects of the A2A adenosine receptor. *Sci. World J.* 11, 320–339. doi: 10.1100/tsw.2011.22

Mittal, P., Klingler-Hoffmann, M., Arentz, G., Winderbaum, L., Kaur, G., Anderson, L., et al. (2017). Annexin A2 and alpha actinin 4 expression correlates with metastatic potential of primary endometrial cancer. *Biochim. Biophys Acta.* 1865, 846–857. doi: 10.1016/j.bbapap.2016.10.010

Morandi, F., Morandi, B., Horenstein, A. L., Chillemi, A., Quarona, V., Zaccarello, G., et al. (2015). A non-canonical adenosinergic pathway led by CD38 in human melanoma cells induces suppression of T cell proliferation. *Oncotarget* 6, 25602–25618. doi: 10.18632/oncotarget.4693

Pievani, A., Borleri, G., Pende, D., Moretta, L., Rambaldi, A., Golay, J., et al. (2011). Dual-functional capability of CD3+CD56+ CIK cells, a T-cell subset that acquires NK function and retains TCR-mediated specific cytotoxicity. *Blood* 118, 3301–3310. doi: 10.1182/blood-2011-02-336321

Plattner, H., and Verkhratsky, A. (2016). Inseparable tandem: evolution chooses ATP and Ca2+ to control life, death and cellular signalling. *Philos. Trans. R Soc. Lond. B Biol. Sci.* 371:20150419. doi: 10.1098/rstb.2015.0419

Praetorius, H. A., and Leipziger, J. (2010). Intrarenal purinergic signaling in the control of renal tubular transport. *Annu. Rev. Physiol.* 72, 377–393. doi: 10.1146/annurev-physiol-021909-135825

Quarona, V., Ferri, V., Chillemi, A., Bolzoni, M., Mancini, C., Zaccarello, G., et al. (2015). Unraveling the contribution of ectoenzymes to myeloma life and survival in the bone marrow niche. *Ann. N.Y. Acad. Sci.* 1335, 10–22. doi: 10.1111/nyas.12485

Sanchez, L., Wang, Y., Siegel, D. S., and Wang, M. L. (2016). Daratumumab: a first-in-class CD38 monoclonal antibody for the treatment of multiple myeloma. *J. Hematol. Oncol.* 9:51. doi: 10.1186/s13045-016-0283-0

Sangiolo, D., Mesiano, G., Gammaitoni, L., Leuci, V., Todorovic, M., Giraudo, L., et al. (2014). Cytokine-induced killer cells eradicate bone and soft-tissue sarcomas. *Cancer Res.* 74, 119–129. doi: 10.1158/0008-5472.CAN-13-1559

Schmid, S., Kübler, M., Korcan Ayata, C., Lazar, Z., Haager, B., Hoßfeld, M., et al. (2015). Altered purinergic signaling in the tumor associated immunologic microenvironment in metastasized non-small-cell lung cancer. *Lung Cancer.* 90, 516–521. doi: 10.1016/j.lungcan.2015.10.005

Schmidt-Wolf, I. G., Negrin, R. S., Kiem, H. P., Blume, K. G., and Weissman, I. L. (1991). Use of a SCID mouse/human lymphoma model to evaluate cytokine-induced killer cells with potent antitumor cell activity. *J. Exp. Med.* 174, 139–149. doi: 10.1084/jem.174.1.139

Shallis, R. M., Terry, C. M., and Lim, S. H. (2017). The multi-faceted potential of CD38 antibody targeting in multiple myeloma. *Cancer Immunol. Immunother.* 66, 697–703. doi: 10.1007/s00262-017-1990-2

Shi, S., Wang, R., Chen, Y., Song, H., Chen, L., and Huang, G. (2013). Combining antiangiogenic therapy with adoptive cell immunotherapy exerts better antitumor effects in non-small cell lung cancer models. *PLoS ONE* 8:e65757. doi: 10.1371/journal.pone.0065757

Shryock, J. C., and Belardinelli, L. (1997). Adenosine and adenosine receptors in the cardiovascular system: biochemistry, physiology, and pharmacology. *Am. J. Cardiol.* 79, 2–10. doi: 10.1016/S0002-9149(97)00256-7

Silva, C. L. M. (2016). Purinergic signaling in schistosomal infection. *Biomed. J.* 39, 316–325. doi: 10.1016/j.bj.2016.06.006

Sitkovsky, M. V., Hatfield, S., Abbott, R., Belikoff, B., Lukashev, D., and Ohta, A. (2014). Hostile, hypoxia-A2-adenosinergic tumor biology as the next barrier to overcome for tumor immunologists. *Cancer Immunol. Res.* 2, 598–605. doi: 10.1158/2326-6066.CIR-14-0075

Stagg, J., and Smyth, M. J. (2010). Extracellular adenosine triphosphate and adenosine in cancer. *Oncogene* 29, 5346–5358. doi: 10.1038/onc.2010.292

Surprenant, A., and North, R. A. (2009). Signaling at purinergic P2X receptors. *Annu. Rev. Physiol.* 71, 333–359. doi: 10.1146/annurev.physiol.70.113006.100630

Valgardsdottir, R., Capitanio, C., Texido, G., Pende, D., Cantoni, C., Pesenti, E., et al. (2014). Direct involvement of CD56 in cytokine-induced killer-mediated lysis of CD56(+) hematopoietic target cells. *Exp. Hematol.* 42, 1013–21.e1. doi: 10.1016/j.exphem.2014.08.005

Vesely, M. D., Kershaw, M. H., Schreiber, R. D., and Smyth, M. J. (2011). Natural innate and adaptive immunity to cancer. *Annu. Rev. Immunol.* 29, 235–271. doi: 10.1146/annurev-immunol-031210-101324

Volonté, C., Amadio, S., D'Ambrosi, N., Colpi, M., and Burnstock, G. (2006). P2 receptor web: complexity and fine-tuning. *Pharmacol. Ther.* 112, 264–280. doi: 10.1016/j.pharmthera.2005.04.012

Wang, L., Zhou, X., Zhou, T., Ma, D., Chen, S., Zhi, X., et al. (2008). Ecto-5′-nucleotidase promotes invasion, migration and adhesion of human breast cancer cells. *J. Cancer Res. Clin. Oncol.* 134, 365–372. doi: 10.1007/s00432-007-0292-z

Wong, H. C., Jeng, E. K., and Rhode, P. R. (2013). The IL-15-based superagonist ALT-803 promotes the antigen-independent conversion of memory CD8(+) T cells into innate-like effector cells with antitumor activity. *Oncoimmunology* 2:e26442. doi: 10.4161/onci.26442

Yegutkin, G. G. (2008). Nucleotide- and nucleoside-converting ectoenzymes: Important modulators of purinergic signalling cascade. *Biochim. Biophys. Acta.* 1783, 673–694. doi: 10.1016/j.bbamcr.2008.01.024

Young, A., Mittal, D., Stannard, K., Yong, M., Teng, M. W., Allard, B., et al. (2014). Co-blockade of immune checkpoints and adenosine A2A receptor suppresses metastasis. *Oncoimmunology* 3:e958952. doi: 10.4161/21624011.2014.958952

Zimmermann, H., Zebisch, M., and Sträter, N. (2012). Cellular function and molecular structure of ecto-nucleotidases. *Purinergic Signal.* 8, 437–502. doi: 10.1007/s11302-012-9309-4

6

Adenosine A_{2A} Receptor Blockade Modulates Glucocorticoid-Induced Morphological Alterations in Axons, but not in Dendrites, of Hippocampal Neurons

Helena Pinheiro[1,2†], Rita Gaspar[1,2†], Filipa I. Baptista[1,2], Carlos A. Fontes-Ribeiro[1,2,3], António F. Ambrósio[1,2,3] and Catarina A. Gomes[1,2,3]*

[1] Coimbra Institute for Clinical and Biomedical Research, Faculty of Medicine, University of Coimbra, Coimbra, Portugal, [2] Center for Innovation in Biomedicine and Biotechnology, University of Coimbra, Coimbra, Portugal, [3] Faculty of Medicine, University of Coimbra, Coimbra, Portugal

***Correspondence:**
Catarina A. Gomes
catarina.gomes@fmed.uc.pt

†Co-authors

The exposure to supra-physiological levels of glucocorticoids in prenatal life can lead to a long-term impact in brain cytoarchitecture, increasing the susceptibility to neuropsychiatric disorders. Dexamethasone, an exogenous glucocorticoid widely used in pregnant women in risk of preterm delivery, is associated with higher rates of neuropsychiatric conditions throughout life of the descendants. In animal models, prenatal dexamethasone exposure leads to anxious-like behavior and increased susceptibility to depressive-like behavior in adulthood, concomitant with alterations in neuronal morphology in brain regions implicated in the control of emotions and mood. The pharmacologic blockade of the purinergic adenosine A_{2A} receptor, which was previously described as anxiolytic, is also able to modulate neuronal morphology, namely in the hippocampus. Additionally, recent observations point to an interaction between glucocorticoid receptors (GRs) and adenosine A_{2A} receptors. In this work, we explored the impact of dexamethasone on neuronal morphology, and the putative implication of adenosine A_{2A} receptor in the mediation of dexamethasone effects. We report that *in vitro* hippocampal neurons exposed to dexamethasone (250 nM), in the early phases of development exhibit a polarized morphology alteration: dendritic atrophy and axonal hypertrophy. While the effect of dexamethasone in the axon is dependent on the activation of adenosine A_{2A} receptor, the effect in the dendrites relies on the activation of GRs, regardless of the activation of adenosine A_{2A} receptor. These results support the hypothesis of the interaction between GRs and adenosine A_{2A} receptors and the potential therapeutic value of modulating adenosine A_{2A} receptors activation in order to prevent glucocorticoid-induced alterations in developing neurons.

Keywords: dexamethasone, adenosine A_{2A} receptor, development, hippocampal neurons, morphology

INTRODUCTION

The regulation of glucocorticoid (GC) levels during pregnancy is a major governing mechanism for the transition of the fetus to the extra-uterine life. During pregnancy, the levels of GC in the fetus are maintained lower than the mother's circulating levels and, toward the delivery, the intrauterine levels of GC rise, inducing fetal maturation (Thorburn et al., 1977). Once in the circulation, GC exerts a plethora of effects at the peripheral level and in the brain, by binding to mineralocorticoid (MR) and glucocorticoid receptors (GRs). Since endogenous GC have a higher affinity to MR, low levels of GC bind preferentially these receptors (Myers et al., 2014). Under stress conditions, the fetal hypothalamic-pituitary-adrenal (HPA) axis is activated in the earlier stages of development, inducing tissue differentiation, with detrimental effects later in life (Fowden and Forhead, 2015).

The administration of GC during prenatal and early life development mimics early-stress effects, being highly concerning. However, synthetic GC, such as dexamethasone (DEX), administrated in women at risk of preterm delivery to accelerate fetal lung maturation, are a crucial clinical tool to increase preterm infants survival (Brownfoot et al., 2008). Nevertheless, synthetic GC are up to 20 times more potent than endogenous GC and have higher affinity to GR (contrasting with endogenous GC), triggering different mechanisms likely implicated in their detrimental effects (Fowden and Forhead, 2015). Indeed, the antenatal exposure to synthetic GC was shown, both in humans and animal models, to have long-term effects on HPA axis regulation (Nagano et al., 2008), brain structure and behavior, neurosensory, neuroendocrine, and cardio-metabolic functions (Constantinof et al., 2016).

A brief antenatal exposure to DEX induces long-term behavioral alterations, such as decreased locomotor activity and exploratory behavior, increased susceptibility to depressive-like behavior (Oliveira et al., 2006), anxious-like behavior (Caetano et al., 2016), and altered fear-response in adulthood (Oliveira et al., 2012). The antenatal exposure to GC affects the normal development of the hippocampus, leading to a decrease in hippocampus size and an increase in the number of apoptotic cells during early life (Noorlander et al., 2014). Alterations in the hippocampal structure were reported also in models of early life stress induced by maternal separation, such as atrophy of mossy fiber density (Huot et al., 2002) and dendrites (Batalha et al., 2013). Thus, cytoarchitecture alterations in neurons due to DEX exposure may underlay the behavioral alterations.

Recent observations of A_{2A} receptor (A_{2A}R)-GR interaction in the hippocampus (Batalha et al., 2016) suggest that that A_{2A}R may be modulating DEX-induced effects in hippocampal neuronal cytoarchitecture during development. Indeed, the modulation of A_{2A}R has been regarded as a valuable therapeutic target in neuropsychiatric disorders (Cunha et al., 2008) and in the regulation of neuron morphology. The activation of A_{2A}R in neuronal differentiated PC12 cells demonstrated that A_{2A}R contributes to the increase in the number and length of neurites (Cheng et al., 2002; Charles et al., 2003). In primary cortical neurons, the activation of A_{2A}R increases axonal elongation and dendritic branching during neuronal development (Ribeiro et al., 2016). The modulation of neuronal morphology by A_{2A}R was also reported *in vivo*. Both the administration of caffeine in early life, a non-selective antagonist (Juárez-Méndez et al., 2006) and the treatment with a specific A_{2A}R antagonist in adulthood (Batalha et al., 2013) lead to alterations in neurons morphology, demonstrating that the blockade of A_{2A}R has an impact *in vivo* throughout all life span.

To test the hypothesis of A_{2A}R-GR interaction in hippocampal neuronal morphology we analyzed the effects of exposure to DEX on the morphology of hippocampal neurons during early development in the presence and absence of an A_{2A}R selective antagonist.

We report that DEX exposure induces a differential effect in the dendrites and axon of developing hippocampal neurons, characterized by dendritic atrophy and axonal hypertrophy. Whereas the effect in the increase in axonal length was dependent on the activation of A_{2A}R, the effect in the dendrites depends on the activation of GR, and not on A_{2A}R. These data suggest that the effects of DEX during development rely on distinct mechanisms in the different neuronal compartments.

MATERIALS AND METHODS

Primary Rat Hippocampal Neuronal Cultures

Primary cultures of hippocampal neurons were obtained from Wistar rats, as previously described (Baptista et al., 2013). Pregnant females (gestational day 18) were anesthetized with isoflurane, and sacrificed by cervical dislocation. Pups were delivered by cesarean operation and sacrificed by decapitation using surgical scissors. Briefly, the hippocampi from each hemisphere were macrodissected and dissociated chemically in a 0.15% trypsin solution (Sigma-Aldrich). Trypsinization reaction was blocked with 10% fetal bovine serum. Then, the hippocampi were mechanically dissociated in Neurobasal medium (Gibco) 0.025 mM glutamate (supplemented with 0.5 mM L-glutamine (Sigma), 2% B27, 0.1% gentamycin (Gibco) and plated at a low density (3000 cells/coverslip) in 16 mm coverslips previously coated with poly-D-lysine (0.1 mg/ml, Sigma). Hippocampal neurons cultures were maintained in an incubator at 37°C, 5% CO_2, until the end of the experiments. Four days after plating, at day *in vitro* (DIV) 4, half of the total medium volume was replaced by supplemented Neurobasal medium without glutamate, to avoid excitotoxicity.

All procedures involving animals were approved by the Animal Welfare Committee of the Faculty of Medicine of the University of Coimbra and were conducted in accordance with the European Community directive guidelines for the use of animals in laboratory (2010/63/EU), transposed into the Portuguese law in 2013 (Decreto-Lei 113/2013).

Pharmacological Treatment

At DIV1, hippocampal neurons were treated with DEX (250 nM, Acros Organics), a concentration that leads to GR nuclear translocation under the control of adenosine A_{2A} receptors (unpublished data), and/or the selective $A_{2A}R$ antagonist SCH58261 (SCH, 50 nM, Tocris) [this concentration is selective for $A_{2A}R$ (Zocchi et al., 1996)], and/or the GR antagonist (RU486) mifepristone (MIF; 1 μM, Tocris) and the selective $A_{2A}R$ agonist CGS21680 (CGS, 30 nM). DEX binds preferentially to GR (Kornel et al., 1982) and this concentration of MIF is able to abolish DEX effects *in vitro* (Kamradt et al., 2000; Kimura et al., 2011). When the effects of DEX were tested in the presence of the $A_{2A}R$ antagonist, SCH was added 15 min before DEX, whereas in the case of the GR antagonist, MIF was added immediately before DEX.

Immunocytochemistry

Hippocampal neurons were fixed in 4% PFA and 4% sucrose in PBS solution (137 mM NaCl, 2.7 mM KCl, 10 mM $NaH_2PO_4.2H_2O$, 1.8 mM KH_2PO_4 in miliQ water, pH = 7.4) for 10 min, at RT. After permeabilization/blocking (PBS 5% BSA, NZYtech, 0.1% Triton X-100, Sigma), coverslips were incubated overnight with the primary antibody (1:1000, polyclonal rabbit anti-TUJ1, Covance), at 4°C, and for 2 h at RT with the secondary antibody (1:1000, polyclonal goat anti-rabbit, Thermo Fisher Scientific) after washing with PBS solution. Then, coverslips were incubated for 10 min with DAPI (1:5000 in PBS, Invitrogen) to stain nuclei, and mounted on microscope slides with glycergel mounting medium (DAKO).

Morphometric Analysis of Hippocampal Neurons

Neuronal morphology was analyzed at DIV2 and DIV5, to evaluate the influence of the pharmacological treatments upon the initial development of the axon at DIV2 and the elongation of the dendrites at DIV5 (Dotti et al., 1988, #438). For naming purposes, in this study, the major processes at DIV2 were solely considered as axons. Images of neurons were acquired in a fluorescence microscope Zeiss Axio Imager 2 linked to Zeiss AxioCam, using a 20× objective lens (Plan Apochromat 20×/0.8) and processed by Zen Blue software (Zeiss). The settings of the acquisition were maintained throughout all experiments. Two main criteria were taken into consideration for the selection of neurons: the acquisition of neurons whose neurites were clearly distinguishable and not overlaid with others, and the proximity to other neurons (in a radius of 1000 μm) to avoid morphologic alterations due to lack of trophic support derived from other neurons.

Images were imported to the Neurolucida software (MBF Bioscience) and distinguished axons and dendrites were manually reconstructed, taking into consideration their morphological differences, by a researcher blinded to the treatment conditions. The major branch in each cell with a constant caliber was regarded as the axon, whereas the smaller neurites with taper ending were considered dendrites. All ramifications were considered, regardless of their length. At DIV2, 180 cells were reconstructed for each condition, in a total of six independent experiments. At DIV5, 120 cells were reconstructed for each condition, in a total of five independent experiments.

Morphometric data (branched structure analysis) was obtained in Neurolucida Explorer software, and the number of axons/dendrites, mean length of axons/dendrites, and total numbers of ramifications of each were analyzed.

Statistical Analysis

Statistical analysis was carried out in GraphPad Prism version 5 (GraphPad Software Inc.). All graphic values are expressed as mean ± standard error of the mean (SEM). Comparison between two independent means was done by Student's *t*-test. To assess differences between three groups, a one-way analysis of variance (ANOVA) was used, followed by a Tukey's Multiple Comparison Test, to compare all groups. Differences were considered significant at $p < 0.05$.

RESULTS

Exposure to DEX Has a Differential Effect in Different Neuronal Compartments, Inducing Axon Hypertrophy and Dendrite Atrophy

To assess the effects of DEX upon neuronal morphogenesis, primary hippocampal neurons were treated with DEX (250 nM) after 24 h in culture and neuronal morphology was analyzed after 2 and 5 days in culture (**Figure 1**), by manual reconstruction, using Neurolucida software. Morphometric data were analyzed considering the number and length of dendrites and axons, and the respective ramification.

We observed that DEX treatment did not alter neuronal morphology after 2 days in culture (Supplementary Figure 1). Contrastingly, at 5 days in culture DEX exposure induced a pronounced decrease in the mean length of the dendrites: 107.6 ± 6.6 μm ($p < 0.001$), as compared with non-treated (NT; 150.7 ± 8.1 μm) (**Figure 1d**). However, no statistical effect was detected upon their number and number of ramifications. In the axon, DEX induced the opposite effect, increasing its length: 1139.2 ± 86.1 μm ($p < 0.01$), as compared with NT (811.5 ± 57.6 μm) (**Figure 1g**).

Thus, exposure of hippocampal neurons to DEX induces a contrasting modulation of neuronal morphology, characterized by axonal hypertrophy and dendritic atrophy.

DEX-Induced Increase in Axon Length Is Dependent on the Activation of Adenosine A_{2A} Receptors

To understand if the activation of $A_{2A}R$ is implicated in the modulation of neuronal morphology induced by DEX, we analyzed the impact of DEX in hippocampal neurons under the pharmacological blockade of $A_{2A}R$, using a selective antagonist (SCH58261) (**Figure 2**). Hence, primary hippocampal neurons were treated with 250 nM DEX in the absence or presence of 50 nM SCH58261, and neuronal morphology was analyzed after 5 days in culture.

The blockade of $A_{2A}R$ was not able to prevent the atrophy in the length of the dendrites induced by DEX (110.0 ± 5.4 μm),

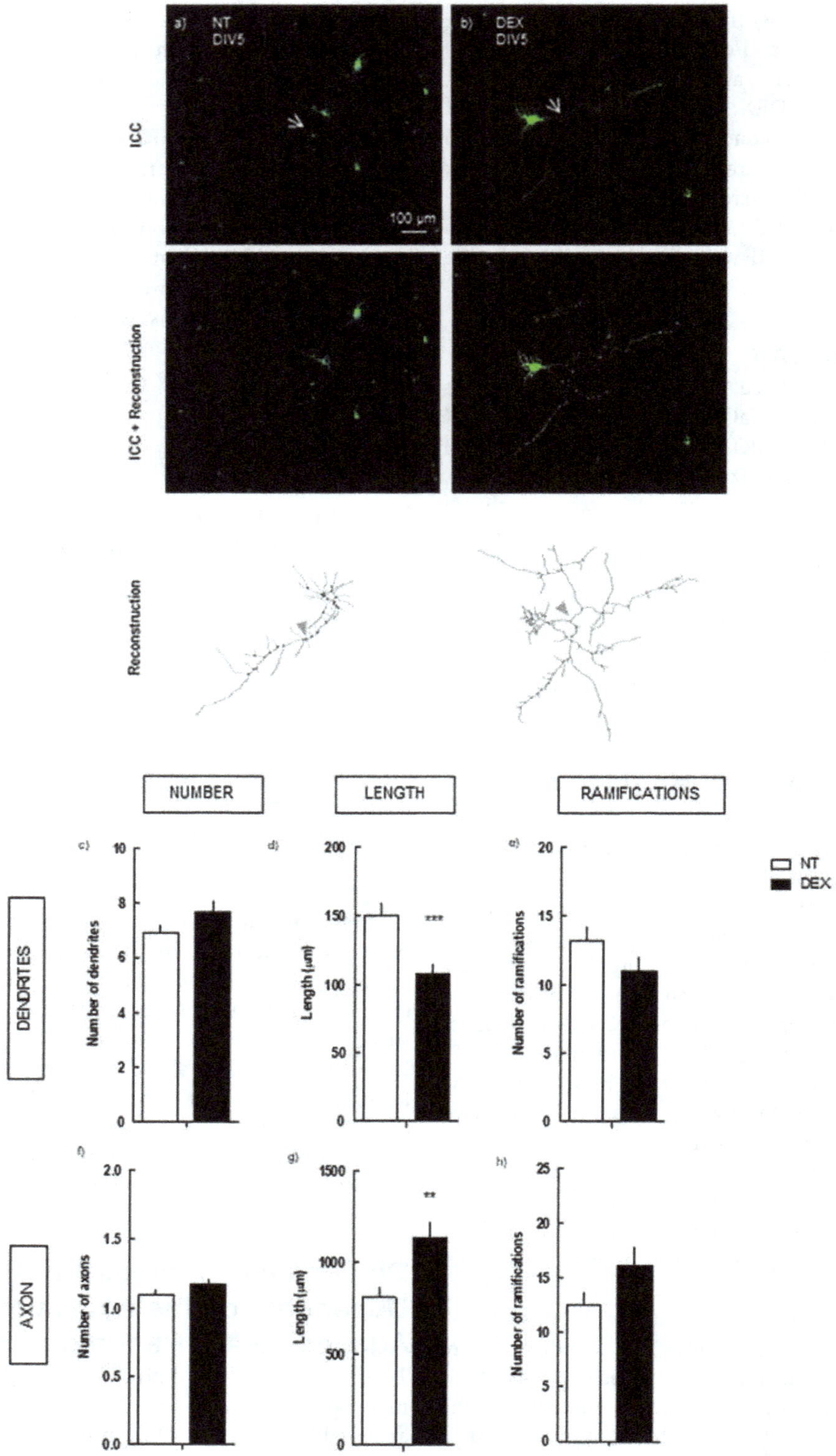

FIGURE 1 | Effect of DEX treatment (4 days treatment) on hippocampal neurons (DIV5). Hippocampal neurons from ED18 rats were cultured *in vitro* for 5 days (DIV5) and treated with DEX (250 nM) at 24 h in culture. Neuronal morphology was assessed by manual reconstruction in Neurolucida software **(a,b)** and morphometric data were acquired in Neurolucida Explorer, regarding the number **(c)**, length **(d)** and number of ramifications **(e)** of dendrites and the number **(f)**, length **(g)**, and number of ramifications **(h)** of axons (identified with an arrow in the representative images). Results are expressed as mean ± SEM of 120 cells, from five independent experiments. Statistical significance was assessed by *t*-student test: $^{**}p < 0.01$, $^{***}p < 0.001$, comparing DEX treatment with NT. ICC, immunocytochemistry; NT, non-treated; DEX, dexamethasone.

comparing with DEX alone (107.6 ± 6.6 μm). Indeed, the effect of $A_{2A}R$ plus DEX, which induced a similar decrease as DEX alone, was significantly different ($p < 0.001$) from NT cells (150.7 ± 8.1 μm). The treatment with SCH *per se* induced a decrease in the length of the dendrites similar to the effect of DEX treatment (**Figure 2f**), indicating that both DEX and SCH induce similar alterations in dendrites' length.

Regarding the number of dendrites, although DEX treatment did not induce a significant alteration, there was a tendency to increase. Regarding the treatment with SCH, there was an increase in the number of dendrites, both in the absence (8.4 ± 0.3; $p < 0.05$) and presence of DEX (9.0 ± 0.4; $p < 0.001$), comparing with NT (6.9 ± 0.3).

Conversely, in the axon, $A_{2A}R$ blockade prevented the increase ($p < 0.001$) in the length induced by DEX (752.4 ± 60.8 μm), comparing with DEX alone (1139.2 ± 86.1 μm; **Figure 2i**), having a similar length as in NT cells (811.5 ± 57.6 μm; n.s.).

These findings show that there is an uncouple in the mechanisms underlying the effect of DEX exposure in dendrites and axon, demonstrating the requirement of the activation of different receptors.

DEX-Mediated Increase in Axon Length Is Not Exclusively Modulated by the Activation of $A_{2A}R$

Given that the blockade of $A_{2A}R$ *per se* led to alterations in neuronal morphology similar to those observed in the blockade of $A_{2A}R$ combined with DEX, we aimed to clarify if the rescue of the axon length is not mediated solely by the blockade of $A_{2A}R$ activation by tonic adenosine, instead of a modulation dependent on GR. Thus, we analyzed the effect of a selective $A_{2A}R$ agonist, 30 nM CGS 21680, in neuronal morphology.

We observed that, in the absence of DEX, the activation of $A_{2A}R$ does not lead to significant alterations in neuronal morphology, not in the dendrites or axon (**Figure 3**).

These results indicate that the DEX-induced axonal hypertrophy, although dependent on the activation of $A_{2A}R$ requires also the activation of GR, indicating a crosstalk between $A_{2A}R$/GR.

Surprisingly, even though the blockade of $A_{2A}R$ *per se* led to alterations in dendrites' morphology, these alterations were not observed by the selective activation of $A_{2A}R$. This indicates that the maintenance of adenosine tonic levels is crucial for neuronal morphology, although the overactivation of $A_{2A}R$ does not alter morphology.

DEX-Induced Decrease in Dendrite Length Is Dependent on the Activation of Glucocorticoids Receptors

Considering that synthetic glucocorticoids, namely DEX, have a high affinity to GR (Kornel et al., 1982), we sought to confirm if the effects of DEX on the morphology of neurons are dependent on the activation of GR. To test this hypothesis, primary hippocampal neurons were treated with 250 nM DEX, in the absence or presence of the antagonist of GR, 1 μM MIF (**Figure 4**).

The blockade of GR prevented the alteration in the length of the dendrites induced by DEX (147.1 ± 8.6 μm; $p < 0.001$) as compared with DEX alone (107.6 ± 6.6 μm) (**Figure 4f**), to values similar to NT cells (150.7 ± 8.1 μm; n.s.). Additionally, the treatment with MIF *per se* led to an increase ($p < 0.01$) in the number of dendrites (8.6 ± 0.4) as compared with NT (6.9 ± 0.3) (**Figure 4e**), demonstrating a hypertrophic effect of the blockade of endogenous glucocorticoids.

The increase in the length of the axon induced by DEX was not prevented by the blockade of GR (1069.1 ± 88.7 μm), as compared with DEX alone (1139.2 ± 86.1 μm, n.s.) (**Figure 4i**). In contrast to the observations in dendrites, the effect of DEX in the presence of MIF in the axon is similar to the effect of DEX alone, indicative of two different mechanisms overriding DEX effects in axon and dendrites.

Indeed, we demonstrate that whereas the effect of DEX in the dendritic morphology depends on the direct activation of GR, the effects on the axon are modulated by the activation of $A_{2A}R$.

The observation that the blockade of GR *per se* leads to an increase ($p < 0.05$) in the number of ramifications in the axon (18.7 ± 2.0) as compared with NT (12.5 ± 1.2), is in line with the possible hypertrophic effect of blocking the action of endogenous glucocorticoids raised above. However, the hypertrophic effect of GR blockade could be also due to an increase in the activation of mineralocorticoid receptors by tonic glucocorticoids, rather than the lack of GR activation.

DISCUSSION

The development of the brain is tightly regulated by environmental factors. Thus, negative environmental stimuli, such as prenatal and early life stress, which lead to increased levels of glucocorticoids can have a long-term impact in the brain cytoarchitecture and function (Oliveira et al., 2006, 2012; Leão et al., 2007). Similarly, glucocorticoid treatments, such as DEX, also lead to detrimental effects in the brain. However, the implementation of these approaches in women in risk of preterm birth was an undoubtable advance in the increase of survival rates of premature newborns (Brownfoot et al., 2008). Therefore, it is crucial to understand the modulating effects of glucocorticoid exposure in the developing brain in order to develop new pharmacological approaches to circumvent their negative effects.

In the present work, we reported that a long-term exposure to DEX in developing hippocampal neurons leads to a differential modulation of neuronal morphology, characterized by dendrites' atrophy and axonal hypertrophy. The observation that DEX did not alter neuronal morphology after 24 h of exposure (Supplementary Figure 1) indicates that DEX-mediated effects in morphology are delayed or restricted to later stages of development.

The delay in DEX effects is in line with previous observations in PC12 cells, in which the treatment with a low dose of DEX leads to an increase in cell growth only after 72 h of exposure, as indicated by the total protein/DNA ratio (Jameson et al., 2006). As that method does not discriminate cell morphology, the results

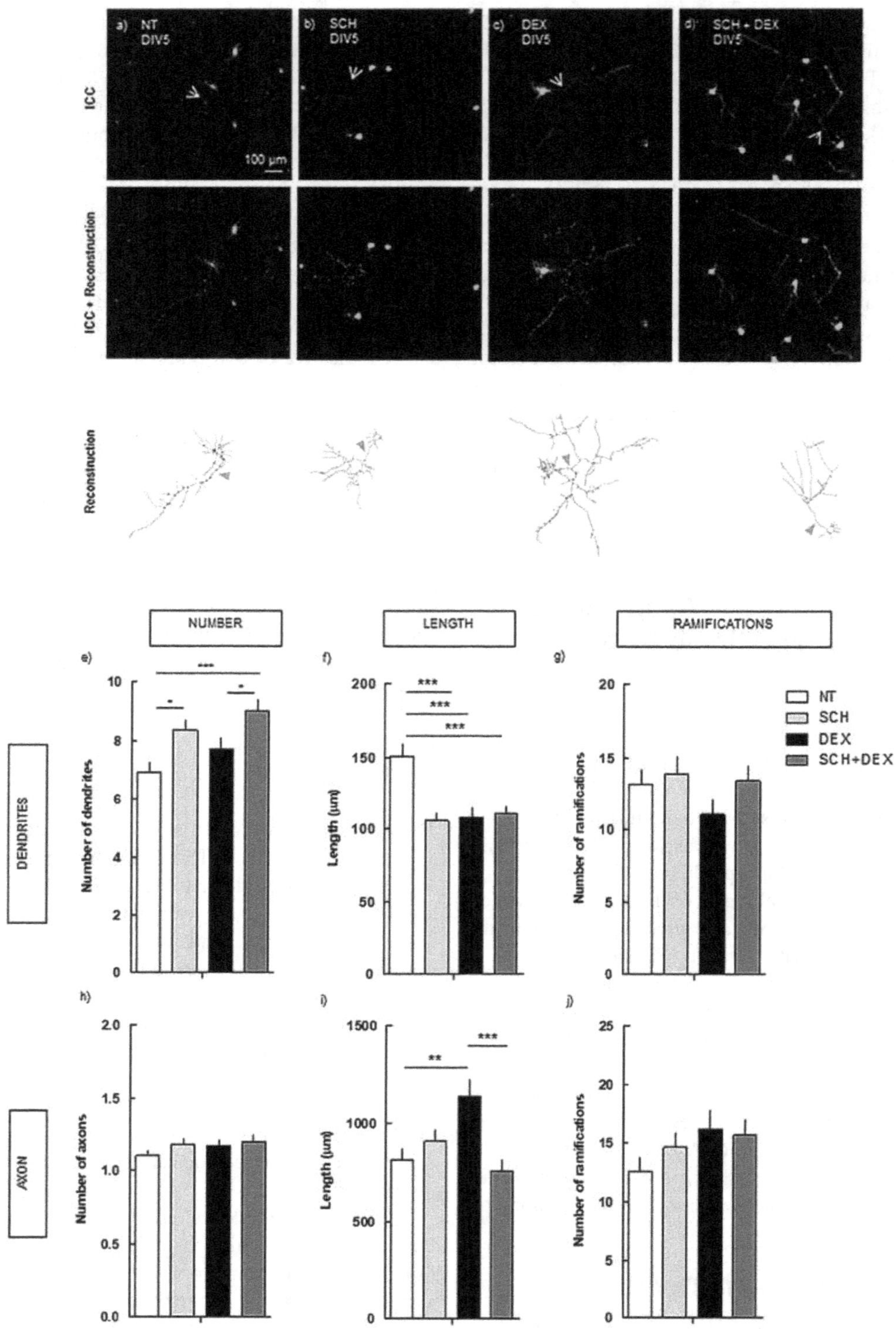

FIGURE 2 | Effect of the blockade of $A_{2A}R$ *per se* and on DEX exposure (4 days treatment) in hippocampal neurons (DIV5). Hippocampal neurons from ED18 rats were cultured *in vitro* for 5 days (DIV5). Cultured neurons were treated with the $A_{2A}R$ antagonist, SCH (50 nM), or with the $A_{2A}R$ antagonist and/or DEX (250 nM; at 24 h in culture). SCH was added 15 min before DEX. Neuronal morphology was assessed by manual reconstruction in Neurolucida software **(a–d)** and morphometric data were acquired in Neurolucida Explorer, regarding the number **(e)**, length **(f)**, and number of ramifications **(g)** of dendrites and the number **(h)**, length **(i)**, and number of ramifications **(j)** of axons (identified with an arrow in the representative images). Results are expressed as mean ± SEM of 120 cells, from five independent experiments. Statistical significance was assessed by one-way ANOVA followed by Tukey's Multiple Comparison Test: $^*p < 0.05$, $^{**}p < 0.01$, $^{***}p < 0.001$, as indicated by the horizontal lines above the columns. ICC, immunocytochemistry; NT, non-treated; SCH, SCH58261, $A_{2A}R$ antagonist; DEX, dexamethasone; SCH+DEX, SCH58261 + Dexamethasone.

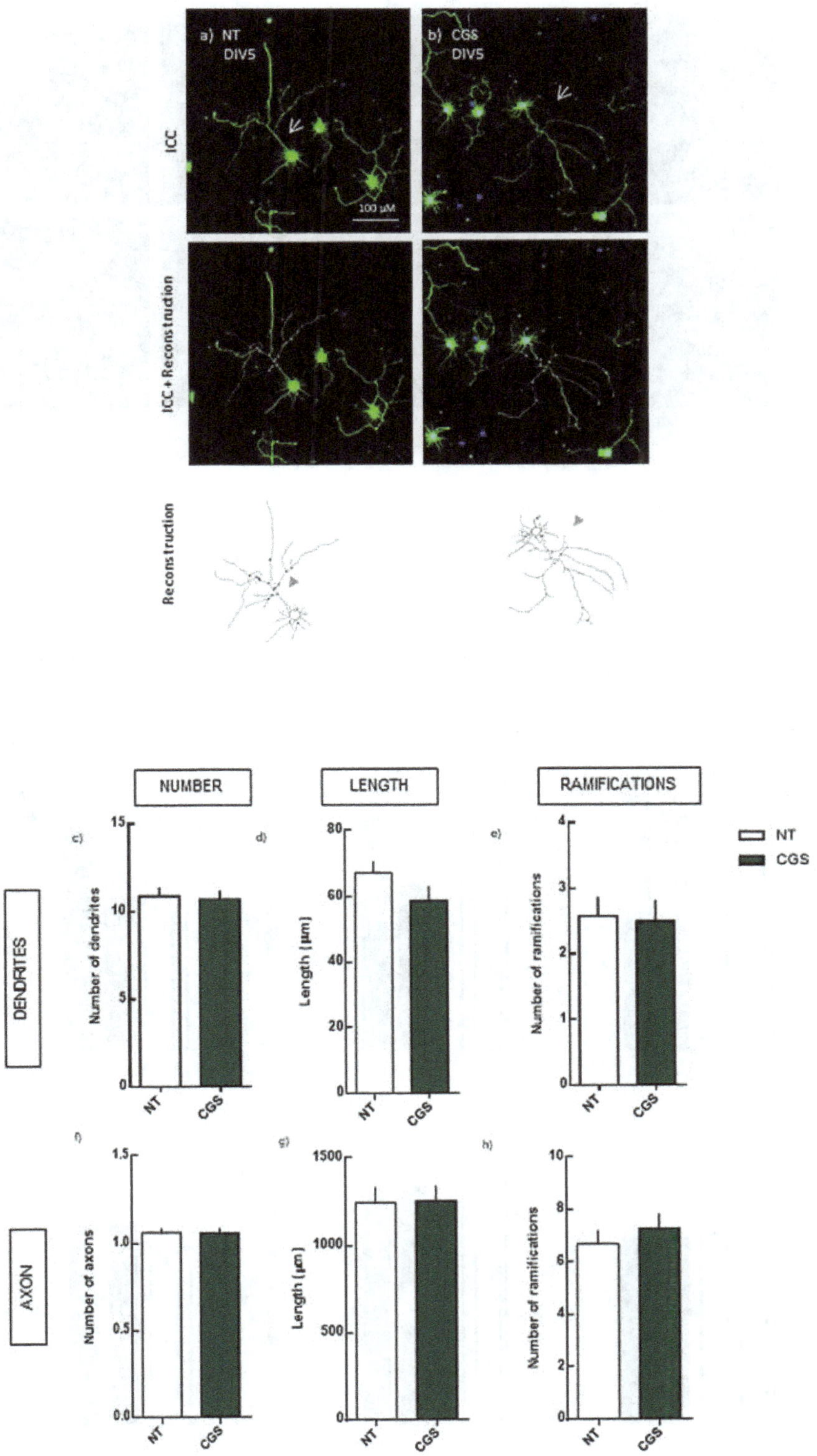

FIGURE 3 | Effect of the selective activation of $A_{2A}R$ (4 days treatment) in hippocampal neurons (DIV5). Hippocampal neurons from ED18 rats were cultured *in vitro* for 5 days (DIV5). Cultured neurons were treated with the $A_{2A}R$ agonist, CGS (30 nM), at 24 h in culture. Neuronal morphology was assessed by manual reconstruction in Neurolucida software **(a,b)** and morphometric data were acquired in Neurolucida Explorer, regarding the number **(c)**, length **(d)**, and number of ramifications **(e)** of dendrites and the number **(f)**, length **(g)**, and number of ramifications **(h)** of axons (identified with an arrow in the representative images). Results are expressed as mean ± SEM of 97–100 cells, from four independent experiments. No statistical significance comparing NT with CGS treatment, assessed by *t*-student test. ICC, immunocytochemistry; NT, non-treated; CGS, CGS21680, $A_{2A}R$ agonist.

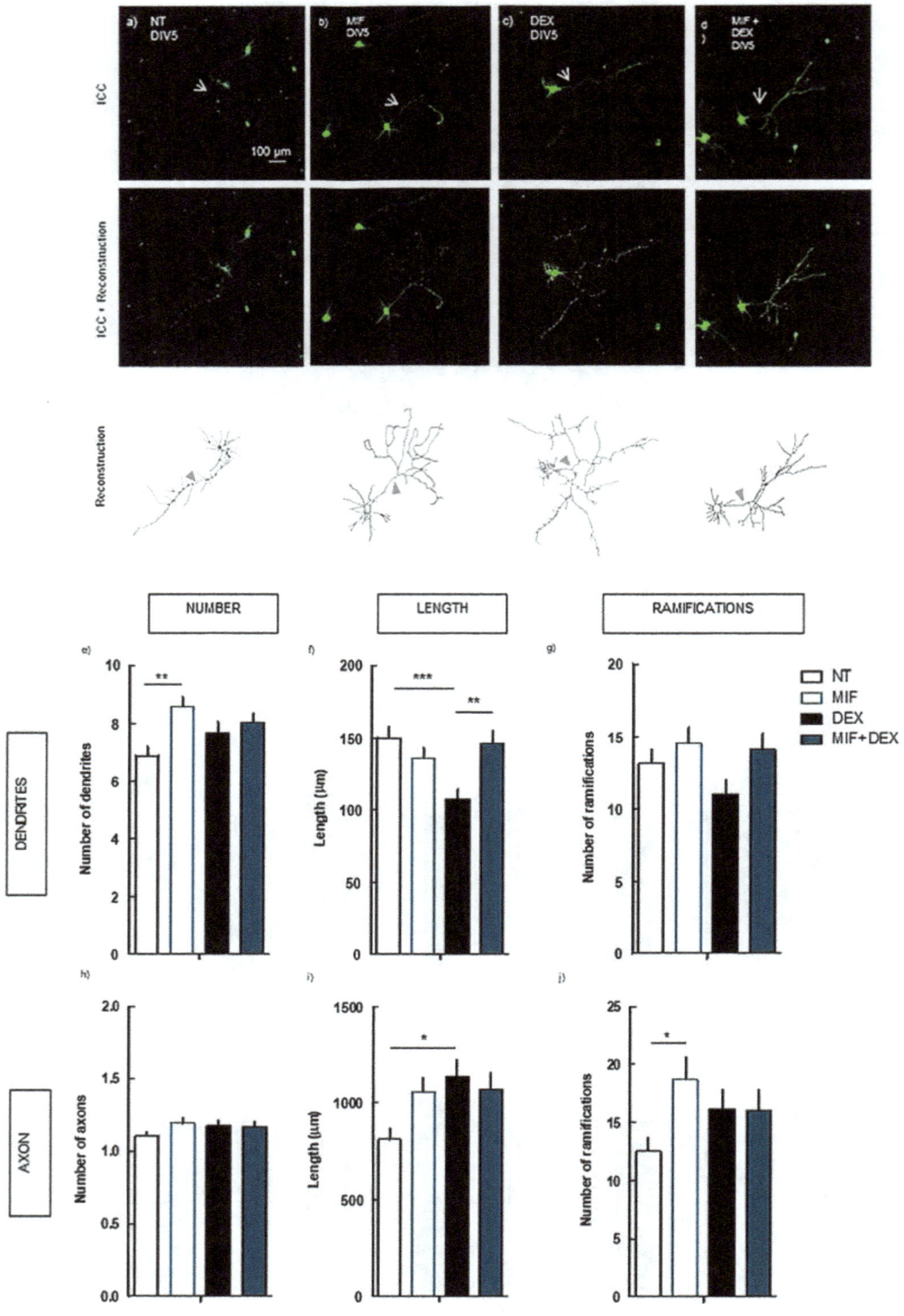

FIGURE 4 | Effect of the blockade of GR *per se* and on DEX exposure (4 days treatment) in hippocampal neurons (DIV5). Hippocampal neurons from ED18 rats were cultured *in vitro* for 5 days (DIV5). Cultured neurons were treated with the GR antagonist, MIF (1 μM), or with the GR antagonist and/or DEX (250 nM; at 24 h in culture). Neuronal morphology was assessed by manual reconstruction in Neurolucida software **(a–d)** and morphometric data were acquired in Neurolucida Explorer, regarding the number **(e)**, length **(f)**, and number of ramifications **(g)** of dendrites and the number **(h)**, length **(i)**, and number of ramifications **(j)** of axons (identified with an arrow in the representative images). Results are expressed as mean ± SEM of 120 cells, from five independent experiments. Statistical significance was assessed by one-way ANOVA followed by Tukey's Multiple Comparison Test: *$p < 0.05$, **$p < 0.01$, ***$p < 0.001$, as indicated by the horizontal lines above the columns. ICC, immunocytochemistry; NT, non-treated; MIF, mifepristone, GR antagonist.; DEX, dexamethasone; MIF+DEX, mifepristone + dexamethasone.

do not oppose our observations, once the differential effect in dendrites and axon may lead to an overall increase in cell area. However, in a different study exploring the effect of high doses of DEX (5 μM) it was observed that DEX exposure for 48 h leads to an overall inhibition of neurite development (Beaujean et al., 2003), contrasting with the present observations that DEX does not induce any effect 24 h after treatment. This discrepancy could be due to the higher concentration of DEX or differences in the susceptibility of the PC12 cell line comparing with cultured hippocampal neurons. In a different cell line, HiB5 cells, it was also observed that the exposure to DEX in a concentration in the same range of the concentration in the present study (10^{-7} M) also inhibits neurite development (Son et al., 2001), which may indicate that cell lines and hippocampal primary neurons may respond differently to DEX exposure.

Overall, there is a lack of understanding regarding the direct effect of DEX in neurons. Over the last two decades, few studies were developed to explore the effects of DEX exposure *in vitro*, which could highly contribute to the dissection of the effects observed at the organism level.

In *in vivo* models, it is interesting to notice that several reports showed dendritic atrophy, resulting from either stress or glucocorticoid exposure in brain regions such as the prefrontal cortex (Brown et al., 2005; Anderson et al., 2016) and the hippocampus (Sousa et al., 1999, 2000; Silva-Gómez et al., 2013). However, alterations in axonal morphology were not yet reported, probably due to the difficulties associated with the analysis of axonal morphology *in vivo* given the higher complexity of this cellular compartment. Nevertheless, alterations in axonal morphology can alter brain connectivity and are implicated in psychiatric disorders. In a genetic model of schizophrenia, it was observed an impair in axonal growth and branching, which leads to cognitive deficits and high incidence of emotional problems (Mukai et al., 2015).

Although the activation of $A_{2A}R$ in the brain is well documented as a modulator of synaptic transmission and plasticity, these receptors are also implicated in neuronal morphologic development *in vivo*. The modulation of $A_{2A}R$ activation was previously reported to impair brain connectivity trough axonal development alterations in a model of *in utero* exposure to an $A_{2A}R$ antagonist. This impairment leads to a delay in axonal migration, which is associated to cognitive deficits in adulthood (Silva et al., 2013). Considering the report that $A_{2A}R$ activation induces axonal elongation *in vitro* by inducing an increase in microtubule dynamics and growth speed (Ribeiro et al., 2016), we speculate that the modulation of DEX axonal effect by $A_{2A}R$ could be due to a similar mechanism.

However, in the present study, the treatment with an $A_{2A}R$ agonist did not alter neuronal morphology, suggesting that the effects of $A_{2A}R$ modulation in hippocampal neurons are different from the ones in cortical neurons, or that the differences in these results are due to the analysis of neuronal morphology in a different time interval in neuronal development, once we analyzed morphology at day 5 in culture whereas in the referred study the analysis of cortical neurons was at day 3. Indeed, it is interesting that although the activation of $A_{2A}R$ is necessary for the effects of DEX in the axon, as seen by the blockade of DEX-effect in the presence of the $A_{2A}R$ antagonist, the activation of $A_{2A}R$ does not alter neuronal morphology. This indicates that DEX-effect is not exclusively mediated by $A_{2A}R$, further supporting the hypothesis of a GR–$A_{2A}R$ crosstalk.

Interestingly, in microglia, we previously described such a putative interaction. It is well documented that $A_{2A}R$ are also important regulators of microglia morphology (Gyoneva et al., 2009, 2014; Orr et al., 2009; Caetano et al., 2016). We described that *in utero* exposure to DEX induces long-term alterations in microglia morphology which correlate with anxiety-like behavior, and that this alterations are recovered by $A_{2A}R$ blockade in a gender-specific manner (Caetano et al., 2016). However, we observed only a partial recovery of microglia morphologic alterations induced by DEX accompanied by a complete recover in behavior might indicate additional targets mediating $A_{2A}R$ blockade effects, namely neurons. This prompted us to understand the direct effects of DEX exposure in neurons, and the therapeutic potential of $A_{2A}R$ blockade.

Although we previously observed a DEX and $A_{2A}R$ gender-specific effect in microglia *in vivo*, in this study, we did not discriminate the sex of the fetuses, due to restrictions in the numbers of animals available to perform neuronal cultures. However, since the neurons suffer a reprogramming upon culture, and are from then on cultured in the same conditions, we do not expect such striking differences in the data obtained.

In what concerns GR–$A_{2A}R$ crosstalk, it was recently described that the blockade of $A_{2A}R$ activation blocks GR translocation to the nucleus, thus impairing GR activation-induced transcriptional alterations (Batalha et al., 2016). Accordingly, the effects of DEX in the axon are blocked by the simultaneous treatment with the $A_{2A}R$ antagonist, suggesting that the axon hypertrophy is dependent on GR transcriptional activity.

However, there is a discrepancy between DEX-effects on dendrites and axons. The dendritic atrophy is independent of the blockade of $A_{2A}R$, which might suggest that the effects on dendrites may be due to GR effects that do not require nuclear translocation and are due to GR non-genomic effects.

On the other hand, the axonal effects were abolished by the blockade of $A_{2A}R$, which disrupts nuclear translocation, indicating that DEX effect on the axon depends on GR genomic action. Although, it is interesting to notice that the DEX effect was not present after 24 h of DEX exposure in either the dendrites or the axon. If the effects in the dendrites are indeed modulated by GR non-genoimc effects, the decrease in dendrites length could potentially be achieved earlier than the increase in the axon, once it would not depend on transcriptional alterations. This point could be clarified by a closer monitoring of the morphological alterations induced by DEX to pinpoint a more accurate moment of the outset of dendritic and axonal alterations.

Additionally, according to this hypothesis, the effect of DEX in the axon should be similarly blocked in the presence of GR antagonist or $A_{2A}R$ antagonist, once both should block the receptor translocation to the nucleus. These results would be explained if the increase of GR nuclear translocation upon activation of $A_{2A}R$ was independent on the presence of GR ligands, as DEX.

It is also possible that the distribution of $A_{2A}R$ is differential in axon and dendrites, leading to a significant effect upon the GR signaling in the axon, but not in the dendrites. It is important to address all these hypotheses to further understand the nature of GR–$A_{2A}R$ interaction and, consequently, the putative pharmacological modulation of $A_{2A}R$ activation.

Furthermore, since the present results indicate that DEX effects on axonal morphology are dependent on the activation of $A_{2A}R$, clarifying the mechanisms underlying these receptors crosstalk can be crucial to understand DEX action on neuronal morphology. As it was previously described, the activation of $A_{2A}R$ in cortical neurons promotes the growth speed of microtubules in the axonal growth cone, leading to axonal elongation (Ribeiro et al., 2016). In future work, it is also important to understand how glucocorticoid exposure modulates neuronal morphology, considering the possibility that the effect of DEX may be as well dependent on microtubule dynamics.

Understanding the mechanistic relation of GR and $A_{2A}R$ and the nature of $A_{2A}R$ morphological modulation in neurons and other cell types is crucial to the further development of $A_{2A}R$ blockade therapies.

The genetic and pharmacological blockade of $A_{2A}R$ was described as anxiolytic in a model of chronic stress in males, both as a preventive and therapeutic tool (Kaster et al., 2015). Additionally, the chronic blockade of $A_{2A}R$ in adulthood is able to revert behavioral, electrophysiological and neuronal morphological alterations induced by maternal separation (Batalha et al., 2013), clearly demonstrating its pharmacological potential in psychiatric pathologies.

However, the response can differ according to gender (Caetano et al., 2016) and it can be prejudicial when administered during development. The blockade of $A_{2A}R$ during development leads to a delay in axonal migration and consequent neuronal excitability, resulting in an increase in the susceptibility to seizures (Silva et al., 2013). Thus, understanding the different pathways induced by $A_{2A}R$ activation in these conditions is essential to further pursue the neuropsychiatric pharmacological advantages of its blockade.

CONCLUSION

Although the use of synthetic GC in clinics is essential due to their beneficial effects in several pathologies, it is important to have a full understanding of their potential deleterious effects, namely in the CNS. The previous described effects of GC exposure in the morphology and physiology of neurons probably underlie the observed neuropsychiatric disturbances. Thus, given the therapeutic potential of $A_{2A}R$ blockade in neuropsychiatric disorders, it is essential to fully comprehend the mechanisms of GR and $A_{2A}R$ interaction, as well as the mechanisms responsible for the modulation of the brain cytoarchitecture by these receptors.

AUTHOR CONTRIBUTIONS

HP designed the experiments with CG, performed the experiments, and wrote the manuscript. RG performed hippocampal neurons primary cultures and immunocytochemistry for the experiment with $A_{2A}R$ agonist treatment. FB assisted in hippocampal neurons primary cultures and revised the manuscript. AA revised the manuscript. CG supervised HP, contributed to the design of the experiments, and revised the manuscript. All authors discussed the results, contributed to and approved the final manuscript.

FUNDING

This work was supported by the Portuguese Foundation for Science and Technology (PEst UID/NEU/04539/2013), COMPETE-FEDER (POCI-01-0145-FEDER-007440), and Centro 2020 Regional Operational Program (CENTRO-01-0145-FEDER-000008: BrainHealth 2020). FB is supported by a fellowship from the Portuguese Foundation for Science and Technology (SFRH/BPD/86830/2012). FB and RG are supported by fellowships from the Portuguese Foundation for Science and Technology (SFRH/BPD/86830/2012 and PD/BD/114116/2015, respectively).

REFERENCES

Anderson, R. M., Glanz, R. M., Johnson, S. B., Miller, M. M., Romig-Martin, S. A., and Radley, J. J. (2016). Prolonged corticosterone exposure induces dendritic spine remodeling and attrition in the rat medial prefrontal cortex. *J. Comp. Neurol.* 524, 3729–3746. doi: 10.1002/cne.24027

Baptista, F. I., Pinto, M. J., Elvas, F., Almeida, R. D., and Ambrósio, A. F. (2013). Diabetes alters KIF1A and KIF5B motor proteins in the hippocampus. *PLoS One* 8:e65515. doi: 10.1371/journal.pone.0065515

Batalha, V. L., Ferreira, D. G., Coelho, J. E., Valadas, J. S., Gomes, R., Temido-Ferreira, M., et al. (2016). The caffeine-binding adenosine A2A receptor induces age-like HPA-axis dysfunction by targeting glucocorticoid receptor function. *Sci. Rep.* 6:31493. doi: 10.1038/srep31493

Batalha, V. L., Pego, J. M., Fontinha, B. M., Costenla, A. R., Valadas, J. S., Baqi, Y., et al. (2013). Adenosine A(2A) receptor blockade reverts hippocampal stress-induced deficits and restores corticosterone circadian oscillation. *Mol. Psychiatry* 18, 320–331. doi: 10.1038/mp.2012.8

Beaujean, D., Rosenbaum, C., Müller, H.-W., Willemsen, J. J., Lenders, J., and Bornstein, S. R. (2003). Combinatorial code of growth factors and neuropeptides define neuroendocrine differentiation in PC12 cells. *Exp. Neurol.* 184, 348–358. doi: 10.1016/j.expneurol.2003.07.007

Brown, S. M., Henning, S., and Wellman, C. L. (2005). Mild, short-term stress alters dendritic morphology in rat medial prefrontal cortex. *Cereb. Cortex* 1991, 1714–1722. doi: 10.1093/cercor/bhi048

Brownfoot, F. C., Crowther, C. A., and Middleton, P. (2008). Different corticosteroids and regimens for accelerating fetal lung maturation for women at risk of preterm birth. *Cochrane Database Syst. Rev.* CD006764. doi: 10.1002/14651858.CD006764.pub2

Caetano, L., Pinheiro, H., Patrício, P., Mateus-Pinheiro, A., Alves, N. D., Coimbra, B., et al. (2016). Adenosine A2A receptor regulation of microglia morphological remodeling-gender bias in physiology and in a model of chronic anxiety. *Mol. Psychiatry* 22, 1035–1043. doi: 10.1038/mp.2016.173

Charles, M.-P., Adamski, D., Kholler, B., Pelletier, L., Berger, F., and Wion, D. (2003). Induction of neurite outgrowth in PC12 cells by the bacterial nucleoside N6-methyldeoxyadenosine is mediated through adenosine A2a receptors and via cAMP and MAPK signaling pathways. *Biochem. Biophys. Res. Commun.* 304, 795–800. doi: 10.1016/S0006-291X(03)00666-1

Cheng, H.-C., Shih, H.-M., and Chern, Y. (2002). Essential role of cAMP-response element-binding protein activation by A2A adenosine receptors in rescuing the nerve growth factor-induced neurite outgrowth impaired by blockage of the MAPK cascade. *J. Biol. Chem.* 277, 33930–33942. doi: 10.1074/jbc.M201206200

Constantinof, A., Moisiadis, V. G., and Matthews, S. G. (2016). Programming of stress pathways: a transgenerational perspective. *J. Steroid Biochem. Mol. Biol.* 160, 175–180. doi: 10.1016/j.jsbmb.2015.10.008

Cunha, R. A., Ferré, S., Vaugeois, J.-M., and Chen, J.-F. (2008). Potential therapeutic interest of adenosine A2A receptors in psychiatric disorders. *Curr. Pharm. Des.* 14, 1512–1524. doi: 10.2174/138161208784480090

Dotti, C. G., Sullivan, C. A., and Banker, G. A. (1988). The establishment of polarity by hippocampal neurons in culture. *J. Neurosci.* 8, 1454–1468.

Fowden, A. L., and Forhead, A. J. (2015). Glucocorticoids as regulatory signals during intrauterine development. *Exp. Physiol.* 100, 1477–1487. doi: 10.1113/EP085212

Gyoneva, S., Orr, A. G., and Traynelis, S. F. (2009). Differential regulation of microglial motility by ATP/ADP and adenosine. *Parkinsonism Relat. Disord.* 15(Suppl. 3), S195–S199. doi: 10.1016/S1353-8020(09)70813-2

Gyoneva, S., Shapiro, L., Lazo, C., Garnier-Amblard, E., Smith, Y., Miller, G. W., et al. (2014). Adenosine A_{2A} receptor antagonism reverses inflammation-induced impairment of microglial process extension in a model of Parkinson's disease. *Neurobiol. Dis.* 67, 191–202. doi: 10.1016/j.nbd.2014.03.004

Huot, R. L., Plotsky, P. M., Lenox, R. H., and McNamara, R. K. (2002). Neonatal maternal separation reduces hippocampal mossy fiber density in adult Long Evans rats. *Brain Res.* 950, 52–63. doi: 10.1016/S0006-8993(02)02985-2

Jameson, R. R., Seidler, F. J., Qiao, D., and Slotkin, T. A. (2006). Adverse neurodevelopmental effects of dexamethasone modeled in PC12 cells: identifying the critical stages and concentration thresholds for the targeting of cell acquisition, differentiation and viability. *Neuropsychopharmacology* 31, 1647–1658. doi: 10.1038/sj.npp.1300967

Juárez-Méndez, S., Carretero, R., Martínez-Tellez, R., Silva-Gómez, A. B., and Flores, G. (2006). Neonatal caffeine administration causes a permanent increase in the dendritic length of prefrontal cortical neurons of rats. *Synapse* 60, 450–455. doi: 10.1002/syn.20318

Kamradt, M. C., Mohideen, N., and Vaughan, A. T. (2000). RU486 increases radiosensitivity and restores apoptosis through modulation of HPV E6/E7 in dexamethasone-treated cervical carcinoma cells. *Gynecol. Oncol.* 77, 177–182. doi: 10.1006/gyno.1999.5724

Kaster, M. P., Machado, N. J., Silva, H. B., Nunes, A., Ardais, A. P., Santana, M., et al. (2015). Caffeine acts through neuronal adenosine A2A receptors to prevent mood and memory dysfunction triggered by chronic stress. *Proc. Natl. Acad. Sci. U.S.A.* 112, 7833–7838. doi: 10.1073/pnas.1423088112

Kimura, M., Moteki, H., and Ogihara, M. (2011). Inhibitory effects of dexamethasone on epidermal growth factor-induced DNA synthesis and proliferation in primary cultures of adult rat hepatocytes. *Biol. Pharm. Bull.* 34, 682–687. doi: 10.1248/bpb.34.682

Kornel, L., Kanamarlapudi, N., Travers, T., Taff, D. J., Patel, N., Chen, C., et al. (1982). Studies on high affinity binding of mineralo- and glucocorticoids in rabbit aorta cytosol. *J. Steroid Biochem.* 16, 245–264. doi: 10.1016/0022-4731(82)90173-X

Leão, P., Sousa, J. C., Oliveira, M., Silva, R., Almeida, O. F. X., and Sousa, N. (2007). Programming effects of antenatal dexamethasone in the developing mesolimbic pathways. *Synapse* 61, 40–49. doi: 10.1002/syn.20341

Mukai, J., Tamura, M., Fénelon, K., Rosen, A. M., Spellman, T. J., Kang, R., et al. (2015). Molecular substrates of altered axonal growth and brain connectivity in a mouse model of schizophrenia. *Neuron* 86, 680–695. doi: 10.1016/j.neuron.2015.04.003

Myers, B., McKlveen, J. M., and Herman, J. P. (2014). Glucocorticoid actions on synapses, circuits, and behavior: implications for the energetics of stress. *Front. Neuroendocrinol.* 35:180–196. doi: 10.1016/j.yfrne.2013.12.003

Nagano, M., Ozawa, H., and Suzuki, H. (2008). Prenatal dexamethasone exposure affects anxiety-like behaviour and neuroendocrine systems in an age-dependent manner. *Neurosci. Res.* 60, 364–371. doi: 10.1016/j.neures.2007.12.005

Noorlander, C. W., Tijsseling, D., Hessel, E. V. S., de Vries, W. B., Derks, J. B., Visser, G. H. A., et al. (2014). Antenatal glucocorticoid treatment affects hippocampal development in mice. *PLoS One* 9:e85671. doi: 10.1371/journal.pone.0085671

Oliveira, M., Bessa, J. M., Mesquita, A., Tavares, H., Carvalho, A., Silva, R., et al. (2006). Induction of a hyperanxious state by antenatal dexamethasone: a case for less detrimental natural corticosteroids. *Biol. Psychiatry* 59, 844–852. doi: 10.1016/j.biopsych.2005.08.020

Oliveira, M., Rodrigues, A.-J., Leão, P., Cardona, D., Pêgo, J. M., and Sousa, N. (2012). The bed nucleus of stria terminalis and the amygdala as targets of antenatal glucocorticoids: implications for fear and anxiety responses. *Psychopharmacology* 220, 443–453. doi: 10.1007/s00213-011-2494-y

Orr, A. G., Orr, A. L., Li, X.-J., Gross, R. E., and Traynelis, S. F. (2009). Adenosine A(2A) receptor mediates microglial process retraction. *Nat. Neurosci.* 12, 872–878. doi: 10.1038/nn.2341

Ribeiro, F. F., Neves-Tomé, R., Assaife-Lopes, N., Santos, T. E., Silva, R. F. M., Brites, D., et al. (2016). Axonal elongation and dendritic branching is enhanced by adenosine A2A receptors activation in cerebral cortical neurons. *Brain Struct. Funct.* 221, 2777–2799. doi: 10.1007/s00429-015-1072-1

Silva, C. G., Métin, C., Fazeli, W., Machado, N. J., Darmopil, S., Launay, P.-S., et al. (2013). Adenosine receptor antagonists including caffeine alter fetal brain development in mice. *Sci. Transl. Med.* 5:197ra104. doi: 10.1126/scitranslmed.3006258

Silva-Gómez, A. B., Aguilar-Salgado, Y., Reyes-Hernández, D. O., and Flores, G. (2013). Dexamethasone induces different morphological changes in the dorsal and ventral hippocampus of rats. *J. Chem. Neuroanat.* 47, 71–78. doi: 10.1016/j.jchemneu.2012.12.004

Son, G. H., Geum, D., Jung, H., and Kim, K. (2001). Glucocorticoid inhibits growth factor-induced differentiation of hippocampal progenitor HiB5 cells. *J. Neurochem.* 79, 1013–1021. doi: 10.1046/j.1471-4159.2001.00634.x

Sousa, N., Lukoyanov, N. V., Madeira, M. D., Almeida, O. F., and Paula-Barbosa, M. M. (2000). Reorganization of the morphology of hippocampal neurites and synapses after stress-induced damage correlates with behavioral improvement. *Neuroscience* 97, 253–266. doi: 10.1016/S0306-4522(00)00050-6

Sousa, N., Paula-Barbosa, M. M., and Almeida, O. F. (1999). Ligand and subfield specificity of corticoid-induced neuronal loss in the rat hippocampal formation. *Neuroscience* 89, 1079–1087. doi: 10.1016/S0306-4522(98)00311-X

Thorburn, G. D., Challis, J. R., and Currie, W. B. (1977). Control of parturition in domestic animals. *Biol. Reprod.* 16, 18–27. doi: 10.1095/biolreprod16.1.18

Zocchi, C., Ongini, E., Conti, A., Monopoli, A., Negretti, A., Baraldi, P. G., et al. (1996). The non-xanthine heterocyclic compound SCH 58261 is a new potent and selective A2a adenosine receptor antagonist. *J. Pharmacol. Exp. Ther.* 276, 398–404.

7

Caffeine and Selective Adenosine Receptor Antagonists as New Therapeutic Tools for the Motivational Symptoms of Depression

Laura López-Cruz[1†], John D. Salamone[2] and Mercè Correa[1,2]*

[1] *Àrea de Psicobiologia, Universitat Jaume I, Castellón de la Plana, Spain,* [2] *Behavioral Neuroscience Division, University of Connecticut, Storrs, CT, United States*

Correspondence:
Mercè Correa
correa@uji.es

†Present address:
Laura López-Cruz,
Department of Psychology and MRC/Wellcome Trust Behavioural and Clinical Neuroscience Institute, University of Cambridge, Cambridge, United Kingdom

Major depressive disorder is one of the most common and debilitating psychiatric disorders. Some of the motivational symptoms of depression, such anergia (lack of self-reported energy) and fatigue are relatively resistant to traditional treatments such as serotonin uptake inhibitors. Thus, new pharmacological targets are being investigated. Epidemiological data suggest that caffeine consumption can have an impact on aspects of depressive symptomatology. Caffeine is a non-selective adenosine antagonist for A_1/A_{2A} receptors, and has been demonstrated to modulate behavior in classical animal models of depression. Moreover, selective adenosine receptor antagonists are being assessed for their antidepressant effects in animal studies. This review focuses on how caffeine and selective adenosine antagonists can improve different aspects of depression in humans, as well as in animal models. The effects on motivational symptoms of depression such as anergia, fatigue, and psychomotor slowing receive particular attention. Thus, the ability of adenosine receptor antagonists to reverse the anergia induced by dopamine antagonism or depletion is of special interest. In conclusion, although further studies are needed, it appears that caffeine and selective adenosine receptor antagonists could be therapeutic agents for the treatment of motivational dysfunction in depression.

Keywords: adenosine receptors, dopamine, caffeine, antidepressants, anergia, fatigue, anxiety

MAJOR DEPRESSION DISORDER: SYMPTOMATOLOGY AND CURRENT TREATMENT

Major depression disorder (MDD) is one of the most debilitating disorders in the world, and the most commonly diagnosed according to the World Health Organization. The Diagnostic and Statistical Manual in its last edition (DMS-5) defines this disorder as a set of symptoms including: depressed mood, decreased interest or pleasure in almost all activities nearly every day, appetite changes (changes in body weight), sleep disturbances, feelings of worthlessness or guilt, diminished ability to concentrate or indecisiveness, psychomotor agitation or retardation and fatigue or loss of energy (American Psychiatric Association, 2013).

Although depression is typically defined as an affective disorder, it also appears that some symptoms such as psychomotor retardation, fatigue, and loss of energy are related to deficits in motivation, specifically in activational aspects of motivation. Motivated behavior is directed toward or away from particular stimuli, but it also is characterized by a high degree of activity, effort, vigor, and persistence (Salamone and Correa, 2002, 2012). People with depression commonly show profound activational impairments, such as lassitude, listlessness, fatigue, and anergia (low self-reported energy) that affect their motivation (Tylee et al., 1999; Stahl, 2002). In fact, among depressed people, energy loss and fatigue are the second most commonly reported symptoms, only behind depressed mood itself (Tylee et al., 1999), and depressed patients with anergia are more common than patients with anxiety related symptoms (Tylee et al., 1999; Drysdale et al., 2017). Furthermore, in depressed patients "lack of energy" was the factor that correlated to problems with fatigability, inability to work, and psychomotor retardation, loading most strongly onto a second order general depression factor (Gullion and Rush, 1998). Many people with MDD have fundamental deficits in reward seeking, exertion of effort, and effort-related decision making that do not simply depend upon any problems that they may have with experiencing pleasure (Treadway et al., 2009). Lack of energy is the symptom most highly correlated with a lack of social function in depressed patients, and is correlated with various work-related impairments such as days in bed, days of lost work, and low work productivity (Swindle et al., 2001). In addition, this cluster of symptoms can be highly resistant to treatment (Stahl, 2002); they are the best predictors of lack of remission after antidepressant drug treatment (Stahl, 2002; Gorwood et al., 2014).

PHARMACOLOGICAL TREATMENTS FOR THE ACTIVATIONAL SYMPTOMS IN DEPRESSION

The severity of effort-related motivational symptoms in depression is related to problems with social function, employment absence, and treatment outcomes (Tylee et al., 1999; Stahl, 2002). Patients with high scores in psychomotor retardation also have longer duration of illness, an earlier age of onset, and more depressive episodes (Calugi et al., 2011; Gorwood et al., 2014). These symptoms are a predictor of delayed response to treatment with either interpersonal psychotherapy or selective serotonin (5-HT) reuptake inhibitor pharmacotherapy (Frank et al., 2011), often remaining as residual symptoms even in patients in remission (Stahl, 2002; Fava et al., 2014; Gorwood et al., 2014).

Most of the present treatment strategies for MDD focus on drugs that block the inactivation (i.e., inhibitors of enzymatic breakdown or uptake) of the monoamine neurotransmitters 5-HT and norepinephrine (NE). The classical antidepressants include monoamine oxidase inhibitors (MAOIs), which affect one of the major catabolic enzymes for monoamines (Quitkin et al., 1979), and drugs that inhibit uptake of one or more monoamines (Feighner, 1999; Yıldız et al., 2002). Although 5-HT and NE reuptake inhibitors have become the most frequently prescribed medications for MDD, they fail to complete symptom remission in 40–60% of all patients (Rush and Trivedi, 1995; Fava et al., 2014), and it is widely accepted that at least 20% of all depressed patients do not respond adequately to most antidepressant drugs (Crown et al., 2002). Many common antidepressants, including 5-HT transport inhibitors such as fluoxetine, are relatively ineffective at treating anergia and fatigue, and in fact, can induce or exacerbate these symptoms (Padala et al., 2012; Stenman and Lilja, 2013; Fava et al., 2014).

Interestingly, some clinical studies suggest that drugs that inhibit dopamine (DA) transport, such as the catecholamine uptake inhibitor bupropion, are relatively more effective than 5-HT uptake inhibitors for treating effort-related motivational symptoms (Rampello et al., 1991; Stahl, 2002; Demyttenaere et al., 2005; Pae et al., 2007). Furthermore, individual differences in behavioral traits can differentiate between depressed patients that are more responsive to bupropion (i.e., motivated, achievement-oriented, active, exercise-oriented people) vs. fluoxetine (people with mood problems, irritability, and rumination) (Bell et al., 2013). Stimulant drugs that are not considered to be antidepressants in the classical sense, such as methylphenidate and modafinil, have been shown to increase energy and motivation in depressed patients (Zisook et al., 2006). Thus, clinical studies, together with preclinical investigations (e.g., Salamone et al., 2006, 2007; Salamone and Correa, 2012; Argyropoulos and Nutt, 2013; Heath et al., 2015), have led to the suggestion that DA systems and related circuits are particularly involved in effort-related motivational symptoms.

ADENOSINE RECEPTORS CO-LOCALIZATION WITH DA RECEPTORS

In addition, another possible therapeutic target for the anergia component of depression is adenosine receptors. Adenosine is a neuromodulator in the central nervous system (CNS) that plays an important role in the regulation of synaptic transmission and neuronal excitability (Cunha, 2001; Sebastião and Ribeiro, 2009). Several subtypes of adenosine receptors are expressed in the brain, with A_1 and A_{2A} G-protein-coupled receptors being the most abundant (Jacobson and Gao, 2006; Fredholm et al., 2011). A_{2A} receptors are expressed at high levels in the striatum and olfactory bulbs and tubercle (Fredholm et al., 2011), but also in areas such as amygdala, hippocampus or prefrontal cortex (Cunha et al., 1994; Pandolfo et al., 2013; Simões et al., 2016). Adenosine A_1 receptors have a higher widespread distribution in the brain, with a somewhat higher concentration in hippocampus (Schwarzschild et al., 2006). All these regions are involved in the regulation of complex processes such as cognition, motivation, and emotion (Hauber and Sommer, 2009; Salamone and Correa, 2012) that seem to be altered in MDD.

The spatial distribution of adenosine receptors within the brain (Fredholm et al., 2011) allows a wide range of effects, including modulation of other neurotransmitter systems (Cunha, 2001). Thus, adenosine A_{2A} receptors are highly expressed postsynaptically in DA rich areas such as neostriatum and accumbens (Acb) (Johansson and Fredholm, 1995; Johansson et al., 1997; DeMet and Chicz-DeMet, 2002; Rebola et al., 2005). In fact, it has been demonstrated that in these areas, there is a functional interaction between DA D_2 and adenosine A_{2A} receptors (see **Figure 1**), which are co-localized on enkephalin-containing medium spiny neurons and converge onto the same signal transduction pathways in an antagonistic way (Ferré et al., 1997, 2008; Fuxe et al., 2003; Ferré, 2008; Beggiato et al., 2014). Similarly, A_1 and D_1 receptors antagonistically interact on substance P-containing medium spiny neurons (Ferré et al., 1997, 2008).

The behavioral significance of this interaction has frequently been studied in the context of neostriatal motor functions and pathologies (Ferré et al., 1997; Correa et al., 2004; Collins et al., 2010). Thus, selective A_{2A} receptor antagonists are being tested in clinical trials for pathologies involving DAergic dysfunctions such as Parkinson disease, and positive results indicate that they can be used as adjuvant therapies (Hung and Schwarzschild, 2014). Caffeine actions on A_1 and A_{2A} adenosine receptors (Ferré, 2008), has promoted its study as an alternative preventive or therapeutic tool for parkinsonian symptoms (Prediger, 2010). Moreover, within the last years, the motivational significance of DA-adenosine receptor interactions has become apparent with regard to processes such as behavioral activation, and effort-related decision-making impaired in depression or other pathologies (Salamone et al., 2006; Salamone and Correa, 2009).

In the present review, we focus on studies that assessed the effect of adenosine antagonists on different aspects of depression in humans, as well as in animal models. Special emphasis will be placed on motivational/psychomotor symptoms induced by DA depletions and studies related to DA-adenosine interactions in pathological symptoms related to effort-related decision-making.

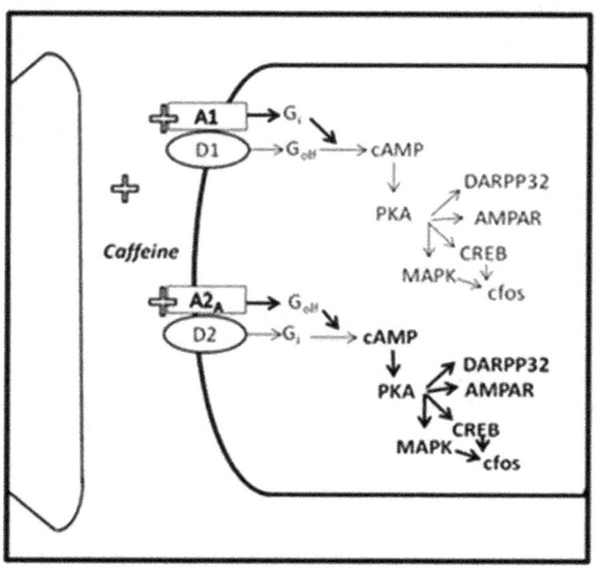

FIGURE 1 | Impact of caffeine on the functional interaction between adenosine and DA receptors. A_1R and $A_{2A}R$, adenosine A_1 and A_{2A} receptors; D_1, DA type 1 receptor; D_2, DA type 2 receptor (adapted from Ferré, 2008).

CAFFEINE CONSUMPTION AND DEPRESSION

Caffeine is a naturally occurring methylxanthine that acts mainly as a non-selective A_1 and A_{2A} adenosine receptor antagonist (Fredholm et al., 1999). This methylxanthine is found in common beverages including coffee, tea, soft drinks, and products containing cocoa, as well as a variety of medications and dietary sources (Barone and Roberts, 1996; Wikoff et al., 2017), ranking as one of the most commonly consumed dietary ingredients throughout the world (Heckman et al., 2010). Daily intake of caffeine among consumers in United States is about 280 mg, and higher intakes are estimated in some European countries (Barone and Roberts, 1996). Caffeine is typically consumed in order to increase alertness, arousal and energy (Malinauskas et al., 2007). Its consumption has been related to changes in cognitive performance and mood in normal population (Smith, 2013; Pasman et al., 2017). However, it enhances performance more in fatigued than well-rested subjects (Lorist et al., 1994; Childs and de Wit, 2008).

There are very few studies on the relation between caffeine consumption and depression-related symptoms, and in many cases, its use is related to self-medication patterns. Some of these studies focus on the role of caffeine as a drug that prevents depression, while others discuss caffeine as a possible treatment for existing depression. Thus, secondary analyses of large epidemiological databases with similar number of men and women indicate that in non-clinical samples that do not work, consumption of caffeine (around 150 mg/day as average) was associated with a reduced risk of depression (Smith, 2009). Also, in a longitudinal study in women free from depressive symptoms at baseline, high levels of caffeine consumption (>550 mg/day) was negatively correlated with the appearance of depressive symptoms (Lucas et al., 2011). In fact, the relative risk for depression was highest for those women with lower caffeine consumption (<100 mg/day) (Lucas et al., 2011). However, in women with multiple sclerosis high doses of caffeine (>400 mg/day) increased the prevalence of MDD (Patten et al., 2000). Moreover, in non-clinical samples, although caffeine consumption at moderate doses was related with decreases in suicide risk (Kawachi et al., 1996; Tanskanen et al., 2000; Lucas et al., 2014), excessive consumption (750 mg/day) was correlated with a higher risk of suicide (Kawachi et al., 1996; Tanskanen, 1997; Lucas et al., 2014). Thus, from the present studies, it seems that intermediate levels of caffeine consumption (300–550 mg/day) produce beneficial effects in non-clinical populations, but not in people with some neurological pathologies. Higher doses will have negative effects, even in non-clinical populations.

Multiple reports have lent support to the idea that depressed people could use caffeine as self-medication. It has been reported that psychiatric patients show a relatively high degree of caffeine consumption compared to the normal population (Greden et al., 1978; Leibenluft et al., 1993; Rihs et al., 1996). This appears to be particularly true in patients that have experienced depressive symptoms (Leibenluft et al., 1993). Different profiles of patients (i.e., with alcohol dependence, seasonal affective disorder, and people with MDD) have been shown to have higher levels of caffeine consumption after experiencing depressive symptoms (as shown by the Hamilton Rating Scale for depression) (Hamilton, 1967; Leibenluft et al., 1993). Specially, among youth with depression, there generally is higher caffeine consumption that in the general population (Whalen et al., 2008). Moreover, the degree of caffeine consumption seems to be a predictor of improvement of somatic symptoms (fatigue among them), and hostility in depressed patients medicated with fluoxetine (Worthington et al., 1996), suggesting that caffeine could be an effective co-treatment for some of the symptoms of depression. However, it is important to note that, at high doses or in people with susceptibility, caffeine is also known to increase anxiety and insomnia (for a review Temple et al., 2017), two side effects that can contribute to worsen MDD. At high doses, however, it has been demonstrated that caffeine may not act as an adenosine receptor antagonist, and other underlying mechanisms seem responsible of its negative effects (for a recent review Fredholm et al., 2017).

IMPACT OF CAFFEINE ON ENERGY/FATIGABILITY AND BEHAVIORAL ACTIVATION IN HUMANS

A wide range of studies demonstrate that caffeine can increase alertness and subjective energy, and also reduce fatigue (Johnson et al., 1990b, 1991; Yu et al., 1991; Smith et al., 1992, 1997; Lieberman, 2001), thus acting as an ergogenic substance. Caffeine has been demonstrated to increase feelings of efficiency, self-confidence, motivation to work (Fredholm et al., 1999), and to improve psychomotor performance (Rees et al., 1999). The behavioral effects of caffeine can be influenced by the baseline arousal levels and also by the nature of the task requirements. It has been argued that the most evident effects of caffeine on fatigue would be expected in situations of low arousal or high fatigue, or in tasks placing high demands on controlled processing (Bachrach, 1966; Lieberman et al., 1987). In fact, beneficial effects of caffeine have been observed in people in low states of alertness, such as after benzodiazepines administration (Johnson et al., 1990b), sleep loss (Childs and de Wit, 2008; Paech et al., 2016), when the person has a cold (Smith et al., 1997), or when the experiment is done in the early morning (Smith et al., 1992). In addition, a broad range of studies have reported effects of caffeine withdrawal on different markers of motivation using descriptors such as fatigue, decreased energy or vigor, lethargy, amotivation for work, etc. (for a review see Juliano and Griffiths, 2004). For example, in controlled studies, after 10 days of high levels of caffeine consumption (1,250 mg/day), withdrawal results in increased subjective ratings of headache, sleepiness, laziness, and fatigue, as well as decreased alertness, activation and vigor (Juliano et al., 2012). Abstinence from intermediate doses in daily coffee and cola consumers (579 mg/day), increased ratings of drowsy/sleepy, fatigue/tired, lazy/sluggy/slow-moving, decreased ratings of active/energetic/excited and motivation to work, and impaired performance on psychomotor tasks (Liguori and Hughes, 1997). Even at low quantities (100 mg/day, in a controlled study), caffeine withdrawal increased ratings of lethargy, fatigue, tiredness, and sluggishness, and decreased ratings of energy, motivation and urge to work (Griffiths et al., 1990).

EFFECT OF CAFFEINE AND ADENOSINE ANTAGONISTS ON CLASSIC ANIMAL MODELS OF DEPRESSION

Preclinical studies have been trying to elucidate the effect of caffeine and selective adenosine antagonists on classical animal models of depression (El Yacoubi et al., 2001). Two of the classic tests for the assessment of antidepressant properties of different substances in rodents are the forced swim test (FST) and the tail suspension test (TST). In the FST animals develop an immobile posture in an inescapable cylinder filled with water (Porsolt et al., 1977; Petit-Demouliere et al., 2005). The TST is based on the observation that a mouse suspended by the tail shows alternating periods of agitation and immobility (Steru et al., 1985). Classical antidepressants reduce immobility time in these paradigms, which have become the gold standard to evaluate antidepressant effects of multiple drugs or to show depressive symptoms induced by behavioral manipulations (Armario and Nadal, 2013). In this regard, learned helplessness has been considered as one of the causes for developing depression in vulnerable individuals that suffer stressful life events. This phenomenon is reproducible in animal models in which the depressive-like state is induced either by chronic uncontrollable and unpredictable stressors (CUS), typically electrical foot-shock (Overmier and Seligman, 1967), but also by chronic mild stress (CMS) induced by irregular exposure to a combination of different types of stressors over a period of weeks (Willner, 2005). In addition, animals that develop learned helplessness show a disruption in escape performance as well as decreases in weight gain, increased immobility in the FST or TST, and reduced locomotion, all symptoms associated to some degree with depression (Seligman, 1972). After the administration of substances with antidepressant properties, animals exposed to CUS or CMS display escape-directed behaviors, reducing time of immobility (Porsolt et al., 1977; Steru et al., 1985).

All these tests and manipulations have been used to study the therapeutic properties of caffeine and selective adenosine antagonists or genetic deletion of adenosine receptors in rodents. In one of the seminal papers, Porsolt et al. (1977) demonstrated that an acute dose of caffeine reduced immobility time in the FST in Sprague-Dawley rats. In later studies, this effect has been confirmed using other strains of rats and mice, after acute or repeated administration of a broad range of doses (3.0–30.0 mg/kg) and using diverse animal tests (FST, TST) (Kulkarni and Mehta, 1985; Kaster et al., 2004, 2015; Robles-Molina et al., 2012; Kale and Addepalli, 2014; Minor and Hanff, 2015; Szopa et al., 2016). In accordance with the effects of caffeine, adenosine A_{2A} receptor antagonists have also been effective in these tests. Thus, SCH58261 and istradefylline (KW6002) reduced total immobility time in both the TST and the FST in mice (El Yacoubi et al., 2001). SCH58261 also reduced immobility time in a selectively bred 'helpless' mice strain in the TST (El Yacoubi et al., 2001). Moreover, A_{2A} receptor knockout (A_{2A}KO) mice showed reductions in immobility time compared to wild type (WT) animals in both tests (El Yacoubi et al., 2001).

Using the learned helplessness model for inducing depressive symptoms, it has been demonstrated that acute doses as well as chronic administration of caffeine can reduce the impact of CUS (Woodson et al., 1998; Hunter et al., 2003; Minor et al., 2008; Pechlivanova et al., 2012; Kaster et al., 2015). Thus, pharmacological or genetic blockade of A_{2A} receptors not only prevented but also reversed CUS-induced behavioral and physiological signs of depression such as decreased weight gain, increased corticosterone levels, escape behavior impairments in a shuttle box, increased immobility time in the FST and TST, increased anxiety, and decreased locomotion and spatial reference memory (Kaster et al., 2015). However, caffeine only reverted the deficits of reference memory but did not reverse mood-related alterations (Machado et al., 2017) in mice genetically selected to display 'depressive'-like symptoms (El Yacoubi et al., 2003). Consistent with these findings, mice that received the selective A_{2A} receptor antagonist istradefylline, as well as the constitutive A_{2A}KO mice, were protected from the CUS-induced behavioral impairments in the FST, TST, and memory tests (Kaster et al., 2004), suggesting a key role for A_{2A} receptors in acute and chronic stress-induced depressive effects.

Based on these results some researchers have focused on adenosine receptor antagonists, including caffeine, as tools to reverse behavioral impairments induced by pharmacological manipulations of the adenosine system (Kulkarni and Mehta, 1985; Minor et al., 1994a, 2008; Woodson et al., 1998; Hunter et al., 2003; Pechlivanova et al., 2012). Thus, high doses of acutely administered adenosine (50.0–100.0 mg/kg, intraperitoneally IP) (Kulkarni and Mehta, 1985), or its analoge 1-chloroadenosine (2.0 mg/kg, IP) induce immobility in the FST in mice, and caffeine as well as theophylline (8.0 mg/kg, IP), reversed this effect (Kulkarni and Mehta, 1985). Theophylline, is a psychoactive methylxanthine found in tea and other substances, and is also a metabolite of caffeine that acts as a non-selective adenosine antagonist for A_1/A_{2A} receptors as well (Gu et al., 1992). Increases of adenosine in the central nervous system have been also associated with escape deficits in the inescapable shock paradigm (Kulkarni and Mehta, 1985; Minor et al., 1994b; Woodson et al., 1998; Minor and Hanff, 2015). Thus, it has been demonstrated that intraventricular (ICV) administration of NBTI [S-(4-nitrobenzyl)-6-theoinosine], an equilibrative nucleoside transporter (ENT) blocker that increases extracellular adenosine levels blocking its reuptake (see **Figure 2**), impaired escape latency in rats (Jacobson et al., 1992; Noji et al., 2004) at the same level that rats preexposed to 100 inescapable tail shocks, and potentiates escape impairments produced by 50 inescapable tail shocks (Minor et al., 2008). Moreover, ICV administration of erytrho-9(2-hydroxy/3/nonyl adenine (ENHA), a selective adenosine deaminase (ADA) inhibitor which blocks adenosine metabolism, mimicked the effect of inescapable shock (Woodson et al., 1998). This manipulation increases the concentration of extracellular adenosine by blocking the major degradation pathway. Low doses of caffeine reversed escape deficits induced by EHNA (Woodson et al., 1998). The reversal effects of caffeine appear to be specific to actions on adenosine receptors, and not as a general stimulant psychomotor effect, since amphetamine exacerbated the behavioral impairments induced by inescapable shocks (Minor et al., 1994a). In addition, caffeine reversed the escape deficit produced by a bilateral injection of glutamate into the prefrontal cortex of rats (Hunter et al., 2003). This escape deficit induced by glutamate in the prefrontal cortex has been also associated with enhanced adenosine (Petty et al., 1985), since increases in glutamate are counterbalanced by an increase in adenosine production and release (Deckert and Gleiter, 1994; Kerkhofs et al., 2018).

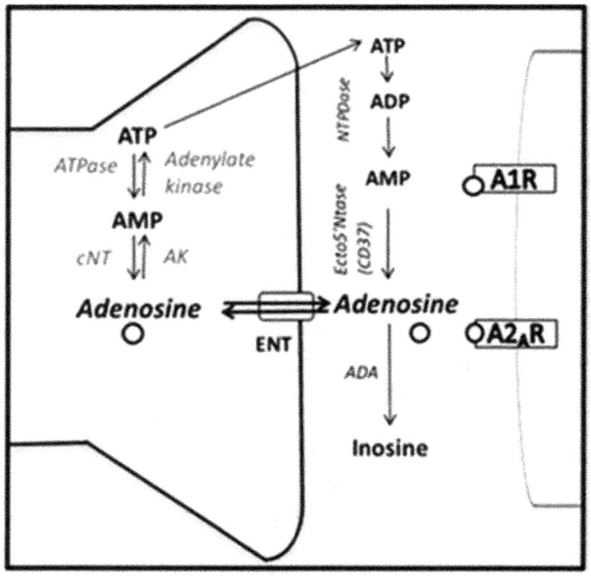

FIGURE 2 | Adenosine synthesis and metabolism. ADA, adenosine deaminase; AK, adenosine kinase; A_1R and A_{2A}R, adenosine A_1 and A_{2A} receptors; cNT, cytosolic endo-nucleotidase; ENT, equilibrative nucleoside transporter; Ecto5′Ntase (CD73), 5′-ectonucleotidase; NTPDase, nucleoside triphosphate dephosphorylase (adapted from Ruby et al., 2011).

Caffeine has also been used to enhance the effect of monoaminergic antidepressants (especially 5-HT/NE uptake inhibitors) that are being used in clinical practice, and have been demonstrated to reduce immobility in classical animal tests of depression. Thus, caffeine at low doses that do not have an effect on their own can potentiate the effects of desipramine, imipramine, duloxetine, fluoxetine and paroxetine, in animals tested on the FST (Robles-Molina et al., 2012; Kale and Addepalli, 2014; Szopa et al., 2016). In addition, a low dose of caffeine can also improve the effect of bupropion (a DA/NE uptake inhibitor), potentiating extracellular levels of DA and NE (Kale and Addepalli, 2014).

IMPACT OF ADENOSINE ANTAGONISTS ON BEHAVIORAL ACTIVATION: PRECLINICAL STUDIES

Tasks measuring behavioral activation and effort-based functions have been suggested as potential animal models for the motivational symptoms of depression (Salamone, 2007; Markou et al., 2013; Salamone et al., 2016). Thus in the animal literature, as in the human data, there are studies showing how caffeine and selective adenosine antagonists affect the willingness to work depending on the demands of the task. In operant tasks with different work demands, caffeine and theophylline produced rate-dependent effects on lever pressing to obtain palatable food in rats (Randall et al., 2011). Moderate doses of caffeine and theophylline (5.0–20.0 mg/kg) increased responding on the low task with low response demands; a fixed interval 240 s (FI-240 s) schedule. However, higher doses (10–40 mg/kg) decreased responding on a fixed ratio 20 (FR20), schedule that typically generates high rates of responding (Randall et al., 2011). A_{2A} receptor antagonists increased lever pressing in the low effort-demanding task (FI-240 s) but did not suppress the high effort task (FR20) in the dose range tested. In fact, there was a tendency for istradefylline to increase FR20 responding at a moderate dose. A_1 antagonists failed to increase lever-pressing rate, but decreased FR20 responding at higher doses. These results suggest that the work potentiating effects of methylxanthines are mediated by their actions on adenosine A_{2A} receptors, while their A_1 receptor antagonistic action could be mediating the suppressant effects.

Progressive ratio (PR) schedules, which require gradually increasing work output, have been also employed to explore the effect of caffeine on motivation to work for sucrose or food in rats and monkeys (Buffalo et al., 1993; Brianna Sheppard et al., 2012; Retzbach et al., 2014). Acutely and chronically moderate doses of caffeine (5–25 mg/kg) elevated PR lever pressing for sucrose (Brianna Sheppard et al., 2012; Retzbach et al., 2014). Caffeine had no effect on inactive lever presses suggesting that this increase was not due to an increase in general motor activity (Retzbach et al., 2014). Recently, our laboratory has demonstrated that caffeine has differential effects on PR performance depending on baseline individual differences (SanMiguel et al., 2018). Caffeine (5.0–10.0 mg/kg) increased responding for a solution containing sucrose in low baseline responders, but decreased lever pressing (10.0–20.0 mg/kg) in high responders (SanMiguel et al., 2018). However, in rhesus monkeys intravenous (IV) caffeine (10.0 mg/kg) decreased percent of task completed, and breakpoint in a PR for palatable food (Buffalo et al., 1993), possibly because this dose directly administered in the blood stream resulted in higher levels in the brain.

Thus, from studies in rats and monkeys it seems that high doses of caffeine have an impairing effect on performance in tasks that evaluate willingness to work for a reinforcer if performance is already high. Methylxanthines can help to increase work output when the requirement of the task is low. However, selective A_{2A} receptor antagonists seem to be beneficial independently of the baseline performance, as demonstrated also in goals directed tasks (Li et al., 2016).

EFFORT BASED DECISION-MAKING DEFICITS INDUCED BY INTERFERENCE WITH DA FUNCTION: POTENTIAL THERAPEUTIC ROLE OF ADENOSINE ANTAGONISTS

Activational aspects of motivation (i.e., vigor, persistence, work output) are highly adaptative because they enable organisms to overcome obstacles or work-related response costs that separate them from significant stimuli (Salamone and Correa, 2002, 2012; van den Bos et al., 2006). An important feature of adaptive behavior, in the face of work-related challenges, is effort-related decision making. Regularly, organisms must make cost/benefit analyses in which they weigh the value of a stimulus relative to the cost of obtaining it (Salamone et al., 2007, 2016). People with MDD show impairments in estimation, anticipation, and recall of reinforcing stimuli (Pizzagalli, 2014), and also show a reduced likelihood of selecting high effort activities in human tasks of effort-related decision making (Treadway et al., 2012; Yang et al., 2014).

Extensive animal data have demonstrated that Acb DA is a key mediator of effort-based decision-making processes (for a review see Salamone et al., 2016). Interference with DA transmission biases behavior toward less valued rewards that involve less effort and less activity. In these preclinical studies addressing the effort-related decision-making process, animals are given a choice between a more valued reinforcer that can only be obtained by engaging in a more demanding (higher effort) activity vs. a low effort/low value option. One such procedure is a T-maze task that provides an effort-related challenge by having a vertical barrier in the arm with the higher reward density (HD) vs. an arm that contains a lower density of reward (LD) and has no barrier (Salamone et al., 1994; Cousins and Salamone, 1996; Cousins et al., 1996; Mott et al., 2009; Pardo et al., 2012). In this procedure, rodents choose to climb the barrier to get more reward in 90% of the trials, once they have been trained (Cousins and Salamone, 1996; Pardo et al., 2012). In operant tasks animals are given a choice between lever pressing for the more preferred reward (in FR5 or PR schedules) vs. approaching and consuming a less preferred reinforcer that is concurrently freely available in the chamber (Salamone et al., 1991; Randall et al., 2012; Pardo et al., 2015). When tested on the concurrent FR5/free reward choice task, rats typically spend most time pressing the lever for the preferred reward and less consuming freely available food or fluids (Salamone et al., 1991; Pardo et al., 2015). In contrast, rats tested on the PR/chow choice task show more individual variability, and tend to disengage more readily from the PR lever pressing component because of the increasing work requirement (Randall et al., 2012, 2014). Research with these concurrent choice tasks has shown that interference with DA transmission via DA depletions or DA receptor antagonism typically biases rodents toward the low effort-low reward option (Salamone et al., 1991; Salamone and Correa, 2009; Worden et al., 2009; Pardo et al., 2012; Randall et al., 2012, 2014; Yohn et al., 2015).

Using these effort related choice procedures, it has been demonstrated that the catecholamine depleting agent and vesicular transport inhibitor (VMAT-2) tetrabenazine (TBZ), reduces selection of high effort alternatives, but animals compensate by increasing the amount of free less preferred reinforcer consumed (Nunes et al., 2013; Randall et al., 2014; Pardo et al., 2015; Yohn et al., 2015, 2017). TBZ depletes monoamines, with its greatest impact being upon striatal DA (Pettibone et al., 1984; Tanra et al., 1995; Nunes et al., 2013). TBZ is used as a therapeutic drug to treat Huntington's disease patients, and it induces symptoms of depression in humans, including fatigue (Frank, 2010; Guay, 2010; Rodrigues et al., 2017). TBZ has also been used in the FST and TST rodent models of depression (Kent et al., 1986; Wang et al., 2010). Although the effort-related effects of TBZ are attenuated by the DA uptake blocker bupropion (Nunes et al., 2013; Randall et al., 2014; Yohn et al., 2015) which is been used as an antidepressant, other classical drugs for the treatment of depression such as the 5-HT uptake inhibitors fluoxetine and citalopram, and the NE uptake inhibitor desipramine, failed to reverse the effects of TBZ, and higher doses even led to further behavioral impairments (Yohn et al., 2015, 2016b,c).

In addition to DA, adenosine also is involved in these effort related decision-making processes (Farrar et al., 2007, 2010; Hauber and Sommer, 2009; Mott et al., 2009; Salamone and Correa, 2009). Microinjections of adenosine A_{2A} receptor agonists into the Acb produced effects on instrumental behavior and effort-related choice that resembled those produced by Acb DA receptor antagonism or depletion (Font et al., 2008; Mingote et al., 2008). In addition, considerable evidence indicates that DA D_2 and adenosine A_{2A} receptors interact to regulate effort-related functions (Salamone and Correa, 2009, 2012). Thus, adenosine A_{2A} receptor antagonists were able to reverse the shift in choice toward a low effort alternative induced by administration of the D_2 antagonists haloperidol and eticlopride (Farrar et al., 2007, 2010; Mott et al., 2009; Salamone et al., 2009; Worden et al., 2009; Pardo et al., 2012, 2013). Moreover, A_{2A} KO mice were resistant to the effects of haloperidol on performance of the T-maze barrier task (Pardo et al., 2012). Recently, it has been demonstrated that A_{2A} KO mice are also resistant to the anergia inducing effects of D_2 antagonism in a paradigm in which animals can choose between exercising on a much preferred running wheel or sedentary consuming sweet food (Correa et al., 2016). In contrast, adenosine A_1 antagonists were ineffective at reversing the effort-related effects of either the D_1 receptor antagonist ecopipam or the D_2 receptor antagonist eticlopride (Salamone and Correa, 2009; Nunes et al., 2010; Pardo et al., 2012).

The therapeutic effect of caffeine and theophylline on effort-related choice behavior after the administration of D_2 antagonists has also been reported in rats tested on the concurrent FR5/chow feeding choice task. Caffeine partially attenuated the effects of haloperidol, increasing the lever pressing and decreasing the free chow intake in haloperidol-treated rats (Salamone et al., 2009) and the same pattern of results were observed in a more recent study in which caffeine reversed the anergia-like effect induced by TBZ in an adapted version of the T-maze task with RW (Correa et al., 2016) increasing the time running (effortful option) and decreasing the time spent eating free available sweet pellets (sedentary option) (López-Cruz et al., 2018). This behavioral effect was supported by changes in an intracellular marker of DA neurotransmission [phosphorylated form of DARPP-32; pDARPP-32(Thr34)] in the striatum (López-Cruz et al., 2018). Similarly, theophylline reversed the effects induced by this D_2 antagonist in mice tested in the T-maze barrier task (Pardo et al., 2012). Furthermore, several papers have reported that the adenosine A_{2A} receptor antagonist MSX-3 can reverse the effort-related effects of TBZ across multiple tasks (Nunes et al., 2013; Randall et al., 2014; Yohn et al., 2015). All these findings suggest that the reversal effects induced by methylxanthines on anergia induced by DA D_1 and D_2 receptor antagonism could be mediated mainly by A_{2A} receptors.

Mental fatigue associated with high attentional demands can also be overcome by the use of psychostimulants such as amphetamine or caffeine (Silber et al., 2006; Peeling and Dawson, 2007). For instance, caffeine restores memory performance in sleep-deprived or aged humans, a finding replicated in rodent animal models (Cunha and Agostinho, 2010). In cost/benefit decision-making tasks involving the evaluation of the costs related to high attention-demands, rats can choose between engaging in hard trials (difficult visuospatial discrimination) leading to more reward versus easy trials leading to less reward (Cocker et al., 2012). Under basal conditions, animals chose high effort/high reward trials more than low-effort/low reward trials. However, there are substantial baseline differences. Amphetamine increases the selection of high effort/high reward trials in animals that usually do not choose this option, but it decreases the selection of the high cognitive demand trials in animals that usually choose them. A high dose of caffeine decreased choice of high effort/high reward trials in animals that usually choose them as did amphetamine, but it did not increase the selection in the ones that usually did not choose them (Cocker et al., 2012).

A_{2A} RECEPTOR ANTAGONISTS HAVE THERAPEUTIC ACTIONS ON CYTOKINE-INDUCED FATIGUE

Cytokines are signaling molecules for the immune system mediating physiological responses to infection (Dantzer, 2001). These molecules also mediate a set of behavioral signs that include depressed activity and loss of interest or motivation (Kent et al., 1992). Compared to the general population, depressed patients have elevated levels of proinflammatory cytokines such as tumor necrosis factor alpha (TN-alpha) interleukin-1β (IL-1β), and IL-6 (Dowlati et al., 2010; Hiles et al., 2012). Fatigue, loss of energy and psychomotor slowing are reported to occurred in patients receiving treatment with IFN-α or with high levels of IL-6 (Miller et al., 2009; Goldsmith et al., 2016b). Moreover, many inflammatory stimuli have been found to target reductions in ventral striatal neural function, and decreased synthesis of striatal DA, which is possibly related to symptoms of reduced motivation and motor retardation (Felger and Treadway, 2017). Studies with IL-6 indicate that this cytokine is responsive to stress, and is implicated in the production of depression-like effects in mice, including actions on traditional tests such as the FST, TST, and social interaction tests (Sukoff Rizzo et al., 2012). In anergia related studies, IL-6 and IL-1β reduced the tendency to work for food when an alternative food source (concurrently available chow) could be obtained through minimal effort (Nunes et al., 2014; Yohn et al., 2016a).

Brain cytokine signaling involves adenosine signaling at adenosine A_{2A} receptors (Hanff et al., 2010). These receptors regulate IL-1β and LPS linked to pathological behavioral and physiological responses such as anxiety (Chiu et al., 2014) or neuroinflammation (Brothers et al., 2010; Simões et al., 2012). Adenosine A_{2A} receptor signaling provides inhibitory feedback on proinflammatory cytokine signaling in peripheral immune cells (Sitkovsky and Ohta, 2005). Thus, the effects of IL-6 and IL-1β were attenuated through co-administration of the adenosine A_{2A} receptor antagonist MSX-3, as well as the major stimulant methylphenidate, which blocks catecholamine uptake (Nunes et al., 2014; Yohn et al., 2016c). Though previous work has shown that MSX-3 had no effect of FR5/chow-feeding choice performance when administered on its own (Farrar et al., 2007), MSX-3 produced a very robust reversal of the behavioral effects of IL-6 and IL-1β, restoring the baseline behavioral pattern of responding (i.e., increasing lever pressing and decreasing chow consumption) to a normal level (Nunes et al., 2014; Yohn et al., 2016c). These results highlight the therapeutic potential of adenosine A_{2A} receptor antagonism for pathologies related to neuroinflammation (Simões et al., 2012; Cunha, 2016).

ANERGIA AND FATIGUE INFLUENCE DECISION-MAKING IN HUMANS WITH DEPRESSION

Translational studies in humans have implemented tasks that evaluate the decision-making process in normal as well as psychiatric patients. The effort expenditure for rewards task (EEfRT; Treadway et al., 2009), is based on the operant lever pressing choice tasks described above (Salamone et al., 1991). In the human version of this task, subjects choose on each trial between a high cost/high reward option (HC/HR) and low cost/low reward option (LC/LR) to obtain different monetary rewards. The HC/HR trials required 100 button presses with the non-dominant pinky finger within 21 s, and subjects were eligible to win higher amounts that varied per trial between $1.24–4.30. In contrast, the LC/LR option only required 30 button presses with the dominant index finger during 7 s, and subjects could win $1.00 for each successfully completed trial.

Patients with MDD were significantly less likely to make HC/HR choices relative to controls, and this result was not related with depression-related differences in psychomotor speed (Treadway et al., 2012). The effect of caffeine on this task in depressed patients has not been explored, but it was assessed in normal subjects. Thus, in the normal population, caffeine (200 mg), significantly increased the speed of responses compared to placebo (Wardle et al., 2012). However, caffeine did not have an effect on percentage of HC/HR choices (Wardle et al., 2012). In fact, it decreased effortful choices in high cardiovascular responders (subjects with high arterial pressure in response to caffeine) (Wardle et al., 2012). These results contrast with studies showing that, during exercise, caffeine decreases the perception of effort in humans (Doherty and Smith, 2005), improving performance particularly for endurance testing (Doherty and Smith, 2004). Thus, caffeine may only improve performance in highly demanding situations.

CONCLUSION AND FURTHER DIRECTIONS

Although many available treatments for MDD provide relief for individuals with depressed mood, no single therapeutic modality provides a full and permanent recovery across all the symptoms of MDD in the majority of patients (McClintock et al., 2011). Clinicians have come to emphasize the importance of taking into account effort-related motivational symptoms in depression (Tylee et al., 1999; Stahl, 2002; Demyttenaere et al., 2005; Salamone et al., 2016). Decreased psychomotor speed, referred to clinically as psychomotor retardation, fatigue and anergia are cardinal symptoms of MDD that have been associated with poor antidepressant treatment response (Goldsmith et al., 2016a). Even among patients in remission, anergia and psychomotor retardation are pervasive symptoms (Gorwood et al., 2014). Thus, novel pharmacological targets are being investigated in clinical and preclinical studies.

There are promising results shown in epidemiological studies as well as in animal models, about the impact of caffeine and selective adenosine receptor antagonists on these symptoms. Is worth noting that the epidemiological studies have revealed a relation between caffeine consumption and decreased risk for developing depression (Lucas et al., 2011), and some reports demonstrate the use of caffeine as a self-medication among depressed patients (Leibenluft et al., 1993). However, it seems clear that more controlled studies are needed to explore the effect of caffeine across a wide variety of depressive symptoms, and it seems necessary to test more selective drugs for A_{2A} receptors.

Systematic studies of the effects of methylxanthines on animal models of depression and anergia have shown efficacy at improving parameters related with initiation and maintenance of behavior in order to escape an aversive situation, but also in order to pursue valued reinforcers and achieve goals (Kulkarni and Mehta, 1985; Woodson et al., 1998; Hunter et al., 2003; Minor et al., 2008; Randall et al., 2011; Pechlivanova et al., 2012). As with the human data, these therapeutic actions depend upon the dose administered, since high doses of caffeine and theophylline not only do not improve depressive symptoms, but can in fact promote anxiety (Correa and Font, 2008; López-Cruz et al., 2014). Moreover, it is important to take into consideration that the use of high doses of caffeine and other methylxanthiness, specially, among the elder, could also have severe side effects such as tachycardia, gastric discomfort, or insomnia (Frozi et al., 2018). All these side effects could in fact worse the symptoms of MDD. Both in humans and in animal studies, the therapeutic actions of methylxanthines also seem to be dependent on the basal estate; for instance they seem to be effective when subjects are in a state or fatigue, tiredness or sleepiness (Johnson et al., 1990a; Smith et al., 1992; Childs and de Wit, 2008), or when the DArgic system is compromised. Such effects are less evident when humans and rodents are under "normal" conditions.

Several A_{2A} selective receptor antagonists have also shown to reverse motivational impairments induced by DA antagonism or depletion in animal models of anergia (Farrar et al., 2007; Mott et al., 2009; Salamone et al., 2009; Pardo et al., 2012; Correa et al., 2016). Furthermore, a recent report indicates that istradefylline can improve fatigue-related symptoms in Parkinson's disease patients (Abe et al., 2016; Sako et al., 2017). Adenosine A_{2A} receptors might be involved in these processes through their interaction with DA D_2 receptors in the Acb, region highly involved in the activational component of motivation (for a review see Salamone and Correa, 2012).

Consistent with these findings, it has been demonstrated that the rank order of clinical effectiveness in depressed patients with psychomotor retardation, paralleled the specificity of antidepressants as DA-mimetic agents (Rampello et al., 1991). Antidepressants such as bupropion have demonstrated to have therapeutical effects on motivational symptoms in humans (Pae et al., 2007) and in animal models or anergia (Nunes et al., 2013; Randall et al., 2014; Yohn et al., 2015). In animal studies, caffeine was shown to improve the effects of antidepressants such as bupropion, duloxetine, and desipramine (Robles-Molina et al., 2012; Kale and Addepalli, 2014; Kale and Addepalli, 2015; Szopa et al., 2016). These studies have led to the suggestion that caffeine could be used as an enhancer of antidepressant pharmacotherapy (for a review see Kale et al., 2010), a suggestion that is consistent with the clinical trials for antiparkinsonian effects showing that A_{2A} receptor antagonists can be a good adjuvant in the treatment of motor symptoms (Hung and Schwarzschild, 2014).

However, determination of the predominant symptomatology is key to therapeutic success. Recent neuroimage data from patients with depression indicate that they can be clustered based on four different connectivity profiles ('biotypes') that are associated with differences in clinical symptoms (Drysdale et al., 2017). Thus, reduced connectivity in anterior cingulate and orbitofrontal areas supporting motivation was most severe in biotypes 1 and 2, which were characterized partly by increased anergia and fatigue (Drysdale et al., 2017). This type of objective diagnostic can help to identify different type of patients that could benefit from different type of antidepressant therapies. For instance, in patients affected by anxious depression a selective inhibitor of 5-HT reuptake appears to be more effective than a selective inhibitor of DA reuptake (Rampello et al., 1995), and caffeine in those type of depressed patients may worsen the anxiety symptomatology. However, adenosine A_{2A} receptor antagonism may offer an alternative therapeutic strategy for treating effort-related motivational dysfunctions in humans, probably with lower abuse liability and fewer major stimulant motor effects compared to DA uptake inhibitors.

AUTHOR CONTRIBUTIONS

All authors listed have made a substantial, direct and intellectual contribution to the work, and approved it for publication.

FUNDING

This research was supported by a grant from MEC (PSI2015-68497-R), ME- FPU (AP2010-3793) Spain, and from NIH/NIMH (R03MH094966-01A1), United States.

REFERENCES

Abe, K., Fujita, M., and Yoshikawa, H. (2016). Effectiveness of istradefylline for fatigue and quality of life in Parkinson's disease patients' and of their caregivers. *APD* 5, 24–28. doi: 10.4236/apd.2016.52004

American Psychiatric Association (2013). *Diagnostic and Statistical Manual of Mental Disorders*, 5th Edn. Washington, DC: American Psychiatric Association. doi: 10.1176/appi.books.9780890425596

Argyropoulos, S. V., and Nutt, D. J. (2013). Anhedonia revisited: is there a role for dopamine-targeting drugs for depression? *J. Psychopharmacol.* 27, 869–877. doi: 10.1177/0269881113494104

Armario, A., and Nadal, R. (2013). Individual differences and the characterization of animal models of psychopathology: a strong challenge and a good opportunity. *Front. Pharmacol.* 4:137. doi: 10.3389/fphar.2013.00137

Bachrach, H. (1966). Note on the psychological effects of caffeine. *Psychol. Rep.* 18:86. doi: 10.2466/pr0.1966.18.1.86

Barone, J. J., and Roberts, H. R. (1996). Caffeine consumption. *Food Chem. Toxicol.* 34, 119–129. doi: 10.1016/0278-6915(95)00093-3

Beggiato, S., Antonelli, T., Tomasini, M. C., Borelli, A. C., Agnati, L. F., Tanganelli, S., et al. (2014). Adenosine A2A-D2 receptor-receptor interactions in putative heteromers in the regulation of the striato-pallidal gaba pathway: possible relevance for Parkinson's disease and its treatment. *Curr. Protein Pept. Sci.* 15, 673–680. doi: 10.2174/1389203715666140901103205

Bell, D. S., Shipman, W. M., Cleves, M. A., and Siegelman, J. (2013). Which drug for which patient? Is there a fluoxetine responding versus a bupropion responding personality profile? *Clin. Pract. Epidemiol. Ment. Health* 9, 142–147. doi: 10.2174/1745017901309010142

Brianna Sheppard, A., Gross, S. C., Pavelka, S. A., Hall, M. J., and Palmatier, M. I. (2012). Caffeine increases the motivation to obtain non-drug reinforcers in rats. *Drug Alcohol Depend.* 124, 216–222. doi: 10.1016/j.drugalcdep.2012.01.008

Brothers, H. M., Marchalant, Y., and Wenk, G. L. (2010). Caffeine attenuates lipopolysaccharide-induced neuroinflammation. *Neurosci. Lett.* 480, 97–100. doi: 10.1016/j.neulet.2010.06.013

Buffalo, E. A., Gillam, M. P., Allen, R. R., and Paule, M. G. (1993). Acute effects of caffeine on several operant behaviors in rhesus monkeys. *Pharmacol. Biochem. Behav.* 46, 733–737. doi: 10.1016/0091-3057(93)90570-J

Calugi, S., Cassano, G. B., Litta, A., Rucci, P., Benvenuti, A., Miniati, M., et al. (2011). Does psychomotor retardation define a clinically relevant phenotype of unipolar depression? *J. Affect. Disord.* 129, 296–300. doi: 10.1016/j.jad.2010.08.004

Childs, E., and de Wit, H. (2008). Enhanced mood and psychomotor performance by a caffeine-containing energy capsule in fatigued individuals. *Exp. Clin. Psychopharmacol.* 16, 13–21. doi: 10.1037/1064-1297.16.1.13

Chiu, G. S., Darmody, P. T., Walsh, J. P., Moon, M. L., Kwakwa, K. A., Bray, J. K., et al. (2014). Adenosine through the A_{2A} adenosine receptor increases

IL-1β in the brain contributing to anxiety. *Brain Behav. Immun.* 41, 218–231. doi: 10.1016/j.bbi.2014.05.018

Cocker, P. J., Hosking, J. G., Benoit, J., and Winstanley, C. A. (2012). Sensitivity to cognitive effort mediates psychostimulant effects on a novel rodent cost/benefit decision-making task. *Neuropsychopharmacology* 37, 1825–1837. doi: 10.1038/npp.2012.30

Collins, L. E., Galtieri, D. J., Collins, P., Jones, S. K., Port, R. G., Paul, N. E., et al. (2010). Interactions between adenosine and dopamine receptor antagonists with different selectivity profiles: effects on locomotor activity. *Behav. Brain Res.* 211, 148–155. doi: 10.1016/j.bbr.2010.03.003

Correa, M., and Font, L. (2008). Is there a major role for adenosine A_{2A} receptors in anxiety? *Front. Biosci.* 13, 4058–4070.

Correa, M., Pardo, M., Bayarri, P., López-Cruz, L., San Miguel, N., Valverde, O., et al. (2016). Choosing voluntary exercise over sucrose consumption depends upon dopamine transmission: effects of haloperidol in wild type and adenosine A2AKO mice. *Psychopharmacology* 233, 393–404. doi: 10.1007/s00213-015-4127-3

Correa, M., Wisniecki, A., Betz, A., Dobson, D. R., O'Neill, M. F., O'Neill, M. J., et al. (2004). The adenosine A_{2A} antagonist KF17837 reverses the locomotor suppression and tremulous jaw movements induced by haloperidol in rats: possible relevance to parkinsonism. *Behav. Brain Res.* 148, 47–54. doi: 10.1016/S0166-4328(03)00178-5

Cousins, M. S., Atherton, A., Turner, L., and Salamone, J. D. (1996). Nucleus accumbens dopamine depletions alter relative response allocation in a T-maze cost/benefit task. *Behav. Brain Res.* 74, 189–197. doi: 10.1016/0166-4328(95)00151-4

Cousins, M. S., and Salamone, J. D. (1996). Skilled motor deficits in rats induced by ventrolateral striatal dopamine depletions: behavioral and pharmacological characterization. *Brain Res.* 732, 186–194. doi: 10.1016/0006-8993(96)00519-7

Crown, W. H., Finkelstein, S., Berndt, E. R., Ling, D., Poret, A. W., Rush, A. J., et al. (2002). The impact of treatment-resistant depression on health care utilization and costs. *J. Clin. Psychiatry* 63, 963–971. doi: 10.4088/JCP.v63n1102

Cunha, R. A. (2001). Adenosine as a neuromodulator and as a homeostatic regulator in the nervous system: different roles, different sources and different receptors. *Neurochem. Int.* 38, 107–125. doi: 10.1016/S0197-0186(00)00034-6

Cunha, R. A. (2016). How does adenosine control neuronal dysfunction and neurodegeneration? *J. Neurochem.* 139, 1019–1055. doi: 10.1111/jnc.13724

Cunha, R. A., and Agostinho, P. M. (2010). Chronic caffeine consumption prevents memory disturbance in different animal models of memory decline. *J. Alzheimers Dis.* 20(Suppl. 1), S95–S116. doi: 10.3233/JAD-2010-1408

Cunha, R. A., Johansson, B., van der Ploeg, I., Sebastião, A. M., Ribeiro, J. A., and Fredholm, B. B. (1994). Evidence for functionally important adenosine A_{2a} receptors in the rat hippocampus. *Brain Res.* 649, 208–216. doi: 10.1016/0006-8993(94)91066-9

Dantzer, R. (2001). Cytokine-induced sickness behavior: mechanisms and implications. *Ann. N. Y. Acad. Sci.* 933, 222–234. doi: 10.1111/j.1749-6632.2001.tb05827.x

Deckert, J., and Gleiter, C. H. (1994). Adenosine–an endogenous neuroprotective metabolite and neuromodulator. *J. Neural Transm. Suppl.* 43, 23–31.

DeMet, E. M., and Chicz-DeMet, A. (2002). Localization of adenosine A_{2A}-receptors in rat brain with [3H]ZM-241385. *Naunyn Schmiedebergs Arch. Pharmacol.* 366, 478–481. doi: 10.1007/s00210-002-0613-3

Demyttenaere, K., De Fruyt, J., and Stahl, S. M. (2005). The many faces of fatigue in major depressive disorder. *Int. J. Neuropsychopharmacol.* 8, 93–105. doi: 10.1017/S1461145704004729

Doherty, M., and Smith, P. M. (2004). Effects of caffeine ingestion on exercise testing: a meta-analysis. *Int. J. Sport Nutr. Exerc. Metab.* 14, 626–646. doi: 10.1123/ijsnem.14.6.626

Doherty, M., and Smith, P. M. (2005). Effects of caffeine ingestion on rating of perceived exertion during and after exercise: a meta-analysis. *Scand. J. Med. Sci. Sports* 15, 69–78. doi: 10.1111/j.1600-0838.2005.00445.x

Dowlati, Y., Herrmann, N., Swardfager, W., Liu, H., Sham, L., Reim, E. K., et al. (2010). A meta-analysis of cytokines in major depression. *Biol. Psychiatry* 67, 446–457. doi: 10.1016/j.biopsych.2009.09.033

Drysdale, A. T., Grosenick, L., Downar, J., Dunlop, K., Mansouri, F., Meng, Y., et al. (2017). Resting-state connectivity biomarkers define neurophysiological subtypes of depression. *Nat. Med.* 23, 28–38. doi: 10.1038/nm.4246

El Yacoubi, M., Bouali, S., Popa, D., Naudon, L., Leroux-Nicollet, I., Hamon, M., et al. (2003). Behavioral, neurochemical, and electrophysiological characterization of a genetic mouse model of depression. *Proc. Natl. Acad. Sci. U.S.A.* 100, 6227–6232. doi: 10.1073/pnas.1034823100

El Yacoubi, M., Ledent, C., Parmentier, M., Bertorelli, R., Ongini, E., Costentin, J., et al. (2001). Adenosine A_{2A} receptor antagonists are potential antidepressants: evidence based on pharmacology and A_{2A} receptor knockout mice. *Br. J. Pharmacol.* 134, 68–77. doi: 10.1038/sj.bjp.0704240

Farrar, A. M., Pereira, M., Velasco, F., Hockemeyer, J., Müller, C. E., and Salamone, J. D. (2007). Adenosine A_{2A} receptor antagonism reverses the effects of dopamine receptor antagonism on instrumental output and effort-related choice in the rat: implications for studies of psychomotor slowing. *Psychopharmacology* 191, 579–586. doi: 10.1007/s00213-006-0554-5

Farrar, A. M., Segovia, K. N., Randall, P. A., Nunes, E. J., Collins, L. E., Stopper, C. M., et al. (2010). Nucleus accumbens and effort-related functions: behavioral and neural markers of the interactions between adenosine A_{2A} and dopamine D_2 receptors. *Neuroscience* 166, 1056–1067. doi: 10.1016/j.neuroscience.2009.12.056

Fava, M., Ball, S., Nelson, J. C., Sparks, J., Konechnik, T., Classi, P., et al. (2014). Clinical relevance of fatigue as a residual symptom in major depressive disorder. *Depress. Anxiety* 31, 250–257. doi: 10.1002/da.22199

Feighner, J. P. (1999). Mechanism of action of antidepressant medications. *J. Clin. Psychiatry* 60(Suppl. 4), 4–11; discussion 12.

Felger, J. C., and Treadway, M. T. (2017). Inflammation effects on motivation and motor activity: role of dopamine. *Neuropsychopharmacology* 42, 216–241. doi: 10.1038/npp.2016.143

Ferré, S. (2008). An update on the mechanisms of the psychostimulant effects of caffeine. *J. Neurochem.* 105, 1067–1079. doi: 10.1111/j.1471-4159.2007.05196.x

Ferré, S., Fredholm, B. B., Morelli, M., Popoli, P., and Fuxe, K. (1997). Adenosine-dopamine receptor-receptor interactions as an integrative mechanism in the basal ganglia. *Trends Neurosci.* 20, 482–487. doi: 10.1016/S0166-2236(97)01096-5

Ferré, S., Quiroz, C., Woods, A. S., Cunha, R., Popoli, P., Ciruela, F., et al. (2008). An update on adenosine A_{2A}-dopamine D_2 receptor interactions: implications for the function of G protein-coupled receptors. *Curr. Pharm. Des.* 14, 1468–1474. doi: 10.2174/138161208784480108

Font, L., Mingote, S., Farrar, A. M., Pereira, M., Worden, L., Stopper, C., et al. (2008). Intra-accumbens injections of the adenosine A_{2A} agonist CGS 21680 affect effort-related choice behavior in rats. *Psychopharmacology* 199, 515–526. doi: 10.1007/s00213-008-1174-z

Frank, E., Cassano, G. B., Rucci, P., Thompson, W. K., Kraemer, H. C., Fagiolini, A., et al. (2011). Predictors and moderators of time to remission of major depression with interpersonal psychotherapy and SSRI pharmacotherapy. *Psychol. Med.* 41, 151–162. doi: 10.1017/S0033291710000553

Frank, S. (2010). Tetrabenazine: the first approved drug for the treatment of chorea in US patients with Huntington disease. *Neuropsychiatr. Dis. Treat.* 6, 657–665. doi: 10.2147/NDT.S6430

Fredholm, B. B., Bättig, K., Holmén, J., Nehlig, A., and Zvartau, E. E. (1999). Actions of caffeine in the brain with special reference to factors that contribute to its widespread use. *Pharmacol. Rev.* 51, 83–133.

Fredholm, B. B., Jzerman, A. P., Jacobson, K. A., Linden, J., and Müller, C. E. (2011). International union of basic and clinical pharmacology. LXXXI. Nomenclature and classification of adenosine receptors–an update. *Pharmacol. Rev.* 63, 1–34. doi: 10.1124/pr.110.003285

Fredholm, B. B., Yang, J., and Wang, Y. (2017). Low, but not high, dose caffeine is a readily available probe for adenosine actions. *Mol. Aspects Med.* 55, 20–25. doi: 10.1016/j.mam.2016.11.011

Frozi, J., de Carvalho, H. W., Ottoni, G. L., Cunha, R. A., and Lara, D. R. (2018). Distinct sensitivity to caffeine-induced insomnia related to age. *J. Psychopharmacol.* 32, 89–95. doi: 10.1177/0269881117722997

Fuxe, K., Agnati, L. F., Jacobsen, K., Hillion, J., Canals, M., Torvinen, M., et al. (2003). Receptor heteromerization in adenosine A_{2A} receptor signaling: relevance for striatal function and Parkinson's disease. *Neurology* 61, S19–S23. doi: 10.1212/01.WNL.0000095206.44418.5C

Goldsmith, D. R., Haroon, E., Woolwine, B. J., Jung, M. Y., Wommack, E. C., Harvey, P. D., et al. (2016a). Inflammatory markers are associated with decreased psychomotor speed in patients with major depressive disorder. *Brain Behav. Immun.* 56, 281–288. doi: 10.1016/j.bbi.2016.03.025

Goldsmith, D. R., Rapaport, M. H., and Miller, B. J. (2016b). A meta-analysis of blood cytokine network alterations in psychiatric patients: comparisons between schizophrenia, bipolar disorder and depression. *Mol. Psychiatry* 21, 1696–1709. doi: 10.1038/mp.2016.3

Gorwood, P., Richard-Devantoy, S., Baylé, F., and Cléry-Melin, M. L. (2014). Psychomotor retardation is a scar of past depressive episodes, revealed by simple cognitive tests. *Eur. Neuropsychopharmacol.* 24, 1630–1640. doi: 10.1016/j.euroneuro.2014.07.013

Greden, J. F., Fontaine, P., Lubetsky, M., and Chamberlin, K. (1978). Anxiety and depression associated with caffeinism among psychiatric inpatients. *Am. J. Psychiatry* 135, 963–966. doi: 10.1176/ajp.135.8.963

Griffiths, R. R., Evans, S. M., Heishman, S. J., Preston, K. L., Sannerud, C. A., Wolf, B., et al. (1990). Low-dose caffeine physical dependence in humans. *J. Pharmacol. Exp. Ther.* 255, 1123–1132.

Gu, L., Gonzalez, F. J., Kalow, W., and Tang, B. K. (1992). Biotransformation of caffeine, paraxanthine, theobromine and theophylline by cDNA-expressed human CYP1A2 and CYP2E1. *Pharmacogenetics* 2, 73–77. doi: 10.1097/00008571-199204000-00004

Guay, D. R. (2010). Tetrabenazine, a monoamine-depleting drug used in the treatment of hyperkinetic movement disorders. *Am. J. Geriatr. Pharmacother.* 8, 331–373. doi: 10.1016/j.amjopharm.2010.08.006

Gullion, C. M., and Rush, A. J. (1998). Toward a generalizable model of symptoms in major depressive disorder. *Biol. Psychiatry* 44, 959–972. doi: 10.1016/S0006-3223(98)00235-2

Hamilton, M. (1967). Development of a rating scale for primary depressive illness. *Br. J. Soc. Clin. Psychol.* 6, 278–296. doi: 10.1111/j.2044-8260.1967.tb00530.x

Hanff, T. C., Furst, S. J., and Minor, T. R. (2010). Biochemical and anatomical substrates of depression and sickness behavior. *Isr. J. Psychiatry Relat. Sci.* 47, 64–71.

Hauber, W., and Sommer, S. (2009). Prefrontostriatal circuitry regulates effort-related decision making. *Cereb. Cortex* 19, 2240–2247. doi: 10.1093/cercor/bhn241

Heath, C. J., Bussey, T. J., and Saksida, L. M. (2015). Motivational assessment of mice using the touchscreen operant testing system: effects of dopaminergic drugs. *Psychopharmacology* 232, 4043–4057. doi: 10.1007/s00213-015-4009-8

Heckman, M. A., Weil, J., and Gonzalez de Mejia, E. (2010). Caffeine (1, 3, 7-trimethylxanthine) in foods: a comprehensive review on consumption, functionality, safety, and regulatory matters. *J. Food Sci.* 75, R77–R87. doi: 10.1111/j.1750-3841.2010.01561.x

Hiles, S. A., Baker, A. L., de Malmanche, T., and Attia, J. (2012). A meta-analysis of differences in IL-6 and IL-10 between people with and without depression: exploring the causes of heterogeneity. *Brain Behav. Immun.* 26, 1180–1188. doi: 10.1016/j.bbi.2012.06.001

Hung, A. Y., and Schwarzschild, M. A. (2014). Treatment of Parkinson's disease: what's in the non-dopaminergic pipeline? *Neurotherapeutics* 11, 34–46. doi: 10.1007/s13311-013-0239-9

Hunter, A. M., Balleine, B. W., and Minor, T. R. (2003). Helplessness and escape performance: glutamate-adenosine interactions in the frontal cortex. *Behav. Neurosci.* 117, 123–135. doi: 10.1037/0735-7044.117.1.123

Jacobson, K. A., and Gao, Z.-G. (2006). Adenosine receptors as therapeutic targets. *Nat. Rev. Drug Discov.* 5, 247–264. doi: 10.1038/nrd1983

Jacobson, K. A., van Galen, P. J., and Williams, M. (1992). Adenosine receptors: pharmacology, structure-activity relationships, and therapeutic potential. *J. Med. Chem.* 35, 407–422. doi: 10.1021/jm00081a001

Johansson, B., and Fredholm, B. B. (1995). Further characterization of the binding of the adenosine receptor agonist [3H]CGS 21680 to rat brain using autoradiography. *Neuropharmacology* 34, 393–403. doi: 10.1016/0028-3908(95)00009-U

Johansson, B., Georgiev, V., and Fredholm, B. B. (1997). Distribution and postnatal ontogeny of adenosine A_{2A} receptors in rat brain: comparison with dopamine receptors. *Neuroscience* 80, 1187–1207. doi: 10.1016/S0306-4522(97)00143-7

Johnson, L. C., Freeman, C. R., Spinweber, C. L., and Gomez, S. A. (1991). Subjective and objective measures of sleepiness: effect of benzodiazepine and caffeine on their relationship. *Psychophysiology* 28, 65–71. doi: 10.1111/j.1469-8986.1991.tb03388.x

Johnson, L. C., Spinweber, C. L., and Gomez, S. A. (1990a). Benzodiazepines and caffeine: effect on daytime sleepiness, performance, and mood. *Psychopharmacology* 101, 160–167.

Johnson, L. C., Spinweber, C. L., Gomez, S. A., and Matteson, L. T. (1990b). Daytime sleepiness, performance, mood, nocturnal sleep: the effect of benzodiazepine and caffeine on their relationship. *Sleep* 13, 121–135.

Juliano, L. M., and Griffiths, R. R. (2004). A critical review of caffeine withdrawal: empirical validation of symptoms and signs, incidence, severity, and associated features. *Psychopharmacology* 176, 1–29. doi: 10.1007/s00213-004-2000-x

Juliano, L. M., Huntley, E. D., Harrell, P. T., and Westerman, A. T. (2012). Development of the caffeine withdrawal symptom questionnaire: caffeine withdrawal symptoms cluster into 7 factors. *Drug Alcohol Depend.* 124, 229–234. doi: 10.1016/j.drugalcdep.2012.01.009

Kale, P. P., and Addepalli, V. (2014). Augmentation of antidepressant effects of duloxetine and bupropion by caffeine in mice. *Pharmacol. Biochem. Behav.* 124, 238–244. doi: 10.1016/j.pbb.2014.06.005

Kale, P. P., and Addepalli, V. (2015). Enhancement of nootropic effect of duloxetine and bupropion by caffeine in mice. *Indian J. Pharmacol.* 47, 199–201. doi: 10.4103/0253-7613.153430

Kale, P. P., Addepalli, V., Bafna, P. A., and Prabhavalkar, K. S. (2010). Caffeine-induced augmentation of antidepressant therapy. *J. Exp. Clin. Med.* 2, 282–286. doi: 10.1016/j.jecm.2010.09.001

Kaster, M. P., Machado, N. J., Silva, H. B., Nunes, A., Ardais, A. P., Santana, M., et al. (2015). Caffeine acts through neuronal adenosine A_{2A} receptors to prevent mood and memory dysfunction triggered by chronic stress. *Proc. Natl. Acad. Sci. U.S.A.* 112, 7833–7838. doi: 10.1073/pnas.1423088112

Kaster, M. P., Rosa, A. O., Rosso, M. M., Goulart, E. C., Santos, A. R., and Rodrigues, A. L. (2004). Adenosine administration produces an antidepressant-like effect in mice: evidence for the involvement of A_1 and A_{2A} receptors. *Neurosci. Lett.* 355, 21–24. doi: 10.1016/j.neulet.2003.10.040

Kawachi, I., Willett, W. C., Colditz, G. A., Stampfer, M. J., and Speizer, F. E. (1996). A prospective study of coffee drinking and suicide in women. *Arch. Intern. Med.* 156, 521–525. doi: 10.1001/archinte.1996.00440050067008

Kent, S., Bluthe, R. M., Dantzer, R., Hardwick, A. J., Kelley, K. W., Rothwell, N. J., et al. (1992). Different receptor mechanisms mediate the pyrogenic and behavioral effects of interleukin 1. *Proc. Natl. Acad. Sci. U.S.A.* 89, 9117–9120. doi: 10.1073/pnas.89.19.9117

Kent, T. A., Preskorn, S. H., Glotzbach, R. K., and Irwin, G. H. (1986). Amitriptyline normalizes tetrabenazine-induced changes in cerebral microcirculation. *Biol. Psychiatry* 21, 483–491. doi: 10.1016/0006-3223(86)90190-3

Kerkhofs, A., Xavier, A. C., da Silva, B. S., Canas, P. M., Idema, S., Baayen, J. C., et al. (2018). Caffeine controls glutamatergic synaptic transmission and pyramidal neuron excitability in human neocortex. *Front. Pharmacol.* 8:899. doi: 10.3389/fphar.2017.00899

Kulkarni, S. K., and Mehta, A. K. (1985). Purine nucleoside–mediated immobility in mice: reversal by antidepressants. *Psychopharmacology* 85, 460–463. doi: 10.1007/BF00429665

Leibenluft, E., Fiero, P. L., Bartko, J. J., Moul, D. E., and Rosenthal, N. E. (1993). Depressive symptoms and the self-reported use of alcohol, caffeine, and carbohydrates in normal volunteers and four groups of psychiatric outpatients. *Am. J. Psychiatry* 150, 294–301. doi: 10.1176/ajp.150.2.294

Li, Y., He, Y., Chen, M., Pu, Z., Chen, L., Li, P., et al. (2016). Optogenetic activation of adenosine A_{2A} receptor signaling in the dorsomedial striatopallidal neurons suppresses goal-directed behavior. *Neuropsychopharmacology* 41, 1003–1013. doi: 10.1038/npp.2015.227

Lieberman, H. R. (2001). The effects of ginseng, ephedrine, and caffeine on cognitive performance, mood and energy. *Nutr. Rev.* 59, 91–102. doi: 10.1111/j.1753-4887.2001.tb06995.x

Lieberman, H. R., Wurtman, R. J., Emde, G. G., and Coviella, I. L. (1987). The effects of caffeine and aspirin on mood and performance. *J. Clin. Psychopharmacol.* 7, 315–320. doi: 10.1097/00004714-198710000-00004

Liguori, A., and Hughes, J. R. (1997). Caffeine self-administration in humans: 2. A within-subjects comparison of coffee and cola vehicles. *Exp. Clin. Psychopharmacol.* 5, 295–303. doi: 10.1037/1064-1297.5.3.295

López-Cruz, L., Pardo, M., Salamone, J. D., and Correa, M. (2014). Differences between the nonselective adenosine receptor antagonists caffeine and theophylline in motor and mood effects: studies using medium to high doses in animal models. *Behav. Brain Res.* 270, 213–222. doi: 10.1016/j.bbr.2014.05.020

López-Cruz, L., SanMiguel, N., Carratalá-Ros, C., Monferrer, L., Salamone, J. D., and Correa, M. (2018). Dopamine depletion shifts behavior from activity based reinforcers to more sedentary ones and adenosine receptor antagonism reverses that shift: relation to ventral striatum DARPP32 phosphorylation patterns. *Neuropharmacology* doi: 10.1016/j.neuropharm.2018.01.034 [Epub ahead of print].

Lorist, M. M., Snel, J., Kok, A., and Mulder, G. (1994). Influence of caffeine on selective attention in well-rested and fatigued subjects. *Psychophysiology* 31, 525–534. doi: 10.1111/j.1469-8986.1994.tb02345.x

Lucas, M., Mirzaei, F., Pan, A., Okereke, O. I., Willett, W. C., O'Reilly, É. J., et al. (2011). Coffee, caffeine, and risk of depression among women. *Arch. Intern. Med.* 171, 1571–1578. doi: 10.1001/archinternmed.2011.393

Lucas, M., O'Reilly, E. J., Pan, A., Mirzaei, F., Willett, W. C., Okereke, O. I., et al. (2014). Coffee, caffeine, and risk of completed suicide: results from three prospective cohorts of American adults. *World J. Biol. Psychiatry* 15, 377–386. doi: 10.3109/15622975.2013.795243

Machado, N. J., Simões, A. P., Silva, H. B., Ardais, A. P., Kaster, M. P., Garção, P., et al. (2017). Caffeine reverts memory but not mood impairment in a depression-prone mouse strain with up-regulated adenosine A_{2A} receptor in hippocampal glutamate synapses. *Mol. Neurobiol.* 54, 1552–1563. doi: 10.1007/s12035-016-9774-9

Malinauskas, B. M., Aeby, V. G., Overton, R. F., Carpenter-Aeby, T., and Barber-Heidal, K. (2007). A survey of energy drink consumption patterns among college students. *Nutr. J.* 6:35. doi: 10.1186/1475-2891-6-35

Markou, A., Salamone, J. D., Bussey, T. J., Mar, A. C., Brunner, D., Gilmour, G., et al. (2013). Measuring reinforcement learning and motivation constructs in experimental animals: relevance to the negative symptoms of schizophrenia. *Neurosci. Biobehav. Rev.* 37, 2149–2165. doi: 10.1016/j.neubiorev.2013.08.007

McClintock, S. M., Husain, M. M., Wisniewski, S. R., Nierenberg, A. A., Stewart, J. W., Trivedi, M. H., et al. (2011). Residual symptoms in depressed outpatients who respond by 50% but do not remit to antidepressant medication. *J. Clin. Psychopharmacol.* 31, 180–186. doi: 10.1097/JCP.0b013e31820ebd2c

Miller, A. H., Maletic, V., and Raison, C. L. (2009). Inflammation and its discontents: the role of cytokines in the pathophysiology of major depression. *Biol. Psychiatry* 65, 732–741. doi: 10.1016/j.biopsych.2008.11.029

Mingote, S., Font, L., Farrar, A. M., Vontell, R., Worden, L. T., Stopper, C. M., et al. (2008). Nucleus accumbens adenosine A_{2A} receptors regulate exertion of effort by acting on the ventral striatopallidal pathway. *J. Neurosci.* 28, 9037–9046. doi: 10.1523/JNEUROSCI.1525-08.2008

Minor, T. R., Chang, W. C., and Winslow, J. L. (1994a). Stress and adenosine: I. Effect of methylxanthine and amphetamine stimulants on learned helplessness in rats. *Behav. Neurosci.* 108, 254–264.

Minor, T. R., and Hanff, T. C. (2015). Adenosine signaling in reserpine-induced depression in rats. *Behav. Brain Res.* 286, 184–191. doi: 10.1016/j.bbr.2015.02.032

Minor, T. R., Rowe, M., Cullen, P. K., and Furst, S. (2008). Enhancing brain adenosine signaling with the nucleoside transport blocker NBTI (S-(4-nitrobenzyl)-6-theoinosine) mimics the effects of inescapable shock on later shuttle-escape performance in rats. *Behav. Neurosci.* 122, 1236–1247. doi: 10.1037/a0013143

Minor, T. R., Winslow, J. L., and Chang, W. C. (1994b). Stress and adenosine: II. Adenosine analogs mimic the effect of inescapable shock on shuttle-escape performance in rats. *Behav. Neurosci.* 108, 265–276.

Mott, A. M., Nunes, E. J., Collins, L. E., Port, R. G., Sink, K. S., Hockemeyer, J., et al. (2009). The adenosine A_{2A} antagonist MSX-3 reverses the effects of the dopamine antagonist haloperidol on effort-related decision making in a T-maze cost/benefit procedure. *Psychopharmacology* 204, 103–112. doi: 10.1007/s00213-008-1441-z

Noji, T., Karasawa, A., and Kusaka, H. (2004). Adenosine uptake inhibitors. *Eur. J. Pharmacol.* 495, 1–16. doi: 10.1016/j.ejphar.2004.05.003

Nunes, E. J., Randall, P. A., Estrada, A., Epling, B., Hart, E. E., Lee, C. A., et al. (2014). Effort-related motivational effects of the pro-inflammatory cytokine interleukin 1-beta: studies with the concurrent fixed ratio 5/ chow feeding choice task. *Psychopharmacology* 231, 727–736. doi: 10.1007/s00213-013-3285-4

Nunes, E. J., Randall, P. A., Hart, E. E., Freeland, C., Yohn, S. E., Baqi, Y., et al. (2013). Effort-related motivational effects of the VMAT-2 inhibitor tetrabenazine: implications for animal models of the motivational symptoms of depression. *J. Neurosci.* 33, 19120–19130. doi: 10.1523/JNEUROSCI.2730-13.2013

Nunes, E. J., Randall, P. A., Santerre, J. L., Given, A. B., Sager, T. N., Correa, M., et al. (2010). Differential effects of selective adenosine antagonists on the effort-related impairments induced by dopamine D1 and D2 antagonism. *Neuroscience* 170, 268–280. doi: 10.1016/j.neuroscience.2010.05.068

Overmier, J. B., and Seligman, M. E. (1967). Effects of inescapable shock upon subsequent escape and avoidance responding. *J. Comp. Physiol. Psychol.* 63, 28–33. doi: 10.1037/h0024166

Padala, P. R., Padala, K. P., Monga, V., Ramirez, D. A., and Sullivan, D. H. (2012). Reversal of SSRI-associated apathy syndrome by discontinuation of therapy. *Ann. Pharmacother.* 46:e8. doi: 10.1345/aph.1Q656

Pae, C. U., Lim, H.-K., Han, C., Patkar, A. A., Steffens, D. C., Masand, P. S., et al. (2007). Fatigue as a core symptom in major depressive disorder: overview and the role of bupropion. *Expert Rev. Neurother.* 7, 1251–1263. doi: 10.1586/14737175.7.10.1251

Paech, G. M., Banks, S., Pajcin, M., Grant, C., Johnson, K., Kamimori, G. H., et al. (2016). Caffeine administration at night during extended wakefulness effectively mitigates performance impairment but not subjective assessments of fatigue and sleepiness. *Pharmacol. Biochem. Behav.* 145, 27–32. doi: 10.1016/j.pbb.2016.03.011

Pandolfo, P., Machado, N. J., Köfalvi, A., Takahashi, R. N., and Cunha, R. A. (2013). Caffeine regulates frontocorticostriatal dopamine transporter density and improves attention and cognitive deficits in an animal model of attention deficit hyperactivity disorder. *Eur. Neuropsychopharmacol.* 23, 317–328. doi: 10.1016/j.euroneuro.2012.04.011

Pardo, M., López-Cruz, L., San Miguel, N., Salamone, J. D., and Correa, M. (2015). Selection of sucrose concentration depends on the effort required to obtain it: studies using tetrabenazine, D1, D2, and D3 receptor antagonists. *Psychopharmacology* 232, 2377–2391. doi: 10.1007/s00213-015-3872-7

Pardo, M., Lopez-Cruz, L., Valverde, O., Ledent, C., Baqi, Y., Müller, C. E., et al. (2012). Adenosine A_{2A} receptor antagonism and genetic deletion attenuate the effects of dopamine D_2 antagonism on effort-based decision making in mice. *Neuropharmacology* 62, 2068–2077. doi: 10.1016/j.neuropharm.2011.12.033

Pardo, M., López-Cruz, L., Valverde, O., Ledent, C., Baqi, Y., Müller, C. E., et al. (2013). Effect of subtype-selective adenosine receptor antagonists on basal or haloperidol-regulated striatal function: studies of exploratory locomotion and c-Fos immunoreactivity in outbred and A_{2A}R KO mice. *Behav. Brain Res.* 247, 217–226. doi: 10.1016/j.bbr.2013.03.035

Pasman, W. J., Boessen, R., Donner, Y., Clabbers, N., and Boorsma, A. (2017). Effect of caffeine on attention and alertness measured in a home-setting, using web-based cognition tests. *JMIR Res. Protoc.* 6:e169. doi: 10.2196/resprot.6727

Patten, S. B., Metz, L. M., and Reimer, M. A. (2000). Biopsychosocial correlates of lifetime major depression in a multiple sclerosis population. *Mult. Scler.* 6, 115–120. doi: 10.1177/135245850000600210

Pechlivanova, D. M., Tchekalarova, J. D., Alova, L. H., Petkov, V. V., Nikolov, R. P., and Yakimova, K. S. (2012). Effect of long-term caffeine administration on depressive-like behavior in rats exposed to chronic unpredictable stress. *Behav. Pharmacol.* 23, 339–347. doi: 10.1097/FBP.0b013e3283564dd9

Peeling, P., and Dawson, B. (2007). Influence of caffeine ingestion on perceived mood states, concentration, and arousal levels during a 75-min university lecture. *Adv. Physiol. Educ.* 31, 332–335. doi: 10.1152/advan.00003.2007

Petit-Demouliere, B., Chenu, F., and Bourin, M. (2005). Forced swimming test in mice: a review of antidepressant activity. *Psychopharmacology* 177, 245–255. doi: 10.1007/s00213-004-2048-7

Pettibone, D. J., Totaro, J. A., and Pflueger, A. B. (1984). Tetrabenazine-induced depletion of brain monoamines: characterization and interaction with selected antidepressants. *Eur. J. Pharmacol.* 102, 425–430. doi: 10.1016/0014-2999(84)90562-4

Petty, F., McChesney, C., and Kramer, G. (1985). Intracortical glutamate injection produces helpless-like behavior in the rat. *Pharmacol. Biochem. Behav.* 22, 531–533. doi: 10.1016/0091-3057(85)90270-9

Pizzagalli, D. A. (2014). Depression, stress, and anhedonia: toward a synthesis and integrated model. *Annu. Rev. Clin. Psychol.* 10, 393–423. doi: 10.1146/annurev-clinpsy-050212-185606

Porsolt, R. D., Le Pichon, M., and Jalfre, M. (1977). Depression: a new animal model sensitive to antidepressant treatments. *Nature* 266, 730–732. doi: 10.1038/266730a0

Prediger, R. D. (2010). Effects of caffeine in Parkinson's disease: from neuroprotection to the management of motor and non-motor symptoms. *J. Alzheimers Dis.* 20(Suppl. 1), S205–S220. doi: 10.3233/JAD-2010-091459

Quitkin, F., Rifkin, A., and Klein, D. F. (1979). Monoamine oxidase inhibitors. A review of antidepressant effectiveness. *Arch. Gen. Psychiatry* 36, 749–760. doi: 10.1001/archpsyc.1979.01780070027003

Rampello, L., Nicoletti, G., and Raffaele, R. (1991). Dopaminergic hypothesis for retarded depression: a symptom profile for predicting therapeutical responses. *Acta Psychiatr. Scand.* 84, 552–554. doi: 10.1111/j.1600-0447.1991.tb03193.x

Rampello, L., Nicoletti, G., Raffaele, R., and Drago, F. (1995). Comparative effects of amitriptyline and amineptine in patients affected by anxious depression. *Neuropsychobiology* 31, 130–134. doi: 10.1159/000119183

Randall, P. A., Lee, C. A., Podurgiel, S. J., Hart, E., Yohn, S. E., Jones, M., et al. (2014). Bupropion increases selection of high effort activity in rats tested on a progressive ratio/chow feeding choice procedure: implications for treatment of effort-related motivational symptoms. *Int. J. Neuropsychopharmacol.* 18:yu017. doi: 10.1093/ijnp/pyu017

Randall, P. A., Nunes, E. J., Janniere, S. L., Stopper, C. M., Farrar, A. M., Sager, T. N., et al. (2011). Stimulant effects of adenosine antagonists on operant behavior: differential actions of selective A_{2A} and A_1 antagonists. *Psychopharmacology* 216, 173–186. doi: 10.1007/s00213-011-2198-3

Randall, P. A., Pardo, M., Nunes, E. J., López Cruz, L., Vemuri, V. K., Makriyannis, A., et al. (2012). Dopaminergic modulation of effort-related choice behavior as assessed by a progressive ratio chow feeding choice task: pharmacological studies and the role of individual differences. *PLoS One* 7:e47934. doi: 10.1371/journal.pone.0047934

Rebola, N., Canas, P. M., Oliveira, C. R., and Cunha, R. A. (2005). Different synaptic and subsynaptic localization of adenosine A_{2A} receptors in the hippocampus and striatum of the rat. *Neuroscience* 132, 893–903. doi: 10.1016/j.neuroscience.2005.01.014

Rees, K., Allen, D., and Lader, M. (1999). The influences of age and caffeine on psychomotor and cognitive function. *Psychopharmacology* 145, 181–188. doi: 10.1007/s002130051047

Retzbach, E. P., Dholakia, P. H., and Duncan-Vaidya, E. A. (2014). The effect of daily caffeine exposure on lever-pressing for sucrose and c-Fos expression in the nucleus accumbens in the rat. *Physiol. Behav.* 135, 1–6. doi: 10.1016/j.physbeh.2014.05.038

Rihs, M., Muller, C., and Baumann, P. (1996). Caffeine consumption in hospitalized psychiatric patients. *Eur. Arch. Psychiatry Clin. Neurosci.* 246, 83–92. doi: 10.1007/BF02274898

Robles-Molina, E., Millán, D., Hong, E., Huang, F., and Villafaña, S. (2012). Increased antidepressant-like effect of desipramine combined with central stimulants (caffeine and amphetamine) in mice. *Open Life Sci.* 7, 391–396. doi: 10.2478/s11535-012-0028-1

Rodrigues, F. B., Duarte, G. S., Costa, J., Ferreira, J. J., and Wild, E. J. (2017). Tetrabenazine versus deutetrabenazine for Huntington's disease: twins or distant cousins? *Mov. Disord. Clin. Pract.* 4, 582–585. doi: 10.1002/mdc3.12483

Ruby, L., Adams, C. A., Mrazeck, A. D., and Choi, D. S. (2011). "Adenosine signaling in anxiety," in *Anxiety Disorders*, ed. V. Kalinin (Rijeka: InTech). doi: 10.5772/19423

Rush, A. J., and Trivedi, M. H. (1995). Treating depression to remission. *Psychiatr. Ann.* 64(Suppl. 15), 7–12. doi: 10.3928/0048-5713-19951201-03

Sako, W., Murakami, N., Motohama, K., Izumi, Y., and Kaji, R. (2017). The effect of istradefylline for Parkinson's disease: a meta-analysis. *Sci. Rep.* 7:18018. doi: 10.1038/s41598-017-18339-1

Salamone, J., Correa, M., Mingote, S., Weber, S., and Farrar, A. (2006). Nucleus accumbens dopamine and the forebrain circuitry involved in behavioral activation and effort-related decision making: implications for understanding anergia and psychomotor slowing in depression. *Curr. Psychiatry Rev.* 2, 267–280. doi: 10.2174/157340006776875914

Salamone, J. D. (2007). Functions of mesolimbic dopamine: changing concepts and shifting paradigms. *Psychopharmacology* 191:389. doi: 10.1007/s00213-006-0623-9

Salamone, J. D., and Correa, M. (2002). Motivational views of reinforcement: implications for understanding the behavioral functions of nucleus accumbens dopamine. *Behav. Brain Res.* 137, 3–25. doi: 10.1016/S0166-4328(02)00282-6

Salamone, J. D., and Correa, M. (2009). Dopamine/adenosine interactions involved in effort-related aspects of food motivation. *Appetite* 53, 422–425. doi: 10.1016/j.appet.2009.07.018

Salamone, J. D., and Correa, M. (2012). The mysterious motivational functions of mesolimbic dopamine. *Neuron* 76, 470–485. doi: 10.1016/j.neuron.2012.10.021

Salamone, J. D., Correa, M., Farrar, A., and Mingote, S. M. (2007). Effort-related functions of nucleus accumbens dopamine and associated forebrain circuits. *Psychopharmacology* 191, 461–482. doi: 10.1007/s00213-006-0668-9

Salamone, J. D., Correa, M., Yohn, S., Lopez Cruz, L., San Miguel, N., and Alatorre, L. (2016). The pharmacology of effort-related choice behavior: dopamine, depression, and individual differences. *Behav. Process.* 127, 3–17. doi: 10.1016/j.beproc.2016.02.008

Salamone, J. D., Cousins, M. S., and Bucher, S. (1994). Anhedonia or anergia? Effects of haloperidol and nucleus accumbens dopamine depletion on instrumental response selection in a T-maze cost/benefit procedure. *Behav. Brain Res.* 65, 221–229. doi: 10.1016/0166-4328(94)90108-2

Salamone, J. D., Farrar, A. M., Font, L., Patel, V., Schlar, D. E., Nunes, E. J., et al. (2009). Differential actions of adenosine A_1 and A_{2A} antagonists on the effort-related effects of dopamine D_2 antagonism. *Behav. Brain Res.* 201, 216–222. doi: 10.1016/j.bbr.2009.02.021

Salamone, J. D., Steinpreis, R. E., McCullough, L. D., Smith, P., Grebel, D., and Mahan, K. (1991). Haloperidol and nucleus accumbens dopamine depletion suppress lever pressing for food but increase free food consumption in a novel food choice procedure. *Psychopharmacology* 104, 515–521. doi: 10.1007/BF02245659

SanMiguel, N., Pardo, M., Carratalá-Ros, C., López-Cruz, L., Salamone, J. D., and Correa, M. (2018). Individual differences in the energizing effects of caffeine on effort-based decision-making tests in rats. *Pharmacol. Biochem. Behav.* 169, 27–34. doi: 10.1016/j.pbb.2018.04.004

Schwarzschild, M. A., Agnati, L., Fuxe, K., Chen, J. F., and Morelli, M. (2006). Targeting adenosine A_{2A} receptors in Parkinson's disease. *Trends Neurosci.* 29, 647–654. doi: 10.1016/j.tins.2006.09.004

Sebastião, A. M., and Ribeiro, J. A. (2009). Tuning and fine-tuning of synapses with adenosine. *Curr. Neuropharmacol.* 7, 180–194. doi: 10.2174/157015909789152128

Seligman, M. E. (1972). Learned helplessness. *Annu. Rev. Med.* 23, 407–412. doi: 10.1146/annurev.me.23.020172.002203

Silber, B. Y., Croft, R. J., Papafotiou, K., and Stough, C. (2006). The acute effects of d-amphetamine and methamphetamine on attention and psychomotor performance. *Psychopharmacology* 187, 154–169. doi: 10.1007/s00213-006-0410-7

Simões, A. P., Duarte, J. A., Agasse, F., Canas, P. M., Tomé, A. R., Agostinho, P., et al. (2012). Blockade of adenosine A_{2A} receptors prevents interleukin-1β-induced exacerbation of neuronal toxicity through a p38 mitogen-activated protein kinase pathway. *J. Neuroinflammation* 9:204. doi: 10.1186/1742-2094-9-204

Simões, A. P., Machado, N. J., Gonçalves, N., Kaster, M. P., Simões, A. T., Nunes, A., et al. (2016). Adenosine A_{2A} receptors in the amygdala control synaptic plasticity and contextual fear memory. *Neuropsychopharmacology* 41, 2862–2871. doi: 10.1038/npp.2016.98

Sitkovsky, M. V., and Ohta, A. (2005). The "danger" sensors that STOP the immune response: the A2 adenosine receptors? *Trends Immunol.* 26, 299–304. doi: 10.1016/j.it.2005.04.004

Smith, A., Thomas, M., Perry, K., and Whitney, H. (1997). Caffeine and the common cold. *J. Psychopharmacol.* 11, 319–324. doi: 10.1177/026988119701100406

Smith, A. P. (2009). Caffeine, cognitive failures and health in a non-working community sample. *Hum. Psychopharmacol.* 24, 29–34. doi: 10.1002/hup.991

Smith, A. P. (2013). Caffeine, extraversion and working memory. *J. Psychopharmacol.* 27, 71–76. doi: 10.1177/0269881112460111

Smith, A. P., Kendrick, A. M., and Maben, A. L. (1992). Effects of breakfast and caffeine on performance and mood in the late morning and after lunch. *Neuropsychobiology* 26, 198–204. doi: 10.1159/000118920

Stahl, S. M. (2002). The psychopharmacology of energy and fatigue. *J. Clin. Psychiatry* 63, 7–8. doi: 10.4088/JCP.v63n0102

Stenman, E., and Lilja, A. (2013). Increased monoaminergic neurotransmission improves compliance with physical activity recommendations in depressed patients with fatigue. *Med. Hypotheses* 80, 47–49. doi: 10.1016/j.mehy.2012.10.007

Steru, L., Chermat, R., Thierry, B., and Simon, P. (1985). The tail suspension test: a new method for screening antidepressants in mice. *Psychopharmacology* 85, 367–370. doi: 10.1007/BF00428203

Sukoff Rizzo, S. J., Neal, S. J., Hughes, Z. A., Beyna, M., Rosenzweig-Lipson, S., Moss, S. J., et al. (2012). Evidence for sustained elevation of IL-6 in the CNS as a key contributor of depressive-like phenotypes. *Transl. Psychiatry* 2:e199. doi: 10.1038/tp.2012.120

Swindle, R., Kroenke, K., and Braun, L. A. (2001). "Energy and improved workplace productivity in depression," in *Investing in Health: The Social and Economic Benefits of Health Care Innovation: Research in Human Capital and Development*, Vol. 14, eds I. Farquhar, K. Summers, and A. Sorkin (Bingley: Emerald Group Publishing Limited), 323–341.

Szopa, A., Poleszak, E., Wyska, E., Serefko, A., Wośko, S., Wlaź, A., et al. (2016). Caffeine enhances the antidepressant-like activity of common antidepressant drugs in the forced swim test in mice. *Naunyn Schmiedebergs Arch. Pharmacol.* 389, 211–221. doi: 10.1007/s00210-015-1189-z

Tanra, A. J., Kagaya, A., Okamoto, Y., Muraoka, M., Motohashi, N., and Yamawaki, S. (1995). TJS-010, a new prescription of oriental medicine, antagonizes tetrabenazine-induced suppression of spontaneous locomotor activity in rats. *Prog. Neuropsychopharmacol. Biol. Psychiatry* 19, 963–971.

Tanskanen, A. (1997). Coffee, caffeine and mental health. *Duodecim* 113, 191–196.

Tanskanen, A., Tuomilehto, J., Viinamäki, H., Vartiainen, E., Lehtonen, J., and Puska, P. (2000). Heavy coffee drinking and the risk of suicide. *Eur. J. Epidemiol.* 16, 789–791. doi: 10.1023/A:1007614714579

Temple, J. L., Bernard, C., Lipshultz, S. E., Czachor, J. D., Westphal, J. A., and Mestre, M. A. (2017). The safety of ingested caffeine: a comprehensive review. *Front. Psychiatry* 8:80. doi: 10.3389/fpsyt.2017.00080

Treadway, M. T., Buckholtz, J. W., Cowan, R. L., Woodward, N. D., Li, R., Ansari, M. S., et al. (2012). Dopaminergic mechanisms of individual differences in human effort-based decision-making. *J. Neurosci.* 32, 6170–6176. doi: 10.1523/JNEUROSCI.6459-11.2012

Treadway, M. T., Buckholtz, J. W., Schwartzman, A. N., Lambert, W. E., and Zald, D. H. (2009). Worth the "EEfRT"? The effort expenditure for rewards task as an objective measure of motivation and anhedonia. *PLoS One* 4:e6598. doi: 10.1371/journal.pone.0006598

Tylee, A., Gastpar, M., Lépine, J. P., and Mendlewicz, J. (1999). DEPRES II (Depression research in European society II): a patient survey of the symptoms, disability and current management of depression in the community. DEPRES steering committee. *Int. Clin. Psychopharmacol.* 14, 139–151. doi: 10.1097/00004850-199905030-00001

van den Bos, R., van der Harst, J., Jonkman, S., Schilders, M., and Spruijt, B. (2006). Rats assess costs and benefits according to an internal standard. *Behav. Brain Res.* 171, 350–354. doi: 10.1016/j.bbr.2006.03.035

Wang, H., Chen, X., Li, Y., Tang, T.-S., and Bezprozvanny, I. (2010). Tetrabenazine is neuroprotective in Huntington's disease mice. *Mol. Neurodegener.* 5:18. doi: 10.1186/1750-1326-5-18

Wardle, M. C., Treadway, M. T., and de Wit, H. (2012). Caffeine increases psychomotor performance on the effort expenditure for rewards task. *Pharmacol. Biochem. Behav.* 102, 526–531. doi: 10.1016/j.pbb.2012.06.016

Whalen, D. J., Silk, J. S., Semel, M., Forbes, E. E., Ryan, N. D., Axelson, D. A., et al. (2008). Caffeine consumption, sleep, and affect in the natural environments of depressed youth and healthy controls. *J. Pediatr. Psychol.* 33, 358–367. doi: 10.1093/jpepsy/jsm086

Wikoff, D., Welsh, B. T., Henderson, R., Brorby, G. P., Britt, J., Myers, E., et al. (2017). Systematic review of the potential adverse effects of caffeine consumption in healthy adults, pregnant women, adolescents, and children. *Food Chem. Toxicol.* 109(Pt 1), 585–648. doi: 10.1016/j.fct.2017.04.002

Willner, P. (2005). Chronic mild stress (CMS) revisited: consistency and behavioural-neurobiological concordance in the effects of CMS. *Neuropsychobiology* 52, 90–110. doi: 10.1159/000087097

Woodson, J. C., Minor, T. R., and Job, R. F. (1998). Inhibition of adenosine deaminase by erythro-9-(2-hydroxy-3-nonyl)adenine (EHNA) mimics the effect of inescapable shock on escape learning in rats. *Behav. Neurosci.* 112, 399–409. doi: 10.1037/0735-7044.112.2.399

Worden, L. T., Shahriari, M., Farrar, A. M., Sink, K. S., Hockemeyer, J., Müller, C. E., et al. (2009). The adenosine A_{2A} antagonist MSX-3 reverses the effort-related effects of dopamine blockade: differential interaction with D_1 and D_2 family antagonists. *Psychopharmacology* 203, 489–499. doi: 10.1007/s00213-008-1396-0

Worthington, J., Fava, M., Agustin, C., Alpert, J., Nierenberg, A. A., Pava, J. A., et al. (1996). Consumption of alcohol, nicotine, and caffeine among depressed outpatients. Relationship with response to treatment. *Psychosomatics* 37, 518–522. doi: 10.1016/S0033-3182(96)71515-3

Yang, X.-H., Huang, J., Zhu, C.-Y., Wang, Y.-F., Cheung, E. F. C., Chan, R. C., et al. (2014). Motivational deficits in effort-based decision making in individuals with subsyndromal depression, first-episode and remitted depression patients. *Psychiatry Res.* 220, 874–882. doi: 10.1016/j.psychres.2014.08.056

Yıldız, A., Gönül, A. S., and Tamam, L. (2002). Mechanism of actions of antidepressants: beyond the receptors. *Bull. Clin. Psychopharmacol.* 12, 194–200.

Yohn, S. E., Arif, Y., Haley, A., Tripodi, G., Baqi, Y., Müller, C. E., et al. (2016a). Effort-related motivational effects of the pro-inflammatory cytokine interleukin-6: pharmacological and neurochemical characterization. *Psychopharmacology* 233, 3575–3586. doi: 10.1007/s00213-016-4392-9

Yohn, S. E., Errante, E. E., Rosenbloom-Snow, A., Somerville, M., Rowland, M., Tokarski, K., et al. (2016b). Blockade of uptake for dopamine, but not norepinephrine or 5-HT, increases selection of high effort instrumental activity: implications for treatment of effort-related motivational symptoms in psychopathology. *Neuropharmacology* 109, 270–280. doi: 10.1016/j.neuropharm.2016.06.018

Yohn, S. E., Lopez-Cruz, L., Hutson, P. H., Correa, M., and Salamone, J. D. (2016c). Effects of lisdexamfetamine and s-citalopram, alone and in combination, on effort-related choice behavior in the rat. *Psychopharmacology* 233, 949–960. doi: 10.1007/s00213-015-4176-7

Yohn, S. E., Gorka, D., Mistry, A., Collins, S., Qian, E., Correa, M., et al. (2017). Oral ingestion and intraventricular injection of curcumin attenuates the effort-related effects of the VMAT-2 inhibitor tetrabenazine: implications for motivational symptoms of depression. *J. Nat. Prod.* 80, 2839–2844. doi: 10.1021/acs.jnatprod.7b00425

Yohn, S. E., Thompson, C., Randall, P. A., Lee, C. A., Müller, C. E., Baqi, Y., et al. (2015). The VMAT-2 inhibitor tetrabenazine alters effort-related decision making as measured by the T-maze barrier choice task: reversal with the adenosine A_{2A} antagonist MSX-3 and the catecholamine uptake blocker bupropion. *Psychopharmacology* 232, 1313–1323. doi: 10.1007/s00213-014-3766-0

Yu, G., Maskray, V., Jackson, S. H., Swift, C. G., and Tiplady, B. (1991). A comparison of the central nervous system effects of caffeine and theophylline in elderly subjects. *Br. J. Clin. Pharmacol.* 32, 341–345. doi: 10.1111/j.1365-2125.1991.tb03909.x

Zisook, S., Rush, A. J., Haight, B. R., Clines, D. C., and Rockett, C. B. (2006). Use of bupropion in combination with serotonin reuptake inhibitors. *Biol. Psychiatry* 59, 203–210. doi: 10.1016/j.biopsych.2005.06.027

8

The P2Y$_{12}$ Receptor Antagonist Ticagrelor Reduces Lysosomal pH and Autofluorescence in Retinal Pigmented Epithelial Cells from the ABCA4$^{-/-}$ Mouse Model of Retinal Degeneration

*Wennan Lu[1], Néstor M. Gómez[1], Jason C. Lim[1], Sonia Guha[1,2], Ann O'Brien-Jenkins[1], Erin E. Coffey[1], Keith E. Campagno[1], Stuart A. McCaughey[1], Alan M. Laties[2], Leif G. Carlsson[3] and Claire H. Mitchell[1,4,5]**

[1] Department of Anatomy and Cell Biology, University of Pennsylvania, Philadelphia, PA, United States, [2] Jules Stein Eye Institute, University of California, Los Angeles, Los Angeles, CA, United States, [3] Department of Bioscience Heart Failure, Cardiovascular, Renal and Metabolic Diseases, IMED Biotech Unit, AstraZeneca, Gothenburg, Sweden, [4] Department of Ophthalmology, University of Pennsylvania, Philadelphia, PA, United States, [5] Department of Physiology, University of Pennsylvania, Philadelphia, PA, United States

***Correspondence:**
Claire H. Mitchell
chm@upenn.edu

The accumulation of partially degraded lipid waste in lysosomal-related organelles may contribute to pathology in many aging diseases. The presence of these lipofuscin granules is particularly evident in the autofluorescent lysosome-associated organelles of the retinal pigmented epithelial (RPE) cells, and may be related to early stages of age-related macular degeneration. While lysosomal enzymes degrade material optimally at acidic pH levels, lysosomal pH is elevated in RPE cells from the ABCA4$^{-/-}$ mouse model of Stargardt's disease, an early onset retinal degeneration. Lowering lysosomal pH through cAMP-dependent pathways decreases accumulation of autofluorescent material in RPE cells *in vitro*, but identification of an appropriate receptor is crucial for manipulating this pathway *in vivo*. As the P2Y$_{12}$ receptor for ADP is coupled to the inhibitory G$_i$ protein, we asked whether blocking the P2Y$_{12}$ receptor with ticagrelor could restore lysosomal acidity and reduce autofluorescence in compromised RPE cells from ABCA4$^{-/-}$ mice. Oral delivery of ticagrelor giving rise to clinically relevant exposure lowered lysosomal pH in these RPE cells. Ticagrelor also partially reduced autofluorescence in the RPE cells of ABCA4$^{-/-}$ mice. *In vitro* studies in ARPE-19 cells using more specific antagonists AR-C69931 and AR-C66096 confirmed the importance of the P2Y$_{12}$ receptor for lowering lysosomal pH and reducing autofluorescence. These observations identify P2Y$_{12}$ receptor blockade as a potential target to lower lysosomal pH and clear lysosomal waste in RPE cells.

Keywords: P2Y$_{12}$ receptor, ticagrelor, age-related macular degeneration, lysosomal pH, retinal pigment epithelium, lysosomal storage diseases

INTRODUCTION

In some aging diseases, the accumulation of autofluorescent lipofuscin granules can signify an impaired clearance of waste material by lysosomes. Many degradative lysosomal enzymes are pH sensitive, with optimal activity in acidic environments. Lysosomal alkalinization has been detected in models of neural degenerative diseases of accumulation, such as early-onset Alzheimer's disease (Lee et al., 2010, 2015; Coffey et al., 2014) and Stargardt's retinal dystrophy (Liu et al., 2008).

Retinal pigmented epithelial (RPE) cells are particularly sensitive to perturbations in lysosomal enzyme activity, as they are responsible for phagocytosing the lipid-rich photoreceptor outer segment (POS) tips that are shed daily. The accumulation of autofluorescent lipofuscin waste may contribute to the early pathological changes leading age-related macular degeneration (AMD); dry geographic atrophy and wet neovascularization forms of AMD are now thought to stem from the intermediate AMD stage, where RPE cells are characterized by the accumulation of intracellular lipofuscin and extracellular drusen debris (Ferris et al., 2013). The accumulation of lipofuscin in RPE cells is associated with increases in the retinoid by-product *N*-retinylidene-*N*-retinylethanolamine (A2E), and A2E levels are increased in RPE cells from the $ABCA4^{-/-}$ mouse model of recessive Stargardt's retinopathy (Charbel Issa et al., 2013). Furthermore, A2E can lead to elevation of lysosomal pH, although the delay between drug application and alkalinization suggests an indirect pathway (Holz et al., 1999; Liu et al., 2008; Toops et al., 2015). This alkalinization may reduce lysosomal activity and contribute to a secondary accumulation of oxidized lipid waste.

Restoring an acidic environment to compromised lysosomes in RPE cells is predicted to enhance activity of pH-sensitive lysosomal enzymes and improve degradation, thus reducing the pathologies associated with accumulation of waste material (Guha et al., 2014a). While several pathways capable of acidifying compromised lysosomes and improving degradative function have been identified in RPE cells, manipulation of cytoplasmic cAMP was particularly effective (Liu et al., 2008). Drugs targeting receptors coupled to stimulatory G protein (G_s) reduced lysosomal pH and enhanced the clearance of lysosomal waste and opsin turnover in RPE cells fed POSs (Liu et al., 2008; Guha et al., 2012). Importantly, this approach was also effective at lowering lysosomal pH when given to RPE cells isolated from $ABCA4^{-/-}$ mice (Liu et al., 2012; Guha et al., 2014a). While these *in vitro* experiments provided proof of concept that drugs linked to cAMP could lower lysosomal pH and enhance lysosomal degradation, the *in vivo* translation of this approach required identification of the appropriate receptor target.

Several factors make the $P2Y_{12}$ receptor antagonist ticagrelor (Brilinta) an attractive choice to target lysosomal accumulations in RPE cells. As the $P2Y_{12}$ receptor for adenosine di-phosphate (ADP) is coupled to G_i, antagonizing the $P2Y_{12}$ raises cAMP (Cattaneo, 2015). Several $P2Y_{12}$ receptor antagonists are widely used as antithrombotic agents and are approved for use in elderly patients (McFadyen et al., 2018). Ticagrelor is a reversible allosteric $P2Y_{12}$ receptor antagonist that does not require hepatic activation, removing complications associated with genetic variants of the enzyme CYP2C19 common with other $P2Y_{12}$ antagonists used clinically (Birkeland et al., 2010; Tantry et al., 2010). Ticagrelor is broadly utilized clinically to reduce the rate of thrombotic cardiovascular events in patients with acute coronary syndrome or a history of myocardial infarction (Storey et al., 2010; Bonaca et al., 2016). Finally, the $P2Y_{12}$ receptor is expressed in cultured human ARPE-19 cells (Reigada et al., 2005). In this initial study, we examined whether ticagrelor lowers lysosomal pH and reduce lysosomal autofluorescence in RPE cells from the $ABCA4^{-/-}$ mouse model of retinal degeneration.

MATERIALS AND METHODS

Animal Care and Use

All procedures were approved by the University of Pennsylvania IACUC in compliance with the Public Health Service Policy on Humane Care and Use of Laboratory Animals. C57BL/6J and $ABCA4^{-/-}$ mice were reared at 5–15 lux and sacrificed using CO_2. C57BL/6J mice were obtained from Jackson Laboratories (Bar Harbor, ME, United States). $ABCA4^{-/-}$ mice were obtained from Dr. Gabriel Travis of UCLA. All mice were negative for the RD8 mutation (Goméz et al., 2018). Mouse eyes were isolated and RPE cells processed as described previously (Liu et al., 2012).

$P2Y_{12}$ Receptor Pharmacological Agents

Ticagrelor was delivered in food or water at concentrations relevant to those used clinically in humans. The recommended maintenance dosage for ticagrelor (AZD6140) in humans of approximate mass of 90 kg is 180 mg per day; thus 2 mg/kg translated to 0.06 mg per diem for a 30 g mouse. Clinically dosed ticagrelor tablets (90 mg, Lot # YK0083 from the University of Pennsylvania pharmacy) were powdered and initially dissolved in water at 12 μg/ml to give 0.06 mg per diem, based on a mean water consumption of 5 ml per diem. (The concentration was adjusted to 10 μg/ml for later experiments to match the stated solubility more precisely, although precipitate was not detected in either concentration.) The solution was administered in tinted light-resistant bottles wrapped with black paper and refreshed every 1–2 days for 5–19 days. No clear correlation was found between exposure time or concentration, and lysosomal pH signal. Ticagrelor was delivered in food using a custom mouse diet containing 0.1% ticagrelor in Purina Lab Meal 5001 was made by MP Biomedicals (Lot #P9748, Santa Ana, CA, United States) from purified drug provided by AstraZeneca. Untreated food pellets or those containing 0.1% ticagrelor were added at 100–200 g every week and the remainder weighed to determine total food consumption. Ticagrelor has a pIC_{50} at the human $P2Y_{12}$ receptor of 8.0 (Nylander and Schulz, 2016). The pIC_{50} of ticagrelor in an ADP-induced whole blood platelet aggregation assay in humans is 6.6, similar to that in mouse. Ticagrelor is reported to be quickly absorbed from the gut, reaching a peak concentration in 1.5 h, with blood plasma levels linearly dependent on the dose (Goel, 2013).

MeS-ADP; 2-(Methylthio)adenosine 5′-diphosphate (catalogue #1624, Tocris Bio-Techne Corporation, Minneapolis, MN, United States), which has a pIC_{50} of 8.2 and 7.9 at the $P2Y_1$ and $P2Y_{12}$ receptors, respectively (Jacobson et al., 2009), was supplied pre-dissolved in water at 10 mM and diluted. AR-C66931; N^6-(2-methylthioethyl)-2-(3,3,3-trifluoropropylthio)-β,γ-dichloromethylene-ATP (a.k.a cangrelor, catalogue #5720 Tocris) with a pIC_{50} of 9.4 (Jacobson et al., 2009), was stored as a 10 mM stock solution in water. AR-C66096; 2-propylthio-betagamma-difluoromethylene ATP tetrasodium salt (catalogue #3321, Tocris) inhibits ADP-induced aggregation of washed human platelets pIC_{50} = 8.16 and was supplied pre-dissolved at a concentration of 10 mM.

Measurement of Lysosomal pH From RPE Cells

Lysosomal pH was measured as described using the dye LysoSensor Yellow/Blue DND-160 (Liu et al., 2012). In brief, RPE cells from pairs of treated and untreated mice were isolated, loaded with LysoSensor Yellow/Blue 160 DSN, washed, and loaded into wells of a plate reader; the autofluorescence in these cells was previously found to be negligible in cells loaded with LysoSensor 160 DSN (Liu et al., 2008). The limited number of cells precluded calibration to absolute pH, so data were analyzed as the ratio of light excited at 340 vs. 380 nm, an index of lysosomal pH (Guha et al., 2014a). Lysosomal pH measurements were made with UV-Star 384-well plates (Grenier Bio One) to minimize the disruption of the signal at 340 nm. As these ratios can vary from experiment to experiment, values were normalized to enable results from multiple trials to be combined. Lysosomal pH was determined from cultured ARPE-19 cells as described (Guha et al., 2013).

Polymerase Chain Reaction (PCR)

Total RNA was isolated from fresh mouse RPE/choroid cells using Trizol and the RNeasy mini kit (Qiagen, Inc.). RNA yield was determined by nanodrop 2000 spectrophotometer; 100 ng of total RNA was converted into cDNA using High Capacity RNA-to-cDNA kit (#4387406, Applied Biosystems). Primer pairs for mouse $P2Y_{12}$: Forward: CATTGCTGTACACCGTCCTG; Reverse: AACTTGGCACACCAAGGTTC; 212-bp product. PCR was performed with 2 μl first-strand DNA synthesis product, 50 mM $MgCl_2$, and10 μM of each primer with the 0.5 μl first recombinant DNA polymerase (Platinum® *Taq* DNA Polymerase; Applied Biosystems) at 95°C for 10 min, followed by 35 cycles at 95°C for 30 s, 60°C for 45 s, and 72°C for 1 min, with a final extension step at 72°C for 10 min. First-strand DNA synthesis was omitted from the negative control. Quantitative PCR (qPCR) was performed on isolated RPE/choroid from 16 month old C57BL6J or $ABCA4^{-/-}$ mice. Total RNA (100 ng) was reverse transcribed and qPCR was performed using SYBR Green and the 7300 RealTimePCR system (Applied Biosystems, Corp.) as described (Lu et al., 2017) using the following primers: A1AR- F: ATCCCTCTCCGGTACAAGACAGT, R: ACTCAGG TTGTTCCAGCCAAAC (Streitova et al., 2010); A3AR- F: AC TTCTATGCCTGCCTTTTCATGT, R: AACCGTTCTATATCTG ACTGTCAGCTT (Streitova et al., 2010); CFH- F:ACCACATGT GCCAAATGCTA; R:TGTTGAGTCTCGGCACTTTG (Radu et al., 2014); ENT1- F:CTTGGGATTCAGGGTCAGAA, R: ATC AGGTCACACGACACCAA (Eckle et al., 2013); P2Y12- F: CA TTGCTGTACACCGTCCTG, R: AACTTGGCACACCAAGG TTC (Veitinger et al., 2011). Data were analyzed using the delta-delta CT approach, with results expressed as fold change in gene expression.

Microscopy and Immunocytochemistry

Freshly isolated RPE cells from C57Bl6J mice were cultured for 1 day and fixed in 4% paraformaldehyde (PFA), rinsed with Duebcco's phosphate buffered saline (DPBS), permeabilized at room temperature in 0.1% Triton X-100 for 10 min, then blocked with 10% goat serum in SuperBlock blocking buffer (#37515, Thermo Fisher Scientific) for 60 min. Anti-mouse $P2Y_{12}$ antibody (1:50 dilution, #AS-55043A, AnaSpec, Inc., Fremont, CA, United States) was added overnight at 4°C, followed by incubation in donkey anti-rabbit Alexa-Fluor 568 (1:500 dilution; Invitrogen, Carlsbad, CA, United States). Slides were mounted in Slow Fade Gold Antifade Mountant (Thermo Fisher Scientific) and imaged using a Nikon Eclipse 600 microscope (Nikon USA, Melville, NY, United States). To quantify the autofluorescence found in RPE whole mounts from $ABCA4^{-/-}$ mice, images were obtained at 488 nm ex/> 540 nm em from 16 regions using a Nikon Eclipse 600 microscope and autofluorescence was measured using the Nikon Elements software. Spectral analysis of RPE cells in $ABCA4^{-/-}$ mice was performed on 7 μm thick sections from the central $1/3^{rd}$ of the retina following standard fixation (Albalawi et al., 2017) using the Nikon A1R Laser Scanning Confocal Microscope and Nikon NIS-Elements software package at the University of Pennsylvania Live Cell Imaging Core. The endogenous autofluorescent spectral profile of $ABCA4^{-/-}$ mouse RPE was collected after excitation by 406, 488, 561, and 639 lasers. The RPE layer was visualized with a 60X objective and emission was determined in 2.5 nm wide bins throughout the spectrum, grouped into 32 bins per sweep. Confocal scan settings were maintained from sample to sample, and pairs of treated and untreated sections were processed in parallel when possible to minimize day-to-day variations. ROI's were drawn along the RPE layer and corresponding emission levels were exported for analysis.

ARPE-19 Cell Culture

ARPE-19 cells (American Tissue Type Collection, Manassas, VA, United States) were grown as described previously (Reigada et al., 2005). In brief, cells were grown in 1:1 mixture of Dulbecco's modified Eagle's medium (DMEM) and Ham's F12 medium with 3 mM L-glutamine, 100 g/ml streptomycin and 10% FBS (all Thermo Fisher Scientific, Inc., Waltham, MA, United States). Cells were incubated at 37°C in 5% CO_2 and subcultured weekly with 0.05% trypsin and 0.02% ethylenediaminetetraacetic acid (EDTA).

In Vitro Autofluorescence Model

ARPE-19 cells were grown to confluence in 6-well plates, then treated with the pulse chase chloroquine/POS protocol as

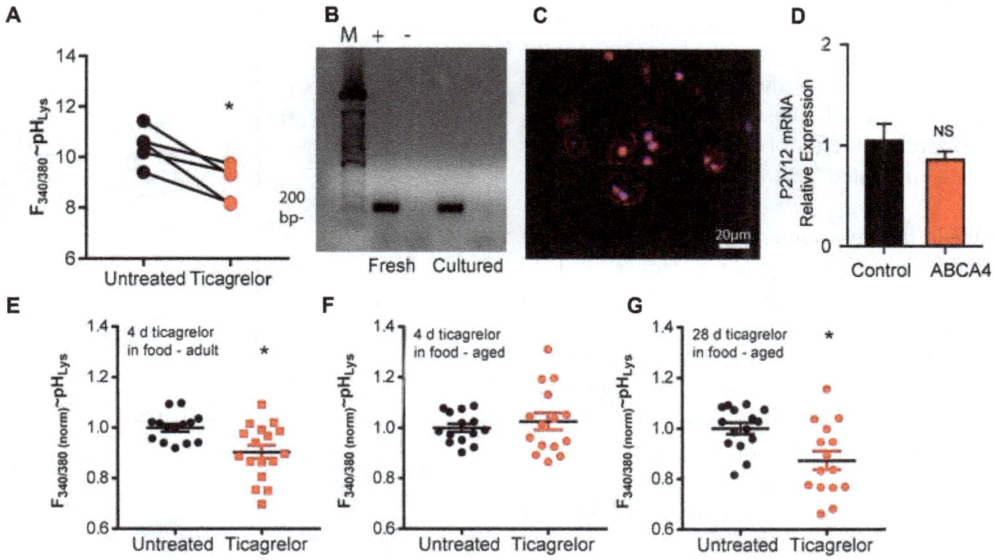

FIGURE 1 | Ticagrelor lowers lysosomal pH in ABCA4$^{-/-}$ mice. **(A)** Decline in the ratio of LysoSensor YellowBlue DNS 160 fluorescence excited at 340 vs. 380 nm in freshly isolated RPE cells from 20-month old untreated ABCA4$^{-/-}$ mice (black circles) and those treated with 10–12 μg/ml ticagrelor in water (red squares). As mice were processed in pairs in individual days, lines connect mean measurements from treated and untreated pairs processed in parallel. *p = 0.029, n = 5, each circle represents the mean of 5–6 wells. **(B)** RT-PCR (+) shows P2Y$_{12}$ receptor expression in RPE cells freshly isolated from mouse eyes (Fresh) or after 3 days in cell culture (Cultured). Bands are at the expected size of 212 bp. No product was detected when reverse transcriptase was omitted from the reaction (–). M-markers at 100 bp (see Supplementary Figure 3 for full gel). **(C)** Immunohistochemistry indicating expression of P2Y$_{12}$ near the cell membrane of freshly isolated RPE cells from 9-month-old C57BL/6J mice. **(D)** Results from quantitative PCR assessment indicating there is no significant (NS) difference between expression of P2Y$_{12}$ receptor mRNA from RPE/choroid of C57BL/6J (n = 4) and ABCA4$^{-/-}$ mice (n = 3). **(E)** Ticagrelor added to a custom diet (0.1%) for 4 days was sufficient to lower lysosomal pH in RPE cells from ABCA4$^{-/-}$ mice 7–8 months old (adult) (*p = 0.0054, n = 14–17 measurements from three mice each condition). **(F)** Exposure to ticagrelor in food for 4 days did not reduce the mean signal in RPE cells from ABCA4$^{-/-}$ mice aged 18–24 months (Old) (p = 0.514, n = 14–15 measures from three mice each condition). **(G)** Extending ticagrelor treatment to 28 days was sufficient to reduce lysosomal pH in the older mice (*p = 0.0066, n = 15 measures from three mice each condition). Throughout, data are expressed as scatter plot with mean ± SEM of the ratio of light excited at 340/380 nm; values were normalized to the mean control for each day to account for differences in LysoSensor dye loading.

described (Guha et al., 2012). Cells were incubated with 2 ml POS for 2 h; POS were isolated as previously described (Liu et al., 2012). Cells were washed thoroughly with medium to remove non-internalized POS followed by a 2 h chase in DMEM/F12. Subsequently, the medium was removed and the cells incubated for 20 h with one of the following solutions: DMEM/F12, 10 μM CHQ, CHQ + 10 μM AR-C66096. This protocol was repeated daily. After 6 days the cells were repeatedly washed, detached with trypsin, and analyzed on a flow cytometer (FACS Calibur; BD Biosciences, Heidelberg, Germany) at the Penn PDM Flow Cytometry Facility. The FITC channel (excitation laser wavelength, 488 nm; detection filter wavelength, 530 nm) was used with a gate set to exclude cell debris and cell clusters.

Magic Red Staining

Magic Red powder was reconstituted as per the manufacturer's instructions (Bio-Rad, Inc., Hercules, CA, United States). ARPE-19 cells grown on coverslips were exposed to 10 μM tamoxifen or control solution. Magic Red was diluted into PBS 1:26 and applied to the cells for 30 min, followed by a 5 min incubation of 50 nM LysoTracker Green. Magic Red was visualized at 540 nm ex and LysoTracker Green at 488 nm using the Nikon Eclipse 600, as above.

Data Analysis

All data are given as mean ± standard error of the mean. Analysis was performed using SigmaStat (Systat Software, Inc., San Jose, CA, United States) and/or GraphPad Software, Inc. (La Jolla, CA, United States). Differences between treatments were analyzed using a one-way analysis of variance (ANOVA) with indicated *post hoc* tests as appropriate, or a Student's t-test using unpaired or paired configuration where appropriate.

RESULTS

Systemic Delivery of P2Y$_{12}$ Antagonist Ticagrelor Lowers Lysosomal pH in RPE Cells From ABCA4$^{-/-}$ Mice

Initial experiments to determine whether ticagrelor decreased lysosomal pH in RPE cells from ABCA4$^{-/-}$ mice were carried out by adding ticagrelor to the drinking water. Mice were given free access to drinking water only or water containing 10–12 μg/ml ticagrelor for 4–19 days. Fresh solution was provided every 1–2 days. Measurements of remaining water suggested ticagrelor did not alter consumption. Age- and gender-matched ABCA4$^{-/-}$ mice used for this experiment examined daily appeared healthy and exhibited normal behavior with no increased bleeding events noted. Previous work suggest lysosomal pH must be measured from freshly isolated RPE cells from ABCA4$^{-/-}$ mice, as the effect of lipofuscin on the lysosomal pH is altered by each cell division (Guha et al., 2014a). As such, lysosomal pH levels could only be determined accurately from only pair of one untreated and one treated mouse per day.

Ticagrelor acidified the lysosomes of RPE cells from ABCA4$^{-/-}$ mice. The lysosomal pH signal was reduced in RPE cells from treated mice as compared to untreated mice in all pairs examined, leading to a significant decline when averaged together (**Figure 1A**). The presence of the P2Y$_{12}$ receptor in mouse RPE cells was confirmed at the mRNA level (**Figure 1B**) and using immunocytochemistry; expression was concentrated near the cell membrane consistent with a membrane-associated receptor (**Figure 1C**). Quantitative PCR indicated no difference in the expression of P2Y$_{12}$ mRNA in RPE cells from C57BL/6J and ABCA4$^{-/-}$ mice (**Figure 1D**).

In a separate study, ticagrelor was added to the mouse chow to confirm the ability of oral delivery to lower lysosomal pH in the RPE cells of ABCA4$^{-/-}$ mice. Four days of exposure lowered the lysosomal pH in 7–8 month-old adult ABCA4$^{-/-}$ mice, as compared to untreated mice (**Figure 1E**). Four days of treatment did not alter the lysosomal pH of RPE cells from 18 to 24 month-old mice compared to untreated controls (**Figure 1F**), but extending treatment to 28 days significantly reduced lysosomal pH in these older mice (**Figure 1G**). Plasma levels of ticagrelor in the mice treated with ticagrelor in food were 0.89 ± 0.07 μM ($n = 13$) and were undetectable in untreated mice.

P2Y$_{12}$ Receptor Regulates Lysosomal pH *in Vitro*

The ability of ticagrelor to lower lysosomal pH was tested directly *in vitro* in the ARPE-19 cultured human cell line. The P2Y$_{12}$ agonist Mes-ADP raised lysosomal pH in these cells (**Figure 2A**). Addition of ticagrelor (**Figure 2B**) or P2Y$_{12}$ receptor antagonist AR-C66931 (**Figure 2C**) to the ARPE-19 cells reduced the lysosomal pH relative to MeS-ADP alone.

P2Y$_{12}$ Receptor Antagonists Reduce Autofluorescence

Lowering lysosomal pH increased clearance of autofluorescent material in prior *in vitro* work (Liu et al., 2008, 2012; Baltazar et al., 2012; Guha et al., 2012). To determine whether ticagrelor could decrease autofluorescence *in vivo*, levels were determined from 16 regions of the RPE whole mount from untreated mice and those receiving ticagrelor in food (**Figure 3A**). There was considerable variation in the autofluorescence values in untreated mice. However, comparing the pattern of autofluorescence across all regions suggested there was a greater difference in autofluorescent levels in samples from the inferior/nasal region (**Figure 3B**). Representative images show the autofluorescence in untreated (**Figure 3C**) and treated mice (**Figure 3D**). Quantification indicated that the autofluorescence

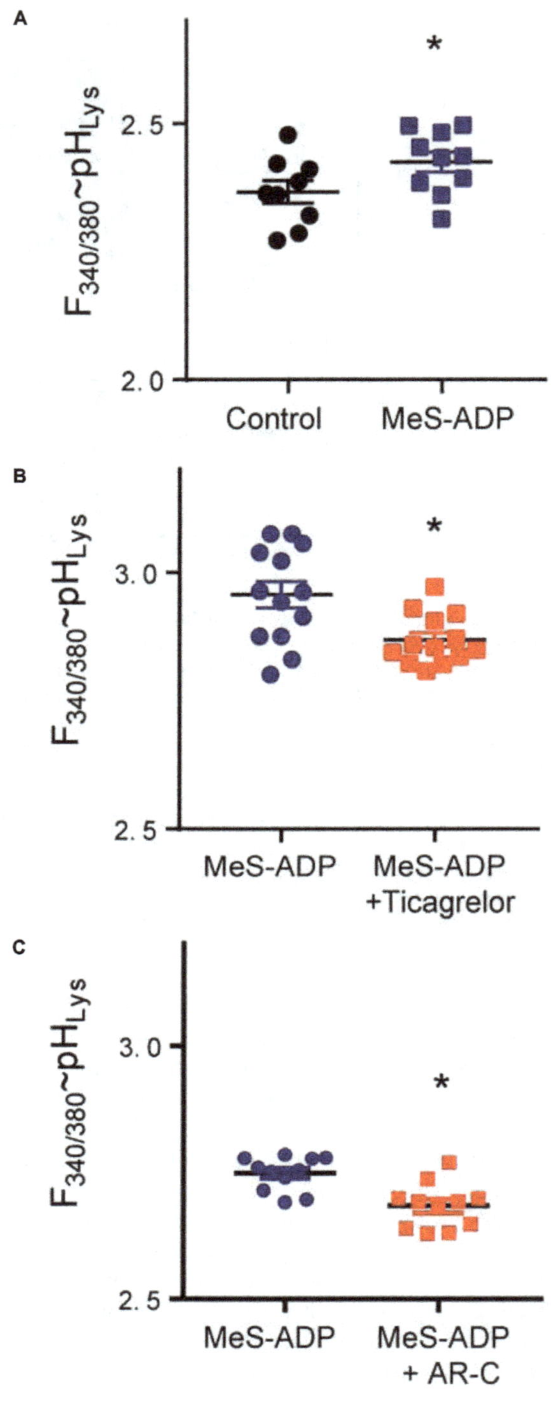

FIGURE 2 | Manipulation of the P2Y$_{12}$ receptor alters lysosomal pH in ARPE-19 cells. **(A)** The lysosomal pH of ARPE-19 cells was elevated by P2Y$_{12}$ receptor agonist methylthio ADP (MeS-ADP, 10 μM). $^*p = 0.002$, $n = 9$–10. **(B)** Ticagrelor (20 μM) lowered the lysosomal pH in cells treated with MeS-ADP ($^*p = 0.006$, $n = 13$). **(C)** The P2Y$_{12}$ receptor antagonist AR-C66931 (ARC, 10 μM) also reduced lysosomal pH in ARPE-19 cells treated with MeS-ADP ($^*p = 0.033$, $n = 10$). Data are expressed as the ratio of fluorescence excited at 340 vs. 380 nm in cells loaded with LysoSensor Yellow/Blue DNS 160; this is indicative of lysosomal pH, although absolute ratios varied with preparation; n represents the number of wells in a single trial with figures representative of 2–4 trials.

from RPE cells in the interior/nasal regions was reduced (**Figure 3E**) in mice treated with ticagrelor. However, there was no difference in mean levels in the superior/temporal regions (**Figure 3F**).

To further characterize the effect of ticagrelor, autofluorescence in RPE cells was analyzed in retinal sections from untreated ABCA4$^{-/-}$ mice and mice treated with ticagrelor. Increased autofluorescence in the RPE cells was detected in many sections from the untreated mice, as compared to those treated with ticagrelor (**Figure 3G**). While variation in autofluorescence levels across regions and mice was considerable, quantification of the autofluorescent output for a broad range of excitation/emission pairs showed a reduction, with emission at 571, 612, and 663 nm particularly effected (**Figure 3H**).

$P2Y_{12}$ Receptor Antagonism Reduces Autofluorescence *in Vitro*

The effect of $P2Y_{12}$ antagonism on autofluorescence was determined *in vitro* using FACS analysis following application of the pulse chase protocol for loading ARPE-19 cells with POSs and alkalinizing lysosomes with chloroquine (see section "Materials and Methods"). Cellular autofluorescence was increased by chloroquine alone, but the addition of POSs increased this autofluorescence substantially (**Figure 4A**). The $P2Y_{12}$ receptor antagonist AR-C66096 reduced the autofluorescence produced by POSs in cells treated with chloroquine (**Figure 4B**). This suggests that blocking the $P2Y_{12}$ receptor reduces lipofuscin accumulation in RPE cells *in vitro*, as it does *in vivo*.

To strengthen the link between lysosomal pH and degradative enzyme activity, ARPE-19 cells were stained with Magic Red to determine cathepsin B activity. The Magic Red substrate releases fluorescent cresyl violet in organelles containing cathepsin B that is catalytically active (Creasy et al., 2007). Magic Red staining was substantial under control conditions; staining colocalized LysoTracker Green, consistent with the lysosomal localization of cathepsin B activity (**Figure 4C**). To determine whether rapid changes in lysosomal pH alter the activity of cathepsin B, cells were treated with tamoxifen, which raises lysosomal pH more rapidly and reproducibly than chloroquine in these cells (**Figure 4D**, Liu et al., 2008). Magic Red staining was absent in cells treated with tamoxifen, consistent with the pH dependence of degradative enzymes in ARPE-19 cells.

Ticagrelor and Gene Expression

The effect of ticagrelor on expression of several key genes in RPE cells was examined. Relative gene expression analysis using quantitative PCR showed a significant downregulation in the expression of the equilibrative nucleoside transporter 1 (ENT1), and complement factor H (CFH) in the RPE of mice treated with 0.1% ticagrelor in food for 14 days. There was no change in expression of mRNA for the $P2Y_{12}$ receptor, the A_1 adenosine receptor or the A_3 adenosine receptor (Supplementary Figure 1).

DISCUSSION

We found that systemic delivery of ticagrelor lowered lysosomal pH in RPE cells of ABCA4$^{-/-}$ mice. Lysosomal pH was reduced both by ticagrelor added to the drinking water, and by addition of ticagrelor to the mouse chow. Results from ticagrelor in food suggest older mice require longer treatment for lysosomal acidification. Ticagrelor, as well as the $P2Y_{12}$ antagonist AR-C66931, lowered lysosomal pH in cultured human ARPE-19 cells, showing receptor block had a direct effect on lysosomal pH in RPE cells. Ticagrelor delivered orally also reduced autofluorescence in the inferior/nasal regions of these RPE cells, while block of the $P2Y_{12}$ receptor reduced autofluorescence *in vitro* in ARPE-19 cells fed POSs. This provides the first evidence that systemic delivery of a $P2Y_{12}$ antagonist improves lysosomal dysregulation in RPE cells.

Contribution of the P2Y12 Receptor

Several observations implicate block of the $P2Y_{12}$ receptor in the lysosomal acidification by ticagrelor. Previous studies indicated that elevation of cAMP, either directly or through drugs known to target the G_s protein that stimulates adenylate cyclase, lowered lysosomal pH in RPE cells from ABCA4$^{-/-}$ mice when applied *ex vivo*, and in compromised ARPE-19 cells (Liu et al., 2008, 2012; Guha et al., 2012, 2014b). This lysosomal acidification was blocked by a protein kinase inhibitor (PKI), implicating protein kinase A in the acidification. As the $P2Y_{12}$ receptor is coupled to the inhibitory G_i protein, $P2Y_{12}$ receptor antagonists will produce similar effects (Supplementary Figure 2). Although ticagrelor can also inhibit the equilibrative nucleoside transporter 1 to raise extracellular adenosine (Nylander et al., 2013; Armstrong et al., 2014; Aungraheeta et al., 2016), it is unlikely adenosine contributes much to the response in this study as plasma levels of ticagrelor in our treated mice were 0.87 ± 0.07 μM, while plasma levels of adenosine reached half -maximal concentrations with ~30 μM ticagrelor (Nylander et al., 2013). In addition, AR-C66931 does not act on ENT1 (Armstrong et al., 2014), and thus the ability of AR-C66931 to acidify lysosomes *in vitro* indicates $P2Y_{12}$ antagonism is sufficient to lower lysosomal pH in these cells. Together, this implicates the $P2Y_{12}$ receptor in mediating the effects of ticagrelor observed in this study.

Mechanisms for Reduced Autofluorescence

Ticagrelor may reduce autofluorescence from RPE cells through multiple pathways. For example, the lysosomal pH in RPE cells from ABCA4$^{-/-}$ mice is alkalinized above age-matched controls (Liu et al., 2008) and lowering lysosomal pH with ticagrelor would enhance the activity of pH sensitive degradative lysosomal enzymes. Data above using Magic Red indicate cathepsin B activity in RPE cells is decreased by moderate elevations in lysosomal pH; this parallels the rise in cathepsin D activity following lysosomal acidification in RPE cells found previously (Guha et al., 2012). Acidifying lysosomal pH in RPE cells also enhanced the turnover of opsin derived from phagocytosed

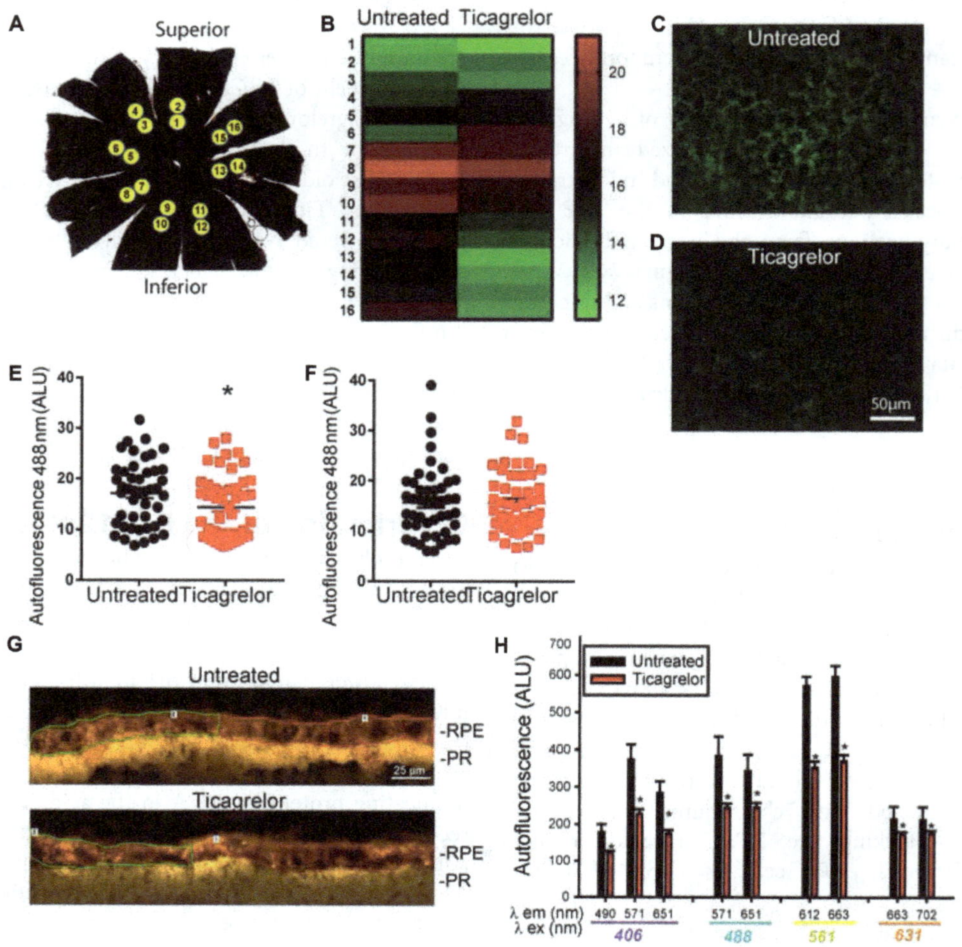

FIGURE 3 | Ticagrelor reduces autofluorescence in RPE cells from ABCA4$^{-/-}$ mice. **(A)** A RPE whole mount preparation indicating the location of images obtained for autofluorescence quantification. **(B)** Heat map illustrating variation in intensity of autofluorescence (488 nm ex/>525 nm em) in regions corresponding to those in "A." Each band is the mean of six untreated mice or mice treated with 0.1% ticagrelor in food for 28 days. Scale at right shows relative intensity. Images of autofluorescence excited at 488 nm in inferior regions of RPE wholemounts from untreated **(C)** and treated **(D)** ABCA4$^{-/-}$ mice. **(E)** Autofluorescence intensity from regions 9–16 of six mice in each condition ($p = 0.039$, $n = 48$ measurements; eight from each mouse). **(F)** Autofluorescence intensity from regions 1–8 of six mice in each condition, $n = 48$). Mice were 257–333 days old after ticagrelor treatment. **(G)** Images from sections of the outer retina showing the RPE and photoreceptor outer segments (POSs) in untreated 20 month old ABCA4$^{-/-}$ mice at 406 nm ex/>409 nm em. The demarcation of two regions of interest (ROI) in the RPE layer are shown. Analogous image for 20 month old ABCA4$^{-/-}$ mouse treated with 10 μg/ml ticagrelor in drinking water for 4 days. **(H)** Mean autofluorescence output for key excitation/emission pairs wavelengths (λ, as indicated; $^*p < 0.05$, $n = 16$ untreated, 10 treated sections from 4 to 5 mice respectively).

POSs, suggesting pH manipulation can enhance turnover of phagocytosed waste (Baltazar et al., 2012).

In addition to modulating the activity of lysosomal enzymes, decreased autofluorescence in RPE cells may reflect an enhanced exocytosis of waste material. The *bis*-retinoid A2E is present in high levels in the RPE cells of ABCA4$^{-/-}$ mice (Mata et al., 2001). Although the endogenous breakdown of A2E is difficult (Wu et al., 2011), A2E shows a peak autofluorescence emission at 570 nm when excited at 380 nm (Sparrow et al., 1999), and the decrease in this emission in mice receiving ticagrelor suggests the A2E may be exocytosed. The TRPML1 channel contributes to the exocytosis of lysosomal waste; TRPML1 activity is pH dependent (Samie et al., 2013; Li et al., 2017), and recent studies suggest the TRPML1 channel is particularly active in RPE cells (Goméz et al., 2018). It is possible that enhanced exocytosis may contribute to the reduced autofluorescence in ABCA4$^{-/-}$ mice receiving ticagrelor, although further experiments are needed to confirm this.

Remaining Issues

Several additional issues remain unresolved in this study. For example, it is not clear why elderly ABCA4$^{-/-}$ mice required an extended treatment with ticagrelor before lysosomal pH was reduced, while there was no detectable trend between treatment length and the lysosomal acidification in mice receiving ticagrelor in their drinking water, especially as plasma concentrations of ticagrelor did not increase with prolonged dosage. Furthermore, it is unclear why the decline in RPE autofluorescence was limited to the inferior/nasal regions of the whole mounts. Regional

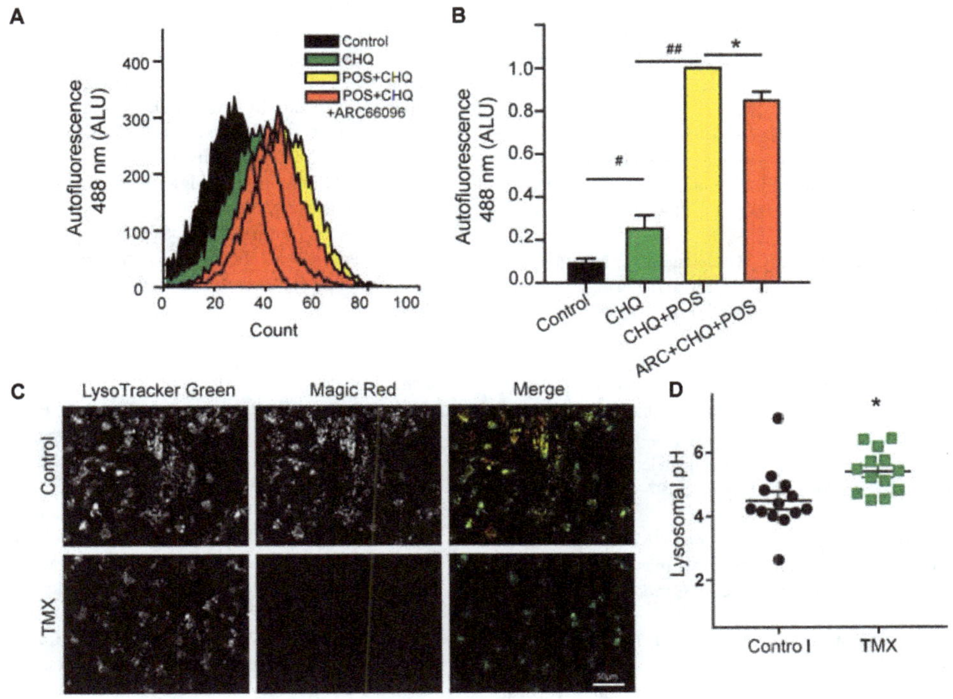

FIGURE 4 | Blocking $P2Y_{12}$ reduces RPE autofluorescence *in vitro*. **(A)** Treatment of ARPE-19 cells with POSs and 10 μM chloroquine (CHQ) using the pulse chase method led to a substantial rise in autofluorescence at 488 nm ex/>525 nm em. FACS analysis demonstrates the increased autofluorescence with the CHQ/POS treatment for >6 days. Treatment of cells with 10 μM $P2Y_{12}$ receptor antagonist AR-C66096 shifted the autofluorescence curve to the left. **(B)** Quantification of the mean autofluorescence from five independent FACS trials showing a significant reduction in POS/CHQ autofluorescence excited at 488 nm in cells treated with 10 μM AR-C66096 (#$p = 0.02$, ##$p < 0.001$, *$p = 0.014$, $n = 5$). **(C)** ARPE-19 cells displaying overlap of Magic Red and LysoTracker Green, suggesting cathepsin B activity in lysosomes under control conditions (top). Magic Red staining was eliminated by elevation of lysosomal pH with 10 μM tamoxifen (bottom). **(D)** Tamoxifen (10 μM) raises lysosomal pH in ARPE-19 cells (*$p = 0.012$, $n = 13$).

differences in photoreceptor death occur with light damage models, with degree of light and differential levels of rhodopsin implicated (Organisciak and Vaughan, 2010); both of these parameters could influence the clearance of autofluorescence by ticagrelor. The mechanisms by which ticagrelor can decrease expression of CFH and ENT1 are also unclear; neither gene is linked to the CLEAR network directly regulated by lysosomal activity suggesting a more indirect connection (Palmieri et al., 2011). As discussed above, the relative effects of ticagrelor on lysosomal degradation versus exocytosis of autofluorescent waste are also relevant. Future work is needed to address these issues.

Relevance to Human Doses

Given that ticagrelor is used in mainly elderly patients, the comparison of doses used here in mice with human dosage is relevant. Plasma levels in mice receiving 0.1% ticagrelor in food were 0.89 μM; this corresponds to 465 ng/mL and is close to levels in mice reported recently on 0.1% ticagrelor (Preusch et al., 2016). In humans receiving the standard dose of 180 mg/day, plasma concentrations of ticagrelor ranged from a maximum of 770 ng/ml 2 h after dosing to a minimum of 227 ng/mL (Storey et al., 2007, 2016). This suggests the levels of ticagrelor that lower lysosomal pH and decrease autofluorescence in mice are within the range found in patients. Whether treatments with ticagrelor can protect vision in $ABCA4^{-/-}$ mice is currently being evaluated.

Portions of this work have previously been presented in abstract form (Lu et al., 2017).

AUTHOR CONTRIBUTIONS

WL, NG, JL, SG, EC, AO, and KC performed the experiments. SM, LC, AL, and CM wrote the manuscript. CM and AL conceived of the idea.

FUNDING

This work was supported by grants from the NIH EY013434 and EY015537 and core grant EY001583 (CM), the Jody Sack Fund (WL), and AstraZeneca.

ACKNOWLEDGMENTS

We would like to thank Gabriel Baltazar for help with lysosomal pH and Magic Red measurements, Bruce Shenker and Ali Zekavat for assistance with the Flow Cytometry, Ann-Sofie Sandinge for the analysis of ticagrelor in plasma and Renato DeRita for his help coordinating with AstraZeneca.

REFERENCES

Albalawi, F., Lu, W., Beckel, J. M., Lim, J. C., McCaughey, S. A., and Mitchell, C. H. (2017). The P2X7 receptor primes IL-1β and the NLRP3 inflammasome in astrocytes exposed to mechanical strain. *Front. Cell. Neurosci.* 11:227. doi: 10.3389/fncel.2017.00227

Armstrong, D., Summers, C., Ewart, L., Nylander, S., Sidaway, J. E., and van Giezen, J. J. (2014). Characterization of the adenosine pharmacology of ticagrelor reveals therapeutically relevant inhibition of equilibrative nucleoside transporter 1. *J. Cardiovasc. Pharmacol. Ther.* 19, 209–219. doi: 10.1177/1074248413511693

Aungraheeta, R., Conibear, A., Butler, M., Kelly, E., Nylander, S., Mumford, A., et al. (2016). Inverse agonism at the P2Y12 receptor and ENT1 transporter blockade contribute to platelet inhibition by ticagrelor. *Blood* 128, 2717–2728. doi: 10.1182/blood-2016-03-707844

Baltazar, G. C., Guha, S., Boesze-Battaglia, K., Laties, A. M., Tyagi, P., Kompella, U. B., et al. (2012). Acidic nanoparticles restore lysosomal pH and degradative function in compromised RPE cells. *PLoS One* 7:e49635. doi: 10.1007/978-1-4614-3209-8_14

Birkeland, K., Parra, D., and Rosenstein, R. (2010). Antiplatelet therapy in acute coronary syndromes: focus on ticagrelor. *J. Blood Med.* 1, 197–219. doi: 10.2147/JBM.S9650

Bonaca, M. P., Bhatt, D. L., Storey, R. F., Steg, P. G., Cohen, M., Kuder, J., et al. (2016). Ticagrelor for prevention of ischemic events after myocardial infarction in patients with peripheral artery disease. *J. Am. Coll. Cardiol.* 67, 2719–2728. doi: 10.1016/j.jacc.2016.03.524

Cattaneo, M. (2015). P2Y12 receptors: structure and function. *J. Thromb. Haemost.* 13(Suppl. 1), S10–S16. doi: 10.1111/jth.12952

Charbel Issa, P., Barnard, A. R., Singh, M. S., Carter, E., Jiang, Z., Radu, R. A., et al. (2013). Fundus autofluorescence in the Abca4(−/−) mouse model of Stargardt disease–correlation with accumulation of A2E, retinal function, and histology. *Invest. Ophthalmol. Vis. Sci.* 54, 5602–5612. doi: 10.1167/iovs.13-11688

Coffey, E. E., Beckel, J. M., Laties, A. M., and Mitchell, C. H. (2014). Lysosomal alkalization and dysfunction in human fibroblasts with the Alzheimer's disease-linked presenilin 1 A246E mutation can be reversed with cAMP. *Neuroscience* 263, 111–124. doi: 10.1016/j.neuroscience.2014.01.001

Creasy, B. M., Hartmann, C. B., White, F. K., and McCoy, K. L. (2007). New assay using fluorogenic substrates and immunofluorescence staining to measure cysteine cathepsin activity in live cell subpopulations. *Cytometry A* 71, 114–123. doi: 10.1002/cyto.a.20365

Eckle, T., Hughes, K., Ehrentraut, H., Brodsky, K. S., Rosenberger, P., Choi, D. S., et al. (2013). Crosstalk between the equilibrative nucleoside transporter ENT2 and alveolar Adora2b adenosine receptors dampens acute lung injury. *FASEB J.* 27, 3078–3089. doi: 10.1096/fj.13-228551

Ferris, F. L. III, Wilkinson, C. P., Bird, A., Chakravarthy, U., Chew, E., Csaky, K., et al. (2013). Clinical classification of age-related macular degeneration. *Ophthalmology* 120, 844–851. doi: 10.1016/j.ophtha.2012.10.036

Goel, D. (2013). Ticagrelor: the first approved reversible oral antiplatelet agent. *Int. J. Appl. Basic Med. Res.* 3, 19–21. doi: 10.4103/2229-516X.112234

Goméz, N. M., Lu, W., Lim, J. C., Kiselyov, K., Campagno, K. E., Grishchuk, Y., et al. (2018). Robust lysosomal calcium signaling through channel TRPML1 is impaired by lipofuscin accumulation. *FASEB J.* 32, 782–794. doi: 10.1096/fj.201700220RR

Guha, S., Baltazar, G. C., Coffey, E. E., Tu, L. A., Lim, J. C., Beckel, J. M., et al. (2013). Lysosomal alkalinization, lipid oxidation, impaired autophagy and reduced phagosome clearance triggered by P2X7 receptor activation in retinal pigmented epithelial cells. *FASEB J.* 27, 4500–4509. doi: 10.1096/fj.13-236166

Guha, S., Baltazar, G. C., Tu, L. A., Liu, J., Lim, J. C., Lu, W., et al. (2012). Stimulation of the D5 dopamine receptor acidifies the lysosomal pH of retinal pigmented epithelial cells and decreases accumulation of autofluorescent photoreceptor debris. *J. Neurochem.* 122, 823–833. doi: 10.1111/j.1471-4159.2012.07804.x

Guha, S., Coffey, E. E., Lu, W., Lim, J. C., Beckel, J. M., Laties, A. M., et al. (2014a). Approaches for detecting lysosomal alkalinization and impaired degradation in fresh and cultured RPE cells: evidence for a role in retinal degenerations. *Exp. Eye Res.* 126, 68–76. doi: 10.1016/j.exer.2014.05.013

Guha, S., Liu, J., Baltazar, G. C., Laties, A. M., and Mitchell, C. H. (2014b). Rescue of compromised lysosomes enhances degradation of photoreceptor outer segments and reduce lipofuscin-like autofluorescence. *Adv. Exp. Med. Biol.* 801, 105–111. doi: 10.1007/978-1-4614-3209-8_14

Holz, F. G., Schutt, F., Kopitz, J., Eldred, G. E., Kruse, F. E., Volcker, H. E., et al. (1999). Inhibition of lysosomal degradative functions in RPE cells by a retinoid component of lipofuscin. *Invest. Ophthalmol. Vis. Sci.* 40, 737–743.

Jacobson, K. A., Ivanov, A. A., de Castro, S., Harden, T. K., and Ko, H. (2009). Development of selective agonists and antagonists of P2Y receptors. *Purinergic Signal.* 5, 75–89. doi: 10.1007/s11302-008-9106-2

Lee, J. H., McBrayer, M. K., Wolfe, D. M., Haslett, L. J., Kumar, A., Sato, Y., et al. (2015). Presenilin 1 maintains lysosomal Ca^{2+} homeostasis via TRPML1 by regulating vATPase-mediated lysosome acidification. *Cell Rep.* 12, 1430–1444. doi: 10.1016/j.celrep.2015.07.050

Lee, J. H., Yu, W. H., Kumar, A., Lee, S., Mohan, P. S., Peterhoff, C. M., et al. (2010). Lysosomal proteolysis and autophagy require presenilin 1 and are disrupted by Alzheimer-related PS1 mutations. *Cell* 141, 1146–1158. doi: 10.1016/j.cell.2010.05.008

Li, M., Zhang, W. K., Benvin, N. M., Zhou, X., Su, D., Li, H., et al. (2017). Structural basis of dual Ca^{2+}/pH regulation of the endolysosomal TRPML1 channel. *Nat. Struct. Mol. Biol.* 24, 205–213. doi: 10.1038/nsmb.3362

Liu, J., Lu, W., Guha, S., Baltazar, G. C., Coffey, E. E., Laties, A. M., et al. (2012). Cystic fibrosis transmembrane conductance regulator (CFTR) contributes to reacidification of alkalinized lysosomes in RPE cells. *Am. J. Physiol. Cell Physiol.* 303, C160–C169. doi: 10.1152/ajpcell.00278.2011

Liu, J., Lu, W., Reigada, D., Nguyen, J., Laties, A. M., and Mitchell, C. H. (2008). Restoration of lysosomal pH in RPE cells from cultured human and ABCA4(−/−) mice: pharmacologic approaches and functional recovery. *Invest. Ophthalmol. Vis. Sci.* 49, 772–780. doi: 10.1167/iovs.07-0675

Lu, W., Albalawi, F., Beckel, J. M., Lim, J. C., Laties, A. M., and Mitchell, C. H. (2017). The P2X7 receptor links mechanical strain to cytokine IL-6 up-regulation and release in neurons and astrocytes. *J. Neurochem.* 141, 436–448. doi: 10.1111/jnc.13998

Mata, N. L., Tzekov, R. T., Liu, X., Weng, J., Birch, D. G., and Travis, G. H. (2001). Delayed dark-adaptation and lipofuscin accumulation in abcr+/− mice: implications for involvement of ABCR in age-related macular degeneration. *Invest. Ophthalmol. Vis. Sci.* 42, 1685–1690.

McFadyen, J. D., Schaff, M., and Peter, K. (2018). Current and future antiplatelet therapies: emphasis on preserving haemostasis. *Nat. Rev. Cardiol.* 15, 181–191. doi: 10.1038/nrcardio.2017.206

Nylander, S., Femia, E. A., Scavone, M., Berntsson, P., Asztely, A. K., Nelander, K., et al. (2013). Ticagrelor inhibits human platelet aggregation via adenosine in addition to P2Y12 antagonism. *J. Thromb. Haemost.* 11, 1867–1876. doi: 10.1111/jth.12360

Nylander, S., and Schulz, R. (2016). Effects of P2Y12 receptor antagonists beyond platelet inhibition–comparison of ticagrelor with thienopyridines. *Br. J. Pharmacol.* 173, 1163–1178. doi: 10.1111/bph.13429

Organisciak, D. T., and Vaughan, D. K. (2010). Retinal light damage: mechanisms and protection. *Prog. Retin. Eye Res.* 29, 113–134. doi: 10.1016/j.preteyeres.2009.11.004

Palmieri, M., Impey, S., Kang, H., di Ronza, A., Pelz, C., Sardiello, M., et al. (2011). Characterization of the CLEAR network reveals an integrated control of cellular clearance pathways. *Hum. Mol. Genet.* 20, 3852–3866. doi: 10.1093/hmg/ddr306

Preusch, M. R., Rusnak, J., Staudacher, K., Mogler, C., Uhlmann, L., Sievers, P., et al. (2016). Ticagrelor promotes atherosclerotic plaque stability in a mouse model of advanced atherosclerosis. *Drug Des. Devel. Ther.* 10, 2691–2699. doi: 10.2147/DDDT.S105718

Radu, R. A., Hu, J., Jiang, Z., and Bok, D. (2014). Bisretinoid-mediated complement activation on retinal pigment epithelial cells is dependent on complement factor H haplotype. *J. Biol. Chem.* 289, 9113–9120. doi: 10.1074/jbc.M114.548669

Reigada, D., Lu, W., Zhang, X., Friedman, C., Pendrak, K., McGlinn, A., et al. (2005). Degradation of extracellular ATP by the retinal pigment epithelium. *Am. J. Physiol. Cell Physiol.* 289, C617–C624. doi: 10.1152/ajpcell.00542.2004

Samie, M., Wang, X., Zhang, X., Goschka, A., Li, X., Cheng, X., et al. (2013). A TRP channel in the lysosome regulates large particle phagocytosis via focal exocytosis. *Dev. Cell* 26, 511–524. doi: 10.1016/j.devcel.2013.08.003

Sparrow, J. R., Parish, C. A., Hashimoto, M., and Nakanishi, K. (1999). A2E, a lipofuscin fluorophore, in human retinal pigmented epithelial cells in culture. *Invest. Ophthalmol. Vis. Sci.* 40, 2988–2995.

Storey, R. F., Angiolillo, D. J., Bonaca, M. P., Thomas, M. R., Judge, H. M., Rollini, F., et al. (2016). Platelet inhibition with ticagrelor 60 mg versus 90 mg twice daily in the PEGASUS-TIMI 54 trial. *J. Am. Coll. Cardiol.* 67, 1145–1154. doi: 10.1016/j.jacc.2015.12.062

Storey, R. F., Angiolillo, D. J., Patil, S. B., Desai, B., Ecob, R., Husted, S., et al. (2010). Inhibitory effects of ticagrelor compared with clopidogrel on platelet function in patients with acute coronary syndromes: the PLATO (PLATelet inhibition and patient Outcomes) PLATELET substudy. *J. Am. Coll. Cardiol.* 56, 1456–1462. doi: 10.1016/j.jacc.2010.03.100

Storey, R. F., Husted, S., Harrington, R. A., Heptinstall, S., Wilcox, R. G., Peters, G., et al. (2007). Inhibition of platelet aggregation by AZD6140, a reversible oral P2Y12 receptor antagonist, compared with clopidogrel in patients with acute coronary syndromes. *J. Am. Coll. Cardiol.* 50, 1852–1856. doi: 10.1016/j.jacc.2007.07.058

Streitova, D., Sefc, L., Savvulidi, F., Pospisil, M., Hola, J., and Hofer, M. (2010). Adenosine A(1), A(2a), A(2b), and A(3) receptors in hematopoiesis. 1. Expression of receptor mRNA in four mouse hematopoietic precursor cells. *Physiol. Res.* 59, 133–137.

Tantry, U. S., Bliden, K. P., Wei, C., Storey, R. F., Armstrong, M., Butler, K., et al. (2010). First analysis of the relation between CYP2C19 genotype and pharmacodynamics in patients treated with ticagrelor versus clopidogrel: the ONSET/OFFSET and RESPOND genotype studies. *Circ. Cardiovasc. Genet.* 3, 556–566. doi: 10.1161/CIRCGENETICS.110.958561

Toops, K. A., Tan, L. X., Jiang, Z., Radu, R. A., and Lakkaraju, A. (2015). Cholesterol-mediated activation of acid sphingomyelinase disrupts autophagy in the retinal pigment epithelium. *Mol. Biol. Cell* 26, 1–14. doi: 10.1091/mbc.E14-05-1028

Veitinger, S., Veitinger, T., Cainarca, S., Fluegge, D., Engelhardt, C. H., Lohmer, S., et al. (2011). Purinergic signalling mobilizes mitochondrial Ca^{2+} in mouse Sertoli cells. *J. Physiol.* 589, 5033–5055. doi: 10.1113/jphysiol.2011.216309

Wu, Y., Zhou, J., Fishkin, N., Rittmann, B. E., and Sparrow, J. R. (2011). Enzymatic degradation of A2E, a retinal pigment epithelial lipofuscin bisretinoid. *J. Am. Chem. Soc.* 133, 849–857. doi: 10.1021/ja107195u

9

Pharmacological Blockade of Adenosine A_{2A} but not A_1 Receptors Enhances Goal-Directed Valuation in Satiety-Based Instrumental Behavior

Yan Li[1†], Xinran Pan[2†], Yan He[2†], Yang Ruan[2], Linshan Huang[2], Yuling Zhou[2], Zhidong Hou[2], Chaoxiang He[2], Zhe Wang[1], Xiong Zhang[1] and Jiang-Fan Chen[2,3*]*

[1] Department of Neurology, The Second Affiliated Hospital and Yuying Children's Hospital of Wenzhou Medical University, Wenzhou, China, [2] School of Optometry and Ophthalmology and Eye Hospital, The Institute of Molecular Medicine, Wenzhou Medical University, Wenzhou, China, [3] Department of Neurology, School of Medicine, Boston University, Boston, MA, United States

***Correspondence:**
Xiong Zhang
zhangxiong98@gmail.com
Jiang-Fan Chen
chenjf@bu.edu

† These authors have contributed equally to this work.

The balance and smooth shift between flexible, goal-directed behaviors and repetitive, habitual actions are critical to optimal performance of behavioral tasks. The striatum plays an essential role in control of goal-directed versus habitual behaviors through a rich interplay of the numerous neurotransmitters and neuromodulators to modify the input, processing and output functions of the striatum. The adenosine receptors (namely $A_{2A}R$ and A_1R), with their high expression pattern in the striatum and abilities to interact and integrate dopamine, glutamate and cannabinoid signals in the striatum, may represent novel therapeutic targets for modulating instrumental behavior. In this study, we examined the effects of pharmacological blockade of the $A_{2A}Rs$ and A_1Rs on goal-directed versus habitual behaviors in different information processing phases of instrumental learning using a satiety-based instrumental behavior procedure. We found that $A_{2A}R$ antagonist acts at the coding, consolidation and expression phases of instrumental learning to modulate animals' sensitivity to goal-directed valuation without modifying action-outcome contingency. However, pharmacological blockade and genetic knockout of A_1Rs did not affect acquisition or sensitivity to goal-valuation of instrumental behavior. These findings provide pharmacological evidence for a potential therapeutic strategy to control abnormal instrumental behaviors associated with drug addiction and obsessive-compulsive disorder by targeting the $A_{2A}R$.

Keywords: adenosine A_{2A} receptor, adenosine A_1 receptor, goal-directed behavior, habit, instrumental behavior

INTRODUCTION

Goal-directed and habitual behaviors are crucial adaptive behaviors for our daily life. Goal-directed behavior evaluates actions prospectively and can flexibly adjust action depending on environmental changes, but this comes at the cost of more cognitive resource. By contrast, habitual behavior is usually developed after repeated overtraining for days and represents automatic responses elicited by external or internal triggers during the performance of routine procedures with less cognitive loads (Dolan and Dayan, 2013). These two behavioral processes can develop in parallel or sequentially and can also reciprocally compete with each other for behavioral control

(Yin and Knowlton, 2006; Balleine and O'Doherty, 2010; Kim and Hikosaka, 2015). The balance between flexible goal-directed actions and repetitive habitual behaviors has an essential role in achieving optimal performance of behavioral task. Dysregulation of goal-directed versus habitual behaviors is considered to be a potential mechanism underlying the relapse of drug addiction (Ostlund and Balleine, 2008), obsessive compulsive disorder (Gillan et al., 2011; Robbins et al., 2012; Burguiere et al., 2015), and may contribute to the executive dysfunction in Parkinson's (Redgrave et al., 2010; de Wit et al., 2011) and Huntington's disease patients (Lawrence et al., 1998).

The striatum plays an essential role in control of goal-directed versus habitual behaviors (Yin and Knowlton, 2006; Graybiel and Grafton, 2015; Kim and Hikosaka, 2015). The dorsal medial striatum (DMS)-connecting orbitofrontal cortex (OFC) is critical for goal-directed valuation (Gremel and Costa, 2013), while the dorsal lateral striatum (DLS) and its connecting infralimbic cortex act as dual operators for habitual behavioral control (Smith and Graybiel, 2013a,b). Additionally, the accumbens nucleus (NAc)-ventral Pallidum (VP) pathway is necessary for goal-directed valuation as inactivation of NAc-VP pathway impairs the predictive learning (Leung and Balleine, 2013). Furthermore, the nigro-striatal dopamine signaling acts as a prediction error and motivational signal to drive instrumental learning (Glimcher, 2011; Rossi et al., 2013; Steinberg et al., 2013). Thus, the striatum acts as a key locus in integrating the cortico-striatal glutamate and the substantia nigra-striatal dopamine signals to control goal-directed and habitual behaviors.

The striatal control of instrumental behaviors is accomplished through a rich interplay of the numerous neurotransmitters and neuromodulators to modify the input, processing and output functions of the striatum (Lovinger, 2010). Several studies have documented the involvement of the D_2 receptor (Kwak et al., 2014), cannabinoid receptor type 1 (CB_1R) (Hilario et al., 2007) and 5-hydroxytryptamine 6 (5-HT_6) receptor (Eskenazi et al., 2015) in control of instrumental behavior. However, pharmacological control of instrumental behaviors is under-explored and the effective pharmacological strategies for the control of goal-directed versus habitual behaviors are lacking. Adenosine A_1 and A_{2A} receptors are highly expressed in the striatum and are increasingly recognized as important pharmacological targets for controlling cognition under normal and disease conditions (Chen et al., 2013; Chen, 2014). The Gs-coupled facilitating A_{2A} receptor ($A_{2A}R$) and Gi-coupled inhibitory A_1 receptor (A_1R) both integrate dopamine (Shen W. et al., 2008), glutamate (Kreitzer and Malenka, 2007), and BNDF (Tebano et al., 2008; Wei et al., 2014) signaling to modulate synaptic plasticity and control cognition. For example, using our newly developed chimeric rhodopsin-$A_{2A}R$ proteins (opto$A_{2A}R$), we recently demonstrated that transient activation of $A_{2A}R$ by light in a time-locked manner with reward delivery is sufficient to impair goal-directed behavior whereas focal knockdown of $A_{2A}R$ in the striatum enhances goal-directed behaviors (Yu et al., 2009; Li et al., 2016). Similarly, pharmacological blockade of $A_{2A}R$ promoted goal-directed seeking for ethanol in ENT1 knockout mice (Nam et al., 2013b) and restored goal-directed sensitivity to negative feedback in the methamphetamine (METH)-paired context (Furlong et al., 2017). These pharmacological, genetic, and optogenetic demonstrations of the cognitive "brake" mechanism of $A_{2A}R$ activation led us to propose that pharmacological blockade of the $A_{2A}R$ represents a promising therapeutic target for controlling goal-directed behaviors.

As the first step in developing an adenosine receptor-based pharmacological approach to control the goal-directed versus habitual behaviors, we coupled the $A_{2A}R$ antagonist (KW6002) and A_1R antagonist (DPCPX) with the satiety-based instrumental learning paradigm to address the effect of pharmacological blockade of the $A_{2A}R$ and A_1R on three aspects of instrumental learning processes: (i) behavioral elements of instrumental behaviors (i.e., acquisition of action-outcome contingency versus goal-evaluation) by acquisition of instrumental behavior, the devaluation test and the omission test; (ii) the instrumental learning processes by administering the $A_{2A}R$ antagonist either prior to the training (learning/encoding) or post-training (consolidation) during the random interval (RI) schedule, or immediately before the devaluation and omission tests (expression/retrieval of instrumental behaviors); (iii) the potential role of the A_1 receptor in control of instrumental learning.

MATERIALS AND METHODS

Animals

Animals were handled in accordance with the protocols approved by the Institutional Ethics Committee for Animal Use in Research and Education at Wenzhou Medical University, China. C57BL/6 male mice at least 8 weeks old (23–27 g each) were used in the experiments. The A_1R knockout mice ($A_1R^{-/-}$=$^{+/+}$) and wild-type littermate controls (A_1RC=C) have been well characterized previously (Johansson et al., 2001) and confirmed by PCR analysis of gene identification before the experiment. Mice were housed in an ambient temperature of 22 ± 0.5°C and a relative humidity of 60 ± 2% with a 12 h light/dark cycle. Mice were single-housed and underwent experiments in the light cycle.

Satiety-Based Instrumental Training and Testing

All instrumental learning experiments were performed in standard operant chambers (Med Associates). Each chamber was equipped with a retractable lever on either side of a pump with a syringe that delivered liquid reward (20% sucrose solution, 20 μl/reinforce which can be suspended from the syringe) and a house light (3 W, 24 V) mounted on the opposite side of the chamber. Training and testing procedures were performed following Rossi et al (Rossi and Yin, 2012) and illustrated in **Figure 1A**. In brief, mice were first given one 30-min magazine training session during which the sucrose solution was delivered on a random time 60 s schedule with the lever removed. Three days of continuous reinforcement (CRF) training sessions were followed to sufficiently establish the initial association between lever press and reward. At the start of the session, the house light was illuminated, and one lever was inserted into

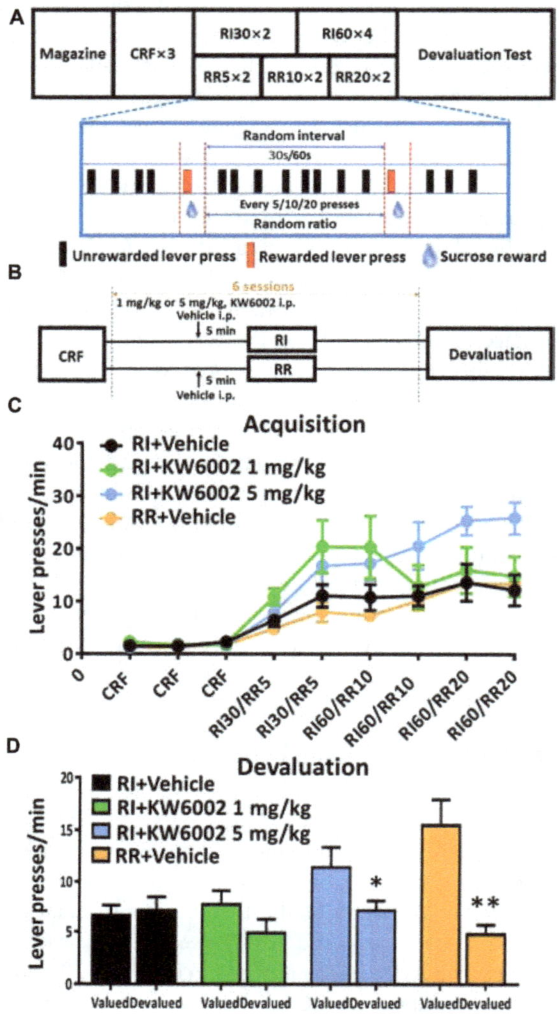

FIGURE 1 | Pharmacological blockade of A_{2A}Rs promoted goal-directed valuation. **(A)** Satiety-based instrumental behavior design schematic. Mice underwent Magazine-CRF-RI/RR-Devaluation procedure sequentially. CRF, continuous reinforcement; RI, random interval; RR, random ratio. **(B)** KW6002 and vehicle were injected intraperitoneally 5 min before daily RI training session at different doses (1 and 5 mg/kg), meanwhile vehicle was administrated 5 min before daily RR training session as another control group to form goal-directed behavior **(C)**. All mice gradually increased their lever presses in the RI/RR training sessions (training main effect: $p < 0.001$). There was the interaction effect of training sessions X drug administration groups ($p = 0.006$) and between subject effect of different drug administration groups ($p = 0.022$). The statistical significance was only observed between RI+KW6002 5 mg/kg and RR + Vehicle groups (*post hoc* by Bonferroni test, $p = 0.035$). **(D)** In the devaluation test, mice trained with RI and RR procedures performed habitual ($p = 0.755$) and goal-directed ($p = 0.002$, $^{**}p < 0.01$) behaviors, respectively, as designed. Mice received 1 mg/kg KW6002 tended to decrease their lever presses in the devalued condition but with no statistical significance ($p = 0.141$), while mice of 5 mg/kg group displayed markedly goal-directed performance in the devaluation test ($p = 0.030$, $^{*}p < 0.05$). All data was analyzed by two-way ANOVA for repeated measurement, followed by *post hoc* comparison with Bonferroni test [RI group, $n = 8$; RI+KW6002 (1 mg/kg) group, $n = 7$; RI+KW6002 (5 mg/kg) group, $n = 8$; RR group, $n = 9$].

the chamber. The house light remained illuminated and the lever remained inserted and active during the entire session. During CRF session, each lever press resulted in the delivery of one drop of 20 μl 20% sucrose solution. Sessions ended after 60 min or when 50 rewards had been earned, whichever came first. After CRF, mice underwent RI schedule which was critical for habitual learning. They were trained 2 days on RI 30 s, with a 0.1 probability of reward availability every 3 s contingent upon lever pressing, followed by 4 days on the 60 s interval schedules (0.1 probability of reward availability every 6 s contingent upon lever pressing). Just as CRF training, RI sessions ended after 60 min or when 50 rewards had been earned, whichever came first. To further confirm goal-directed behavioral pattern, we also employed random ratio (RR) training paradigm as control which contributed to goal-directed behavior. Progressively leaner schedules of reinforcement were used: CRF for 3 days, then RR 5 for 2 days (RR5; each response was rewarded at a probability of 0.2 on average), RR10 for 2 days and finally RR20 for 2 days. In the training sessions, home chows were given 1.5–2g daily to maintain 80–85% of their free-feeding weight.

Following the RI/RR training sessions, a 2-day devaluation test was conducted. A specific satiety procedure was applied to alter the current value of a specific reward. On each day the mice were allowed to have free access to home chows, which were used for maintaining their weights in the training sessions or sucrose solution which was earned by their lever pressing for at least an hour to achieve sensory-specific satiety. Immediately after the unlimited pre-feeding session, mice were given a 5-min extinction test during which the lever was inserted and pressing times were recorded without reward delivery. The order of the valued and devalued condition tests (day 1 or day 2) was counterbalanced across animals. Mice sensitive to manipulation of outcome value would significantly reduce their lever presses on the devalued condition compared with the valued condition. Then after two supplementary RI60 training sessions, mice were further evaluated by a 30-min omission test in which action-outcome contingency was altered. In the omission test, mice had to control their lever-press impulsion formed by previous training sessions for 20 s to obtain the reward. Any lever press would reset the time counter and mice would hold another 20 s not to press the lever for reward delivery.

Drug Administration

The following drugs were used in the present study: KW-6002 ((E)-1,3-diethyl-8-(3,4-dimethoxystyryl)-7-methyl-3,7-dihydro-1H-purine-2,6-dione, a selective adenosine A_{2A}R antagonist) and DPCPX (8-cyclopentyl-1,3-dipropylxanthine, a selective adenosine A_1R antagonist). KW-6002 (1 mg/kg, 5 mg/kg, Sundia, United States) was suspended in dimethyl sulfoxide (DMSO, sigma), ethoxylated castor oil (Sigma) and water with a proportion of 15%:15%:70%. DPCPX (6 mg/kg, Abcam) was dissolved in 0.9% NaCl with 5% DMSO. The control mice were treated with corresponding vehicles. All the solutions were prepared immediately before administration. The administered doses of KW-6002 and DPCPX referred to previous researches (Chen et al., 2001; Prediger et al., 2004; Nguyen et al., 2014). Drugs were injected intraperitoneally (i.p.) routinely in a volume of 0.1 ml/10 g of body weight. The specific drug administration time course depended on experimental designs: prior to (30 min before) and post (10 min after) everyday RI training for learning and consolidation periods of instrumental learning, respectively (**Figure 2A**), while treated 30 min before devaluation test/omission test, but not available in the RI training sessions for expression of instrumental behavior (**Figure 3A**).

DPCPX Concentration Detection

Considering the critical role of the striatum in control of instrumental behavior, we measured the concentration of DPCPX in the striatum of mice after intraperitoneal injection to verify the effective concentration of DPCPX. 30 min after DPCPX (6 mg/kg, i.p.) administration, the striata of mice were collected and homogenized. 0.1 ml of collected homogenate was added to a 1.5 ml centrifuge tube and followed by the addition of 0.01 ml methanol and 0.3ml of acetonitrile. The tubes were vortex mixed for 0.5 min. After centrifugation at 13,000 rpm for 10 min, 100 μl of supernatant was transferred to an autosampler vial. Next, 2 μl of the mixture was injected into the LC-MS/MS system for analysis. DCPCX concentrations were determined by ultrahigh performance liquid chromatography with mass spectrometry method (UHPLC-MS/MS). UHPLC-MS/MS analyses were performed by an Agilent UHPLC unit (Agilent Corporation, MA, United States) with a ZORBAX Eclipse Plus C18 column (1.8 μm, 2.1 × 50 mm, I.D. Agilent

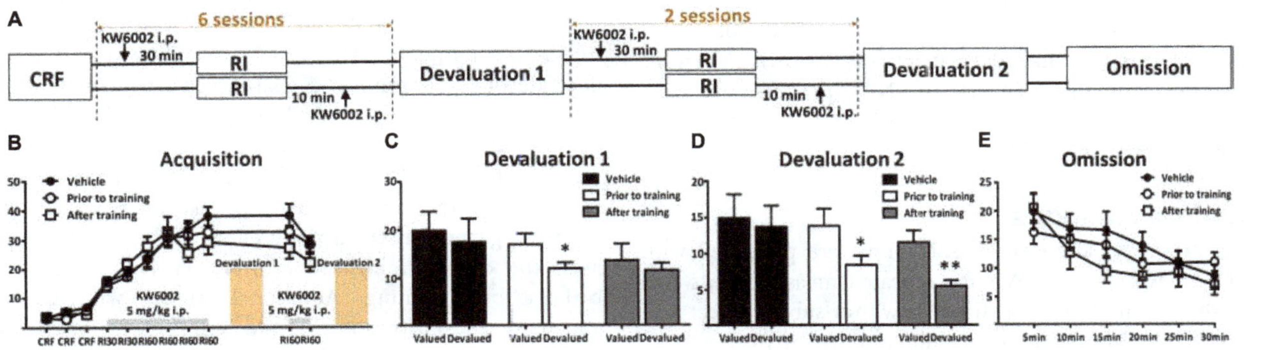

FIGURE 2 | Pharmacological blockade of $A_{2A}Rs$ prior to and post daily training session promoted goal-directed seeking but not acquisition of instrumental conditioning. **(A)** Experimental design schematic with KW6002 injected intraperitoneally prior to and post-training. **(B)** There was no significant difference in acquisition of instrumental learning among these groups for lack of between groups effect ($p = 0.593$) and training X drug administration groups interaction effect ($p = 0.108$). **(C)** In the first devaluation test, mice with KW6002 injected prior to training showed sensitive to outcome devaluation ($p = 0.021$, $^*p < 0.05$), compared to vehicle ($p = 0.223$) and that with KW6002 treated post-training ($p = 0.539$). **(D)** Then after two additional days of RI60 training, whatever KW6002 administered prior to ($p = 0.034$, $^*p < 0.05$) or post ($p = 0.008$, $^{**}p < 0.01$) training, mice displayed sensitive to outcome devaluation in the second devaluation test compared to the vehicle group ($p = 0.482$). **(E)** All mice decreased their lever presses indistinctively in the omission test in which the action-outcome contingency was reversed, showing neither testing time X drug administration groups interaction effect ($p = 0.359$) nor between-subject effect of drug administered groups ($p = 0.836$). All data was analyzed by two-way ANOVA for repeated measurement, followed by *post hoc* comparison with Bonferroni test ($n = 8$/group).

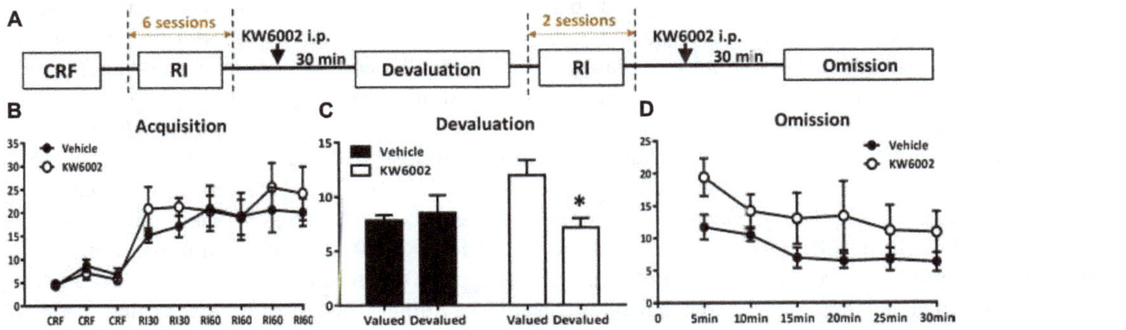

FIGURE 3 | Pharmacological blockade of $A_{2A}Rs$ specifically in the expression phase of instrumental conditioning selectively promote goal-directed valuation but not action-outcome contingency. **(A)** Experimental design schematic with KW6002 injected intraperitoneally in the expression phase (i.e., devaluation and omission test) of instrumental behavior but not available in the training sessions. **(B)** Mice established instrumental conditioning indistinctively in the acquisition phase without between pre-manipulation groups effect ($p = 0.541$) and interaction effect of training sessions X pre-manipulation groups ($p = 0.608$). **(C)** KW6002 5 mg/kg or vehicle was administered 30 min before reward/home chow condition (i.e., devalued/valued condition). After 1-h exposure to devalued/valued condition at liberty, the devaluation test was proceeded in which reward delivery was absent and lever presses was recorded. Mice with KW6002 injected performed more goal-directed ($p = 0.017$, $^*p < 0.05$), compared to that injected with vehicle ($p = 0.710$). **(D)** After 2-day extended RI60 training sessions, KW6002 5 mg/kg or vehicle was injected 30 min before omission test. Mice of both groups significant decreased their lever presses (time main effect, $p = 0.020$). But there was neither between-subject effect of drug treatments ($p = 0.089$) nor drug treatments X testing time interaction effect ($p = 0.728$). All data was analyzed by two-way ANOVA for repeated measurement, followed by *post hoc* comparison with Bonferroni test (vehicle group, $n = 8$; KW6002 group, $n = 7$).

Corporation, MA, United States) thermostated at 25°C. The mobile phase was composed of 0.1% formic acid (A) and acetonitrile (B) with gradient as follows: 0.0 min at 50% B, 0.0–2.0 min linear increase to 98% B, and 2.0–3.5 min at 50% B and the flow rate was 0.4 ml/min. The total run time was 3.5 min. The electrospray interface was maintained at 500°C. Nitrogen nebulization was performed with a nitrogen flow of 800 l/h. Argon was used as the collision gas. DPCPX was detected in multiple reaction monitoring (MRM) scan mode with positive ion detection. The precursor-product ion pairs used for the MRM detection were m/z 305.4 → 178.1 for DCPCX.

Quantitative PCR of A_1R mRNA

Striatal tissues from A_1R KO mice and their WT littermates were analyzed by the quantitative real-time polymerase chain reaction (qPCR) procedure as we have described previously (Zhang et al., 2015) using the following forward and reverse primers for A_1R mRNA: primers: forward, 5′-CATCCTGGCTC TGCTTGCTATT-3′; reverse and 5′-TTGGCTATCCAGGCTTGTTCC-3′.

Statistical Analysis

All data presented as mean ± SEM and were processed with SPSS 17.0. Two-way ANOVA for repeated measurements was used with training/testing sessions as within-subject effect and different drug administrations/genotypes as between-subject effect, followed by *post hoc* comparison by Bonferroni test, and with $p < 0.05$ as statistical significance.

RESULTS

Pharmacological Blockade of $A_{2A}Rs$ Promoted Goal-Directed Valuation

To perform flexible, goal-directed actions, animals must acquire the ability to encode both the *contingency* between a specific action and its outcome, and the current *value* of the outcome during instrumental conditioning (Balleine and Dickinson, 1998). We administered KW6002 (i.p. at 1 mg/kg or 5 mg/kg or vehicle) 5 min prior to everyday RI training session which was critical for establishment of habitual action (**Figure 1B**) to investigate the modulatory effect of $A_{2A}R$ blockade on the acquisition of instrumental behaviors. To better identify goal-directed behavioral pattern, we have also included another group of mice that were trained in parallel with RR paradigm which led to goal-directed behavior as control (**Figure 1B**). All mice gradually increased their lever presses and reached a platform eventually, indicating the successful training paradigm (**Figure 1C**). Mice treated with KW6002 at 5 mg/kg significantly elevated lever presses rate (interaction effect of training sessions X drug administration groups: $F_{5,140} = 2.659$, $p = 0.006$; between-subject effect of drug administration groups: $F_{3,28} = 3.740, p = 0.022$): the statistical significance was observed between the RI + KW6002 5 mg/kg and the RR + Vehicle groups (Bonferroni *post hoc* test, $p = 0.035$) but absent in any other comparison pairs including RI+KW6002 5 mg/kg versus RI + Vehicle groups (*post hoc* by Bonferroni test, $p = 0.116$).

The outcome devaluation procedure was used to demonstrate the importance of the evaluative components of goal-directed actions by $A_{2A}R$ blockade. In the devaluation test, lever presses rates between the valued and devalued conditions were compared (**Figure 1D**). Mice in the RI + Vehicle training group did not decrease lever presses in the devalued condition, showing no devaluation effect and indicating a habitual behavior ($F_{1,7} = 0.105$, $p = 0.755$), while the RR + Vehicle training group significantly decreased their lever presses ($F_{1,8} = 20.865$, $p = 0.002$), demonstrating goal-directed behavior. Notably, KW6002 at 1 mg/kg tended to decrease lever pressing rate in devalued condition compared to valued condition ($F_{1,6} = 2.867$, $p = 0.141$), whereas KW6002 at 5 mg/kg group showed markedly sensitive to outcome devaluation with decreased level pressing rate ($F_{1,7} = 7.418$, $p = 0.030$). Thus, pharmacological blockade of $A_{2A}R$ promoted goal-directed valuation. Whether the $A_{2A}R$ antagonist influence the acquisition of the instrumental learning need further clarification since the increased lever presses rate by KW6002 in the acquisition phase might be attributed to the improvement in instrumental learning or enhanced general motor activity effect of the $A_{2A}R$ antagonist given the drug administration immediately (~5 min) prior to behavioral training. Additional studies with the $A_{2A}R$ antagonist administration 30 min prior to or post training might better dissociate the learning from motor effect of $A_{2A}R$ antagonist.

Pharmacological Blockade of $A_{2A}R$ at the Coding, Consolidation and Expression Phases of Instrumental Behavior Exerted Its Enhanced Effect on Goal-Directed Valuation but Not on Action-Outcome Contingency

To further determine the modulatory effect of $A_{2A}R$ on the distinct processes of instrumental behavior (i.e., learning/coding, consolidation and expression phases), we administered KW6002 at specific time course of instrumental learning processes. Based on our previous study showing the effective biological (i.e., motor) effect of KW6002 5 mg/kg maintained for 150–170 min (Shen H.Y. et al., 2008; Yu et al., 2008), we selected the specific three time points for KW6002/vehicle administration (**Figures 2A, 3A**): (a) prior to training (30 min before RI training) or (b) post training (10 min after RI training) or (c) prior to behavioral testing (30 min before devaluation/omission test but not available in the RI training sessions) to determine the modulatory effects of KW6002 on coding and consolidation phases as well as the expression of instrumental behavior, respectively.

Figure 2B shows that KW6002 treatment either at the prior to-training phase or post-training phase did not affect the performance of mice during the RI sessions (main effect between drug administration groups, $F_{2,21} = 0.536$, $p = 0.593$ and training sessions X drug administration groups interaction effect, $F_{14,147} = 2.480$, $p = 0.108$). In the first devaluation test (**Figure 2C**), mice with vehicle injection formed a stable habitual behavior ($F_{1,7} = 1.787$, $p = 0.223$) as expected. Importantly, mice injected with KW6002 prior to everyday RI training session, which is the coding period, decreased their lever presses rate remarkably in the devalued condition ($F_{1,7} = 8.779, p = 0.021$), indicating blockade of $A_{2A}R$ enhanced goal-directed coding. However, since KW6002 post-training group did show some trend in decreasing lever pressing rate in the devaluation test, albeit not reaching statistical significance ($F_{1,7} = 0.417$, $p = 0.539$), we further explore the goal-directness promoting effect by KW6002 in the consolidation phase, by proceeding a 2-day complementary RI60 training sessions after the first devaluation test. Then we performed second devaluation test as illustrated in **Figure 2A**. After 2 additional days of RI training, both prior to-training and post-training groups significantly reduced lever presses in the devalued condition (prior to-training group, $F_{1,7} = 6.931$, $p = 0.034$; post-training group, $F_{1,7} = 13.413$, $p = 0.008$), i.e., goal-directed behavior, while control group (i.e., injected with vehicle) showed the characteristics of habitual behavior ($F_{1,7} = 0.552$, $p = 0.482$) (**Figure 2D**). Thus, KW6002 treatment in the consolidation phase of instrumental behavior promoted goal-directed behavior as well. Lastly, we performed the omission test during which the established lever press-reward association was reversed, so reward delivery depended on withholding the lever press action. As illustrated in **Figure 2E**, all mice decreased lever presses rate indistinctively in the omission test. Neither interaction effect of testing time X drug administration groups ($F_{10,105} = 1.124$, $p = 0.359$) nor main effect between drug administration groups ($F_{2,21} = 0.997$, $p = 0.836$) were detected. Thus, blockade of $A_{2A}Rs$ at the coding or consolidation phases of instrumental behavior enhanced goal-directed valuation but did not affect action-outcome association.

We then sought to investigate whether $A_{2A}R$ exerted its effect by acting on expression phase of instrumental behavior. In this experiment, KW6002 was administered 30 min before behavioral tests (devaluation and omission tests), but unavailable in all of the RI training sessions (**Figure 3A**). As expected, both pre-manipulation groups gradually increased lever presses rate and reached the platform and didn't show any difference between each other (between groups effect, $F_{1,13} = 0.395$, $p = 0.541$; interaction effect of training sessions X pre-manipulation groups, $F_{5,65} = 0.554$, $p = 0.608$) (**Figure 3B**). As **Figure 3C** shows, mice with KW6002 treatment at the expression phase displayed markedly sensitivity to outcome devaluation ($F_{1,6} = 10.857$, $p = 0.017$) compared with the controls ($F_{1,7} = 0.150, p = 0.710$) in the devaluation test. Thus, blockade of $A_{2A}R$ facilitated expression of goal-directed behavior. In the omission test (**Figure 3D**), both groups decreased their lever presses gradually over testing time (testing time main effect: $F_{5,65} = 4.226$, $p = 0.020$), indicating the timing effectiveness of the omission test. But the tendencies of lever-press decrease rate for the two groups were parallel as indicated by the absent of the drug treatments X testing time interaction effect ($F_{5,65} = 0.365$, $p = 0.728$), though mice injected with KW6002 apparently pressed more than that of the vehicle-treated mice (between-subject effect of drug treatments, $F_{1,13} = 3.369$, $p = 0.089$). The increased lever presses rate by KW6002 in the omission test might attribute to general motor but not learning effect of $A_{2A}R$ antagonist, for drug administration was 30 min before the test. Therefore, the action-outcome contingency may not be affected by $A_{2A}R$ antagonist.

Pharmacological Blockade and Genetic Knockout of A_1Rs Did Not Affect Acquisition or Goal-Evaluation of Instrumental Behavior

Adenosine acts on facilitating $A_{2A}R$ and inhibitory A_1R to integrate dopamine, glutamate, and BNDF signaling to modulate synaptic plasticity. We next investigated the possible involvement of A_1Rs in the modulation of instrumental behavior. To ensure the effective DPCPX drug concentration in the striatum after our A_1R pharmacological treatment paradigm, we determined the pharmacokinetic characteristic of DPCPX (**Figure 4A**) and showed the effective concentration of DPCPX in accordance with its biological effect as described previously (Baumgold et al., 1992). The A_1R antagonist DPCPX (6 mg/kg) did not affect lever pressing performance during instrumental training sessions (**Figure 4B**, main effect between drug administration groups, $F_{1,14} = 0.293$, $p = 0.597$; interaction effect of drug administration groups X training sessions, $F_{5,70} = 0.371$, $p = 0.867$). The devaluation test proceeded in drug-free condition (**Figure 4C**) revealed that mice with or without DPCPX treatment responded insensitively to satiety devaluation (DPCPX group, $F_{1,7} = 2.922$, $p = 0.131$; vehicle group, $F_{1,7} = 0.916$, $p = 0.370$). In addition, both groups of mice reduced lever presses indistinguishably in the omission test (**Figure 4D**, main effect between drug administration groups, $F_{1,14} = 0.129$, $p = 0.724$; interaction effect of drug administration groups X testing time, $F_{5,70} = 0.610$, $p = 0.580$).

To further confirm this finding by pharmacological blockade of A_1Rs, we determined the effect of genetic knockout of the A_1R on acquisition and goal-evaluation using A_1R knockout mice and their wild-type littermates. The nearly complete deletion of A_1Rs was verified by qPCR (**Figure 4E**). All mice, regardless of genotypes, increased their rate of lever pressing during the training sessions (**Figure 4F**) with no significant difference between genotypes ($F_{1,13} = 1.669$, $p = 0.219$) or interaction between training sessions and genotypes ($F_{5,65} = 1.105$, $p = 0.355$). During the devaluation test (**Figure 4G**), both A_1R KO and WT mice similarly showed insensitive to outcome devaluation (A_1R KO group, $F_{1,6} = 1.802$, $p = 0.228$; WT group, $F_{1,7} = 1.483, p = 0.263$), indicating that their responding was habitual. The omission test (**Figure 4H**) further confirmed the results of pharmacological blockade of A_1R by genetic knockout approach: there was neither main (genotypes) effect ($F_{1,13} = 1.521$, $p = 0.239$) nor the interaction of genotypes X testing time ($F_{5,65} = 0.260$, $p = 0.817$). This finding suggested that A_1R exerted limited effect on the control of instrumental behavior.

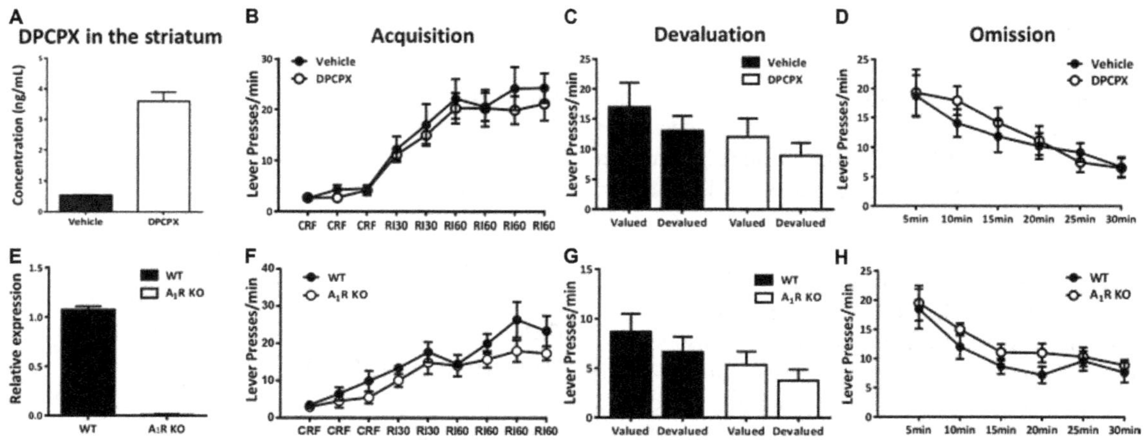

FIGURE 4 | Pharmacological blockade and genetic knockout of A_1Rs did not affect action-outcome association or goal-evaluation of instrumental behavior. **(A)** The concentration of DPCPX was detected in the striatum of mice 30 min after drug administration (n = 3/group), demonstrating the effectiveness of drug level we used. **(B)** Mice with and without DPCPX manipulation performed analogical learning curves in the acquisition of instrumental conditioning (between-subject effect, $p = 0.597$; drug administration X training interaction effect, $p = 0.867$). **(C)** Both DPCPX ($p = 0.131$) and vehicle ($p = 0.370$) groups displayed insensitive to outcome devaluation. **(D)** There didn't show any difference between DPCPX and vehicle groups in the omission test (between-subject effect, $p = 0.724$; drug administration X testing time interaction effect, $p = 0.580$). **(E)** The knockout efficiency of A_1R KO mice was confirmed by qPCR. **(F)** A_1R knockout did not affect acquisition of instrumental behavior since there lack of main effect of genotypes ($p = 0.219$) and training sessions X genotypes interaction effect ($p = 0.355$). **(G)** A_1R knockout mice and their littermates did not significantly decrease lever presses rate in the devalued condition (A_1R KO group, $p = 0.228$; WT group, $p = 0.263$). **(H)** Both groups decreased their lever presses indistinctively in the omission test (genotypes main effect, $p = 0.239$; genotypes X testing time interaction effect, $p = 0.817$). All data was analyzed by two-way ANOVA for repeated measurement.

DISCUSSION

A_{2A}R Antagonist Modulate Animals' Sensitivity to Goal-Directed Valuation Without Modifying Action-Outcome Contingency

Action-outcome contingency and goal-directed valuation are two cognitive components involved in instrumental conditioning (Balleine and Dickinson, 1998). Action-outcome contingency is determined by the causal relationship between the particular actions and outcomes, while goal-directed valuation depends on the anticipation or desire for the outcome (Yin and Knowlton, 2006). Both components were acquired in the training sessions of instrumental behavior. Thus, outcome devaluation procedure was specialized to probe the importance of the evaluative component of goal-directed actions. We found that pharmacological blockade of A_{2A}Rs critically promoted animals' sensitivity to outcome value (by the devaluation test) but did not affect action-outcome relationship (as manifested by similar performance in the training sessions and in the omission test). When administering 5 min prior to the training, KW6002 at 5 mg/kg apparently elevated the acquisition of learning curve. This enhancement is, however, potentially confounded by the enhanced general motor activity effect of the A_{2A}R antagonist. Additional studies with the A_{2A}R antagonist administering 30 min prior to or post-training can better dissociate the learning process from motor effect and clarify this issue. The selective modulation of animals' sensitivity to outcome devaluation by A_{2A}R antagonist is in agreement with our recent finding that optogenetic activation of striatopallidal A_{2A}R signaling in DMS alters goal-valuation as evident by the devaluation test (Li et al., 2016). On the other hand, the lack of the effect of A_{2A}R antagonist on the acquisition of instrumental behaviors collaborates with similar findings by genetic inactivation of striatal A_{2A}Rs (Yu et al., 2009) and optogenetic activation of striatopallidal A_{2A}R signaling (Li et al., 2016).

The mechanism underlying the selective modulation of goal-valuation by the A_{2A}R is not clear. The previous study that overexpression of the D_2R in the striatopallidal pathway is associated with a shift in behavioral control from habitual action to goal-directed responding but did not affect acquisition phase of instrumental learning (Kwak et al., 2014). Also, loss of striatal endocannabinoid-mediated long-term depression selectively in DLS striatopallidal neurons prevent the transition from goal-directed seeking to habitual responding behavior but did not interfere lever-press performance in the acquisition phase (Gremel et al., 2016). Given the documented antagonistic interaction of the A_{2A}R-D_2R and the A_{2A}R-CB_1R in the striatum by possibly the A_{2A}R-D_2R heterodimers (He et al., 2016) and A_{2A}R-CB_1R heterodimers (Moreno et al., 2017), these findings suggest that A_{2A}R may selectively influence coding of the current value of the outcome (but not the contingency association) by the A_{2A}R interaction with the D_2R and CB_1R functions in the striatum.

Moreover, this selective control of animals' sensitivity to reward valuation by A_{2A}Rs might be related to a motivation factor, as A_{2A}R (Mingote et al., 2008; Nam et al., 2013a) and D_2R (Trifilieff et al., 2013) activities in the striatum contribute to motivational control of behaviors. Lastly, since the A_{2A}R are predominantly expressed in the striatopallidal neurons, the A_{2A}R control of goal-directed valuation is further supported by the finding from the striatal circuit studies showing that as pharmacogenetic inactivation of the striatopallidal pathway enhanced motivation by energizing the initiation of goal-directed behavior (Carvalho Poyraz et al., 2016), while optogenetic stimulation of the striatopallidal pathway suppressed motivational behavior (O'Hare et al., 2016; Vicente et al., 2016).

$A_{2A}R$ Antagonist Acts at the Coding, Consolidation and Expression Phases of Instrumental Learning to Promote Goal-Directed Behavior

Defining the specific information processing phases (i.e., learning/coding, consolidation and expression of instrumental behaviors) for $A_{2A}R$ antagonist control of goal-directed versus habitual behaviors is critical for our understanding of the neurotransmitter modulatory mechanisms and for the development of effective pharmacological strategy to control aberrant habit formation and drug addiction. Our demonstration of the enhanced goal-directed behavior by administration of KW6002 at the pre-training or post-training or expression phases suggests that $A_{2A}R$ acts at the coding, consolidation and expression phases of instrumental learning to promote animals' sensitivity to goal-directed valuation. It should be noted that the influence of the pre-training treatment paradigm on the goal-directed behavior might be partly attributed to its effect on the consolidation phase due to the relatively long-lasting effect (>2 h) of the $A_{2A}R$ antagonist KW6002. The similar control of instrumental behaviors by multiple treatment paradigms of KW6002 indicate that $A_{2A}R$ control of instrumental behaviors is largely independent of the confounding motor activity.

Various neurotransmitter systems have been implicated in control of the distinct phases of instrumental conditioning. For example, NMDA receptor signaling preferentially affected the coding (by administering NMDA antagonist at the pre-training phase) but not the expression (by administering NMDA antagonist at the post-training phase) of the instrumental conditioning (Yin et al., 2005). Furthermore, virus-induced overexpression of D_2R (Trifilieff et al., 2013) and 5-HT_6 receptor (Eskenazi and Neumaier, 2011; Eskenazi et al., 2015) preferentially affect the coding course of operant conditioning. Additionally, optogenetic activation of endocannabinoid signaling in the training session and pharmacogenetic suppression of endocannabinoid signaling in the devaluation test gated habit formation (Gremel et al., 2016), indicating that endocannabinoid modulated instrumental learning in both coding and expression sessions, consistent with the CB_1R knockout study (Hilario et al., 2007). Thus, the $A_{2A}R$ may interact with multiple neurotransmitter systems in the cortico-striatal projection pathways to integrate/modulate glutamate, dopamine and endocannabinoid signaling for instrumental behavioral control at multiple phases of information processing. Furthermore, cognitive control and working memory processes are important for the efficient control of goal-directed behavior (Buschman and Miller, 2014). We and others have documented that the $A_{2A}R$ antagonists or focal $A_{2A}R$ knockdown in the DMS significantly enhance working memory (Wei et al., 2014; Kaster et al., 2015; Li et al., 2018). Thus, it is possible that when KW6002 is administered prior to the training phase, the $A_{2A}R$ antagonist may enhance goal-directed behavior by improving working memory. On the other hand, other mechanisms (such as "off-line" processing during sleep) may contribute to the $A_{2A}R$ antagonist-mediated enhancement of goal-directed behavior when $A_{2A}R$ antagonists are administered after the training or during the expression/retrieval phase.

Pharmacological Blockade and Genetic Knockout of A_1Rs Did Not Affect Acquisition or Goal-Evaluation of Instrumental Behavior

Adenosine signaling acts at the facilitating $A_{2A}R$ and inhibitory A_1R to exert its homeostatic control of brain function. However, very limited information is available regarding the A_1R control of cognition, particularly instrumental behaviors. With its relatively high expression in the cerebral cortex, hippocampus and striatum (Reppert et al., 1991; Dixon et al., 1996), A_1R activation has a profound inhibitory control of excitatory transmission by presynaptic and post-synaptic mechanisms (Dunwiddie and Masino, 2001; Ribeiro et al., 2002). Striatal A_1Rs can preferentially interact with the striatal D_1Rs via possible A_1R-D_1R heterodimers in the striatonigral neurons to control striatal signaling and behavior (Gines et al., 2000). Accordingly, A_1Rs modulate striatal synaptic plasticity, and prevent scopolamine- and morphine-induced impairment in working memory (Hooper et al., 1996; Lu et al., 2010). However, in the fix-interval and fix-ratio operant training paradigms, A_1R antagonist failed to increase lever pressing rate, but decreased fix ratio 20 (FR20, every 20 lever presses resulted in one reward) responding at higher doses (Randall et al., 2011). Operant performance alone was insufficient to define instrumental learning modes as goal-directed or habitual actions without devaluation and omission test (Yin and Knowlton, 2006). Thus, the role of the A_1R in goal-directed versus habitual behaviors is still unknown. Our study demonstrated that pharmacological blockade or global knockout of A_1R did not affect the acquisition of instrumental learning or sensitivity to reward value or reversal of action-outcome relationship. This finding is in agreement with a recent study that DPCPX failed to reverse the effect of D_2R antagonist on effort-relevant tasks but KW6002 and caffeine (a non-selective adenosine antagonist) can (Salamone et al., 2009). These findings suggest that A_1R plays limited modulatory role in control of instrumental behavior and adenosine predominantly acts on A_{2A}Rs but not A_1Rs to modulate instrumental learning.

In summary, our study demonstrated that pharmacological blockade of $A_{2A}R$ but not A_1R promote goal-directed behaviors by enhancing goal-directed valuation without affecting the action-outcome contingency and by acting at the coding, consolidation, and expression phases of goal-directed learning processes. These findings collaborates with our previous genetic and optogenetic studies, and with recent pharmacological studies of $A_{2A}R$ antagonists to control abnormal instrumental behavior in drug addiction paradigms (Nam et al., 2013a;

Pintsuk et al., 2016), providing pharmacological evidence for a therapeutic strategy to enhance goal-directed behaviors in neuropsychiatric disorders. The translational potential of $A_{2A}R$ antagonists is further enhanced by the recent demonstration of the safety profiles of the $A_{2A}R$ antagonist KW6002 in clinical phase III trials for motor benefit in >3500 Parkinson's disease patients (Chen et al., 2013) and by regular consumption of caffeine (a non-specific adenosine $A_{2A}R$ and A_1R antagonist) by 50% world population.

AUTHOR CONTRIBUTIONS

YL, YH, XZ, and J-FC designed the experiments. YL, XP, YH, YR, LH, ZW, and CH collected the data. YL, XP, YH, YZ, and ZH analyzed the data. YL, XZ, and J-FC wrote the manuscript.

FUNDING

This study was sponsored by the National Natural Science Foundation of China (Grant Nos. 81600983, 31771178, and 81600991), by the Start-up Fund from Wenzhou Medical University (Grant Nos. 89211010 and 89212012), the Zhejiang Provincial Special Funds (Grant No. 604161241), the Natural Science Foundation of Zhejiang Province of China (Grant Nos. LY15H090020, LQ16H090006, and LQ17H090005), and the Wenzhou Science and Technology Program (Grant Nos. 2016Y0725 and 2016Y0613).

REFERENCES

Balleine, B. W., and Dickinson, A. (1998). Goal-directed instrumental action: contingency and incentive learning and their cortical substrates. *Neuropharmacology* 37, 407–419. doi: 10.1016/S0028-3908(98)00033-1

Balleine, B. W., and O'Doherty, J. P. (2010). Human and rodent homologies in action control: corticostriatal determinants of goal-directed and habitual action. *Neuropsychopharmacology* 35, 48–69. doi: 10.1038/npp.2009.131

Baumgold, J., Nikodijevic, O., and Jacobson, K. A. (1992). Penetration of adenosine antagonists into mouse brain as determined by ex vivo binding. *Biochem. Pharmacol.* 43, 889–894. doi: 10.1016/0006-2952(92)90257-J

Burguiere, E., Monteiro, P., Mallet, L., Feng, G., and Graybiel, A. M. (2015). Striatal circuits, habits, and implications for obsessive-compulsive disorder. *Curr. Opin. Neurobiol.* 30, 59–65. doi: 10.1016/j.conb.2014.08.008

Buschman, T. J., and Miller, E. K. (2014). Goal-direction and top-down control. *Philos. Trans. R. Soc. Lond. B Biol. Sci.* 369:20130471. doi: 10.1098/rstb.2013.0471

Carvalho Poyraz, F., Holzner, E., Bailey, M. R., Meszaros, J., Kenney, L., Kheirbek, M. A., et al. (2016). Decreasing striatopallidal pathway function enhances motivation by energizing the initiation of goal-directed action. *J. Neurosci.* 36, 5988–6001. doi: 10.1523/JNEUROSCI.0444-16.2016

Chen, J. F. (2014). Adenosine receptor control of cognition in normal and disease. *Int. Rev. Neurobiol.* 119, 257–307. doi: 10.1016/B978-0-12-801022-8.00012-X

Chen, J. F., Eltzschig, H. K., and Fredholm, B. B. (2013). Adenosine receptors as drug targets–what are the challenges? *Nat. Rev. Drug Discov.* 12, 265–286. doi: 10.1038/nrd3955

Chen, J.-F., Xu, K., Petzer, J. P., Staal, R., Xu, Y. H., Beilstein, M., et al. (2001). Neuroprotection by caffeine and A2A adenosine receptor inactivation in a model of Parkinson's disease. *J. Neurosci.* 21:RC143.

de Wit, S., Barker, R. A., Dickinson, A. D., and Cools, R. (2011). Habitual versus goal-directed action control in Parkinson disease. *J. Cogn. Neurosci.* 23, 1218–1229. doi: 10.1162/jocn.2010.21514

Dixon, A. K., Gubitz, A. K., Sirinathsinghji, D. J., Richardson, P. J., and Freeman, T. C. (1996). Tissue distribution of adenosine receptor mRNAs in the rat. *Br. J. Pharmacol.* 118, 1461–1468. doi: 10.1111/j.1476-5381.1996.tb15561.x

Dolan, R. J., and Dayan, P. (2013). Goals and habits in the brain. *Neuron* 80, 312–325. doi: 10.1016/j.neuron.2013.09.007

Dunwiddie, T. V., and Masino, S. A. (2001). The role and regulation of adenosine in the central nervous system. *Annu. Rev. Neurosci.* 24, 31–55. doi: 10.1146/annurev.neuro.24.1.31

Eskenazi, D., Brodsky, M., and Neumaier, J. F. (2015). Deconstructing 5-HT6 receptor effects on striatal circuit function. *Neuroscience* 299, 97–106. doi: 10.1016/j.neuroscience.2015.04.046

Eskenazi, D., and Neumaier, J. F. (2011). Increased expression of the 5-HT6 receptor by viral mediated gene transfer into posterior but not anterior dorsomedial striatum interferes with acquisition of a discrete action-outcome task. *J. Psychopharmacol.* 25, 944–951. doi: 10.1177/0269881110388330

Furlong, T. M., Supit, A. S., Corbit, L. H., Killcross, S., and Balleine, B. W. (2017). Pulling habits out of rats: adenosine 2A receptor antagonism in dorsomedial striatum rescues meth-amphetamine-induced deficits in goal-directed action. *Addict. Biol.* 22, 172–183. doi: 10.1111/adb.12316

Gillan, C. M., Papmeyer, M., Morein-Zamir, S., Sahakian, B. J., Fineberg, N. A., Robbins, T. W., et al. (2011). Disruption in the balance between goal-directed behavior and habit learning in obsessive-compulsive disorder. *Am. J. Psychiatry* 168, 718–726. doi: 10.1176/appi.ajp.2011.10071062

Gines, S., Hillion, J., Torvinen, M., Le Crom, S., Casado, V., Canela, E. I., et al. (2000). Dopamine D1 and adenosine A1 receptors form functionally interacting heteromeric complexes. *Proc. Natl. Acad. Sci. U.S.A.* 97, 8606–8611. doi: 10.1073/pnas.150241097

Glimcher, P. W. (2011). Understanding dopamine and reinforcement learning: the dopamine reward prediction error hypothesis. *Proc. Natl. Acad. Sci. U.S.A.* 108(Suppl. 3), 15647–15654. doi: 10.1073/pnas.1014269108

Graybiel, A. M., and Grafton, S. T. (2015). The striatum: where skills and habits meet. *Cold Spring Harb. Perspect. Biol.* 7:a021691. doi: 10.1101/cshperspect.a021691

Gremel, C. M., Chancey, J. H., Atwood, B. K., Luo, G., Neve, R., Ramakrishnan, C., et al. (2016). Endocannabinoid modulation of orbitostriatal circuits gates habit formation. *Neuron* 90, 1312–1324. doi: 10.1016/j.neuron.2016.04.043

Gremel, C. M., and Costa, R. M. (2013). Orbitofrontal and striatal circuits dynamically encode the shift between goal-directed and habitual actions. *Nat. Commun.* 4:2264. doi: 10.1038/ncomms3264

He, Y., Li, Y., Chen, M., Pu, Z., Zhang, F., Chen, L., et al. (2016). Habit formation after random interval training is associated with increased adenosine A2A receptor and dopamine D2 receptor heterodimers in the striatum. *Front. Mol. Neurosci.* 9:151. doi: 10.3389/fnmol.2016.00151

Hilario, M. R., Clouse, E., Yin, H. H., and Costa, R. M. (2007). Endocannabinoid signaling is critical for habit formation. *Front. Integr. Neurosci.* 1:6. doi: 10.3389/neuro.07.006.2007

Hooper, N., Fraser, C., and Stone, T. W. (1996). Effects of purine analogues on spontaneous alternation in mice. *Psychopharmacology (Berl)* 123, 250–257. doi: 10.1007/BF02246579

Johansson, B., Halldner, L., Dunwiddie, T. V., Masino, S. A., Poelchen, W., Gimenez-Llort, L., et al. (2001). Hyperalgesia, anxiety, and decreased hypoxic neuroprotection in mice lacking the adenosine A1 receptor. *Proc. Natl. Acad. Sci. U.S.A.* 98, 9407–9412. doi: 10.1073/pnas.161292398

Kaster, M. P., Machado, N. J., Silva, H. B., Nunes, A., Ardais, A. P., Santana, M., et al. (2015). Caffeine acts through neuronal adenosine A2A receptors to prevent mood and memory dysfunction triggered by chronic stress. *Proc. Natl. Acad. Sci. U.S.A.* 112, 7833–7838. doi: 10.1073/pnas.1423088112

Kim, H. F., and Hikosaka, O. (2015). Parallel basal ganglia circuits for voluntary and automatic behaviour to reach rewards. *Brain* 138, 1776–1800. doi: 10.1093/brain/awv134

Kreitzer, A. C., and Malenka, R. C. (2007). Endocannabinoid-mediated rescue of striatal LTD and motor deficits in Parkinson's disease models. *Nature* 445, 643–647. doi: 10.1038/nature05506

Kwak, S., Huh, N., Seo, J. S., Lee, J. E., Han, P. L., and Jung, M. W. (2014). Role of dopamine D2 receptors in optimizing choice strategy in a dynamic and uncertain environment. *Front. Behav. Neurosci.* 8:368. doi: 10.3389/fnbeh.2014.00368

Lawrence, A. D., Sahakian, B. J., and Robbins, T. W. (1998). Cognitive functions and corticostriatal circuits: insights from Huntington's disease. *Trends Cogn. Sci.* 2, 379–388. doi: 10.1016/S1364-6613(98)01231-5

Leung, B. K., and Balleine, B. W. (2013). The ventral striato-pallidal pathway mediates the effect of predictive learning on choice between goal-directed actions. *J. Neurosci.* 33, 13848–13860. doi: 10.1523/JNEUROSCI.1697-13.2013

Li, Y., He, Y., Chen, M., Pu, Z., Chen, L., Li, P., et al. (2016). Optogenetic activation of adenosine A2A receptor signaling in the dorsomedial striatopallidal neurons suppresses goal-directed behavior. *Neuropsychopharmacology* 41, 1003–1013. doi: 10.1038/npp.2015.227

Li, Z., Chen, X., Wang, T., Gao, Y., Li, F., Chen, L., et al. (2018). The corticostriatal adenosine A2A receptor controls maintenance and retrieval of spatial working memory. *Biol. Psychiatry* 83, 530–541. doi: 10.1016/j.biopsych.2017.07.017

Lovinger, D. M. (2010). Neurotransmitter roles in synaptic modulation, plasticity and learning in the dorsal striatum. *Neuropharmacology* 58, 951–961. doi: 10.1016/j.neuropharm.2010.01.008

Lu, G., Zhou, Q. X., Kang, S., Li, Q. L., Zhao, L. C., Chen, J. D., et al. (2010). Chronic morphine treatment impaired hippocampal long-term potentiation and spatial memory via accumulation of extracellular adenosine acting on adenosine A1 receptors. *J. Neurosci.* 30, 5058–5070. doi: 10.1523/JNEUROSCI.0148-10.2010

Mingote, S., Font, L., Farrar, A. M., Vontell, R., Worden, L. T., Stopper, C. M., et al. (2008). Nucleus accumbens adenosine A2A receptors regulate exertion of effort by acting on the ventral striatopallidal pathway. *J. Neurosci.* 28, 9037–9046. doi: 10.1523/JNEUROSCI.1525-08.2008

Moreno, E., Chiarlone, A., Medrano, M., Puigdellivol, M., Bibic, L., Howell, L. A., et al. (2017). Singular location and signaling profile of adenosine A2A-cannabinoid CB1 receptor heteromers in the dorsal striatum. *Neuropsychopharmacology* 43, 964–977. doi: 10.1038/npp.2017.12

Nam, H. W., Bruner, R. C., and Choi, D. S. (2013a). Adenosine signaling in striatal circuits and alcohol use disorders. *Mol. Cells* 36, 195–202. doi: 10.1007/s10059-013-0192-9

Nam, H. W., Hinton, D. J., Kang, N. Y., Kim, T., Lee, M. R., Oliveros, A., et al. (2013b). Adenosine transporter ENT1 regulates the acquisition of goal-directed behavior and ethanol drinking through A2A receptor in the dorsomedial striatum. *J. Neurosci.* 33, 4329–4338. doi: 10.1523/JNEUROSCI.3094-12.2013

Nguyen, M. D., Lee, S. T., Ross, A. E., Ryals, M., Choudhry, V. I., and Venton, B. J. (2014). Characterization of spontaneous, transient adenosine release in the caudate-putamen and prefrontal cortex. *PLoS One* 9:e87165. doi: 10.1371/journal.pone.0087165

O'Hare, J. K., Ade, K. K., Sukharnikova, T., Van Hooser, S. D., Palmeri, M. L., Yin, H. H., et al. (2016). Pathway-specific striatal substrates for habitual behavior. *Neuron* 89, 472–479. doi: 10.1016/j.neuron.2015.12.032

Ostlund, S. B., and Balleine, B. W. (2008). On habits and addiction: an associative analysis of compulsive drug seeking. *Drug. Discov. Today Dis. Models* 5, 235–245. doi: 10.1016/j.ddmod.2009.07.004

Pintsuk, J., Borroto-Escuela, D. O., Pomierny, B., Wydra, K., Zaniewska, M., Filip, M., et al. (2016). Cocaine self-administration differentially affects allosteric A2A-D2 receptor-receptor interactions in the striatum. Relevance for cocaine use disorder. *Pharmacol. Biochem. Behav.* 144, 85–91. doi: 10.1016/j.pbb.2016.03.004

Prediger, R. D., Batista, L. C., and Takahashi, R. N. (2004). Adenosine A1 receptors modulate the anxiolytic-like effect of ethanol in the elevated plus-maze in mice. *Eur. J. Pharmacol.* 499, 147–154. doi: 10.1016/j.ejphar.2004.07.106

Randall, P. A., Nunes, E. J., Janniere, S. L., Stopper, C. M., Farrar, A. M., Sager, T. N., et al. (2011). Stimulant effects of adenosine antagonists on operant behavior: differential actions of selective A2A and A1 antagonists. *Psychopharmacology (Berl)* 216, 173–186. doi: 10.1007/s00213-011-2198-3

Redgrave, P., Rodriguez, M., Smith, Y., Rodriguez-Oroz, M. C., Lehericy, S., Bergman, H., et al. (2010). Goal-directed and habitual control in the basal ganglia: implications for Parkinson's disease. *Nat. Rev. Neurosci.* 11, 760–772. doi: 10.1038/nrn2915

Reppert, S. M., Weaver, D. R., Stehle, J. H., and Rivkees, S. A. (1991). Molecular cloning and characterization of a rat A1-adenosine receptor that is widely expressed in brain and spinal cord. *Mol. Endocrinol.* 5, 1037–1048. doi: 10.1210/mend-5-8-1037

Ribeiro, J. A., Sebastiao, A. M., and De Mendonca, A. (2002). Adenosine receptors in the nervous system: pathophysiological implications. *Prog. Neurobiol.* 68, 377–392. doi: 10.1016/S0301-0082(02)00155-7

Robbins, T. W., Gillan, C. M., Smith, D. G., De Wit, S., and Ersche, K. D. (2012). Neurocognitive endophenotypes of impulsivity and compulsivity: towards dimensional psychiatry. *Trends Cogn. Sci.* 16, 81–91. doi: 10.1016/j.tics.2011.11.009

Rossi, M. A., Sukharnikova, T., Hayrapetyan, V. Y., Yang, L., and Yin, H. H. (2013). Operant self-stimulation of dopamine neurons in the substantia nigra. *PLoS One* 8:e65799. doi: 10.1371/journal.pone.0065799

Rossi, M. A., and Yin, H. H. (2012). Methods for studying habitual behavior in mice. *Curr. Protoc. Neurosci.* 60, 8.29.1–8.29.9. doi: 10.1002/0471142301.ns0829s60

Salamone, J. D., Farrar, A. M., Font, L., Patel, V., Schlar, D. E., Nunes, E. J., et al. (2009). Differential actions of adenosine A1 and A2A antagonists on the effort-related effects of dopamine D2 antagonism. *Behav. Brain Res.* 201, 216–222. doi: 10.1016/j.bbr.2009.02.021

Shen, H. Y., Coelho, J. E., Ohtsuka, N., Canas, P. M., Day, Y. J., Huang, Q. Y., et al. (2008). A critical role of the adenosine A2A receptor in extrastriatal neurons in modulating psychomotor activity as revealed by opposite phenotypes of striatum and forebrain A2A receptor knock-outs. *J. Neurosci.* 28, 2970–2975. doi: 10.1523/JNEUROSCI.5255-07.2008

Shen, W., Flajolet, M., Greengard, P., and Surmeier, D. J. (2008). Dichotomous dopaminergic control of striatal synaptic plasticity. *Science* 321, 848–851. doi: 10.1126/science.1160575

Smith, K. S., and Graybiel, A. M. (2013a). A dual operator view of habitual behavior reflecting cortical and striatal dynamics. *Neuron* 79, 361–374. doi: 10.1016/j.neuron.2013.05.038

Smith, K. S., and Graybiel, A. M. (2013b). Using optogenetics to study habits. *Brain Res.* 1511, 102–114. doi: 10.1016/j.brainres.2013.01.008

Steinberg, E. E., Keiflin, R., Boivin, J. R., Witten, I. B., Deisseroth, K., and Janak, P. H. (2013). A causal link between prediction errors, dopamine neurons and learning. *Nat. Neurosci.* 16, 966–973. doi: 10.1038/nn.3413

Tebano, M. T., Martire, A., Potenza, R. L., Gro, C., Pepponi, R., Armida, M., et al. (2008). Adenosine A(2A) receptors are required for normal BDNF levels and BDNF-induced potentiation of synaptic transmission in the mouse hippocampus. *J. Neurochem.* 104, 279–286.

Trifilieff, P., Feng, B., Urizar, E., Winiger, V., Ward, R. D., Taylor, K. M., et al. (2013). Increasing dopamine D2 receptor expression in the adult nucleus accumbens enhances motivation. *Mol. Psychiatry* 18, 1025–1033. doi: 10.1038/mp.2013.57

Vicente, A. M., Galvao-Ferreira, P., Tecuapetla, F., and Costa, R. M. (2016). Direct and indirect dorsolateral striatum pathways reinforce different action strategies. *Curr. Biol.* 26, R267–R269. doi: 10.1016/j.cub.2016.02.036

Wei, C. J., Augusto, E., Gomes, C. A., Singer, P., Wang, Y., Boison, D., et al. (2014). Regulation of fear responses by striatal and extrastriatal adenosine A2A receptors in forebrain. *Biol. Psychiatry* 75, 855–863. doi: 10.1016/j.biopsych.2013.05.003

Yin, H. H., and Knowlton, B. J. (2006). The role of the basal ganglia in habit formation. *Nat. Rev. Neurosci.* 7, 464–476. doi: 10.1038/nrn1919

Yin, H. H., Knowlton, B. J., and Balleine, B. W. (2005). Blockade of NMDA receptors in the dorsomedial striatum prevents action-outcome learning in instrumental conditioning. *Eur. J. Neurosci.* 22, 505–512. doi: 10.1111/j.1460-9568.2005.04219.x

Yu, C., Gupta, J., Chen, J. F., and Yin, H. H. (2009). Genetic deletion of A2A adenosine receptors in the striatum selectively impairs habit formation. *J. Neurosci.* 29, 15100–15103. doi: 10.1523/JNEUROSCI.4215-09.2009

Yu, L., Shen, H. Y., Coelho, J. E., Araujo, I. M., Huang, Q. Y., Day, Y. J., et al. (2008). Adenosine A2A receptor antagonists exert motor and neuroprotective effects by distinct cellular mechanisms. *Ann. Neurol.* 63, 338–346. doi: 10.1002/ana.21313

Zhang, S., Li, H., Li, B., Zhong, D., Gu, X., Tang, L., et al. (2015). Adenosine A1 receptors selectively modulate oxygen-induced retinopathy at the hyperoxic and hypoxic phases by distinct cellular mechanisms. *Invest. Ophthalmol. Vis. Sci.* 56, 8108–8119. doi: 10.1167/iovs.15-17202

10

Adenosine Receptor-Mediated Cardioprotection —Current Limitations and Future Directions

*Robert D. Lasley**

Department of Physiology, Wayne State University School of Medicine, Detroit, MI, United States

Correspondence:
Robert D. Lasley
rlasley@med.wayne.edu

Since the seminal reports of adenosine receptor-mediated cardioprotection in the early 1990s, there have been a multitude of such reports in various species and preparations. Original observations of the beneficial effects of A_1 receptor agonists have been followed up with numerous reports also implicating A_{2A}, A_3, and most recently A_{2B}, receptor agonists as cardioprotective agents. Although adenosine has been approved for clinical use in the United States for the treatment of supraventricular tachycardia and coronary artery imaging, and the selective A_{2A} agonist, regadenoson, for the latter, clinical use of adenosine receptor agonists for protecting the ischemic heart has not advanced beyond early trials. An examination of the literature indicates that existing experimental studies have several limitations in terms of clinical relevance, as well as lacking incorporation of recent new insights into adenosine receptor signaling. Such deficiencies include the lack of experimental studies in models that most closely mimic human cardiovascular disease. In addition, there have been very few studies in chronic models of myocardial ischemia, where limiting myocardial remodeling and heart failure, not reduction of infarct size, are the primary endpoints. Despite an increasing number of reports of the beneficial effects of adenosine receptor antagonists, not agonists, in chronic diseases, this idea has not been well-studied in experimental myocardial ischemia. There have also been few studies examining adenosine receptor subtype interactions as well as receptor heterodimerization. The purpose of this Perspective article is to discuss these deficiencies to highlight future directions of research in the field of adenosine receptor-mediated protection of ischemic myocardium.

Keywords: adenosine receptor subtypes, cardioprotection, chronic myocardial ischemia, co-morbidities, clinical trials

Although the hypothesis that adenosine could be cardioprotective first became recognized in the early to mid-1980s, it started inauspiciously. Based on observations that the post-ischemic heart was characterized by both decreased ATP content and reduced ventricular function, Reibel and Rovetto (1978) reported that a reperfusion infusion of adenosine (50 μM) in isolated perfused rat hearts did not improve ATP content, although ventricular function was not measured (Reibel and Rovetto, 1978). Several subsequent studies did yield beneficial effects of exogenous and endogenous adenosine on post-ischemic ATP content and ventricular function, but these results were based in large part on initiating treatment prior to the onset of ischemia (Humphrey and Seelye, 1982; Dhasmana et al., 1983; Ely et al., 1985). Initial reports that reperfusion infusions of adenosine could reduce infarct size (Olafsson et al., 1987; Pitarys et al., 1991), could not be replicated in subsequent studies (Homeister et al., 1990; Goto et al., 1991; Vander Heide and Reimer, 1996). Interest in adenosine's effects in protecting the ischemic heart did not gain widespread acceptance until early 1990 when our laboratory first reported an A_1 receptor cardioprotective effect (Lasley et al., 1990). A year later Liu et al. (1991) reported a role for A_1 receptors in ischemic preconditioning to reduce myocardial infarct size. Over the next 30 years there has been an explosion in the number of adenosine receptor cardioprotection studies, primarily focusing on infarct size reduction, with all four adenosine receptor subtypes (A_1, A_{2A}, A_3, A_{2B}) being implicated (Headrick and Lasley, 2009; McIntosh and Lasley, 2012).

Despite these numerous reports in experimental models, there have been few, if any, clinical trials of adenosine receptor cardioprotection in humans. Searching the database at "ClinicalTrials.gov" with the terms "ischemic heart disease" and "adenosine" yields 192 trials; changing the disease/condition to myocardial infarction (MI) yields only 40 trials. Nearly all of these trials have related to adenosine's effects on arrhythmias, coronary blood flow, and platelets. When searching this database with "adenosine receptor" 582 trials are shown, but combining with "myocardial infarction" only 9 trials are cited, and the majority of these trials used adenosine, not a receptor analog thereof. The only adenosine receptor agonists used in cardiac related clinical trials have been the A_1 agonists Selodenoson (DTI-0009) and Capadenoson (BAY68-4986) for controlling ventricular rate in atrial fibrillation, the A_{2A} agonist regadeson and related agents for coronary imaging, and most recently the partial A_1 agonist Neladenoson bialanate (BAY1067197) for heart failure.

This limited translation of hundreds of experimental studies, in every animal species tested to date, to the clinical arena raises the question of whether the past 30 years of adenosine receptor cardioprotection investigations have been for naught. This perspective will examine limitations of our existing knowledge of adenosine-mediated protection of the ischemic heart to help guide future studies to fully understand the cardioprotective effects of adenosine therapeutics and harness its potential in humans.

LACK OF CLINICALLY RELEVANT ANIMAL MODELS

Nearly all experimental studies on adenosine receptor cardioprotection have been conducted in normal, healthy adult animals. In contrast cardioprotective interventions in humans occur in the presence of various co-morbidities, such as arterial hypertension, obesity, diabetes, hypercholesterolemia, and often advanced age. Although there are numerous reports examining the role of adenosine and its receptors in these pathologies (Long et al., 2010; Wang et al., 2010; Bot et al., 2012; Koupenova et al., 2012; Sangsiri et al., 2013; Zhang et al., 2013; Teng et al., 2014; Nayak et al., 2015; Yang et al., 2016), the only one of these areas in which adenosine cardioprotection has been examined is in healthy aged rats and mice, and results have been conflicting. Isolated heart studies in 16–18 month old mice indicate a loss in the ability of adenosine and the A_1 and A_3 adenosine receptor agonists CPA and Cl-IB-MECA to reduce ischemia-reperfusion injury (Headrick et al., 2003; Peart et al., 2014). Two studies in rat hearts have led to contradictory findings as Schulman et al. (2001) reported a loss of adenosine A_1 agonist (CCPA) preconditioning in 18–20 month-old Wistar rats, whereas Kristo et al. (2005) reported enhanced infarct size reduction in 24–26 months Fischer 344 × Brown Norway hybrid (F344 × BN) rats with the mixed (A_1 and A_{2A}) agonist AMP579. A major difference in these rat studies is that the former was conducted in an isolated perfused heart preparation, whereas the latter was conducted *in vivo*, where the effects of the circulating agonist continued into reperfusion. Interestingly in both rat and mouse studies the effects of A_1 and A_{2A} agonists on heart rate and coronary flow in aged hearts were similar to those in young adult hearts. These findings are consistent with the reports of unaltered A_{2A} agonist (regadenoson) increases in coronary flow in aged human hearts (Cerqueira et al., 2008). One of the major limitations in the field of adenosine receptor cardioprotection is the lack of studies in animal models with clinically relevant morbidities. It is likely that these co-morbidities will alter myocardial adenosine receptor subtype expression and/or signaling mechanisms, as has been reported in models of atherosclerosis and diabetes (Long et al., 2010; Cabiati et al., 2015).

TREATMENT PARADIGMS

Another deficiency in the literature, related to current experimental studies, are the experimental treatment paradigms that are typically used. The majority of experimental studies on adenosine A_1 and A_3 receptors, as well as several studies A_{2B} receptors, have involved administration of agonists prior to ischemia to reduce ischemia-reperfusion injury (Headrick and Lasley, 2009; McIntosh and Lasley, 2012). Such a treatment paradigm has relevance to open heart surgery and preservation solutions for cardiac transplantation, but there have been no clinical trials to date, even assessing safety, for the use of adenosine receptor agonists. In contrast experimental studies on adenosine A_{2A} and A_{2B} agonists have focused on reperfusion treatments for the reduction of myocardial infarct size (Headrick and Lasley, 2009; McIntosh and Lasley, 2012), which upon initial review would appear to have some clinical relevance. Initial animal studies with adenosine A_{2A} agonist reperfusion treatment, which were all successful, occurred soon after the controversial experimental results with adenosine (Olafsson et al., 1987; Homeister et al., 1990; Goto et al., 1991; Pitarys et al., 1991; Vander Heide and Reimer, 1996) and the equivocal results of the acute myocardial infarction study of adenosine (AMISTAD) trial published in 1999 (Mahaffey et al., 1999).

However, the vast majority of experimental studies have initiated treatments during late ischemia or at the onset of reperfusion. Such early reperfusion treatments in the setting of acute myocardial infarction (MI) are not feasible given the time involved from the onset of patient symptoms to the diagnosis of MI and initiation of reperfusion therapy. In fact the results of the AMISTAD-II trial indicated that patients [particularly those receiving thrombolytic therapy, rather than percutaneous coronary intervention (PCI)] receiving intravenous adenosine within 3 h of symptom onset showed significantly reduced 1 and 6 months mortality compared with placebo (Kloner et al., 2006). Patients obtaining adenosine reperfusion treatment later than 3 h of symptom onset received no beneficial effect. These clinical observations were similar to those by (Toufektsian et al., 2006), who reported that a 1 h delay in the reperfusion administration of the highly selective A_{2A} agonist, ATL146e, failed to reduce 24 h infarct size in mice (Toufektsian et al., 2006). Interestingly, the delayed treatment did increase post-MI cardiac function and reduce inflammation. We previously reported (Lasley et al., 2001) that an intracoronary infusion of the A_{2A} agonist CGS21680, 2 h after reperfusion, increased regional preload-recruitable stroke work and stroke work area (load-insensitive parameters of cardiac contractility) in a porcine model of reversible myocardial ischemia-reperfusion injury. This effect was determined to be independent of effects on coronary blood flow, and the same infusion in normal myocardium had no effect on regional contractile function. In summary, the lack of experimental studies in clinically relevant models with appropriate treatment protocols, is likely to have contributed to the lack of clinical trials examining the efficacy of adenosine or receptor agonists for treating acute MI. The primary focus on reduction of acute injury is not only inconsistent with clinical trends of more patients living with chronic myocardial ischemia, but it also neglects some of the other recognized beneficial effects of adenosine receptors.

CHRONIC MYOCARDIAL ISCHEMIA MODELS

Another weakness in experimental models of adenosine receptor cardioprotection is the primary focus on acute cardioprotection. This is an inherent limitation of *in vitro* models, but this continues to be a significant weakness of *in vivo* models, in which the study endpoint is typically infarct size after 2–3 h of reperfusion, with only a limited number of studies extending reperfusion to 24 h. Data from the National Heart, Lung and Blood Institute (NHLBI) and other sources indicate that over the past 40 years, deaths from acute MI have decreased significantly, whereas the incidence of heart failure and deaths from heart failure have increased (Krumholz et al., 2009). Experimental studies with short durations of reperfusion exclude significant components of the post-ischemic inflammatory process, which is a primary contributor to post-MI ventricular remodeling and subsequent heart failure. Such studies also exclude the well-known modulatory effects of adenosine receptors on inflammatory processes. It is also well-recognized that adenosine receptor expression and adenosine formation are increased in chronic inflammation, similar to that seen in chronically ischemic hearts (Xaus et al., 1999; Sun et al., 2006; Hasko et al., 2008; Feoktistov and Biaggioni, 2011; Belikoff et al., 2012).

Unfortunately, there have only been a very limited number of experimental studies assessing the cardioprotective effects of adenosine and/or receptor agonists in chronic models of myocardial ischemia. In what appears to be the first such study, Villarreal et al. (2003) reported that a 2 h intravenous infusion of an adenosine kinase inhibitor, which increases endogenous adenosine levels, but not adenosine itself, in rats just prior to reperfusion (following a 2 h occlusion) increased 2 week post-MI ischemic zone wall thickness, consistent with reduced ventricular remodeling (Villarreal et al., 2003). Wakeno et al. subsequently reported that a 3 weeks treatment (twice daily intraperitoneal injections) with the non-selective agonist, 2-chloroadenosine, starting at 7-day post-MI in rats reduced cardiac remodeling and cardiac fibrosis (Wakeno et al., 2006). Based on results with multiple adenosine receptor antagonists, the authors concluded that this protective effect was due to adenosine A_{2B} receptor stimulation. More recently Sabbah et al. reported that chronic treatment with a partial A_1 receptor agonist (capadenoson), in a coronary microembolization-induced model of heart failure in canines, improved left ventricular function, decreased fibrosis, and reduced plasma n-terminal pro-brain natriuretic peptide concentrations (Sabbah et al., 2013). These beneficial effects observed in the absence of changes in heart rate, blood pressure, or renal function, but were accompanied by increased expression of left ventricular sarcoplasmic reticulum calcium ATPase activity, mitochondrial uncoupling proteins (UCP) and glucose transporters. These latter observations suggest that capadenoson's beneficial effects were due to direct effects on the heart, although the specific mechanism remains unknown.

Despite the lack of chronic experimental myocardial ischemia studies, there is evidence suggesting that adenosine may exert beneficial effects in patients with chronic myocardial ischemia. Bulluck et al. (2016) conducted a meta-analysis on the results of 13 randomized clinical trials using intracoronary or intravenous adenosine in patients with ST-segment elevation MI (STEMI). They concluded that intracoronary adenosine therapy in the presence of primary percutaneous coronary intervention (PPCI) was effective in reducing post-STEMI heart failure, but not in terms of other end-points such as death, non-fatal MI, or revascularization. They also concluded that these effects were most likely due to infarct size reduction via less reperfusion injury, although they could not exclude a role in reducing ventricular remodeling. A double blinded, placebo controlled Phase 2 clinical trial (7 days of treatment) with the A_1 partial agonist BAY1067197 (neladenoson bialanate) in patients with heart failure with reduced ejection fraction indicated that this agent was safe, although no beneficial effects on cardiac function were observed (Voors et al., 2017).

The possibility that adenosine receptors may modulate post-MI remodeling in patients highlights/emphasizes the need to conduct clinically relevant experimental chronic studies, rather than acute studies. Cardiac remodeling is due to chronic inflammation and fibrosis, mediated by immune cells and fibroblasts, both of which express at least two adenosine receptors. Adenosine A_{2A} receptors are well recognized for their anti-inflammatory effects, and there are reports that A_{2B} receptors may exert both anti- and pro-inflammatory effects (Hasko et al., 2008; Csoka et al., 2010; Feoktistov and Biaggioni, 2011; Linden, 2011; Haskó and Cronstein, 2013). Likewise, there is evidence that both A_{2A} and A_{2B} receptors regulate fibroblast function, including cardiac fibroblasts, although there are conflicting reports on their specific effects (Zhong et al., 2005; Villarreal et al., 2009; Zhang et al., 2014; Karmouty-Quintana et al., 2015; Shaikh and Cronstein, 2016). These observations and reports of adenosine receptor involvement in various chronic diseases (Long et al., 2010; Wang et al., 2010; Bot et al., 2012; Koupenova et al., 2012; Sangsiri et al., 2013; Zhang et al., 2013; Teng et al., 2014; Nayak et al., 2015; Yang et al., 2016), clearly warrant more studies on adenosine receptor modulation of chronic myocardial ischemia.

RECEPTOR AGONISTS OR ANTAGONISTS?

One aspect related to the lack of studies on adenosine receptor modulation of chronic myocardial ischemia, which has only recently been recognized, is the issue of receptor agonism vs. antagonism. All studies examining acute myocardial ischemia models have focused on treatment with receptor agonists, and in these studies blockade or deletion of any of the four adenosine receptor subtypes has resulted in little exacerbation of ischemia-reperfusion injury. However, there are numerous reports that antagonism or deletion of adenosine receptor subtypes is protective in models of both arterial and pulmonary hypertension, pulmonary and renal fibrosis, and sepsis (Sun et al., 2006; Kolachala et al., 2008; Zhou et al., 2011; Belikoff et al., 2012; Karmouty-Quintana et al., 2012, 2013a; Zhang et al., 2013; Nayak et al., 2015). The majority of these studies have focused on the anti-inflammatory and/or anti-fibrotic effects of A_{2B} receptor blockade.

At first glance, reports that A_{2B} antagonism is beneficial in chronic disease would appear to be contradictory to the reports of beneficial effects of A_{2B} agonism in the acute phase of myocardial ischemia. However, a review of the literature indicates there is substantial evidence for adenosine receptors playing dual roles in acute vs. chronic pathologies. For example, although the anti-inflammatory role of A_{2A} receptors has been recognized for years, there are more recent reports that A_{2A} receptor stimulation prolong IL-1β release and caspase-1 activity, consistent with inflammasome activation, in murine macrophages (Ouyang et al., 2013) and brain (Chiu et al., 2014). Ingwersen et al. (2016) also reported that while A_{2A} receptor stimulation was acutely beneficial in a murine model of autoimmune neuroinflammation, chronic inflammation was reduced in A_{2A} KO mice (Ingwersen et al., 2016). The time-dependent, opposing effects of adenosine A_{2A} and A_{2B} receptors are in fact consistent with the dual role of inflammation in the post-ischemic heart. Macrophages participate in both the initial pro-inflammatory phase to remove dead and dying tissue, but the subsequent anti-inflammatory period is necessary in order for cardiac fibroblasts to differentiate into myofibroblasts, which then deposit collagen (Nahrendorf et al., 2010; Frangogiannis, 2012; Prabhu and Frangogiannis, 2016). Collagen deposition is critical for maintaining scar thickness and strength in the infarct zone, but prolonged inflammation and excess collagen deposition lead to adverse ventricular remodeling (Nahrendorf et al., 2010; Frangogiannis, 2012; Prabhu and Frangogiannis, 2016).

To date there are only a very limited number of studies assessing potential beneficial effects of adenosine receptor blockade in chronic heart disease, both in experimental models and in clinical trials. Beneficial effects of A_1 receptor antagonists in experimental models of acute heart failure have been reported going back well over a decade (Nagashima et al., 1995; Givertz et al., 2007; Greenberg et al., 2007; Slawsky and Givertz, 2009). These beneficial effects were thought to be due primarily to blockade of A_1 receptor-mediated vasoconstriction of the renal afferent artery as well as proximal tubule reabsorption of sodium. Despite these positive findings in initial small trials, a large, randomized, placebo controlled Phase 3 trial (PROTECT) with the A_1 antagonist, rolofylline, failed to significantly impact cardiac or renal primary or secondary end points (Massie et al., 2010). More recently, the beneficial effects of A_{2B} receptor antagonism in experimental models of post-MI remodeling have been reported. Toldo et al. (2012) reported that the administration of the A_{2B} antagonist, GS-6201, immediately following a permanent occlusion in mice resulted in a thicker scar, less LV hypertrophy and improved post-MI cardiac function after 4 weeks. Similar findings were reported with the same A_{2B} antagonist in a chronic occlusion-reperfusion model in rats (Zhang et al., 2014). Thus, despite numerous experimental studies reporting beneficial effects of adenosine receptor antagonists in multiple non-cardiac pathologies, there remains a paucity of similar studies in chronic heart disease.

ADDITIONAL UNRESOLVED ISSUES

In addition to the above clinical-relevance issues, there are some unresolved basic science matters related to adenosine receptor-mediated cardioprotection. Adenosine receptors are differentially expressed on multiple cells types, thus altering the tissue and organ response to even selective agonists or antagonists (Chen et al., 2013; Sheth et al., 2014). This may explain, in part, the reported time-dependent differences in acute vs. chronic effects of adenosine receptor antagonists (Karmouty-Quintana et al., 2013b). As stated earlier, all four adenosine receptors have been implicated in protection against acute myocardial ischemia-reperfusion injury, and there are multiple reports that this is mediated by all four receptor subtypes modulating the same signaling pathways, presumably in cardiomyocytes (McIntosh and Lasley, 2012). There has yet to be an explanation why cardiomyocytes would express four different adenosine receptor subtypes exerting the same effect via the same signaling pathways. As discussed previously, the lack of studies addressing adenosine receptor effects in models of chronic myocardial ischemia have hindered our knowledge of the roles of specific adenosine receptors in non-cardiomyocytes, such as endothelial cells, immune cells and cardiac fibroblasts. Species-dependent differences in the selectivity of adenosine receptor agonists and antagonists have been recognized for many years, and this topic has most recently been addressed by Alnouri et al. (2015) and Jacobson and Müller (2016). This issue has undoubtedly had effects on the interpretation of numerous experimental studies, but its biggest impact has probably been on clinical trials, where despite reports of safety and tolerance, there remain few reports on the efficacy of adenosine receptor analogs in treating ischemic heart disease (Massie et al., 2010; Voors et al., 2017). Finally, there is increasing evidence in multiple tissues, that adenosine receptors may exert their effects, in part, via receptor dimerization (Zhan et al., 2011; McIntosh and Lasley, 2012; Chandrasekera et al., 2013; Chen et al., 2013). This aspect of adenosine receptor modulation of myocardial ischemia-reperfusion injury needs to be further explored, as this may lead to new, clinically relevant therapies.

In conclusion, nearly 30 years of experimental findings support the hypothesis that adenosine receptors modulate acute myocardial ischemia-reperfusion injury. Despite this evidence, the use of adenosine, adenosine modulators, or adenosine analogs for treatment of cardiac injury has not been accepted clinically, nor have there been many clinical trials. Clearly the next phase of research on adenosine receptor cardioprotection needs to establish the role of adenosine receptor agonists and antagonists in more clinically relevant models of myocardial ischemia.

AUTHOR CONTRIBUTIONS

The author confirms being the sole contributor of this work and approved it for publication.

REFERENCES

Alnouri, M. W., Jepards, S., Casari, A., Schiedel, A. C., Hinz, S., and Müller, C. E. (2015). Selectivity is species-dependent: characterization of standard agonists and antagonists at human, rat, and mouse adenosine receptors. *Purinergic Signal.* 11, 389–407. doi: 10.1007/s11302-015-9460-9

Belikoff, B. G., Vaickus, L. J., Sitkovsky, M., and Remick, D. G. (2012). A2B adenosine receptor expression by myeloid cells is proinflammatory in murine allergic-airway inflammation. *J. Immunol.* 189, 3707–3713. doi: 10.4049/jimmunol.1201207

Bot, I., de Vries, H., Korporaal, S. J., Foks, A. C., Bot, M., van Veldhoven, J., et al. (2012). Adenosine A2B receptor agonism inhibits neointimal lesion development after arterial injury in apolipoprotein E-deficient mice. *Arterioscler. Thromb. Vasc. Biol.* 32, 2197–2205. doi: 10.1161/ATVBAHA.112.252924

Bulluck, H., Sirker, A., Loke, Y. K., Garcia-Dorado, D., and Hausenloy, D. J. (2016). Clinical benefit of adenosine as an adjunct to reperfusion in ST-elevation myocardial infarction patients: an updated meta-analysis of randomized controlled trials. *Int. J. Cardiol.* 202, 228–237. doi: 10.1016/j.ijcard.2015.09.005

Cabiati, M., Svezia, B., Guzzardi, M. A., Mattii, L., D'Amico, A., Caselli, C., Prescimone, T., et al. (2015). Adenosine receptor transcriptomic profile in cardiac tissue of a Zucker rat model. *DNA Cell Biol.* 34, 333–341. doi: 10.1089/dna.2014.2770

Cerqueira, M. D., Nguyen, P., Staehr, P., Underwood, S. R., Iskandrian, A. E., and ADVANCE-MPI Trial Investigators (2008). Effects of age, gender, obesity, and diabetes on the efficacy and safety of the selective A2A agonist regadenoson versus adenosine in myocardial perfusion imaging integrated ADVANCE-MPI trial results. *JACC Cardiovasc. Imaging* 1, 307–316. doi: 10.1016/j.jcmg.2008.02.003

Chandrasekera, P. C., Wan, T. C., Gizewski, E. T., Auchampach, J. A., and Lasley, R. D. (2013). Adenosine A1 receptors heterodimerize with β1- and β2-adrenergic receptors creating novel receptor complexes with altered G protein coupling and signaling. *Cell. Signal.* 25, 736–742. doi: 10.1016/j.cellsig.2012.12.022

Chen, J. F., Eltzschig, H. K., and Fredholm, B. B. (2013). Adenosine receptors as drug targets–what are the challenges? *Nat. Rev. Drug Discov.* 12, 265–286. doi: 10.1038/nrd3955

Chiu, G. S., Darmody, P. T., Walsh, J. P., Moon, M. L., Kwakwa, K. A., Bray, J. K., et al. (2014). Adenosine through the A2A adenosine receptor increases IL-1β in the brain contributing to anxiety. *Brain Behav. Immun.* 41, 218–231. doi: 10.1016/j.bbi.2014.05.018

Csoka, B., Nemeth, Z. H., Rosenberger, P., Eltzschig, H. K., Spolarics, Z., Pacher, P., et al. (2010). A2B adenosine receptors protect against sepsis-induced mortality by dampening excessive inflammation. *J. Immunol.* 185, 542–550. doi: 10.4049/jimmunol.0901295

Dhasmana, J. P., Digerness, S. B., Geckle, J. M., Ng, T. C., Glickson, J. D., and Blackstone, E. H. (1983). Effect of adenosine deaminase inhibitors on the heart's functional and biochemical recovery from ischemia: a study utilizing the isolated rat heart adapted to ^{31}P nuclear magnetic resonance. *J. Cardiovasc. Pharmacol.* 5, 1040–1047. doi: 10.1097/00005344-198311000-00019

Ely, S. W., Mentzer, R. M., Lasley, R. D., Lee, B. K., and Berne, R. M. (1985). Functional and metabolic evidence of enhanced myocardial tolerance to ischemia and reperfusion with adenosine. *J. Thorac. Cardiovasc. Surg.* 90, 549–556.

Feoktistov, I., and Biaggioni, I. (2011). Role of adenosine A(2B) receptors in inflammation. *Adv Pharmacol.* 61, 115–144. doi: 10.1016/B978-0-12-385526-8.00005-9

Frangogiannis, N. G. (2012). Regulation of the inflammatory response in cardiac repair. *Circ. Res.* 110, 159–173. doi: 10.1161/CIRCRESAHA.111.243162

Givertz, M., Massie, B., Fields, T., Pearson, L., and Dittrich, H. (2007). The effects of KW-3902, an adenosine A1-receptor antagonist, on diuresis and renal function in patients with acute decompensated heart failure and renal impairment or diuretic resistance. *J. Am. Coll. Cardiol.* 50, 1551–1560. doi: 10.1016/j.jacc.2007.07.019

Goto, M., Miura, T., Iliodoromitis, E. K., O'Leary, E. L., Ishimoto, R., Yellon, D. M., et al. (1991). Adenosine infusion during early reperfusion failed to limit myocardial infarct size in a collateral deficient species. *Cardiovasc. Res.* 25, 943–949.

Greenberg, B., Thomas, I., Banish, D., et al. (2007). Effects of multiple oral doses of an A1 adenosine antagonist, BG9928, in patients with heart failure: results of a placebo-controlled, dose-escalation study. *J. Am. Coll. Cardiol.* 50, 600–606. doi: 10.1016/j.jacc.2007.03.059

Haskó, G., and Cronstein, B. (2013). Regulation of inflammation by adenosine. *Front. Immunol.* 4:85. doi: 10.3389/fimmu.2013.00085

Hasko, G., Linden, J., Cronstein, B., and Pacher, P. (2008). Adenosine receptors: therapeutic aspects for inflammatory and immune diseases. *Nature Rev. Drug Disc.* 7, 759–770. doi: 10.1038/nrd2638

Headrick, J. P., and Lasley, R. D. (2009). Adenosine receptors and reperfusion injury of the heart. *Handb. Exp. Pharmacol.* 193, 189–214. doi: 10.1007/978-3-540-89615-9_7

Headrick, J. P., Willems, L., Ashton, K. J., Holmgren, K., Peart, J., and Matherne, G. P. (2003). Ischaemic tolerance in aged mouse myocardium: the role of adenosine and effects of A1 adenosine receptor overexpression. *J. Physiol.* 549, 823–833. doi: 10.1113/jphysiol.2003.041541

Homeister, J. W., Hoff, P. T., Fletcher, D. D., and Lucchesi, B. R. (1990). Combined adenosine and lidocaine administration limits myocardial reperfusion injury. *Circulation* 82, 595–608. doi: 10.1161/01.CIR.82.2.595

Humphrey, S. M., and Seelye, R. N. (1982). Improved functional recovery of ischemic myocardium by suppression of adenosine catabolism. *J. Thorac. Cardiovasc. Surg.* 84, 16–22.

Ingwersen, J., Wingerath, B., Graf, J., Lepka, K., Hofrichter, M., Schröter, F., et al. (2016). Dual roles of the adenosine A2a receptor in autoimmune neuroinflammation. *J. Neuroinflammation.* 13:48. doi: 10.1186/s12974-016-0512-z

Jacobson, K. A., and Müller, C. E. (2016). Medicinal chemistry of adenosine, P2Y and P2X receptors. *Neuropharmacology* 104, 31–49. doi: 10.1016/j.neuropharm.2015.12.001

Karmouty-Quintana, H., Philip, K., Acero, L. F., Chen, N. Y., Weng, T., Molina, J. G., et al. (2015). Deletion of ADORA2B from myeloid cells dampens lung fibrosis and pulmonary hypertension. *FASEB J.* 29, 50–60. doi: 10.1096/fj.14-260182

Karmouty-Quintana, H., Weng, T., Garcia-Morales, L. J., Chen, N. Y., Pedroza, M., Zhong, H., et al. (2013a). Adenosine A2B receptor and hyaluronan modulate pulmonary hypertension associated with chronic obstructive pulmonary disease. *Am. J. Respir. Cell Mol. Biol.* 49, 1038–1047. doi: 10.1165/rcmb.2013-0089OC

Karmouty-Quintana, H., Xia, Y., and Blackburn, M. R. (2013b). Adenosine signaling during acute and chronic disease states. *J. Mol. Med.* 91, 173–181. doi: 10.1007/s00109-013-0997-1

Karmouty-Quintana, H., Zhong, H., Acero, L., Weng, T., Melicoff, E., West, J. D., et al. (2012). The A2B adenosine receptor modulates pulmonary hypertension associated with interstitial lung disease. *FASEB J.* 26, 2546–2557. doi: 10.1096/fj.11-200907

Kloner, R. A., Forman, M. B., Gibbons, R. J., Ross, A. M., Alexander, R. W., and Stone, G. W. (2006). Impact of time to therapy and reperfusion modality on the efficacy of adenosine in acute myocardial infarction: the AMISTAD-2 trial. *Eur. Heart J.* 27, 2400–2405. doi: 10.1093/eurheartj/ehl094

Kolachala, V., Ruble, B., Vijay-Kumar, M., Wang, L., Mwangi, S., Figler, H., et al. (2008). Blockade of adenosine A2B receptors ameliorates murine colitis. *Br. J. Pharmacol.* 155, 127–137. doi: 10.1038/bjp.2008.227

Koupenova, M., Johnston-Cox, H., Vezeridis, A., Gavras, H., Yang, D., Zannis, V., et al. (2012). A2b adenosine receptor regulates hyperlipidemia and atherosclerosis. *Circulation.* 125, 354–363. doi: 10.1161/CIRCULATIONAHA.111.057596

Kristo, G., Yoshimura, Y., Keith, B. J., Mentzer, R. M. Jr., and Lasley, R. D. (2005). Aged rat myocardium exhibits normal adenosine receptor-mediated bradycardia and coronary vasodilation but increased adenosine agonist-mediated cardioprotection. *J. Gerontol. A Biol. Sci. Med. Sci.* 60, 1399–1404. doi: 10.1093/gerona/60.11.1399

Krumholz, H. M., Wang, Y., Chen, J., Drye, E. E., Spertus, J. A., Ross, J. S., et al. (2009). Reduction in acute myocardial infarction mortality in the United States: risk-standardized mortality rates from 1995-2006. *JAMA* 302, 767–773. doi: 10.1001/jama.2009.1178

Lasley, R. D., Jahania, M. S. A., Mentzer, R. M. Jr. (2001). Beneficial effects of the adenosine A_{2a} agonist CGS 21680 in infarcted and stunned porcine myocardium. *Am. J. Physiol.* 280, H1660–H1666. doi: 10.1152/ajpheart.2001.280.4.H1660

Lasley, R. D., Rhee, J. W., Van Wylen, D. G., and Mentzer, R. M. Jr. (1990). Adenosine A_1 receptor mediated protection of the globally ischemic isolated rat heart. *J. Mol. Cell. Cardiol.* 22, 39–47. doi: 10.1016/0022-2828(90)90970-D

Linden, J. (2011). Regulation of leukocyte function by adenosine receptors. *Adv Pharmacol.* 61, 95–114. doi: 10.1016/B978-0-12-385526-8.00004-7

Liu, G. S., Thornton, J., Van Winkle, D. M., Stanley, A. W., Olsson, R. A., and Downey, J. M. (1991). Protection against infarction afforded by preconditioning is mediated by A1 adenosine receptors in rabbit heart. *Circulation* 84, 350–356. doi: 10.1161/01.CIR.84.1.350

Long, X., Mokelke, E. A., Neeb, Z. P., Alloosh, M., Edwards, J. M., and Sturek, M. (2010). Adenosine receptor regulation of coronary blood flow in Ossabaw miniature swine. *J. Pharmacol. Exp. Ther.* 335, 781–787. doi: 10.1124/jpet.110.170803

Mahaffey, K. W., Puma, J. A., Barbagelata, N. A., DiCarli, M. F., Leesar, M. A., Browne, K. F., et al. (1999). Adenosine as an adjunct to thrombolytic therapy for acute myocardial infarction: results of a multicenter, randomized, placebo-controlled trial: the Acute Myocardial Infarction STudy of ADenosine (AMISTAD) trial. *J. Am. Coll. Cardiol.* 34, 1711–1720. doi: 10.1016/S0735-1097(99)00418-0

Massie, B. M., O'Connor, C. M., Metra, M., Ponikowski, P., Teerlink, J. R., Cotter, G., et al. (2010). Rolofylline, an adenosine A1-receptor antagonist, in acute heart failure. *N. Engl. J. Med.* 363, 1419–1428. doi: 10.1056/NEJMoa0912613

McIntosh, V. J., and Lasley, R. D. (2012). Adenosine receptor-mediated cardioprotection: are all 4 subtypes required or redundant? *J. Cardiovasc. Pharmacol. Ther.* 17, 21–33. doi: 10.1177/1074248410396877

Nagashima, K., Kusaka, H., and Karasawa, A. (1995). Protective effects of KW-3902, an adenosine A1-receptor antagonist, against cisplatin-induced acute renal failure in rats. *Jpn. J. Pharmacol.* 67, 349–357. doi: 10.1254/jjp.67.349

Nahrendorf, M., Pittet, M. J., and Swirski, F. K. (2010). Monocytes: protagonists of infarct inflammation and repair after myocardial infarction. *Circulation* 121, 2437–2445. doi: 10.1161/CIRCULATIONAHA.109.916346

Nayak, S., Khan, M. A., Wan, T. C., Pei, H., Linden, J., Dwinell, M. R., et al. (2015). Characterization of Dahl salt-sensitive rats with genetic disruption of the A2B adenosine receptor gene: implications for A2B adenosine receptor signaling during hypertension. *Purinergic Signal.* 11, 519–531. doi: 10.1007/s11302-015-9470-7

Olafsson, B., Forman, M. B., Puett, D. W., Pou, A., Cates, C. U., Friesinger, G. C., et al. (1987). Reduction of reperfusion injury in the canine preparation by intracoronary adenosine: importance of the endothelium and the no-reflow phenomenon. *Circulation* 76, 1135–1145. doi: 10.1161/01.CIR.76.5.1135

Ouyang, X., Ghani, A., Malik, A., Wilder, T., Colegio, O. R., Flavell, R. A., et al. (2013). Adenosine is required for sustained inflammasome activation via the A2A receptor and the HIF-1α pathway. *Nat. Commun.* 4:2909. doi: 10.1038/ncomms3909

Peart, J. N., Pepe, S., Reichelt, M. E., Beckett, N., See Hoe, L., Ozberk, V., et al. (2014). Dysfunctional survival-signaling and stress-intolerance in aged murine and human myocardium. *Exp. Gerontol.* 50, 72–81. doi: 10.1016/j.exger.2013.11.015

Pitarys, C. J., Virmani, R., Vildibill, H. D. Jr., Jackson, E. K., and Forman, M. B. (1991). Reduction of myocardial reperfusion injury by intravenous adenosine administered during the early reperfusion period. *Circulation* 83, 237–247. doi: 10.1161/01.CIR.83.1.237

Prabhu, S. D., and Frangogiannis, N. G. (2016). The biological basis for cardiac repair after myocardial infarction: from inflammation to fibrosis. *Circ. Res.* 119, 91–112. doi: 10.1161/CIRCRESAHA.116.303577

Reibel, D. K., and Rovetto, M. J. (1978). Myocardial ATP synthesis and mechanical function following oxygen deficiency. *Am. J. Physiol.* 234, H620–H624. doi: 10.1152/ajpheart.1978.234.5.H620

Sabbah, H. N., Gupta, R. C., Kohli, S., Wang, M., Rastogi, S., Zhang, K., et al. (2013). Chronic therapy with a partial adenosine A1-receptor agonist improves left ventricular function and remodeling in dogs with advanced heart failure. *Circ. Heart Fail.* 6, 563–571. doi: 10.1161/CIRCHEARTFAILURE.112.000208

Sangsiri, S., Dong, H., Swain, G. M., Galligan, J. J., and Xu, H. (2013). Impaired function of prejunctional adenosine A1 receptors expressed by perivascular sympathetic nerves in DOCA-salt hypertensive rats. *J. Pharmacol. Exp. Ther.* 345, 32–40. doi: 10.1124/jpet.112.199612

Schulman, D., Latchman, D. S., and Yellon, D. M. (2001). Effect of aging on the ability of preconditioning to protect rat hearts from ischemia-reperfusion injury. *Am. J. Physiol. Heart Circ. Physiol.* 281, H1630–H1636. doi: 10.1152/ajpheart.2001.281.4.H1630

Shaikh, G., and Cronstein, B. (2016). Signaling pathways involving adenosine A2A and A2B receptors in wound healing and fibrosis. *Purinergic Signal.* 12, 191–197. doi: 10.1007/s11302-016-9498-3

Sheth, S., Brito, R., Mukherjea, D., Rybak, L. P., and Ramkumar, V. (2014). Adenosine receptors: expression, function and regulation. *Int. J. Mol. Sci.* 28, 2024–2052. doi: 10.3390/ijms15022024

Slawsky, M. T., and Givertz, M. M. (2009). Rolofylline: a selective adenosine 1 receptor antagonist for the treatment of heart failure. *Expert Opin. Pharmacother.* 10, 311–322. doi: 10.1517/14656560802682213

Sun, C. X., Zhong, H., Mohsenin, A., Morschl, E., Chunn, J. L., Molina, J. G., et al. (2006). Role of A2B adenosine receptor signaling in adenosine-dependent pulmonary inflammation and injury. *J. Clin. Invest.* 116, 2173–2182. doi: 10.1172/JCI27303

Teng, B., Smith, J. D., Rosenfeld, M. E., Robinet, P., Davis, M. E., Morrison, R. R., et al. (2014). A1 adenosine receptor deficiency or inhibition reduces atherosclerotic lesions in apolipoprotein E deficient mice. *Cardiovasc. Res.* 102, 157–165. doi: 10.1093/cvr/cvu033

Toldo, S., Zhong, H., Mezzaroma, E., Van Tassell, B. W., Kannan, H., Zeng, D., et al. (2012). GS-6201, a selective blocker of the A2B adenosine receptor, attenuates cardiac remodeling after acute myocardial infarction in the mouse. *J. Pharmacol. Exp. Therap.* 343, 587–595. doi: 10.1124/jpet.111.191288

Toufektsian, M. C., Yang, Z., Prasad, K. M., Overbergh, L., Ramos, S. I, Mathieu, C., et al. (2006). Stimulation of A2A-adenosine receptors after myocardial infarction suppresses inflammatory activation and attenuates contractile dysfunction in the remote left ventricle. *Am. J. Physiol.* 290, H1410–H1418. doi: 10.1152/ajpheart.00860.2005

Vander Heide, R. S., and Reimer, K. A. (1996). Effect of adenosine therapy at reperfusion on myocardial infarct size in dogs. *Cardiovasc. Res.* 31, 711–718. doi: 10.1016/S0008-6363(95)00235-9

Villarreal, F., Epperson, S. A., Ramirez-Sanchez, I., Yamazaki, K. G., and Brunton, L. L. (2009). Regulation of cardiac fibroblast collagen synthesis by adenosine: roles for Epac and PI3K. *Am. J. Physiol. Cell Physiol.* 296, C1178–C1184. doi: 10.1152/ajpcell.00291.2008

Villarreal, F., Zimmermann, S., Makhsudova, L., Montag, A. C., Erion, M. D., Bullough, D. A., et al. (2003). Modulation of cardiac remodeling by adenosine: *in vitro* and *in vivo* effects. *Mol. Cell. Biochem.* 251, 17–26. doi: 10.1023/A:1025401026441

Voors, A. A., Düngen, H. D., Senni, M., Nodari, S., Agostoni, P., Ponikowski, P., et al. (2017). Safety and tolerability of neladenoson bialanate, a novel oral partial adenosine A1 receptor agonist, in patients with chronic heart failure. *J. Clin. Pharmacol.* 57, 440–451. doi: 10.1002/jcph.828

Wakeno, M., Minamino, T., Seguchi, O., Okazaki, H., Tsukamoto, O., Okada, K., et al. (2006). Long-term stimulation of adenosine A2b receptors begun after myocardial infarction prevents cardiac remodeling in rats. *Circulation* 114, 1923–1932. doi: 10.1161/CIRCULATIONAHA.106.630087

Wang, H., Zhang, W., Tang, R., Zhu, C., Bucher, C., Blazar, B. R., et al. (2010). Adenosine receptor A2A deficiency in leukocytes increases arterial neointima formation in apolipoprotein E-deficient mice. *Arterioscler. Thromb. Vasc. Biol.* 30, 915–922. doi: 10.1161/ATVBAHA.109.202572

Xaus, J., Mirabet, M., Lloberas, J., Soler, C., Lluis, C., Franco, R., et al. (1999). IFN-gamma up-regulates the A2B adenosine receptor expression in macrophages: a mechanism of macrophage deactivation. *J. Immunol.* 162, 3607–3614.

Yang, T., Zollbrecht, C., Winerdal, M. E., Zhuge, Z., Zhang, X. M., Terrando, N., et al. (2016). Genetic abrogation of adenosine A3 receptor prevents uninephrectomy and high salt-induced hypertension. *J. Am. Heart Assoc.* 5:7. doi: 10.1161/JAHA.116.003868

Zhan, E., McIntosh, V. J., and Lasley, R. D. (2011). Adenosine A2A and A2B receptors are both required for adenosine A1 receptor-mediated cardioprotection. *Am. J. Physiol.* 301, H1183–H1189. doi: 10.1152/ajpheart.00264.2011

Zhang, H., Zhong, H., Everett, T. H., Wilson, E., Chang, R., Zeng, D., et al. (2014). Blockade of A2B adenosine receptor reduces left ventricular dysfunction and ventricular arrhythmias 1 week after myocardial infarction in the rat model. *Heart Rhythm* 11, 101–109. doi: 10.1016/j.hrthm.2013.10.023

Zhang, W., Zhang, Y., Wang, W., Dai, Y., Ning, C., Luo, R., et al. (2013). Elevated ecto-5′-nucleotidase-mediated increased renal adenosine signaling via A2B adenosine receptor contributes to chronic hypertension. *Circ. Res.* 112, 1466–1478. doi: 10.1161/CIRCRESAHA.111.300166

Zhong, H., Belardinelli, L., Maa, T., and Zeng, D. (2005). Synergy between A2B adenosine receptors and hypoxia in activating human lung fibroblasts. *Am. J. Respir. Cell. Mol. Biol.* 32, 2–8. doi: 10.1165/rcmb.2004-0103OC

Zhou, Y., Schneider, D. J, Morschl, E, Song, L, Pedroza, M., Karmouty-Quintana, H., et al. (2011). Distinct roles for the A2B adenosine receptor in acute and chronic stages of bleomycin-induced lung injury. *J. Immunol.* 186, 1097–1106. doi: 10.4049/jimmunol.1002907

11

Amyotrophic Lateral Sclerosis (ALS) and Adenosine Receptors

Ana M. Sebastião[1,2], Nádia Rei[1,2] and Joaquim A. Ribeiro[1,2]*

[1] *Instituto de Farmacologia e Neurociências, Faculdade de Medicina, Universidade de Lisboa, Lisbon, Portugal,* [2] *Instituto de Medicina Molecular, Universidade de Lisboa, Lisbon, Portugal*

Correspondence:
Ana M. Sebastião
anaseb@medicina.ulisboa.pt

In the present review we discuss the potential involvement of adenosinergic signaling, in particular the role of adenosine receptors, in amyotrophic lateral sclerosis (ALS). Though the literature on this topic is not abundant, the information so far available on adenosine receptors in animal models of ALS highlights the interest to continue to explore the role of these receptors in this neurodegenerative disease. Indeed, all motor neurons affected in ALS are responsive to adenosine receptor ligands but interestingly, there are alterations in pre-symptomatic or early symptomatic stages that mirror those in advanced disease stages. Information starts to emerge pointing toward a beneficial role of A_{2A} receptors ($A_{2A}R$), most probably at early disease states, and a detrimental role of caffeine, in clear contrast with what occurs in other neurodegenerative diseases. However, some evidence also exists on a beneficial action of $A_{2A}R$ antagonists. It may happen that there are time windows where $A_{2A}R$ prove beneficial and others where their blockade is required. Furthermore, the same changes may not occur simultaneously at the different synapses. In line with this, it is not fully understood if ALS is a dying back disease or if it propagates in a centrifugal way. It thus seems crucial to understand how motor neuron dysfunction occurs, how adenosine receptors are involved in those dysfunctions and whether the early changes in purinergic signaling are compensatory or triggers for the disease. Getting this information is crucial before starting the design of purinergic based strategies to halt or delay disease progression.

Keywords: adenosine receptors, amyotrophic lateral sclerosis (ALS), spinal cord motor neurons, neuromuscular junction, glial cells

INTRODUCTION

In the present review, we will address the potential role of adenosine on amyotrophic lateral sclerosis (ALS), also known as Lou Gehrig's disease. This is one of the most devastating neurodegenerative disorders and is the most common form of Motor Neuron Diseases group. During ALS progression, both the upper motor neurons (motor neurons in the cortex) and the lower motor neurons (motor neurons in the spinal cord) degenerate or die. As a consequence of deficient input from the motor neuron, there is a progressive and terminal atrophy of skeletal muscles. All muscles under voluntary control are affected, and individuals lose their strength and the ability to move their arms, legs and body. When diaphragm and the muscles in the chest wall fail, people lose the ability to breathe without ventilation support (Nichols et al., 2013).

The incidence of this disease is 2–3/100,000 and the prevalence 4–7/100,000 (Nalini et al., 2008). The onset of symptoms is predominantly between 55 and 65 years old and the median survival of ALS patients, after the diagnosis, is 3–5 years; however, about 10% of the patients survive for 10 or more years (Wijesekera and Leigh, 2009).

The majority of cases of ALS are sporadic (sALS) (90–95%), but some cases have a positive familial history (fALS) (5–10%) (Kiernan et al., 2011). Both forms, sALS and fALS, present similar pathological and clinical features. In the case of fALS, the inheritance is autossomal dominant, but the penetrance is variable. About 20% of fALS are caused by a missense mutation in *SOD1* gene, encoding for the Cu/Zn superoxide dismutase 1 enzyme. This finding led to the first and most used rodent model for ALS, the $SOD1^{G93A}$ mouse, which in the symptomatic phase recapitulate most features of the disease, including neuromuscular dysfunction (Naumenko et al., 2011). There is still a debate whether motor neuron degeneration initially results from failure of enzymatic machinery at the level of the cell body and proximal parts of the axon that then propagates in a centrifugal way due to impaired axonal transport (Braak et al., 2013), or results from an early dysfunction at the level of the nerve terminals, with consequent synaptic dysfunction and then progressing in a 'dying back' process (Frey et al., 2000; Dadon-Nachum et al., 2011), or both (Baker, 2014). As pointed out (Dadon-Nachum et al., 2011), if cell nerve terminal degeneration precedes with axonal and cell body degeneration, early intervention focusing on motor neurons terminals could potentially delay or prevent the progressive loss of motor neurons. A functional study focusing on the activity of single end-plates demonstrated that neuromuscular transmission impairment starts long before symptomatic onset (Rocha et al., 2013). Importantly, in pre-symptomatic SOD^{G92A} mice there are functional hallmarks of dysregulated intraterminal calcium levels (Rocha et al., 2013) in consonance with the hypothesis that nerve terminal machinery designed to buffer calcium might be impaired at very early disease stages. The pathophysiological alterations at the neuromuscular junction of SOD^{G92A} mice are accompanied with alterations in the activity of adenosine receptors at the motor nerve terminals in these mice (Nascimento et al., 2014, 2015).

Mutations in the gene coding for a nuclear protein, TAR DNA-binding protein-43 are also frequent in fALS (Leblond et al., 2014). This protein has several functions in regulation of gene expression, which thus indicates a clear dysfunction at the level of the neuronal soma in some forms of ALS. ROS induce the mislocalization of TAR-DNA binding protein 43 (TDP-43) from the nucleus into the cytoplasm (Ayala et al., 2011), where it forms aggregates, an early hallmark of ALS (Neumann et al., 2006; Chou et al., 2018). Cytoplasmic mislocalization of TDP-43 is accompanied by further ROS production and overactivation AMP kinase (AMPK), an action suppressed by $A_{2A}R$ activation (Liu et al., 2015a). Importantly, $A_{2A}R$ activation in a TDP-43Tg mouse model of ALS, improved motor function (Liu et al., 2015a). Interestingly also, activation of AMPK changed the location of a mRNA stabilizer in the motor neurons of ALS patients, in mouse motor neurons, and in a motor neuron cell line, and this mislocalization was also suppressed by activation of $A_{2A}Rs$ (Liu et al., 2015b). This again reinforces the idea of a putative neuroprotective role of $A_{2A}Rs$ in ALS since impaired RNA homeostasis is a major pathway for ALS pathogenesis (Liu et al., 2017).

Mutations in *C9ORF72* are also frequently found in fALS and accounts for 10% of the sporadic cases (DeJesus-Hernandez et al., 2011; Smith et al., 2013). Motor neurons with *C9ORF72* mutations have increased expression and activity of NMDA receptors and calcium permeable AMPA receptors (Selvaraj et al., 2018; Shi et al., 2018), known to be targets for adenosine receptor-mediated modulation (Dias et al., 2012, 2013). No information so far exists on the possibility that adenosine receptor ligands may influence motor neuronal survival in this model of ALS.

Being adenosine a ubiquitous neuromodulator, affecting synaptic transmission at pre- post and non-synaptic levels, having adenosine receptors not only neuroprotective but also excitotoxic and neuroinflammatory actions, it is somehow unexpected that only relatively few studies concentrated their attention on the influence of adenosine on ALS progression. Evidence so far available highlights early dysfunctions of neuromodulation by adenosine and the ability to influence those dysfunctions through manipulation of adenosine receptors. In this review we will critically analyze data so far available.

PATHOPHYSIOLOGY OF ALS

ALS is a complex, multifactorial and multi-systemic disease, the pathophysiological mechanisms of motor neurons degeneration remaining yet incompletely known. Some of these mechanisms include RNA dysfunction, protein misfolding and aggregation, marked neuromuscular junction abnormalities, immune system deficiency, mitochondrial dysfunction, neuroinflammation, cytoskeletal derangements, desregulation of growth factors, oxidative stress, axonal disruption and apoptosis, excitotoxity (induced by glutamate), activation of nucleases and proteases and abnormal calcium metabolism (Pasinelli and Brown, 2006; Costa et al., 2010; Chou et al., 2018). It is becoming clear that ALS is a disease that involves different cell types and the communication between them, the damage that occurs in each cell population contributing to ALS pathogenicity and phenotype, thus to the progression of the disease (Taylor et al., 2016). Indeed, non-motor neuron cells, like interneurons, astrocytes, microglia, Schwann cells, skeletal muscle cells and oligodendrocytes play a crucial role in motor neuron survival, and their dysfunction impact upon motor neuron degeneration. In practical terms, a major problem that is shared with many neurodegenerative diseases is that when patients are diagnosed, the neuronal degeneration, in the case of ALS motor neuron degeneration, has already started and progressed.

Functional and structural changes at the level of the endplate are major events in ALS. It has now been realized that the functional changes may precede not only the structural ones but also the onset of symptoms. Studies conducted in our lab (Rocha et al., 2013) to investigate transmission at the diaphragm neuromuscular junction in $SOD1^{G93A}$ mice revealed that the during the pre-symptomatic phase there is an enhanced release of ACh from nerve terminals, as determined by the mean quantal content of end-plate potentials. Also in these neuromuscular junctions the frequency of giant miniature endplate potentials (GMEPPs) was markedly increased, suggesting that the ability of the nerve terminal machinery to control cytoplasmatic $[Ca^{2+}]$ is dysregulated. In early symptomatic (defined as moderate changes performance in the RotaRod test) SOD1^{G93A} mice two groups of neuromuscular junctions were identified, both of them co-existing in the same innervated diaphragm (Rocha et al., 2013): one group, designated as group A (SOD1a group), presented significant reduction of the mean amplitude of EPP, a significant reduction of the mean amplitude of MEPPS, and a slight but not significant reduction of the quantal content of EPPs. All these changes indicate a predominant post-synaptic impairment. The frequency of GMEPPs was significantly reduced in SOD1a neuromuscular junctions, even as compared with wild type siblings, indicating that presynaptic calcium dysregulations persisted, though with opposite signal in pre-symptomatic and in symptomatic mice. The other group of neuromuscular junctions, designated as group B (SOD1b) (Rocha et al., 2013) displayed electrophysiological characteristics somehow in between those of age-matched wild type and pre-symptomatic mice, being not significantly different from any of these groups. Summarizing, data suggest (Rocha et al., 2013) an exacerbated, but already dysregulated, presynaptic activity at the mice neuromuscular junctions that do not yet display motor symptoms; once symptoms start to appear some neuromuscular junctions are already hypofunctional, some others being probably in a transition between hyper and hypofunction.

Presynaptic facilitation of neuromuscular transmission preceding motor symptoms was further confirmed in using a late onset slow progressing disease model, the SOD1^{G37R} mice (Arbour et al., 2015). A recent study (Arbour et al., 2017) taking advantage of this late onset slow progressing disease model, systematically analyzed the changes in synaptic properties over the course of the disease progression and as a function of the motor unit type. Indeed, different motor units have different susceptibility to the disease, and it became clear the time course and the sequence of events associated with neuromuscular transmission dysfunction depend on the motor unit type (Arbour et al., 2017). The slow motor neurons are those that degenerate later and interestingly, they display an early and transient increase in the quantal content of endplate potentials that disappear at disease onset. In contrast, fast fatigue motor neurons, those that degenerate first, have reduced quantal content even before disease onset. Somehow in the between, fatigue resistant motor units only evidence neuromuscular transmission dysfunction after disease onset (Arbour et al., 2017). Interestingly only slow-type motor neurons display intrinsic hyperexcitability in pre-symptomatic mice (Leroy et al., 2014), pointing toward the possibility that early intrinsic hyperexcitability does not contribute to motor neuron degeneration, but rather represents an early compensatory process. It is worthwhile to note that as previously seen while using the SOD1^{G93A} mice (Rocha et al., 2013), in SOD1^{G37R} mice the neuromuscular transmission alterations precede the onset of motor symptoms, as well as precede motor neuron loss, axonal degeneration, and NMJ structural changes (Arbour et al., 2017).

It is nowadays clear that motor neuron degeneration in ALS also involves glial cells, namely astrocytes, oligodendrocytes, microglia, Schwann Cells and, in the case of the neuromuscular junction, perisynaptic Schwann cells (PSCs). PSCs have neuromodulatory properties close to those of astrocytes in the central nervous system, closely interacting with nerve terminals. Thus, PSCs respond to ATP and ACh released during nerve activity, which act through P2Y and muscarinic ACh receptors (mAChRs) coupled to transient increases in intracellular calcium concentration, a process that has to be kept under proper control to keep PSCs competent for their functions to modulate and to repair neuromuscular transmission (Son et al., 1996; Georgiou et al., 1999; Feng and Ko, 2008a,b). Interestingly, PSC of SOD1 mice displayed exacerbated mAChR responses and exacerbated calcium signaling, which precede functional and morphological changes at the neuromuscular junction, suggesting that the impairments of PSC functions may contribute to NMJ dysfunction and ALS pathogenesis (Arbour et al., 2015).

At the level of spinal cord and focusing in neuroinflammatory and cellular intercommunication hallmarks, it has recently been also shown a clear difference between pre-symptomatic and symptomatic stages (Cunha et al., 2017). Thus, before onset of motor symptoms, alterations in both astrocytes and microglia have been detected in the spinal cord of SOD1^{G93A} mice, which comprise decreased expression of astrocytic, microglia, inflammatory and cell communication markers together with upregulation of a glutamate transporter-1 marker. In contrast, in the symptomatic stage, increased markers of inflammation became evident (Cunha et al., 2017). Microglia activation, suggestive of a switch from M1 to M2-like microglia subpopulations, have been detected in control cells exposed to exosomes derived from motor neuron-like cells transfected with mutant SOD1^{G93A} (Cunha et al., 2017), thus suggesting that disease progression is promoted by cell to cell communication events. There is also a growing body of evidence showing that astrocytes expressing ALS-associated proteins impair motor neuron survival and potentiate ALS progression (Di Giorgio et al., 2007; Nagai et al., 2007; Marchetto et al., 2008; Qian et al., 2017).

Recent attention has been paid to two other ALS-related dysfunctions, TDP-43 aggregation and *C9ORF72* repeated expansion. Mutations in the gene that codes for TDP-43, *TARDBP*, may favor TDP-43 aggregation but phosphorylated TDP-43 containing aggregates also occur in sALS (Neumann et al., 2006; Chou et al., 2018). Indeed, TDP-43 aggregates are found in 97% of ALS cases of diverse etiology and constitute a major component of protein inclusions in this disease (Arai et al., 2006; Maekawa et al., 2009). TDP-43 is a nuclear protein that interacts with RNA molecules and is involved in a wide variety of relevant cellular pathways related to RNA and protein homeostasis. TDP-43 C-terminal missense mutations have been identified in ALS patients, which promote mislocalization of TDP-43 from the nucleus to the cytoplasm and lead to neurotoxicity (Gitcho et al., 2008; Nonaka et al., 2009;

Guo et al., 2011). Oxidative stress and ROS formation also favor mislocalization of TDP-43, from the nucleus to the cytoplasm (Ayala et al., 2011), being thus not surprising that SOD mutations also lead to TDP-43 pathology in mice and humans (Shan et al., 2009; Pokrishevsky et al., 2012). ROS upregulates AMP kinase (AMPK) and abnormal AMPK activity has been shown to induce TDP-43 mislocalization in a motor neuron cell line and in the spinal cord of ALS patients (Liu et al., 2015a). Interestingly, mislocalized TDP-43 in the cytoplasm triggers a positive feedback loop, leading to further ROS production and AMPK activation (Liu et al., 2015a).

The present understanding of the mechanisms that underlie motor neuron degeneration associated to expansion of a G4C2 intronic hexanucleotide of the *C9ORF72* gene, is scarce. This mutation is a common cause of fALS but also accounts for near 10% of sALS cases (DeJesus-Hernandez et al., 2011; Smith et al., 2013). A recent study has shown that the *C9ORF72* mutation is associated with an increase in GluA1 AMPA receptor subunit expression, functional expression of Ca^{2+}-permeable AMPA receptors and motor neuron vulnerability to excitotoxicity (Selvaraj et al., 2018). Interestingly, early intrinsic hyperexcitability has been detected in mixed cultures of neurons and glia derived from *C9ORF72* repeat expansion patient iPSCs (Wainger et al., 2014), but not in neuronal cultures with negligible number of glial cells (Selvaraj et al., 2018). Also, conditional medium from astrocytes expressing mutant SOD1 can induce motor neuron hyperexcitability (Fritz et al., 2013). Altogether these studies reinforce the idea that diseased astrocytes trigger excitotoxicity.

Motor neurons, astrocytes, microglia and perisynaptic Schwann cells are known to release and respond to purines, namely ATP and adenosine. Adenosine, by activating membrane receptors (A_1, A_{2A}, A_{2B}, A_3), is an endogenous and ubiquitous modulator of synaptic signaling. Released ATP is a source for extracellular adenosine, but acts on its own purinergic P2 (P2Y and P2X) receptors. So the challenging question is: How purinergic receptors affect the motor neurons and how this impacts in ALS? In this review we will only refer to adenosine receptors since the putative involvement of ATP receptors in the pathophysiology of ALS has been matter of a recent review (Volonté et al., 2016).

ADENOSINE AND ADENOSINE RECEPTORS

Adenosine is a ubiquitous endogenous neuroprotective agent, which has a central role as a neuromodulator of synaptic transmission at the central and peripheral nervous systems, protecting organs and tissues at both physiological and pathophysiological conditions. Adenosine exerts its biological effect via a class of purinergic G protein coupled receptors, which includes A_1R, $A_{2A}R$, $A_{2B}R$ and A_3R, all belonging to family of receptors named by Burnstock (1976) as P_1 purinoceptors (adenosine-sensitive) as opposed to the ATP-sensitive P2 purinoceptors. The A_1R couple to $G_{i/o}$ proteins, inhibiting the production of cyclic AMP. The A_{2A} and A_2B receptors couple to G_s, stimulating the production of cyclic AMP, whereas the A_3R may couple to $G_{i/o}$ or G_q proteins. Adenosine acts like an extracellular signaling molecule, modulating the action of several neurotransmitters (Ribeiro et al., 2003).

Adenosine A_1R are widely distributed in the brain having a widely recognized inhibitory action in synaptic transmission associated to a neuroprotective role, while $A_{2A}R$ have more restrict localizations, being predominant at the basal ganglia. However, both receptors are present in the cortex, the A_1R being the predominant in this brain area (Dunwiddie and Masino, 2001; Sebastião and Ribeiro, 2009a). $A_{2A}R$ may exacerbate excitotoxicity in several brain areas (Ribeiro et al., 2016b) as well as in motor neurons (Mojsilovic-Petrovic et al., 2006). However, $A_{2A}R$ are also able to gate the action of neuroprotective molecules as the neurotrophic factors, a mechanism known to occur in the brain (Diógenes et al., 2004) as well as in motor neurons (Wiese et al., 2007). Trophic actions of $A_{2A}R$ in cortical neurons, some of them being independent of the interplay with neurotrophic factors, have been recently identified (Ribeiro et al., 2016a). Expression of $A_{2A}R$ in spinal motor neurons is intense, being higher than that of A_1R (Kaelin-Lang et al., 1999; Ng et al., 2015).

A_1R in the spinal cord inhibit excitatory inputs (Deuchars et al., 2001) whereas $A_{2A}R$ facilitate inhibitory inputs (Brooke et al., 2004) to sympathetic preganglonic neurons, suggesting that at least in what concerns autonomic nervous system control, the opposing actions of A_1R and $A_{2A}R$ at the synaptic level may both contribute to a common outcome – a decrease in preganglionic neuron activity. The antinociceptic actions of adenosine A_1R are widely known, which involve A_1R at the dorsal horn of the spinal cord. A_3R receptors also mediate antinociception through spinal and supraspinal mechanisms (Little et al., 2015) that also involve anti-inflammation (Janes et al., 2015).

Concerning motor pattern generation, it has been for a long time described that ATP and adenosine have opposite actions in motor pattern generation, the adenosine actions being inhibitory, lowering the excitability of motor circuits (Dale and Gilday, 1996). Recent studies have shown that adenosine, via A_1R, has a general inhibitory action on ventral horn interneurons while potentially maintaining motor neuron excitability (Witts et al., 2015). Interestingly, glial cells are a predominant source of adenosine at to control motor neuron networks at the spinal cord (Witts et al., 2012; Carlsen and Perrier, 2014; Acton and Miles, 2015).

The motor nerve terminals at the neuromuscular junction have served as a model to the pioneer studies on the inhibitory action of adenosine and ATP on neurotransmitter release (Ginsborg and Hirst, 1972; Ribeiro and Walker, 1973, 1975), being now well known that endogenous adenosine inhibits neuromuscular transmission (Sebastião and Ribeiro, 1985), that ATP is a source of extracellular adenosine at the endplate (Ribeiro and Sebastião, 1987), and that adenosine can also be independently released from stimulated motor nerve endings (Cunha and Sebastião, 1993). Motor nerve terminals at the mammalian skeletal neuromuscular junction possess both inhibitory A_1R (Sebastião et al., 1990) and excitatory $A_{2A}R$ (Correia-de-Sá et al., 1991), the $A_{2A}R$ gaining particular relevance at high frequencies of nerve stimulation

(Correia-de-Sá et al., 1996). A_{2B} and A_3 receptors were also more recently detected at the mammalian neuromuscular junction (Garcia et al., 2014).

Adenosine Receptors in Health and Disease

At physiological conditions, the adenosine exerts its neuromodulation action by the activation of A_1 and $A_{2A}R$ high affinity receptors (Sebastião and Ribeiro, 2009a), which mediate dual actions of adenosine both in health and disease (Fredholm, 2014). At pre-synaptic level, adenosine can inhibit or facilitate transmitter release through A_1R and $A_{2A}R$ respectively; at post-synaptic level, it can modulate the actions of several neurotransmitters and it can hyperpolarize or depolarize neurons. All these receptors can be found in neurons and glia cells. While the A_1R is frequently associated to neuroprotective actions, which extend to conditions as hyperexcitability, seizures and ischemia/hypoxia, protecting neurons in response to excitotoxic injury (Boison, 2016; Cunha, 2016; Ribeiro et al., 2016b), the $A_{2A}R$ is often associated to enhancement of excitotoxicity, since these receptors facilitate glutamate release and inhibit glutamate uptake (Popoli et al., 2003; Matos et al., 2012). However, through their ability to gate the actions of neurotrophic factors, $A_{2A}R$ may confer a protective role under specific pathologic conditions (Sebastião and Ribeiro, 2009b; Rodrigues et al., 2014). A_1R, $A_{2A}R$ and $A_{2B}R$ can also influence oxygen deliver into the brain due to their influence in neurovascular coupling (Pelligrino et al., 2010).

Concerning inflammation, $A_{2A}R$ have a duality of actions, depending on the cell type and inflammatory conditions (Haskó et al., 2008). In immune cells the global trend for $A_{2A}R$-mediated actions is to interrupt the proinflammatory cascade and hence limiting tissue inflammation (Sitkovsky et al., 2004; Haskó et al., 2008), contrasting with A_2B receptors that may promote overproduction of proinflammatory cytokines (Haskó et al., 2008). In the central nervous system, however, $A_{2A}R$ mediate anti-inflammatory effects on T cells, and thus protection at early stages of inflammatory diseases; during later stages of disease, however, may contribute to sustained tissue damage within the inflamed central nervous system (Ingwersen et al., 2016). In microglia, $A_{2A}R$ activation leads to their activation, and in such way contributing to foster neuroinflamatory cascades, thus to neurodegeneration (Dai and Zhou, 2011; Rebola et al., 2011; Santiago et al., 2014). Similarly, $A_{2B}R$ and A_3R may mediate either anti-inflammatory or pro-inflammatory actions (Borea et al., 2017).

Adenosine Receptors in ALS

Adenosine Receptors at Spinal Cord: Implications for ALS

In accordance with the expected facilitatory influence of $A_{2A}R$ upon excitotoxicity, $A_{2A}R$ antagonists protect against excitotoxicity-induced motor neuron death (Mojsilovic-Petrovic et al., 2006). However, motor neuron survival after mechanical lesioning has also been shown to be increased by an $A_{2A}R$ activation, through a mechanism that involves interplay with neurotrophines (Wiese et al., 2007). Survival of motor neurons in culture is also facilitated by $A_{2A}R$ activation, this mechanism requiring the activity of the canonical $A_{2A}R$ signaling pathway, cyclic AMP/protein kinase activity, as well as the activity of neurotrophin receptors, again highlighting an interplay between $A_{2A}R$ and neurotrophins to promote motor neuron survival (Komaki et al., 2012). The apparent discrepancies between the neuroprotective actions of $A_{2A}R$ antagonists and $A_{2A}R$ agonists probably result from the diversity of actions that the $A_{2A}R$ have, namely modulation of neuronal activity, neuronal survival, excitotoxicity, neuroinflammation. While facilitating the actions of neurotrophic factors $A_{2A}R$ may promote survival and regeneration, but while enhancing excitotoxicity phenomena $A_{2A}R$ will favor neuronal death. In addition, if neuroinflammation interferes with in the regeneration/degeneration balance $A_{2A}R$ may again have a dual role, depending on the degree and characteristics of the inflammatory process, that it to say, if activation of the inflammatory cascade is beneficial or detrimental. Unraveling all these aspects by taking into consideration the nature of the insult and the time window for treatment is of uttermost importance to understand the role of adenosine receptors in neurodegeneration and in particular in ALS. Our poor understanding of the pathophysiology of the disease itself makes it more difficult to understand the role of adenosine receptors in this disease.

Adenosine levels are significantly elevated in the cerebrospinal fluid of ALS patients (Yoshida et al., 1999), a finding that raised the interest on the understanding the role of adenosine and adenosine receptors in ALS. The expression of A_{2A} receptors is also enhanced in lymphocytes of ALS patients (Vincenzi et al., 2013) as well as in post-mortem spinal cord of ALS patients (Ng et al., 2015). $A_{2A}R$ expression in the spinal cord of early symptomatic $SOD1^{G93A}$ mice was also markedly increased (Ng et al., 2015), but in end-stage $SOD1^{G93A}$ mice a marked decrease was reported (Potenza et al., 2013). Mice data thus may suggest that there is an early enhancement of $A_{2A}R$ expression in the spinal cord, followed by a decrease in latter disease states. A comparison of data obtained in the same laboratory conditions and same animal housing conditions is, however, needed to firmly conclude on biphasic changes in $A_{2A}R$ expression during disease progression. Post-mortem human data (Ng et al., 2015), by definition related to end-stages of the disease, seems to contradict the conclusion of a late-phase decrease in $A_{2A}R$ expression in the spinal cord. Whether the discrepancy arrives from methodological issues (post-mortem time of analysis, tissue collection procedures), species differences (mice vs. human) or from inappropriate disease model, is unknown.

Caffeine is a non-selective adenosine receptors antagonist (Pelligrino et al., 2010; Ribeiro and Sebastião, 2010; Fredholm et al., 2017) and is one of the most consumable psychoactive substances of the western diet. There is thus high interest in understanding the actions of caffeine in neurodegenerative diseases. Indeed, caffeine consumption in humans has been negatively associated with the incidence of some neurodegenerative diseases, as Alzheimer's Disease and Parkinson's Disease (de Mendonça and Cunha, 2010; Flaten et al., 2014; Laurent et al., 2014; Ascherio and Schwarzschild, 2016).

Accordingly, chronic caffeine consumption has been shown to protect several hallmarks of neurodegeneration in animal models of disease, these actions being frequently mimicked by selective $A_{2A}R$ antagonists or $A_{2A}R$ deletion (Canas et al., 2009; Kachroo and Schwarzschild, 2012; Laurent et al., 2016; Ferreira et al., 2017). Concerning ALS, however, conflicting data had recently emerged in the literature, and there are several points that are far from being understood. In clear contrast to what could be expected from previous evidence in other neurodegenerative diseases, chronic administration of caffeine significantly shortens the survival of $SOD1^{G93A}$ mice (Potenza et al., 2013). Also somehow unexpected, chronic administration of caffeine caused a marked decrease in $A_{2A}R$ levels in the spinal cord (Potenza et al., 2013) and in this aspect seems to mimic the disease itself since $SOD1^{G93A}$ mice also displayed a strong reduction in $A_{2A}R$ in the spinal cord. Both conditions (caffeine treatment and SOD^{G93A} mutation) were not additive since there were no further reduction in spinal cord $A_{2A}R$ levels in $SOD1^{G93A}$ mice treated with caffeine (Potenza et al., 2013). Caffeine can inhibit all adenosine receptors, and thus one cannot preclude that those actions of caffeine were due to antagonism of the usually neuroprotective A_1R rather than antagonism of the $A_{2A}R$. Indeed, A_1 and $A_{2A}R$ are known to strongly interact with each other (Ferre et al., 2008), including in motor neurons (Pousinha et al., 2010, 2012), and the loss of inhibitory control of A_1R upon $A_{2A}R$ may cause marked unbalance of the fine-tuning of neuronal function exerted by adenosine receptors. A selective $A_{2A}R$ antagonist, KW6002, administered daily, was recently reported to increase of motor neuron survival, delay the onset of disease and increase in the lifespan that $SOD1^{G93A}$ mice (Ng et al., 2015), which is in accordance with the usual finding that $A_{2A}R$ may exacerbate excitotoxicity.

Concerning the influence of $A_{2A}R$ agonists in ALS progression, it has been shown that treatment of $SOD1^{G93A}$ mice with CGS21680 at a very early symptomatic stage of the disease, delayed disease onset of motor symptoms and enhanced motor neuron survival (Yanpallewar et al., 2012). Interestingly, the effect of the $A_{2A}R$ agonist was similar to that resulting from genetic deletion of the truncated form of the TrkB receptor, TrkB.T1, which is overexpressed in the spinal cord of the $SOD1^{G93A}$ mice. The TrkB.T1 act as negative regulator of full-length TrkB receptor signaling, impairing the ability of its ligand, the neurotrophin Brain Derived Neurotrophic factor (BDNF), to promote neuronal survival, neuronal maturation and neuronal plasticity. Most of the actions of BDNF at synapses are triggered by $A_{2A}R$ activation (Diógenes et al., 2004; Sebastião et al., 2011; Ribeiro et al., 2016b). It is thus likely that the protective influence of $A_{2A}R$ receptor agonist in very early stages of ALS progression in SOD^{G93A} mice results from the ability of $A_{2A}R$ to facilitate full length TrkB receptor activation, thus compensating the negative influence the TrkB.T1 receptor overexpression. That $A_{2A}R$ and $A_{2A}R$ antagonists may have strict time windows to exert its beneficial influences in neurodegeneration has been already proposed (Sebastião and Ribeiro, 2009b) but data from experiments specifically addressing this point have not yet appeared.

Also particularly relevant in the context of understanding the role of $A_{2A}R$ in ALS progression was the finding that $A_{2A}R$ activation, through PKA signaling, suppresses aberrant AMPK activity as well as suppresses mislocalization of TDP-43, in the TDP-43 mouse model of ALS (Liu et al., 2015a). Taking into consideration that mislocalization of TDP-43 from the nucleus to the cytoplasm can be induced not only by mutations in the gene that codes for TDP-43 but also by ROS production, there is some overlap in the disease triggering mechanisms in the SOD mouse models and in the TDP-43 model.

Summarizing, in two models of ALS ($SOD1^{G93A}$ and TDP-43), two different $A_{2A}R$ agonists proved beneficial to improve motor neuron survival (Yanpallewar et al., 2012; Liu et al., 2015a). One study clearly showed detrimental effects of the adenosine receptor antagonist, caffeine in the survival of $SOD1^{G93A}$ mice (Potenza et al., 2013). Thus, as whole and in the specific context of ALS, $A_{2A}R$ activation seems beneficial. Importantly, $A_{2A}R$, through cAMP/PKA signaling and subsequent inhibition of AMPK may contribute to cut the positive feedback mechanism where AMPK activation by ROS leads to further mislocalization of TDP-43, which leads to further ROS production, thus to further AMPK activation. In this way, $A_{2A}R$ activation may hit a key pathophysiologic mechanism of ALS, thus reducing or even halting disease progression. Unfortunately, in the study by Liu et al. (2015a), the influence of $A_{2A}R$ activation in the time of appearance of first symptoms or in the life-span of ALS mice was not assessed. Results from such studies would indeed complement the evidence already obtained on enhancement of motor neuron survival by $A_{2A}R$ activation in two models of ALS (Yanpallewar et al., 2012; Liu et al., 2015a). Also, and taking into consideration that the agonist used by Liu et al. (2015a) already entered clinical trials for other neurodegenerative diseases, a clinical trial specifically designed for a fast devastating disease as ALS, would be of high relevance.

$A_{2A}R$ and D_2 dopamine receptors (D_2R) co-exist in motor neurons of the spinal cord of normal subjects and ALS patients (Chern et al., 2017). Activation of D_2R reverse the $A_{2A}R$-mediated prevention of ROS-induced AMPK activation and TDP-43 mislocalization in cells co-transfected with D_2R and $A_{2A}R$ (Chern et al., 2017). A_{2A}/D_2 negative interactions are well known in the basal ganglia (Fuxe et al., 2007). The evidence that they also exist at the level of the spinal cord and in a context of ALS pathophysiology (Chern et al., 2017), point toward the need of care in the use of D_2R agonists in ALS patients, as well as may suggest a beneficial role of D_2R antagonists in this disease.

From the studies mentioned above, it appears that $A_{2A}R$ agonists may prove of therapeutic value in ALS. Yet, there are several discrepancies in the literature, as the report that a selective $A_{2A}R$ antagonist may delay disease progression. To solve some discrepancies, it will be important to compare in the same colony and under the same experimental conditions, and always against age-matched control littermates, time-dependent and disease state-dependent changes in the activity and expression of adenosine receptors. The comparisons among different mouse models are also of uttermost importance to allow starting to understand the different roles of $A_{2A}R$ as a function of the etiology of the disease itself. It will be also necessary to follow those changes in mice treated with either selective receptor ligands as well as with caffeine. Since ALS progression may not be similar at different synaptic levels, a better understanding of the time-dependent changes in $A_{2A}R$ signaling at upper and lower motor neuron levels would also allow a better understanding in the role of $A_{2A}R$ in ALS. Information of the role of A_1R in this neurodegenerative disease is scarce, which is somehow surprising on the light of the known neuroprotection exerted by these receptors. Their ability to inhibit synaptic transmission, may, however, exert a negative influence in a degenerative disease that markedly compromises information flow in the motor circuit.

Adenosine Receptors at the Neuromuscular Junction: Implications for ALS

The neuromuscular junction early served as a model to understand synaptic transmission mechanisms (Katz and Miledi, 1965), as model to understand neuromodulation by adenosine (Ginsborg and Hirst, 1972), as a model to understand the relevance of endogenous adenosine to control synaptic transmission (Ribeiro and Sebastião, 1987), and as a model to start identifying $A_{2A}R$ at synapses outside the basal ganglia (Correia-de-Sá et al., 1991; Correia-de-Sá and Ribeiro, 1994). Reasons for this are the simplicity of the model, allowing to record from a single synapse receiving input from only one nerve terminal, with a clearly identified neurotransmitter - acetylcholine. In spite of this simplicity, there are several neuromodulators released by either the pre-synaptic, the post-synaptic, the muscle itself and the perisynaptic Schwann cells, which finely tune synaptic transmission and synaptic maintenance. As widely known, ATP and adenosine are among such neuromodulators. Neurotrophic factors are also present at the neuromuscular junction and $A_{2A}R$ are also indispensable promoters of the facilitatory action BDNF, upon neuromuscular transmission (Pousinha et al., 2006), as it was firstly observed hippocampal synapses (Diógenes et al., 2004).

Having studied the action of adenosine for more than 40 years, using the neuromuscular junction as a model, and considering that this simple synaptic model could be as a sort of key (Arbour et al., 2017) to investigate novel approaches for disease therapy, and also that this particular synapse is compromised in ALS, we hypothesized (Nascimento et al., 2014, 2015) that ALS progression could be accompanied by changes in the functioning of adenosine A_1R and $A_{2A}R$, the two high affinity adenosine receptors known to be expressed at motor nerve endings (Correia-de-Sá and Ribeiro, 1994). We used a functional approach, recording endplate potentials (EPPs) and miniature endplate potentials (MEPPs), and quantifying quantal content of EPPs, from Mg^{2+}-paralyzed hemidiaphragm preparations of $SOD1^{G93A}$ mice at pre-symptomatic (absence of motor symptoms assessed by the Rota-Rod) and early symptomatic (mild but significant dysfunction at the Rota-Rod) phases of the disease. We found that at the pre-symptomatic stage the $A_{2A}R$-mediated presynaptic facilitatory action on neuromuscular transmission is exacerbated, whereas in the early symptomatic phase, this excitatory action disappears, indicating that indeed that $A_{2A}R$ function changes upon ALS progression. We then further investigated the role of A_1R in ALS using the same approach and the same disease model (Nascimento et al., 2015) and found that the $A_1R/A_{2A}R$ functional cross-talk is lost in the pre-symptomatic phase, so that the ability of A_1R to brake the action of $A_{2A}R$ is lost, which might explain the exacerbation of the $A_{2A}R$ signaling at this disease state. In addition, there was an increase of A_1R tonic activation in the symptomatic phase, suggesting that the changes adenosine modulation mediated by A_1R may be contributing to disease progression and aggravating symptoms in late disease stage. Whether the lack of A_1R-mediated inhibition of $A_{2A}R$ function, with the corresponding exacerbation of $A_{2A}R$-mediated function, corresponds to an early compensatory process that may facilitate neuromuscular transmission and confer some neuroprotection through an enhancement of the action of neurotrophic factors, remains unknown. Also unknown is if these early excitatory changes, accompanied by dysruptions of the calcium buffering at the nerve terminal (Rocha et al., 2013) and at perisynaptic Schwann Cells (Arbour et al., 2015), are a fast-track to neurodegeneration.

Summarizing, data (Nascimento et al., 2014, 2015) suggest that in ALS there is an unbalanced adenosine receptors modulation at the neuromuscular junction (**Figure 1**) that may start before first signs of motor impairment. We anticipate early compensatory alterations followed by a disruption of neuromodulatory control that may then act as an aggravating factor to exacerbate excitotoxicity, fasting neuronal death. A clear identification of the nature of these adenosine receptors changes, at different diseases states, would allow to identify new therapeutic targets based on the cause of neurodegeneration and thus to halt it.

Interestingly, adenosine A_1R at motor nerve endings, besides inhibiting the release probability, also synchronize release by removing quantal events with long latencies, an action that is sensitive to the redox potential, being abolished by oxidants (Tsentsevitsky et al., 2013). How this impacts in oxidative-stress related motor neuron diseases, as ALS, is yet unknown.

CONCLUSION AND PERSPECTIVES

A major finding in what concerns adenosinergic signaling in ALS is the existence of very early synaptic alterations, which precede motor symptoms and which are evident at the level of the neuromuscular junction as well as, most probably, at central synapses. Whether those changes are triggers for the disease or represent early compensatory modifications is yet unknown. The evidence of a positive influence of $A_{2A}R$ agonists and negative influence of caffeine, may suggest that an early enhancement of $A_{2A}R$ functioning may represent an endogenous attempt to fight the disease. The positive influence of a selective $A_{2A}R$ antagonist may, however, contradict this possibility. A better clarification of the nature of the purinergic signaling dysfunctions, their implications and their time-windows, is for sure relevant not only for a better understanding of the pathophysiology of the disease and the implications of caffeine intake, but also to guide the design of putative therapeutic strategies to halt disease progression. Specifically, it is important to know if the early exacerbation of $A_{2A}R$ signaling detected at the motor nerve endings also occurs at central synapses, in particular, at the spinal

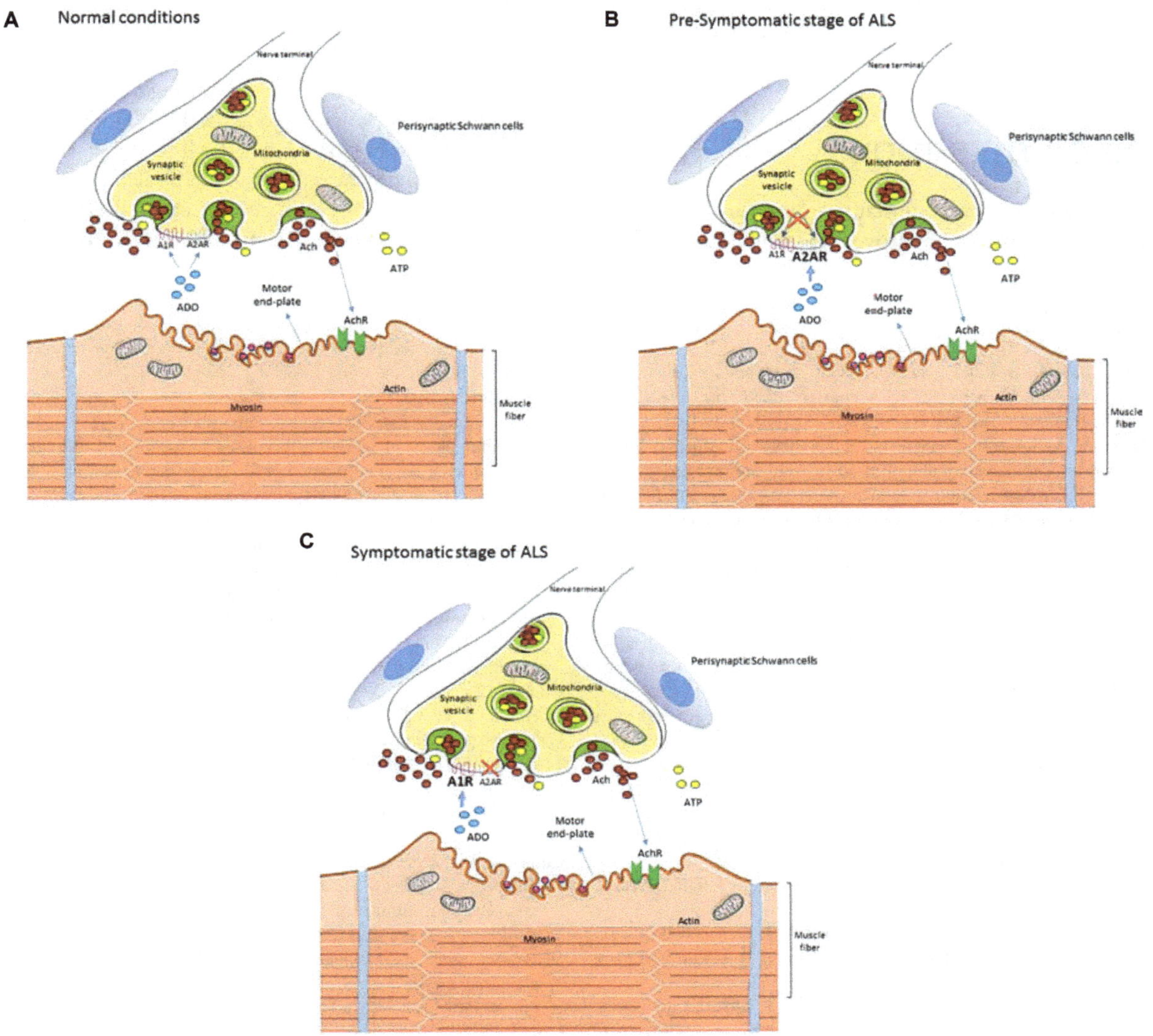

FIGURE 1 | Schematic diagram of the reported changes in adenosine signaling at the neuromuscular junction in an ALS mice model. In wild type **(A)** neuromuscular junctions, adenosine activates both inhibitory A_1R and excitatory $A_{2A}R$, modulating acetylcholine release from motor nerve terminals. In ALS mice at the pre-symptomatic stage **(B)** there is a loss of $A_1R/A_{2A}R$ functional cross-talk at the neuromuscular junction and the excitatory action of $A_{2A}R$ is exacerbated. At the symptomatic stage **(C)** there is an increase of A_1R tonic activation, which may be contributing to neurotransmission failure on late disease stages, whereas the excitatory action of $A_{2A}R$ disappears. For details see Nascimento et al. (2014, 2015). Perisynaptic Schwann cells contribute to the pool of ATP at the synaptic cleft but ATP signaling in these cells seems unchanged in ALS, in contrast with mACh signaling (Arbour et al., 2015). Interestingly, the exacerbated $A_{2A}R$ signaling at the pre-symptomatic stage correlates with an enhanced release of ACh from nerve terminals and with signs of dysregulated calcium buffering at motor nerve endings (Rocha et al., 2013; Arbour et al., 2017).

cord and motor cortex, and how selective blockade of these receptors at different disease states affects disease progression. Keeping in mind the intriguing data reported while testing the influence of caffeine in animal models, it is also of uttermost importance to understand the molecular basis of this action of caffeine, whether it has an impact in the signaling of other neuroprotective molecules, or in the signaling mediated by other adenosine receptors. This knowledge is not only important for the design of future drugs but also to guide research in patients since caffeine is present in many widely consumed beverages and is usually regarded as protective against other neurodegenerative diseases. Lastly, the putative influence of $A_{2A}R$ and A_3R in the inflammatory cascade associated to ALS has to be better understood. Indeed, recent studies have demonstrated the presence of inflammation propagating substrates in the central nervous system of patients afflicted with ALS (Khalid et al., 2017). $A_{2A}R$ receptors mediate anti-inflammatory actions and are up-regulated in lymphocytes from ALS patients(Vincenzi et al., 2013). The A_3R is a promising therapeutic target for inflammatory diseases (Jacobson et al., 2017) but these receptors have been mostly disregarded in what concerns ALS.

In conclusion, though one starts to envisage changes in the adenosinergic system at different stages of ALS progression, much more needs to be known before understanding the causal relationship of those changes and which of them can be targeted to develop novel therapeutics toward this devastating disease.

AUTHOR CONTRIBUTIONS

All authors listed have made a substantial, direct and intellectual contribution to the work, and approved it for publication.

FUNDING

This work was supported by LISBOA-01-0145-FEDER-007391, project co-funded by FEDER through POR Lisboa 2020 (Programa Operacional Regional de Lisboa) from PORTUGAL 2020 and Fundação para a Ciência e Tecnologia (FCT) and by a Twinning action (SynaNet) from the EU H2020 program (Project Number: 692340). NR is in receipt of an FCT fellowship (PD /BD/113463/2015) and is a fellow of the M2B-Ph.D. Program.

REFERENCES

Acton, D., and Miles, G. B. (2015). Stimulation of glia reveals modulation of mammalian spinal motor networks by adenosine. *PLoS One* 10:e0134488. doi: 10.1371/journal.pone.0134488

Arai, T., Hasegawa, M., Akiyama, H., Ikeda, K., Nonaka, T., Mori, H., et al. (2006). TDP-43 is a component of ubiquitin-positive tau-negative inclusions in frontotemporal lobar degeneration and amyotrophic lateral sclerosis. *Biochem. Biophys. Res. Commun.* 351, 602–611. doi: 10.1016/j.bbrc.2006.10.093

Arbour, D., Tremblay, E., Martineau, E., Julien, J. P., and Robitaille, R. (2015). Early and persistent abnormal decoding by glial cells at the neuromuscular junction in an ALS model. *J. Neurosci.* 35, 688–706. doi: 10.1523/JNEUROSCI.1379-14.2015

Arbour, D., Vande Velde, C., and Robitaille, R. (2017). New perspectives on amyotrophic lateral sclerosis: the role of glial cells at the neuromuscular junction. *J. Physiol.* 595, 647–661. doi: 10.1113/JP270213

Ascherio, A., and Schwarzschild, M. A. (2016). The epidemiology of Parkinson's disease: risk factors and prevention. *Lancet Neurol.* 15, 1257–1272. doi: 10.1016/S1474-4422(16)30230-7

Ayala, V., Granado-Serrano, A. B., Cacabelos, D., Naudí, A., Ilieva, E. V., Boada, J., et al. (2011). Cell stress induces TDP-43 pathological changes associated with ERK1/2 dysfunction: implications in ALS. *Acta Neuropathol.* 122, 259–270. doi: 10.1007/s00401-011-0850-y

Baker, M. R. (2014). ALS—dying forward, backward or outward? *Nat. Rev. Neurol.* 10:660. doi: 10.1038/nrneurol.2013.221-c1

Boison, D. (2016). The biochemistry and epigenetics of epilepsy: focus on adenosine and glycine. *Front. Mol. Neurosci.* 9:26. doi: 10.3389/fnmol.2016.00026

Borea, P. A., Gessi, S., Merighi, S., Vincenzi, F., and Varani, K. (2017). Pathological overproduction: the bad side of adenosine. *Br. J. Pharmacol.* 174, 1945–1960. doi: 10.1111/bph.13763

Braak, H., Brettschneider, J., Ludolph, A. C., Lee, V. M., Trojanowski, J. Q., and Del Tredici, K. (2013). Amyotrophic lateral sclerosis–a model of corticofugal axonal spread. *Nat. Rev. Neurol.* 9, 708–714. doi: 10.1038/nrneurol.2013.221

Brooke, R. E., Deuchars, J., and Deuchars, S. A. (2004). Input-specific modulation of neurotransmitter release in the lateral horn of the spinal cord via adenosine receptors. *J. Neurosci.* 24, 127–137. doi: 10.1523/JNEUROSCI.4591-03.2004

Burnstock, G. (1976). Do some nerve cells release more than one transmitter? *Neuroscience* 1, 239–248.

Canas, P. M., Porciúncula, L. O., Cunha, G. M., Silva, C. G., Machado, N. J., Oliveira, J. M., et al. (2009). Adenosine A_{2A} receptor blockade prevents synaptotoxicity and memory dysfunction caused by beta-amyloid peptides via p38 mitogen-activated protein kinase pathway. *J. Neurosci.* 29, 14741–14751. doi: 10.1523/JNEUROSCI.3728-09.2009

Carlsen, E. M., and Perrier, J. F. (2014). Purines released from astrocytes inhibit excitatory synaptic transmission in the ventral horn of the spinal cord. *Front. Neural Circuits* 8:60. doi: 10.3389/fncir.2014.00060

Chern, Y., Lai, C., Liu, Y., and Lai, H. (2017). Activation of the D2 dopamine receptor hampers the protective effect of the A2A adenosine receptor on TDP-43 mislocalization. *FASEB J.* 31:LB140.

Chou, C. C., Zhang, Y., Umoh, M. E., Vaughan, S. W., Lorenzini, I., Liu, F., et al. (2018). TDP-43 pathology disrupts nuclear pore complexes and nucleocytoplasmic transport in ALS/FTD. *Nat. Neurosci.* 21, 228–239. doi: 10.1038/s41593-017-0047-3

Correia-de-Sá, P., and Ribeiro, J. A. (1994). Evidence that the presynaptic A_{2a}-adenosine receptor of the rat motor nerve endings is positively coupled to adenylate cyclase. *Naunyn Schmiedebergs Arch. Pharmacol.* 350, 514–522. doi: 10.1007/BF00173021

Correia-de-Sá, P., Sebastião, A. M., and Ribeiro, J. A. (1991). Inhibitory and excitatory effects of adenosine receptor agonists on evoked transmitter release from phrenic nerve endings of the rat. *Br. J. Pharmacol.* 103, 1614–1620. doi: 10.1111/j.1476-5381.1991.tb09836.x

Correia-de-Sá, P., Timóteo, M. A., and Ribeiro, J. A. (1996). Presynaptic A_1 inhibitory/A_{2A} facilitatory adenosine receptor activation balance depends on motor nerve stimulation paradigm at the rat hemidiaphragm. *J. Neurophysiol.* 76, 3910–3919. doi: 10.1152/jn.1996.76.6.3910

Costa, J., Gomes, C., and de Carvalho, M. (2010). Diagnosis, pathogenesis and therapeutic targets in amyotrophic lateral sclerosis, CNS and neurological disorders. *Drug Targets* 9, 764–778. doi: 10.2174/187152710793237502

Cunha, C., Santos, C., Gomes, C., Fernandes, A., Correia, A. M., Sebastião, A. M., et al. (2017). Downregulated glia interplay and increased miRNA-155 as promising markers to track ALS at an early stage. *Mol. Neurobiol.* doi: 10.1007/s12035-017-0631-2 [Epub ahead of print].

Cunha, R. A. (2016). How does adenosine control neuronal dysfunction and neurodegeneration? *J. Neurochem.* 139, 1019–1055. doi: 10.1111/jnc.13724

Cunha, R. A., and Sebastião, A. M. (1993). Adenosine and adenine nucleotides are independently released from both the nerve terminals and the muscle fibres upon electrical stimulation of the innervated skeletal muscle of the frog. *Pflugers Arch.* 424, 503–510. doi: 10.1007/BF00374914

Dadon-Nachum, M., Melamed, E., and Offen, D. (2011). The "dying-back" phenomenon of motor neurons in ALS. *J. Mol. Neurosci.* 43, 470–477. doi: 10.1007/s12031-010-9467-1

Dai, S. S., and Zhou, Y. G. (2011). Adenosine 2A receptor: a crucial neuromodulator with bidirectional effect in neuroinflammation and brain injury. *Rev. Neurosci.* 22, 231–239. doi: 10.1515/RNS.2011.020

Dale, N., and Gilday, D. (1996). Regulation of rhythmic movements by purinergic neurotransmitters in frog embryos. *Nature* 383, 259–263. doi: 10.1038/383259a0

de Mendonça, A., and Cunha, R. A. (2010). Putative neuroprotective effects of caffeine in clinical trials. Concluding remarks. *J. Alzheimers Dis.* 20(Suppl. 1), S249–S252.

DeJesus-Hernandez, M., Mackenzie, I. R., Boeve, B. F., Boxer, A. L., Baker, M., Rutherford, N. J., et al. (2011). Expanded GGGGCC hexanucleotide repeat in noncoding region of C9ORF72 causes chromosome 9p-linked FTD and ALS. *Neuron* 72, 245–256. doi: 10.1016/j.neuron.2011.09.011

Deuchars, S. A., Brooke, R. E., and Deuchars, J. (2001). Adenosine A_1 receptors reduce release from excitatory but not inhibitory synaptic inputs onto lateral horn neurons. *J. Neurosci.* 21, 6308–6320.

Di Giorgio, F. P., Carrasco, M. A., Siao, M. C., Maniatis, T., and Eggan, K. (2007). Non-cell autonomous effect of glia on motor neurons in an embryonic stem cell-based ALS model. *Nat. Neurosci.* 10, 608–614. doi: 10.1038/nn1885

Dias, R. B., Ribeiro, J. A., and Sebastião, A. M. (2012). Enhancement of AMPA currents and GluR1 membrane expression through PKA- coupled adenosine A_{2A} receptors. *Hippocampus* 22, 276–291. doi: 10.1002/hipo.20894

Dias, R. B., Rombo, D. M., Ribeiro, J. A., and Sebastião, A. M. (2013). Ischemia-induced synaptic plasticity drives sustained expression of calcium-permeable AMPA receptors in the hippocampus. *Neuropharmacology* 65, 114–122. doi: 10.1016/j.neuropharm.2012.09.016

Diógenes, M. J., Fernandes, C. C., Sebastião, A. M., and Ribeiro, J. A. (2004). Activation of adenosine A_{2A} receptor facilitates brain-derived neurotrophic factor modulation of synaptic transmission in hippocampal slices. *J. Neurosci.* 24, 2905–2913. doi: 10.1523/JNEUROSCI.4454-03.2004

Dunwiddie, T. V., and Masino, S. A. (2001). The role and regulation of adenosine in the central nervous system. *Annu. Rev. Neurosci.* 24, 31–55. doi: 10.1146/annurev.neuro.24.1.31

Feng, Z., and Ko, C. P. (2008a). Schwann cells promote synaptogenesis at the neuromuscular junction via transforming growth factor-β1. *J. Neurosci.* 28, 9599–9609. doi: 10.1523/JNEUROSCI.2589-08.2008

Feng, Z., and Ko, C. P. (2008b). The role of glial cells in the formation and maintenance of the neuromuscular junction. *Ann. N. Y. Acad. Sci.* 1132, 19–28. doi: 10.1196/annals.1405.016

Ferre, S., Ciruela, F., Borycz, J., Solinas, M., Quarta, D., Antoniou, K., et al. (2008). Adenosine A_1-A_{2A} receptor heteromers: new targets for caffeine in the brain. *Front. Biosci.* 13, 2391–2399. doi: 10.2741/2852

Ferreira, D. G., Batalha, V. L., Vicente Miranda, H., Coelho, J. E., Gomes, R., Gonçalves, F. Q., et al. (2017). Adenosine A_{2A} receptors modulate α-synuclein aggregation and toxicity. *Cereb. Cortex* 27, 718–730.

Flaten, V., Laurent, C., Coelho, J. E., Sandau, U., Batalha, V. L., Burnouf, S., et al. (2014). From epidemiology to pathophysiology: what about caffeine in Alzheimer's disease? *Biochem. Soc. Trans.* 42, 587–592. doi: 10.1042/BST20130229

Fredholm, B. B. (2014). Adenosine–a physiological or pathophysiological agent? *J. Mol. Med.* 92, 201–206. doi: 10.1007/s00109-013-1101-6

Fredholm, B. B., Yang, J., and Wang, Y. (2017). Low, but not high, dose caffeine is a readily available probe for adenosine actions. *Mol. Aspects Med.* 55, 20–25. doi: 10.1016/j.mam.2016.11.011

Frey, D., Schneider, C., Xu, L., Borg, J., Spooren, W. I., and Caroni, P. (2000). Early and selective loss of neuromuscular synapse subtypes with low sprouting competence in motoneuron diseases. *J. Neurosci.* 20, 2534–2542.

Fritz, E., Izaurieta, P., Weiss, A., Mir, F. R., Rojas, P., Gonzalez, D., et al. (2013). Mutant SOD1-expressing astrocytes release toxic factors that trigger motoneuron death by inducing hyperexcitability. *J. Neurophysiol.* 109, 2803–2814. doi: 10.1152/jn.00500.2012

Fuxe, K., Ferré, S., Genedani, S., Franco, R., and Agnati, L. F. (2007). Adenosine receptor-dopamine receptor interactions in the basal ganglia and their relevance for brain function. *Physiol. Behav.* 92, 210–217. doi: 10.1016/j.physbeh.2007.05.034

Garcia, N., Priego, M., Hurtado, E., Obis, T., Santafe, M. M., Tomàs, M., et al. (2014). Adenosine A2B and A3 receptor location at the mouse neuromuscular junction. *J. Anat.* 225, 109–117. doi: 10.1111/joa.12188

Georgiou, J., Robitaille, R., and Charlton, M. P. (1999). Muscarinic control of cytoskeleton in perisynaptic glia. *J. Neurosci.* 19, 3836–3846.

Ginsborg, B. L., and Hirst, G. D. S. (1972). The effect of adenosine on the release of the transmitter from the phrenic nerve of the rat. *J. Physiol.* 224, 629–645. doi: 10.1113/jphysiol.1972.sp009916

Gitcho, M. A., Baloh, R. H., Chakraverty, S., Mayo, K., Norton, J. B., Levitch, D., et al. (2008). TDP-43 A315T mutation in familial motor neuron disease. *Ann. Neurol.* 63, 535–538. doi: 10.1002/ana.21344

Guo, W., Chen, Y., Zhou, X., Kar, A., Ray, P., Chen, X., et al. (2011). An ALS associated mutation affecting TDP-43 enhances protein aggregation, fibril formation and neurotoxicity. *Nat. Struct. Mol. Biol.* 18, 822–830. doi: 10.1038/nsmb.2053

Haskó, G., Linden, J., Cronstein, B., and Pacher, P. (2008). Adenosine receptors: therapeutic aspects for inflammatory and immune diseases. *Nat. Rev. Drug Discov.* 7, 759–770. doi: 10.1038/nrd2638

Ingwersen, J., Wingerath, B., Graf, J., Lepka, K., Hofrichter, M., Schröter, F., et al. (2016). Dual roles of the adenosine A2a receptor in autoimmune neuroinflammation. *J. Neuroinflammation* 13:48. doi: 10.1186/s12974-016-0512-z

Jacobson, K. A., Merighi, S., Varani, K., Borea, P. A., Baraldi, S., Aghazadeh Tabrizi, M., et al. (2017). A_3 adenosine receptors as modulators of inflammation: from medicinal chemistry to therapy. *Med. Res. Rev.* doi: 10.1002/med.21456 [Epub ahead of print].

Janes, K., Wahlman, C., Little, J. W., Doyle, T., Tosh, D. K., Jacobson, K. A., et al. (2015). Spinal neuroimmune activation is independent of T-cell infiltration and attenuated by A_3 adenosine receptor agonists in a model of oxaliplatin-induced peripheral neuropathy. *Brain Behav. Immun.* 44, 91–99. doi: 10.1016/j.bbi.2014.08.010

Kachroo, A., and Schwarzschild, M. A. (2012). Adenosine A_{2A} receptor gene disruption protects in an α-synuclein model of Parkinson's disease. *Ann. Neurol.* 71, 278–282. doi: 10.1002/ana.22630

Kaelin-Lang, A., Lauterburg, T., and Burgunder, J. M. (1999). Expression of adenosine A2a receptors gene in the olfactory bulb and spinal cord of rat and mouse. *Neurosci. Lett.* 261, 189–191. doi: 10.1016/S0304-3940(99)00022-1

Katz, B., and Miledi, R. (1965). Release of acetylcholine from a nerve terminal by electric pulses of variable strength and duration. *Nature* 207, 1097–1098. doi: 10.1038/2071097a0

Khalid, S. I., Ampie, L., Kelly, R., Ladha, S. S., and Dardis, C. (2017). Immune modulation in the treatment of amyotrophic lateral sclerosis: a review of clinical trials. *Front. Neurol.* 8:486. doi: 10.3389/fneur.2017.00486

Kiernan, M. C., Vucic, S., Cheah, B. C., Turner, M. R., Eisen, A., Hardiman, O., et al. (2011). Amyotrophic lateral sclerosis. *Lancet* 377, 942–955. doi: 10.1016/S0140-6736(10)61156-7

Komaki, S., Ishikawa, K., and Arakawa, Y. (2012). Trk and cAMP-dependent survival activity of adenosine A_{2A} agonist CGS21680 on rat motoneurons in culture. *Neurosci. Lett.* 522, 21–24. doi: 10.1016/j.neulet.2012.06.003

Laurent, C., Burnouf, S., Ferry, B., Batalha, V. L., Coelho, J. E., Baqi, Y., et al. (2016). A_{2A} adenosine receptor deletion is protective in a mouse model of Tauopathy. *Mol. Psychiatry* 21, 97–107. doi: 10.1038/mp.2014.151

Laurent, C., Eddarkaoui, S., Derisbourg, M., Leboucher, A., Demeyer, D., Carrier, S., et al. (2014). Beneficial effects of caffeine in a transgenic model of Alzheimer's disease-like tau pathology. *Neurobiol. Aging* 35, 2079–2090. doi: 10.1016/j.neurobiolaging.2014.03.027

Leblond, C. S., Kaneb, H. M., Dion, P. A., and Rouleau, G. A. (2014). Dissection of genetic factors associated with amyotrophic lateral sclerosis. *Exp. Neurol.* 262, 91–101. doi: 10.1016/j.expneurol.2014.04.013

Leroy, F., Lamotte d'Incamps, B., Imhoff-Manuel, R. D., and Zytnicki, D. (2014). Early intrinsic hyperexcitability does not contribute to motoneuron degeneration in amyotrophic lateral sclerosis. *eLife* 3:e04046. doi: 10.7554/eLife.04046

Little, J. W., Ford, A., Symons-Liguori, A. M., Chen, Z., Janes, K., Doyle, T., et al. (2015). Endogenous adenosine A3 receptor activation selectively alleviates persistent pain states. *Brain* 138, 28–35. doi: 10.1093/brain/awu330

Liu, Y. J., Ju, T. C., Chen, H. M., Jang, Y. S., Lee, L. M., Lai, H. L., et al. (2015a). Activation of AMP-activated protein kinase α1 mediates mislocalization of TDP-43 in amyotrophic lateral sclerosis. *Hum. Mol. Genet.* 24, 787–801. doi: 10.1093/hmg/ddu497

Liu, Y. J., Lee, L. M., Lai, H. L., and Chern, Y. (2015b). Aberrant activation of AMP-activated protein kinase contributes to the abnormal distribution of HuR in amyotrophic lateral sclerosis. *FEBS Lett.* 589, 432–439. doi: 10.1016/j.febslet.2014.12.029

Liu, Y. J., Tsai, P. Y., and Chern, Y. (2017). Energy homeostasis and abnormal RNA metabolism in amyotrophic lateral sclerosis. *Front. Cell. Neurosci.* 11:126. doi: 10.3389/fncel.2017.00126

Maekawa, S., Leigh, P. N., King, A., Jones, E., Steele, J. C., Bodi, I., et al. (2009). TDP-43 is consistently co-localized with ubiquitinated inclusions in sporadic and Guam amyotrophic lateral sclerosis but not in familial amyotrophic lateral sclerosis with and without SOD1 mutations. *Neuropathology* 29, 672–683. doi: 10.1111/j.1440-1789.2009.01029.x

Marchetto, M. C., Muotri, A. R, Mu, Y., Smith, A. M., Cezar, G. G., and Gage, F. H. (2008). Non-cell-autonomous effect of human SOD1 G37R astrocytes on motor neurons derived from human embryonic stem cells. *Cell Stem Cell* 3, 649–657. doi: 10.1016/j.stem.2008.10.001

Matos, M., Augusto, E., Santos-Rodrigues, A. D., Schwarzschild, M. A., Chen, J. F., Cunha, R. A., et al. (2012). Adenosine A_{2A} receptors modulate glutamate uptake in cultured astrocytes and gliosomes. *Glia* 60, 702–716. doi: 10.1002/glia.22290

Mojsilovic-Petrovic, J., Jeong, G. B., Crocker, A., Arneja, A., David, S., Russell, D., et al. (2006). Protecting motor neurons from toxic insult by antagonism of adenosine A2a and Trk receptors. *J. Neurosci.* 26, 9250–9263. doi: 10.1523/JNEUROSCI.1856-06.2006

Nagai, M., Re, D. B., Nagata, T., Chalazonitis, A., Jessell, T. M., Wichterle, H., et al. (2007). Astrocytes expressing ALS-linked mutated SOD1 release factors selectively toxic to motor neurons. *Nat. Neurosci.* 10, 615–622. doi: 10.1038/nn1876

Nalini, A., Thennarasu, K., Gourie-Devi, M., Shenoy, S., and Kulshreshtha, D. (2008). Clinical characteristics and survival pattern of 1,153 patients with amyotrophic lateral sclerosis: experience over 30 years from India. *J. Neurol. Sci.* 272, 60–70. doi: 10.1016/j.jns.2008.04.034

Nascimento, F., Pousinha, P. A., Correia, A. M., Gomes, R., Sebastião, A. M., and Ribeiro, J. A. (2014). Adenosine A_{2A} receptors activation facilitates neuromuscular transmission in the pre-symptomatic phase of the SOD1(G93A) ALS mice, but not in the symptomatic phase. *PLoS One* 9:e104081. doi: 10.1371/journal.pone.0104081

Nascimento, F., Sebastiao, A. M., and Ribeiro, J. A. (2015). Presymptomatic and symptomatic ALS SOD1 (G93A) mice differ in adenosine A_1 and A_{2A} receptor-mediated tonic modulation of neuromuscular transmission. *Purinergic Signal.* 11, 471–480. doi: 10.1007/s11302-015-9465-4

Naumenko, N., Pollari, E., Kurronen, A., Giniatullina, R., Shakirzyanova, A., Magga, J., et al. (2011). Gender-specific mechanism of synaptic impairment and its prevention by GCSF in a mouse model of ALS. *Front. Cell. Neurosci.* 5:26. doi: 10.3389/fncel.2011.00026

Neumann, M., Sampathu, D. M., Kwong, L. K., Truax, A. C., Micsenyi, M. C., Chou, T. T., et al. (2006). Ubiquitinated TDP-43 in frontotemporal lobar degeneration and amyotrophic lateral sclerosis. *Science* 314, 130–133. doi: 10.1126/science.1134108

Nichols, N. L., Van Dyke, J., Nashold, L., Satriotomo, I., Suzuki, M., and Mitchell, G. S. (2013). Ventilatory control in ALS. *Respir. Physiol. Neurobiol.* 189, 429–437. doi: 10.1016/j.resp.2013.05.016

Ng, S. K., Higashimori, H., Tolman, M., and Yang, Y. (2015). Suppression of adenosine 2a receptor (A_{2A}R)-mediated adenosine signaling improves disease phenotypes in a mouse model of amyotrophic lateral sclerosis. *Exp. Neurol.* 267, 115–122. doi: 10.1016/j.expneurol.2015.03.004

Nonaka, T., Kametani, F., Arai, T., Akiyama, H., and Hasegawa, M. (2009). Truncation and pathogenic mutations facilitate the formation of intracellular aggregates of TDP-43. *Hum. Mol. Genet.* 18, 3353–3364. doi: 10.1093/hmg/ddp275

Pasinelli, P., and Brown, R. H. (2006). Molecular biology of amyotrophic lateral sclerosis: insights from genetics. *Nat. Rev. Neurosci.* 7, 710–723. doi: 10.1038/nrn1971

Pelligrino, D. A., Xu, H. L., and Vetri, F. (2010). Caffeine and the control of cerebral hemodynamics. *J. Alzheimers Dis.* 20(Suppl. 1), S51–S62. doi: 10.3233/JAD-2010-091261

Pokrishevsky, E., Grad, L. I., Yousefi, M., Wang, J., Mackenzie, I. R., and Cashman, N. R. (2012). Aberrant localization of FUS and TDP43 is associated with misfolding of SOD1 in amyotrophic lateral sclerosis. *PLoS One* 7:e35050. doi: 10.1371/journal.pone.0035050

Popoli, P., Frank, C., Tebano, M. T., Potenza, R. L., Pintor, A., Domenici, M. R., et al. (2003). Modulation of glutamate release and excitotoxicity by adenosine A_{2A} receptors. *Neurology* 61(11 Suppl. 6), S69–S71. doi: 10.1212/01.WNL.0000095216.89483.A2

Potenza, R. L., Armida, M., Ferrante, A., Pèzzola, A., Matteucci, A., Puopolo, M., et al. (2013). Effects of chronic caffeine intake in a mouse model of amyotrophic lateral sclerosis. *J. Neurosci. Res.* 91, 585–592. doi: 10.1002/jnr.23185

Pousinha, P. A., Correia, A. M., Sebastião, A. M., and Ribeiro, J. A. (2010). Predominance of adenosine excitatory over inhibitory effects on transmission at the neuromuscular junction of infant rats. *J. Pharmacol. Exp. Ther.* 332, 153–163. doi: 10.1124/jpet.109.157255

Pousinha, P. A., Correia, A. M., Sebastião, A. M., and Ribeiro, J. A. (2012). Neuromuscular transmission modulation by adenosine upon aging. *Neurobiol. Aging* 33, 2869–2880. doi: 10.1016/j.neurobiolaging.2012.01.008

Pousinha, P. A., Diogenes, M. J., Ribeiro, J. A., and Sebastião, A. M. (2006). Triggering of BDNF facilitatory action on neuromuscular transmission by adenosine A_{2A} receptors. *Neurosci. Lett.* 404, 143–147. doi: 10.1016/j.neulet.2006.05.036

Qian, K., Huang, H., Peterson, A., Hu, B., Maragakis, N. J., Ming, G. L., et al. (2017). Sporadic ALS astrocytes induce neuronal degeneration in vivo. *Stem Cell Rep.* 8, 843–855. doi: 10.1016/j.stemcr.2017.03.003

Rebola, N., Simões, A. P., Canas, P. M., Tomé, A. R., Andrade, G. M., Barry, C. E., et al. (2011). Adenosine A_{2A} receptors control neuroinflammation and consequent hippocampal neuronal dysfunction. *J. Neurochem.* 117, 100–111. doi: 10.1111/j.1471-4159.2011.07178.x

Ribeiro, F. F., Neves-Tomé, R., Assaife-Lopes, N., Santos, T. E., Silva, R. F. M., Brites, D., et al. (2016a). Axonal elongation and dendritic branching is enhanced by adenosine A_{2A} receptors activation in cerebral cortical neurons. *Brain Struct. Funct.* 221, 2777–2799. doi: 10.1007/s00429-015-1072-1

Ribeiro, F. F., Xapelli, S., Miranda-Lourenço, C., Tanqueiro, S. R., Fonseca-Gomes, J., Diógenes, M. J., et al. (2016b). Purine nucleosides in neuroregeneration and neuroprotection. *Neuropharmacology* 104, 226–242. doi: 10.1016/j.neuropharm.2015.11.006

Ribeiro, J. A., and Sebastião, A. M. (1987). On the role, inactivation and origin of endogenous adenosine at the frog neuromuscular junction. *J. Physiol.* 384, 571–585. doi: 10.1113/jphysiol.1987.sp016470

Ribeiro, J. A., and Sebastião, A. M. (2010). Caffeine and adenosine. *J. Alzheimers Dis.* 20(Suppl. 1), S3–S15. doi: 10.3233/JAD-2010-1379

Ribeiro, J. A., Sebastião, A. M., and De Mendonça, A. (2003). Adenosine receptors in the nervous system: pathophysiological implications. *Prog. Neurobiol.* 68, 377–392. doi: 10.1016/S0301-0082(02)00155-7

Ribeiro, J. A., and Walker, J. (1973). Action of adenosine triphosphate on endplate potentials recorded from muscle fibres of the rat-diaphragm and frog sartorius. *Br. J. Pharmacol.* 49, 724–725. doi: 10.1111/j.1476-5381.1973.tb08555.x

Ribeiro, J. A., and Walker, J. (1975). The effects of adenosine triphosphate and adenosine diphosphate on transmission at the rat and frog neuromuscular junctions. *Br. J. Pharmacol.* 54, 213–218. doi: 10.1111/j.1476-5381.1975.tb06931.x

Rocha, M. C., Pousinha, P. A., Correia, A. M., Sebastião, A. M., and Ribeiro, J. A. (2013). Early changes of neuromuscular transmission in the SOD1(G93A) mice model of ALS start long before motor symptoms onset. *PLoS One* 8:e73846. doi: 10.1371/journal.pone.0073846

Rodrigues, T. M., Jerónimo-Santos, A., Outeiro, T. F., Sebastião, A. M., and Diógenes, M. J. (2014). Challenges and promises in the development of neurotrophic factor-based therapies for Parkinson's disease. *Drugs Aging* 31, 239–261. doi: 10.1007/s40266-014-0160-x

Santiago, A. R., Baptista, F. I., Santos, P. F., Cristóvão, G., Ambrósio, A. F., Cunha, R. A., et al. (2014). Role of microglia adenosine A_{2A} receptors in retinal and brain neurodegenerative diseases. *Mediators Inflamm.* 2014:465694. doi: 10.1155/2014/465694

Sebastião, A. M., Assaife-Lopes, N., Diógenes, M. J., Vaz, S. H., and Ribeiro, J. A. (2011). Modulation of brain-derived neurotrophic factor (BDNF) actions in the nervous system by adenosine A_{2A} receptors and the role of lipid rafts. *Biochim. Biophys. Acta* 1808, 1340–1349. doi: 10.1016/j.bbamem.2010.06.028

Sebastião, A. M., and Ribeiro, J. A. (1985). Enhancement of transmission at the frog neuromuscular junction by adenosine deaminase: evidence for an inhibitory role of endogenous adenosine on neuromuscular transmission. *Neurosci. Lett.* 62, 267–270. doi: 10.1016/0304-3940(85)90366-0

Sebastião, A. M., and Ribeiro, J. A. (2009a). Adenosine receptors and the central nervous system. *Handb. Exp. Pharmacol.* 193, 471–534. doi: 10.1007/978-3-540-89615-9_16

Sebastião, A. M., and Ribeiro, J. A. (2009b). Triggering neurotrophic factor actions through adenosine A_{2A} receptor activation: implications for neuroprotection. *Br. J. Pharmacol.* 158, 15–22. doi: 10.1111/j.1476-5381.2009.00157.x

Sebastião, A. M., Stone, T. W., and Ribeiro, J. A. (1990). On the inhibitory adenosine receptor at the neuromuscular junction and hippocampus of the rat: antagonism by 1,3,8-substituted xanthines. *Br. J. Pharmacol.* 101, 453–459. doi: 10.1111/j.1476-5381.1990.tb12729.x

Selvaraj, B. T., Livesey, M. R., Zhao, C., Gregory, J. M., James, O. T., Cleary, E. M., et al. (2018). *C9ORF72* repeat expansion causes vulnerability of motor neurons to Ca^{2+}-permeable AMPA receptor-mediated excitotoxicity. *Nat. Commun.* 9:347. doi: 10.1038/s41467-017-02729-0

Shan, X., Vocadlo, D., and Krieger, C. (2009). Mislocalization of TDP-43 in the G93A mutant SOD1 transgenic mouse model of ALS. *Neurosci. Lett.* 458, 70–74. doi: 10.1016/j.neulet.2009.04.031

Shi, Y., Lin, S., Staats, K. A., Li, Y., Chang, W. H., Hung, S. T., et al. (2018). Haploinsufficiency leads to neurodegeneration in C9ORF72 ALS/FTD human induced motorneurons. *Nat. Med.* 24, 313–325. doi: 10.1038/nm.4490

Sitkovsky, M. V., Lukashev, D., Apasov, S., Kojima, H., Koshiba, M., Caldwell, C., et al. (2004). Physiological control of immune response and inflammatory tissue damage by hypoxia-inducible factors and adenosine A_{2A} receptors. *Annu. Rev. Immunol.* 22, 657–682. doi: 10.1146/annurev.immunol.22.012703.104731

Smith, B. N., Newhouse, S., Shatunov, A., Vance, C., Topp, S., Johnson, L., et al. (2013). The C9ORF72 expansion mutation is a common cause of ALS+/-FTD in Europe and has a single founder. *Eur. J. Hum. Genet.* 21, 102–108. doi: 10.1038/ejhg.2012.98

Son, Y. J., Trachtenberg, J. T., and Thompson, W. J. (1996). Schwann cells induce and guide sprouting and reinnervation of neuromuscular junctions. *Trends Neurosci.* 19, 280–285. doi: 10.1016/S0166-2236(96)10032-1

Taylor, J. P., Brown, R. H. Jr., and Cleveland, D. W. (2016). Decoding ALS: from genes to mechanism. *Nature* 539, 197–206. doi: 10.1038/nature20413

Tsentsevitsky, A., Kovyazina, I., Nikolsky, E., Bukharaeva, E., and Giniatullin, R. (2013). Redox-sensitive synchronizing action of adenosine on transmitter release at the neuromuscular junction. *Neuroscience* 248, 699–707. doi: 10.1016/j.neuroscience.2013.05.065

Vincenzi, F., Corciulo, C., Targa, M., Casetta, I., Gentile, M., Granieri, E., et al. (2013). A_{2A} adenosine receptors are up-regulated in lymphocytes from amyotrophic lateral sclerosis patients. *Amyotroph. Lateral Scler. Frontotemporal Degener.* 14, 406–413. doi: 10.3109/21678421.2013.793358

Volonté, C., Apolloni, S., Parisi, C., and Amadio, S. (2016). Purinergic contribution to amyotrophic lateral sclerosis. *Neuropharmacology* 104, 180–193. doi: 10.1016/j.neuropharm.2015.10.026

Wainger, B. J., Kiskinis, E., Mellin, C., Wiskow, O., Han, S. S., Sandoe, J., et al. (2014). Intrinsic membrane hyperexcitability of amyotrophic lateral sclerosis patient-derived motorneurons. *Cell Rep.* 7, 1–11. doi: 10.1016/j.celrep.2014.03.019

Wiese, S., Jablonka, S., Holtmann, B., Orel, N., Rajagopal, R., Chao, M. V., et al. (2007). Adenosine receptor A_{2A}-R contributes to motoneuron survival by transactivating the tyrosine kinase receptor TrkB. *Proc. Natl. Acad. Sci. U.S.A.* 104, 17210–17215. doi: 10.1073/pnas.0705267104

Wijesekera, L. C., and Leigh, P. N. (2009). Amyotrophic lateral sclerosis. *Orphanet J. Rare Dis.* 4:3. doi: 10.1186/1750-1172-4-3

Witts, E. C., Nascimento, F., and Miles, G. B. (2015). Adenosine-mediated modulation of ventral horn interneurons and spinal motoneurons in neonatal mice. *J. Neurophysiol.* 114, 2305–2315. doi: 10.1152/jn.00574.2014

Witts, E. C., Panetta, K. M., and Miles, G. B. (2012). Glial-derived adenosine modulates spinal motor networks in mice. *J. Neurophysiol.* 107, 1925–1934. doi: 10.1152/jn.00513.2011

Yanpallewar, S. U., Barrick, C. A., Buckley, H., Becker, J., and Tessarollo, L. (2012). Deletion of the BDNF truncated receptor TrkB.T1 delays disease onset in a mouse model of amyotrophic lateral sclerosis. *PLoS One* 7:e39946. doi: 10.1371/journal.pone.0039946

Yoshida, Y., Une, F., Utatsu, Y., Nomoto, M., Furukawa, Y., Maruyama, Y., et al. (1999). Adenosine and neopterin levels in cerebrospinal fluid of patients with neurological disorders. *Intern. Med.* 38, 133–139. doi: 10.2169/internalmedicine.38.133

12

Adenosine Receptors in Developing and Adult Mouse Neuromuscular Junctions and Functional Links with other Metabotropic Receptor Pathways

Josep Tomàs†, Neus Garcia*†, Maria A. Lanuza*†, Manel M. Santafé, Marta Tomàs, Laura Nadal, Erica Hurtado, Anna Simó-Ollé, Víctor Cilleros-Mañé and Laia Just-Borràs*

Unitat d'Histologia i Neurobiologia, Facultat de Medicina i Ciències de la Salut, Universitat Rovira i Virgili, Reus, Spain

***Correspondence:**
Josep Tomàs
josepmaria.tomas@urv.cat
Neus Garcia
mariadelesneus.garcia@urv.cat
Maria A. Lanuza
mariaangel.lanuza@urv.cat

†These authors have contributed equally to this work.

In the last few years, we have studied the presence and involvement in synaptogenesis and mature transmitter release of the adenosine autoreceptors (AR) in the mammalian neuromuscular junction (NMJ). Here, we review and bring together the previously published data to emphasize the relevance of these receptors for developmental axonal competition, synaptic loss and mature NMJ functional modulation. However, in addition to AR, activity-dependent mediators originating from any of the three cells that make the synapse (nerve, muscle, and glial cells) cross the extracellular cleft to generate signals in target metabotropic receptors. Thus, the integrated interpretation of the complementary function of all these receptors is needed. We previously studied, in the NMJ, the links of AR with mAChR and the neurotrophin receptor TrkB in the control of synapse elimination and transmitter release. We conclude that AR cooperate with these receptors through synergistic and antagonistic effects in the developmental synapse elimination process. In the adult NMJ, this cooperation is manifested so as that the functional integrity of a given receptor group depends on the other receptors operating normally (i.e., the functional integrity of mAChR depends on AR operating normally). These observations underlie the relevance of AR in the NMJ function.

Keywords: motor end-plate, postnatal synapse elimination, axonal competition, acetylcholine release, muscarinic acetylcholine receptors, adenosine receptors, neurotrophins, TrkB

INTRODUCTION

In addition to the main neurotransmitter-receptor signal, several signaling pathways coordinate the pre- and postsynaptic cells and associated glia in the tripartite synapses in accordance with functional demands. In the NMJ, presynaptic mAChRs directly couple ACh secretion to the regulation of the release mechanism itself (Caulfield and Birdsall, 1998; Slutsky et al., 2001; Minic et al., 2002; Santafé et al., 2003, 2004; Garcia et al., 2005). Moreover, presynaptic nicotinic ACh autoreceptors (nAChRs) are also present at the NMJ

Abbreviations: ACh, acetylcholine; AR, adenosine autoreceptors; ATP, adenosine triphosphate; EPP, evoked endplate potentials; LAL, Levator auris longus muscle; mAChR, muscarinic acetylcholine receptor; M_1, M_1-type muscarinic acetylcholine receptor; M_2, M_2-type muscarinic acetylcholine receptor; M_4, M_4-type muscarinic acetylcholine receptor; NMJ, neuromuscular junction; TrkB, tropomyosin-related kinase B receptor; TrkB-Fc, inhibitor recombinant human TrkB-Fc Chimera.

(Correia-de-Sá, 1994; Salgado et al., 2000). Also, at the NMJ, the presynaptic neurotrophin and cytokine receptors can be influenced by target-derived signals (Bibel and Barde, 2000; Roux and Barker, 2002; Pitts et al., 2006), and glutamate together with mGluR1 also mediate the signaling in this synapse (Waerhaug and Ottersen, 1993; Lück et al., 2000; Malomouzh et al., 2011; Marmiroli and Cavaletti, 2012; Walder et al., 2013).

Studies in the early 1970s Ribeiro and Walker (1973) showed that adenosine and ATP modulate the presynaptic component through purinergic receptors (adenosine P1Rs and ATP P2Rs) (Correia-de-Sá et al., 1991; Ribeiro et al., 1996). The first authors describing adenosine effects at the mammalian NMJ were (Ginsborg and Hirst, 1971, 1972; see also Singh et al., 1986). It is known that both nerve and muscle cell activity can contribute to the extracellular adenosine release (Cunha and Sebastião, 1993; Ribeiro et al., 1996).

In the last few years, we have studied the presence and involvement of AR in the synaptogenesis and transmitter release in the developing and mature mammalian NMJ (Garcia et al., 2013; Tomàs et al., 2014; Tomàs J. et al., 2017; Santafé et al., 2015; Nadal et al., 2016a,b, 2017). Here, we review and bring together previously published data to contribute to emphasizing the relevance of these receptors in this synapse. Moreover, we also discuss our previous studies in relation with the interaction between AR, mAChR and the TrkB in the control of synapse elimination during development and transmitter release in the adult NMJ.

Our results indicate that during NMJ synaptogenesis, AR (A_1R and $A_{2A}R$ subtypes) contribute to the developmental synapse elimination process, helping to define the winner of the competition between axon terminals. In the adult, AR help to modulate transmitter release by limiting spontaneous quantal leak of ACh and preserve synaptic function by reducing depression during repetitive activity. To realize these functions, several synergistic and antagonistic relations exist between AR and, at least, the mAChR subtypes (M_1, M_2, and M_4) and the TrkB receptor. These observations underlie the relevance of AR in the NMJ function.

ADENOSINE RECEPTORS LOCALIZATION IN THE NMJ

Four subtypes of AR have been cloned (A_1R, $A_{2A}R$, $A_{2B}R$, and A_3R) and despite the fact that there was some uncertainty about how they were distributed in the cells of the paradigmatic NMJ (Lynge and Hellsten, 2000; Baxter et al., 2005), some of them have been localized in the mouse synapse with confocal immunohistochemistry (Garcia et al., 2005, 2013, 2014; Wright et al., 2009). The confidence of protein localization by immunohistochemistry lies in the specificity of the antibodies used. Though the lack of signal in knockout animals was not investigated, we made an effort to characterize the commercially available antibodies by Western blotting. Our results have shown that the A_1R receptor is more abundant in adult animals, whereas the $A_{2A}R$ receptor predominates in the newborn ones (Garcia et al., 2013). Moreover, the $A_{2B}R$ and A_3R receptors are more expressed in the adult muscles than in the younger ones (Tomàs et al., 2014).

Immunofluorescence staining coupled with confocal microscopy analysis was performed to determine the localization of A_1R, $A_{2A}R$ (whose function has been further investigated) in P6 and P30 NMJ (**Figure 1**). Moreover, localization of $A_{2B}R$, and A_3R has been determined in P30 NMJ. By triple labeling of NMJ we stained each one of these protein receptors in green fluorescence together with Syntaxin or S-100 (blue fluorescence) and nAChR (red fluorescence) and we saw that

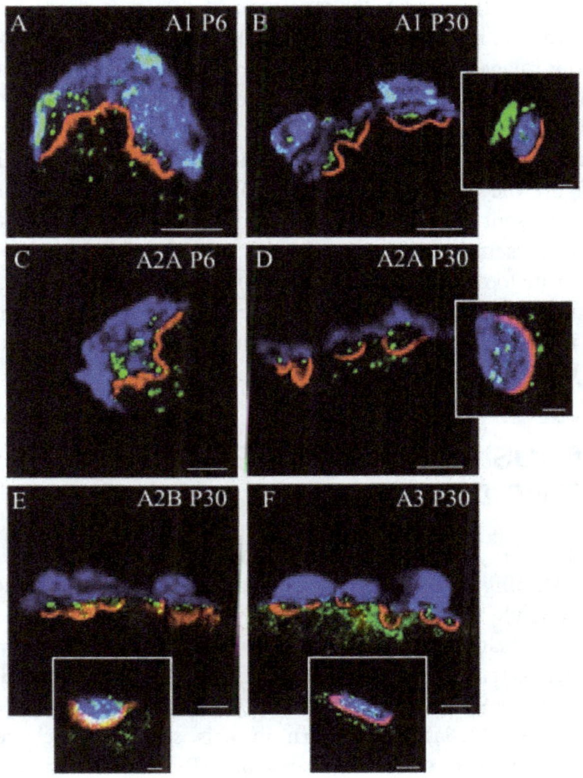

FIGURE 1 | Immunolocalization of A_1R, $A_{2A}R$, $A_{2B}R$, and A_3R receptors in the motor nerve terminals on neuromuscular synapses. Immunofluorescence staining and confocal microscopy analysis in newborn (P6) and mature (P30) mice. Triple labeling of the corresponding receptor proteins (green fluorescence) with S-100 (blue fluorescence) and rhodamine-alpha-bungarotoxin (red fluorescence). In the insets (scale bar, 1 μm), Syntaxin labeling (in blue) is showed instead of S-100. **(A–D)** Are single confocal planes from NMJs obtained using plastic embedded semithin cross-sections (0.5–0.7 μm). **(E,F)** Are single confocal planes from a projection image. In the cross-sections of the synaptic boutons, all receptors are present as a fine granular labeling in the space of the nerve terminals between the blue Schwann cell and the red postsynaptic line. In all cases, (see the insets showed as examples), the receptor proteins colocalize with Syntaxin. The bar indicates 10 μm. The images are illustrative examples of the original studies published in Garcia et al. (2014) (Garcia N., Priego M., Hurtado E., Obis T., Santafe M. M., Tomàs M., Lanuza M. A., Tomàs J. Adenosine A2B and A3 receptor location at the mouse neuromuscular junction. *J. Anat.* 225:109–117) and Garcia et al. (2013) (Garcia N., Priego M., Obis T., Santafe M. M., Tomàs M., Besalduch N., Lanuza M. A., Tomàs J. Adenosine A1 and A2A receptor-mediated modulation of acetylcholine release in the mice neuromuscular junction. *Eur. J. Neurosci.* 38:2229–2241).

the molecules were present. However, since the components of the NMJ (the nerve terminal, the Schwann cell and the muscle fiber) are juxtaposed, it is not always easy to locate the proteins with precision. Thus, in some cases, to better determine A_1R and $A_{2A}R$ localization, we used plastic embedded semithin cross-sections as a tool for high-resolution together with the triple-labeling immunofluorescence analysis. Briefly, after conventional immunohistochemistry the samples were dehydrated with increasing concentrations of ethanol and acetone, the tissue fragments were embedded in Spurr's resin in transverse orientation and sections (0.5–0.7 μm thick) were obtained (Lanuza et al., 2007; Garcia et al., 2010c; Besalduch et al., 2013). Images (A–D) correspond to a single image made in a confocal microscope from a 0,5 μm muscle semithin cross section. Images (E–F) show localization of A2BR and A3R using single confocal Z planes from a projection image of at least 10 confocal Z planes obtained every 0,5 μm. As shown in **Figure 1**, these receptors are differentially located in the three cells that configure the NMJs (Garcia et al., 2013, 2014). To the purpose of the present review, it can be noted that the four subtypes of AR are present in the motor endings, which is understood to be a requisite to modulate presynaptic function. However, some AR are localized also in the other synaptic components (for instance A_3R in the postsynaptic site) and the interpretation of the results here is not a full representation of the AR physiology.

ADENOSINE RECEPTORS ROLE DURING DEVELOPMENT

During the nervous system development there is an overwhelming production of synapses (that may promote connectiviy), followed by an activity-dependent reduction of them. Hebbian competition between axons refines connectivity and increases specificity (Purves and Lichtman, 1980; Jansen and Fladby, 1990; Sanes and Lichtman, 1999; Chen and Regehr, 2000; Nadal et al., 2016a). In newborn animals, skeletal muscle cells are innervated by various motor axons (Ribchester and Barry, 1994) but when the competition ends, the NMJs retain only one axon (Liu et al., 1994; Nguyen and Lichtman, 1996; Chang and Balice-Gordon, 1997; Sanes and Lichtman, 1999; Herrera and Zeng, 2003; Nelson et al., 2003; Wyatt and Balice-Gordon, 2003; Buffelli et al., 2004).

The postsynaptic cell and the terminal Schwann cells may be intermediary in axonal competition. A decrement in polyneuronal innervation occurs at a time when relatively little loss of the nAChR postsynaptic receptors was observed (Lanuza et al., 2002). However, in some cases, local receptor loss has been observed before the corresponding axon loss (Balice-Gordon and Lichtman, 1993). This suggest that pre- and postsynaptic changes are coordinated. Non-myelinating terminal Schwann cells at the NMJ play a role in synapse elimination (reviewed by Lee et al., 2017). A model has been proposed in which the activity of the Schwann cells promote synapse elimination by creating vacant synaptic sites that can be reoccupied by the competing axon terminals.

At the time this process occurs, several signaling mechanisms coordinate the pre- and postsynaptic cell function. First of all, presynaptic mAChR receptors allow direct competitive interaction between nerve endings because of their different activity-dependent ACh secretion (Santafé et al., 2004, 2007, 2009; Nadal et al., 2016a,b; Tomàs J. et al., 2017). Moreover, we also investigated the involvement of presynaptic AR (A_1R and $A_{2A}R$), which monitor both nerve- and muscle-derived adenosine release during the complex period of axonal elimination around P5-P9 (Garcia et al., 2013; Nadal et al., 2016a,b).

We evaluated the average number of axonal connections per NMJ from B6.Cg-Tg (Thy1-YFP) (from now YFP) and C57BL/J6 mice. To the flat and accessible mouse LAL muscle, we subcutaneously applied the unselective AR inhibitor 8-(p-sulfophenyl) theophylline (8SPT) and the agonist adenosine between P5-P15 (**Figure 2**). At P7, after the inhibition with 8SPT of the AR, we observed an acceleration of the axonal elimination on the NMJ indicating that, at this point of development, the role of AR is to delay axonal loss (Nadal et al., 2016a). In accordance, exposure to the physiological agonist adenosine resulted in a retardation of axonal elimination (i.e., a significant high number of triple innervated NMJ and a reduction in the number of dual innervated NMJ, **Figure 2Aa**). We also analyzed axonal loss after selectively blocking A_1R with 8-cyclopentyl-1,3-dipropylxanthine (DPCPX) or $A_{2A}R$ with 2-(2-furanyl)-7-(2-phenylethyl)-7H-pyrazolo[4,3-e] [1, 2, 4] triazolo[1,5-c]pyrimidin-5-amine (SCH-58261) (Nadal et al., 2016a,b). Results showed that axonal loss is accelerated by both inhibitors indicating that, in normal conditions, both receptors A_1R and $A_{2A}R$ are related with delaying axonal elimination. However, at P9 (**Figure 2Ab**), the purinergic function accelerates axonal loss to the maximum rate. Therefore, an initial delay in axonal loss at P7 (an A_1R- and $A_{2A}R$-mediated effect which can be reinforced by exogenously added adenosine) is followed by an A_1R- and $A_{2A}R$-mediated tonic acceleration of axonal loss at P9 (green arrows in **Figure 3** left, Nadal et al., 2016a). We also investigated the effect of long-term AR perturbation with 8SPT over axon number at P15. Despite the continued presence of the inhibitor, monoinnervation is achieved in about 90% of NMJ at P15 (**Figure 2Ac**) suggesting that axonal competition and loss are differentially modulated (Nadal et al., 2016a).

Axonal elimination is accompanied by changes in the structure of the nicotinic ACh receptor (nAChR) clusters in the postsynaptic site (**Figure 2B**). Based on criteria from previous studies on developing mammalian NMJ (Steinbach, 1981; Slater, 1982a,b; Bewick et al., 1996; Lanuza et al., 2002; Garcia et al., 2011), we defined several maturation stages (MS1–MS4). Changes in nAChR distribution transform the uniform nAChR oval cluster at birth (MS1) into an elongated plaque with some heterogeneities in the density of receptors (MS2). Later, they become into clusters with small zones of low receptor density (MS3) that are not innervated that lead to a mature pattern of independent primary gutters (MS4) (Nadal et al., 2016a). In relation with these changes, we found that the antagonist 8SPT, applied in the period P5–P8, had

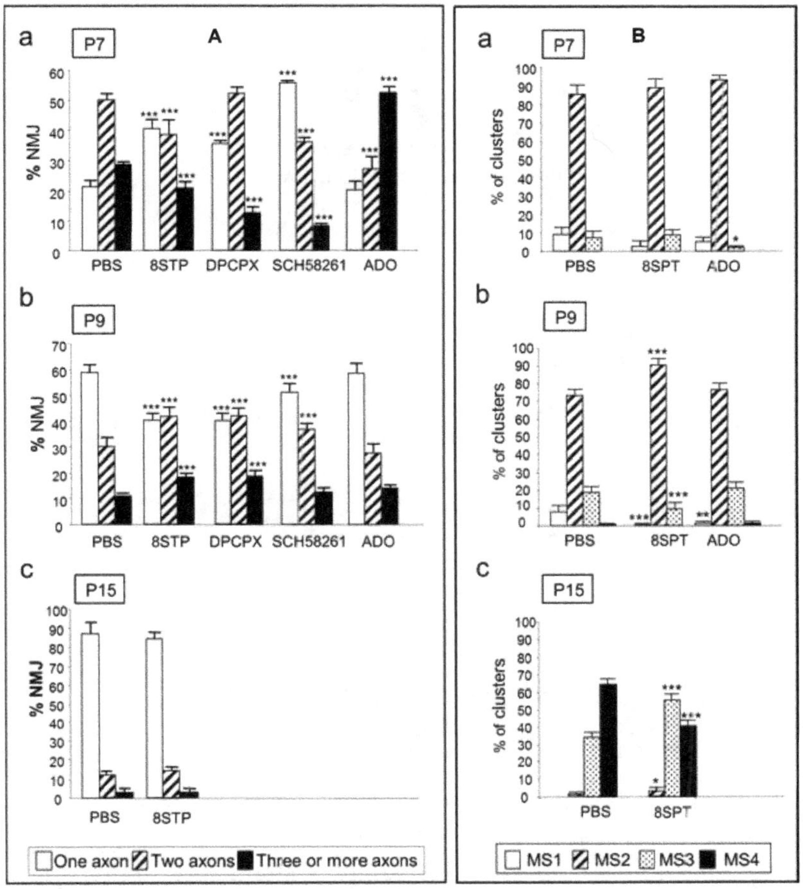

FIGURE 2 | Involvement of AR in axonal elimination and in the morphological maturation of the postsynaptic apparatus. The **(A)** shows the percentage of the singly-, dually-, and triply- (or more) innervated NMJs in the YFP control mice exposed to PBS, and after 2 (P7 in **a**), 4 (P9, in **b**) and in some cases 10 (P15, in **c**) applications (one application every day after P5) of the AR pan-inhibitor 8SPT and the AR agonist adenosine (ADO). We also studied axonal elimination after selectively blocking A_1R with the antagonist DPCPX and inhibiting $A_{2A}R$ with SCH-58261. The **(B)** shows the percentage of the MS1–MS4 maturation stages in the NMJ of the untreated YFP control mice (exposed to PBS), and after 2 (P7 in **a**), 4 (P9, in **b**), and in some cases 10 (P15, in **c**) applications of the 8SPT and ADO. Fisher's test: *$p < 0.05$, **$p < 0.01$, ***$p < 0.005$. This Figure has been adapted and redraw from the Figures 4, 8 in the original article "[Presynaptic muscarinic acetylcholine autoreceptors (M_1, M_2, and M_4 subtypes), adenosine receptors (A_1 and A_{2A}) and tropomyosin-related kinase B receptor (TrkB) modulate the developmental synapse elimination process at the neuromuscular junction]" by [Nadal, L., N. Garcia, E. Hurtado, A. Simó, M. Tomàs, M. A. Lanuza, M. Santafé, and J. Tomàs]." *Mol. Brain.* 2016, 9: 67 (doi: 10.1186/s13041-016-0248-9).

no effect on the clusters morphology when observed at P7 (**Figure 2Ba**). However, at P9 we found that MS2clusters were increased while the MS1 and MS3 ones decreased (**Figure 2Bb**), which indicates a delay in the transition from MS2 to MS3. At P15 (**Figure 2Bc**) the postsynaptic maturation is partially retained at the MS3 stage. Thus, AR are able to accelerate maturation during the P7–P15 period. Interestingly, the agonist adenosine does not unambiguously change the cluster maturation indicating that the tonic effect of the AR evidenced by using 8SPT is close to their maximum (Nadal et al., 2016a).

In summary, AR are involved in the control of the competitive interactions between nerve endings, possibly helping to determine the winner or the losers but, thereafter, axon loss seems to occur with autonomy.

ADENOSINE RECEPTORS ROLE IN THE ADULT NEUROTRANSMISSION

Once a NMJ becomes mature and monoinnervated, AR continue modulating neurotransmission. By measuring the activity-dependent efflux of radiolabelled ACh incorporated in nerve endings, Correia-de-Sá et al. (1991) showed that AR control their nerve-stimulated release. Micromolar adenosine levels reduced evoked and/or spontaneous ACh release in frog NMJs (Searl and Silinsky, 2005; Shakirzyanova et al., 2006; Adámek et al., 2010) and also in rat NMJs (Silinsky et al., 1989; De Lorenzo et al., 2006; Pousinha et al., 2010). However, in rat NMJs, submicromolar adenosine concentrations has the opposite effect (Pousinha et al., 2010). Moreover, in other studies done in mice, only very high doses of adenosine (in

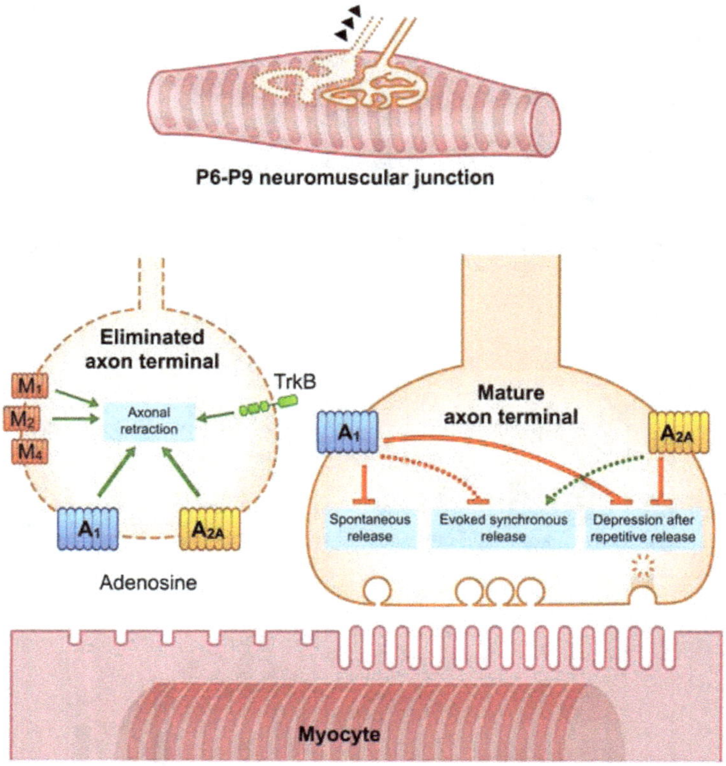

FIGURE 3 | Diagrams showing an overall representation of the data. Between P6-P9 several nerve endings are eliminated and retract whereas one nerve terminal is stabilized. Green arrows indicate stimulation or promotion; red lines indicate inhibition. During the 1st week postnatal an A_1R- and $A_{2A}R$-mediated tonic acceleration of axonal retraction is observed (green arrows in the eliminated axon terminal). In addition to the role of AR, at least mAChR M_1-, M_2-, and M_4-subtypes and the TrkB receptor are also involved. The downstream pathways integrate the signals related with the competitive interactions and accelerate axonal loss. In the adult NMJ, most experiments on transmitter release have been done in recording conditions that interfere with the synapse function to prevent muscle contraction. In these conditions A_1R reduces it whereas $A_{2A}R$ increases it. Discontinuous lines in the mature axon terminal indicate these changes in conditions of safety factor reduction. In experiments with μ-CgTx-GIIIB only the voltage-dependent sodium channel of the muscle cells was shut-down, thus resulting in non-contractile muscles which have well preserved NMJ physiology and safety factor. In these conditions AR are not coupled to any immediate modulation of evoked neurotransmission. However, AR can restrict spontaneous quantal leak of ACh (A_1R) and protect synaptic function by reducing the magnitude of depression during repetitive activity (an A_1R- and $A_{2A}R$-mediated effect).

the range of millimolar) affected neurotransmission (Silinsky, 2004) and, in concordance, some mammalian endplates were insensitive to adenosine (Ginsborg and Hirst, 1972). Therefore, it remains unclear how and when adenosine and AR modulate neurotransmission. The majority of experiments have been done in electrophysiological recording conditions that interfere with the normal function of the NMJ to prevent muscle contraction. For example, in the ACh efflux experiments hemicholinium-3 prevents choline reuptake, high Mg^{2+} concentrations reduce ACh release and d-tubocurarine reduces postsynaptic response. In these conditions, selective agonists and antagonists of the A_1R and $A_{2A}R$ modify ACh release. On the one hand, the A_1R agonist 2-Chloro-N^6-cyclopentyladenosine, 1 μM (CCPA) reduces it (Veggetti et al., 2008) whereas the $A_{2A}R$ agonist 2-p-(2-Carboxyethyl)- phenethylamino-5′-N-ethylcarboxamidoadenosine hydrochloride hydrate, 1 μM (CGS-21680) increases it (Pousinha et al., 2010). However, A_1R reduces release (in high Mg^{2+} and curare blockade) when the NMJ is already weakened and because of that, the meaning of this regulation seems unclear (Garcia et al., 2013).

Because of these uncertainties, we induced muscle paralysis with μ-CgTx-GIIIB (Garcia et al., 2013; Tomàs et al., 2014; Obis et al., 2015; Santafé et al., 2015; Hurtado et al., 2017a,b), a specific inhibitor of the sodium channel of the muscle cells which preserves NMJ function (Garcia et al., 2013) and its safety factor. This experimental condition mimics the physiological conditions of this synapse in the living animals except for the absence of the contraction-dependent retrograde influence of the muscle cells (Besalduch et al., 2011; Hurtado et al., 2017a,b). We observed that 25 μM adenosine reduced (50%) the quantal content of ACh release in agreement with other authors (Ginsborg and Hirst, 1972; Ribeiro and Walker, 1975). However, in the nearly normal basal conditions (only test stimulations of 70 pulses at 0.5 Hz every 5 min in the presence of μ-CgTx-GIIIB), none of the purinergic agonists or antagonists had any effect on the evoked ACh release. In particular, we tested non-selective AR agonists and antagonists (adenosine and 8SPT, respectively), A_1R-selective agonists and antagonists (CCPA 1 μM and DPCPX 100 nM, respectively) and $A_{2A}R$-selective agonists and antagonists (CGS-21680 1 μM and SCH-58261 50 nM, respectively) (Garcia et al., 2013; Tomàs et al., 2014). However, we detected that AR were still functional in reducing the spontaneous release because miniature endplate potentials (MEPP) frequency was increased by SPT8 blockade and decreased by adenosine stimulation, with A_1Rs playing the main role because only DPCPX increased MEPP frequency (Garcia et al., 2013). In addition, imposed synaptic activity (40Hz for 2 min of supramaximal stimuli) resulted in synaptic depression, an effect reduced by micromolar adenosine but potentiated by blocking AR with 8SPT. Depression in control muscles represents a ~50% reduction of the endplate potentials (EPP) amplitude and 10 μM adenosine reduces it to a half (Garcia et al., 2013). Surprisingly, we found that depression was not affected by any selective agent, which suggested that both A_1R and A_{2A}R need to collaborate (Garcia et al., 2013; Tomàs et al., 2014). In perspective, the fact that adenosine and 8SPT modified synaptic depression, whereas A_1R and A_{2A}R ligands did not, suggested us that A_{2B}R and/or A_3R could be implicated. Thus, we investigated the A_{2B}R-selective antagonist MRS1706 (N-(4-Acetylphenyl)-2-[4-(2,3,6,7-tetrahydro-2,6-dioxo-1,3-dipropyl-1H-purin-8-yl)phenoxy]acetamide, 100 nM) and the A_3R-selective antagonist MRS1334 (1,4-Dihydro -2-methyl-6-phenyl-4-(phenylethynyl)-3,5-pyridinedicarboxylic acid 3-ethyl-5-[(3nitrophenyl)methyl] ester, 100 nM). We unexpectedly found that A_{2B}R and A_3R neither had any effect on depression (just as the A_1R and A_{2A}R selective antagonists). Thus, we concluded that two or more AR are necessary to protect against depression (Garcia et al., 2013; Tomàs et al., 2014).

In summary, these findings confirmed that in basal conditions AR are not coupled to any immediate modulation of evoked neurotransmission. However, these receptors are still crucial to preserve resources by avoiding the leak of spontaneous quantal ACh, an action which is probably implicated in their protective role against synaptic depression after repetitive activity (Tomàs et al., 2014), (the mature axonal terminal in **Figure 3**).

LINKS OF AR WITH OTHER METABOTROPIC RECEPTORS (DEVELOPMENT AND ADULTHOOD)

Activity-dependent mediators derived from the three cells of the synapse cross the extracellular cleft in all directions to generate signals in target metabotropic receptors. In the NMJ, there are other purinergic receptors apart from AR (Tsim and Barnard, 2002; Todd and Robitaille, 2006), several mAChR (Santafé et al., 2007, 2009; Wright et al., 2009; Garcia et al., 2010b), neurotrophin receptors (Gonzalez et al., 1999; Garcia et al., 2011; Santafé et al., 2015; Nadal et al., 2016a,b) cytokine receptors (Ribchester et al., 1998; Wang et al., 2002; Garcia et al., 2010a, 2012), calcitonin gene-related peptide receptors (Changeux et al., 1992; Lu and Fu, 1995; Gaydukov et al., 2016), glutamate receptors (Thomas and Sigrist, 2012; Personius et al., 2016; Tsentsevitsky et al., 2017) and neuregulin receptors (Loeb, 2003; Kummer et al., 2006; Simeone et al., 2010; Schmidt et al., 2011; Wang et al., 2017). The way a synapse operates is largely the outcome of the confluence of several signaling pathways on intracellular kinases, which phosphorylate protein targets and materialize adaptive changes to modulate transmitter release and the stability of the connection. Therefore, the appropriate knowledge of synaptic behavior needs the integrated albeit complex interpretation of the complementary function of these receptors. Thus, we studied the link and interaction of AR with mAChR and the neurotrophin receptor TrkB in the control of synapse elimination during development and transmitter release in the adult NMJ (Nadal et al., 2016a,b, 2017).

In relation with the synapse elimination process during development, in addition to the role of AR subtypes (A_1R and A_{2A}R) described above, we investigated the involvement of individual mAChR M_1-, M_2-, and M_4-subtypes and the TrkB receptor (Garcia et al., 2010b; Nadal et al., 2016a,b, 2017). Our data indicated that the three receptor sets and all subtypes considered could affect the competition between axon terminals. At P7, for instance, all these receptors taken individually (analyzed through selective inhibition) are involved in favoring initial competition and thus delaying axonal loss. The confluence of the respective downstream pathways can integrate the signals related with the competitive interactions and possibly helps to determine the nerve ending that finally wins and/or the ones that are lost. This competition concludes with the acceleration of the

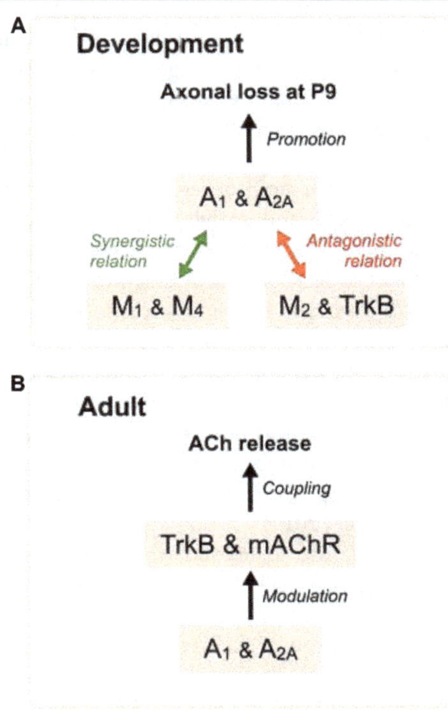

FIGURE 4 | Diagrams showing relations of AR with mAChR and TrkB receptors. In **(A)**, synergistic and antagonistic roles of the AR, mAChR and TrkB receptor during development. AR are necessary to modulate axonal loss and several synergistic (green arrows) and antagonistic (red arrows) relations are clearly observed between all receptors, which affect synapse elimination. In **(B)**, the diagram indicates that the functional integrity of the AR favors the normal operation of the mAChR and the TrkB pathways in the control of the neurotransmitter release in the adulthood.

axonal loss 2 days later (around P9; see the eliminated axonal terminal in **Figure 3**).

To study the collaboration of the AR with mAChR and TrkB, we applied two selective antagonists from two different receptors to see the additive or occlusive effects between them at P9 (Nadal et al., 2016a,b, 2017; Tomàs J. et al., 2017; Tomàs J.M. et al., 2017). These experiments showed the existence of a synergistic role between M_1 and M_4 mAChR, which potentiates the effect of both AR on axonal elimination. Contrarily, the M_2 subtype and the TrkB receptor fully occlude the effects of both A_1R and $A_{2A}R$. Interestingly, when both A_1R and $A_{2A}R$ are blocked at the same time, a mutual occlusion occurs, and the result does not differ from untreated control (Tomàs J.M. et al., 2017).

Thus, both AR are necessary to modulate synapse elimination and several synergistic and antagonistic links are observed between all receptors, which regulate axonal loss (**Figure 4A**). A_1, M_1, and TrkB are coupled to stimulate PKC whereas A_{2A}, M_2, and M_4 inhibit PKA. We hypothesize that a membrane receptor-induced shifting in the protein kinases A and C activity in some nerve endings may play an important role in promoting developmental NMJ maturation.

In the adult NMJ, it is also known that A_1R and $A_{2A}R$ as well as the M_1-, M_2-, and M_4-subtypes of mAChR and the TrkB receptor play several roles in the regulation of transmitter release (Minic et al., 2002; Santafé et al., 2003, 2004, 2007, 2009; Garcia et al., 2010b; Tomàs et al., 2011). By using selective agonists and antagonists we observed that, some receptors (i.e., A_1R as previously stated) produce minor changes in spontaneous quantal output (see **Figure 3**, right) whereas other receptors (i.e., mAChR) induce major changes in evoked release. Thus, each receptor regulates a given combination of spontaneous, evoked and activity-dependent ACh release. As it has been mentioned before, AR preserve resources by reducing spontaneous leak of neurotransmitter (an A_1R effect) and normalize the synapse function because stimulation with adenosine reduces the magnitude of depression during repetitive activity. mAChR stabilize the spontaneous quantal output of ACh and also preserve the synapse function by decreasing evoked release (mainly an M_2 action) and reducing depression. A role for the TrkB receptor is to stabilize the spontaneous quantal leak of ACh but it mainly potentiates evoked release and synaptic potentials (Tomàs et al., 2014).

We also studied the consecutive incubation with two inhibitors affecting two different receptors to see their collaboration in neurotransmission. Adenosine outflow from nerve endings may, through A_1R, reduce M_2 effect on ACh release and adenylyl cyclase may be the shared intracellular node between both pathways (Oliveira et al., 2009). We observed that non-specific AR modulation with 8SPT or adenosine abolishes the effect of a second exposure to the unselective mAChR blocker atropine, but also the effect of the M_1-selective inhibitor pirenzepine and M_2-selective blocker methoctramine. Thus, the normal operation of the AR is necessary for the normal function of the mAChRs (Tomàs et al., 2014) (**Figure 4B**). However, the same effect is observed in the other way around: a previous blockade of mAChR does not allow applied adenosine to change the above described effect on ACh release in our conditions.

Finally, it has also been reported that adenosine acting through A_{2A} receptors is able to transactivate the TrkB receptor without the need of neurotrophin binding (Lee and Chao, 2001; Lee et al., 2002; Wiese et al., 2007). Thus, AR are also implicated in the neurotrophic TrkB signaling (**Figure 4B**).

CONCLUDING REMARKS

Autoreceptors subtypes are present in the motor nerve endings in the NMJ. During development, AR modulate the competition between axon terminals, helping to define the winner and the losers (Nadal et al., 2016b). To accomplish this function, AR establish several synergistic and antagonistic relations with, at least, the mAChR subtypes and the TrkB receptor which affect synapse elimination. In the mature NMJ, AR help transmitter release by limiting the spontaneous quantal leak of ACh, which mitigates depression during repetitive activity and preserves synaptic function (Tomàs et al., 2014). In addition, the functional integrity of the AR is crucial for the normal operation of the mAChR and the TrkB pathways. These observations underlie the relevance of AR in the NMJ function.

AUTHOR CONTRIBUTIONS

LN, EH, AS-O, VC-M, LJ-B, MS, and MT: data collection, quantitative analysis, literature search, data interpretation, and graphic design. NG and ML: statistics. JT, NG, and ML: conception and design, literature search, data interpretation, and manuscript preparation.

FUNDING

This work was supported by a grant from the Catalan Government (2014SGR344 and 2017SGR704) and a grant from MINECO (SAF2015-67143-P).

ACKNOWLEDGMENTS

We thank the reviewers for their careful reading of our manuscript and their many insightful comments.

REFERENCES

Adámek, S., Shakirzyanova, A. V., Malomouzh, A. I., Naumenko, N. V., and Vyskočil, F. (2010). Interaction of glutamate- and adenosine-induced decrease of acetylcholine quantal release at frog neuromuscular junction. *Physiol. Res.* 59, 803–810.

Balice-Gordon, R., and Lichtman, J. (1993). In vivo observations of pre- and postsynaptic changes during the transition from multiple to single innervation at developing neuromuscular junctions. - Semantic Scholar. *J. Neurosci.* 13, 834–855. doi: 10.1523/JNEUROSCI.13-02-00834.1993

Baxter, R. L., Vega-Riveroll, L. J., Deuchars, J., and Parson, S. H. (2005). A_{2A} adenosine receptors are located on presynaptic motor nerve terminals in the mouse. *Synapse* 57, 229–234. doi: 10.1002/syn.20173

Besalduch, N., Lanuza, M. A., Garcia, N., Obis, T., Santafe, M. M., Tomàs, M., et al. (2013). Cellular localization of the atypical isoforms of protein kinase C (aPKCζ/PKMζ and aPKCλ/ι) on the neuromuscular synapse. *Neurosci. Lett.* 556, 166–169. doi: 10.1016/j.neulet.2013.10.006

Besalduch, N., Santafé, M. M., Garcia, N., Gonzalez, C., Tomás, M., Tomás, J., et al. (2011). Transmitter release in the neuromuscular synapse of the protein kinase C theta-deficient adult mouse. *J. Comp. Neurol.* 519, 849–855. doi: 10.1002/cne.22551

Bewick, G. S., Young, C., and Slater, C. R. (1996). Spatial relationships of utrophin, dystrophin, beta-dystroglycan and beta-spectrin to acetylcholine receptor clusters during postnatal maturation of the rat neuromuscular junction. *J. Neurocytol.* 25, 367–379.

Bibel, M., and Barde, Y.-A. (2000). Neurotrophins: key regulators of cell fate and cell shape in the vertebrate nervous system. *Genes Dev.* 14, 2919–2937. doi: 10.1101/gad.841400

Buffelli, M., Busetto, G., Bidoia, C., Favero, M., and Cangiano, A. (2004). Activity-dependent synaptic competition at mammalian neuromuscular junctions. *Physiology* 19, 85–91. doi: 10.1152/nips.01464.2003

Caulfield, M. P., and Birdsall, N. J. (1998). International Union of Pharmacology. XVII. Classification of muscarinic acetylcholine receptors. *Pharmacol. Rev.* 50, 279–290.

Chang, Q., and Balice-Gordon, R. J. (1997). Nip and tuck at the neuromuscular junction: a role for proteases in developmental synapse elimination. *BioEssays* 19, 271–275. doi: 10.1002/bies.950190402

Changeux, J. P., Duclert, A., and Sekine, S. (1992). Calcitonin gene-related peptides and neuromuscular interactions. *Ann. N. Y. Acad. Sci.* 657, 361–378. doi: 10.1111/j.1749-6632.1992.tb22783.x

Chen, C., and Regehr, W. G. (2000). Developmental remodeling of the retinogeniculate synapse. *Neuron* 28, 955–966. doi: 10.1016/S0896-6273(00)00166-5

Correia-de-Sá, P., and Ribeiro, J. A. (1994). Potentiation by tonic A2a-adenosine receptor activation of CGRP-facilitated [3H]-ACh release from rat motor nerve endings. *Br. J. Pharmacol.* 111, 582–588. doi: 10.1111/j.1476-5381.1994.tb14777.x

Correia-de-Sá, P., Sebastião, A. M., and Ribeiro, J. A. (1991). Inhibitory and excitatory effects of adenosine receptor agonists on evoked transmitter release from phrenic nerve ending of the rat. *Br. J. Pharmacol.* 103, 1614–1620. doi: 10.1111/j.1476-5381.1991.tb09836.x

Cunha, R. A., and Sebastião, A. M. (1993). Adenosine and adenine nucleotides are independently released from both the nerve terminals and the muscle fibres upon electrical stimulation of the innervated skeletal muscle of the frog. *Pflugers Arch.* 424, 503–510. doi: 10.1007/BF00374914

De Lorenzo, S., Veggetti, M., Muchnik, S., and Losavio, A. (2006). Presynaptic inhibition of spontaneous acetylcholine release mediated by P2Y receptors at the mouse neuromuscular junction. *Neuroscience* 142, 71–85. doi: 10.1016/j.neuroscience.2006.05.062

Garcia, N., Priego, M., Hurtado, E., Obis, T., Santafe, M. M., Tomàs, M., et al. (2014). Adenosine A2B and A3 receptor location at the mouse neuromuscular junction. *J. Anat.* 225, 109–117. doi: 10.1111/joa.12188

Garcia, N., Priego, M., Obis, T., Santafe, M. M., Tomàs, M., Besalduch, N., et al. (2013). Adenosine A1 and A2A receptor-mediated modulation of acetylcholine release in the mice neuromuscular junction. *Eur. J. Neurosci.* 38, 2229–2241. doi: 10.1111/ejn.12220

Garcia, N., Santafé, M. M., Salon, I., Lanuza, M. A., and Tomàs, J. (2005). Expression of muscarinic acetylcholine receptors (M1-, M2-, M3- and M4-type) in the neuromuscular junction of the newborn and adult rat. *Histol. Histopathol.* 20, 733–743. doi: 10.14670/HH-20.733

Garcia, N., Santafé, M. M., Tomàs, M., Lanuza, M. A., Besalduch, N., Priego, M., et al. (2010a). The glial cell line-derived neurotrophic factor (GDNF) does not acutely change acetylcholine release in developing and adult neuromuscular junction. *Neurosci. Lett.* 480, 127–131. doi: 10.1016/j.neulet.2010.06.022

Garcia, N., Santafé, M. M., Tomàs, M., Priego, M., Obis, T., Lanuza, M. A., et al. (2012). Exogenous ciliary neurotrophic factor (CNTF) reduces synaptic depression during repetitive stimulation. *J. Peripher. Nerv. Syst.* 17, 312–323. doi: 10.1111/j.1529-8027.2012.00419.x

Garcia, N., Tomàs, M., Santafé, M. M., Besalduch, N., Lanuza, M. A., and Tomàs, J. (2010b). The interaction between tropomyosin-related kinase B receptors and presynaptic muscarinic receptors modulates transmitter release in adult rodent motor nerve terminals. *J. Neurosci.* 30, 16514–16522. doi: 10.1523/JNEUROSCI.2676-10.2010

Garcia, N., Tomàs, M., Santafe, M. M., Lanuza, M. A., Besalduch, N., and Tomàs, J. (2010c). Localization of brain-derived neurotrophic factor, neurotrophin-4, tropomyosin-related kinase b receptor, and p75NTR receptor by high-resolution immunohistochemistry on the adult mouse neuromuscular junction. *J. Peripher. Nerv. Syst.* 15, 40–49. doi: 10.1111/j.1529-8027.2010.00250.x

Garcia, N., Tomàs, M., Santafe, M. M., Lanuza, M. A., Besalduch, N., and Tomàs, J. (2011). Blocking p75NTR receptors alters polyinnervation of neuromuscular synapses during development. *J. Neurosci. Res.* 89, 1331–1341. doi: 10.1002/jnr.22620

Gaydukov, A. E., Bogacheva, P. O., and Balezina, O. P. (2016). Calcitonin gene-related peptide increases acetylcholine quantal size in neuromuscular junctions of mice. *Neurosci. Lett.* 628, 17–23. doi: 10.1016/j.neulet.2016.06.014

Ginsborg, B. L., and Hirst, G. (1971). Cyclic AMP, transmitter release and the effect of adenosine on neuromuscular transmission. *Nat. New Biol.* 232, 63–64. doi: 10.1038/newbio232063a0

Ginsborg, B. L., and Hirst, G. D. (1972). The effect of adenosine on the release of the transmitter from the phrenic nerve of the rat. *J. Physiol.* 224, 629–645. doi: 10.1113/jphysiol.1972.sp009916

Gonzalez, M., Ruggiero, F. P., Chang, Q., Shi, Y. J., Rich, M. M., Kraner, S., et al. (1999). Disruption of Trkb-mediated signaling induces disassembly of postsynaptic receptor clusters at neuromuscular junctions. *Neuron* 24, 567–583. doi: 10.1016/S0896-6273(00)81113-7

Herrera, A. A., and Zeng, Y. (2003). Activity-dependent switch from synapse formation to synapse elimination during development of neuromuscular junctions. *J. Neurocytol.* 32, 817–833. doi: 10.1023/B:NEUR.0000020626.29900.fb

Hurtado, E., Cilleros, V., Just, L., Simó, A., Nadal, L., Tomàs, M., et al. (2017a). Synaptic activity and muscle contraction increases PDK1 and PKCβI phosphorylation in the presynaptic membrane of the neuromuscular junction. *Front. Mol. Neurosci.* 10:270. doi: 10.3389/fnmol.2017.00270

Hurtado, E., Cilleros, V., Nadal, L., Simó, A., Obis, T., Garcia, N., et al. (2017b). Muscle contraction regulates BDNF/TrkB signaling to modulate synaptic function through presynaptic cPKCα and cPKCβI. *Front. Mol. Neurosci.* 10:147. doi: 10.3389/fnmol.2017.00147

Jansen, J. K., and Fladby, T. (1990). The perinatal reorganization of the innervation of skeletal muscle in mammals. *Prog. Neurobiol.* 34, 39–90. doi: 10.1016/0301-0082(90)90025-C

Kummer, T. T., Misgeld, T., and Sanes, J. R. (2006). Assembly of the postsynaptic membrane at the neuromuscular junction: paradigm lost. *Curr. Opin. Neurobiol.* 16, 74–82. doi: 10.1016/j.conb.2005.12.003

Lanuza, M. A., Besalduch, N., Garcia, N., Sabaté, M., Santafé, M. M., and Tomàs, J. (2007). Plastic-embedded semithin cross-sections as a tool for high-resolution immunofluorescence analysis of the neuromuscular junction molecules: specific cellular location of protease-activated receptor-1. *J. Neurosci. Res.* 85, 748–756. doi: 10.1002/jnr.21192

Lanuza, M. A., Garcia, N., Santafé, M., González, C. M., Alonso, I., Nelson, P. G., et al. (2002). Pre- and postsynaptic maturation of the neuromuscular junction during neonatal synapse elimination depends on protein kinase C. *J. Neurosci. Res.* 67, 607–617. doi: 10.1002/jnr.10122

Lee, F. S., and Chao, M. V. (2001). Activation of Trk neurotrophin receptors in the absence of neurotrophins. *Proc. Natl. Acad. Sci. U.S.A.* 98, 3555–3560. doi: 10.1073/pnas.061020198

Lee, F. S., Rajagopal, R., Kim, A. H., Chang, P. C., and Chao, M. V. (2002). Activation of trk neurotrophin receptor signaling by pituitary adenylate cyclase-activating polypeptides. *J. Biol. Chem.* 277, 9096–9102. doi: 10.1074/jbc.M107421200

Lee, Y. I., Thompson, W. J., and Harlow, M. L. (2017). Schwann cells participate in synapse elimination at the developing neuromuscular junction. *Curr. Opin. Neurobiol.* 47, 176–181. doi: 10.1016/j.conb.2017.10.010

Liu, Y., Fields, R. D., Festoff, B. W., and Nelson, P. G. (1994). Proteolytic action of thrombin is required for electrical activity-dependent synapse reduction. *Proc. Natl. Acad. Sci. U.S.A.* 91, 10300–10304. doi: 10.1073/pnas.91.22.10300

Loeb, J. A. (2003). Neuregulin: an activity-dependent synaptic modulator at the neuromuscular junction. *J. Neurocytol.* 32, 649–664. doi: 10.1023/B:NEUR.0000020640.84708.35

Lu, B., and Fu, W.-M. (1995). Regulation of postsynaptic responses by calcitonin gene related peptide and ATP at developing neuromuscular junctions. *Can. J. Physiol. Pharmacol.* 73, 1050–1056. doi: 10.1139/y95-149

Lück, G., Hoch, W., Hopf, C., and Blottner, D. (2000). Nitric oxide synthase (NOS-1) coclustered with agrin-induced AChR-specializations on cultured skeletal myotubes. *Mol. Cell. Neurosci.* 16, 269–281. doi: 10.1006/mcne.2000.0873

Lynge, J., and Hellsten, Y. (2000). Distribution of adenosine A_1, A_{2A} and A_{2B} receptors in human skeletal muscle. *Acta Physiol. Scand.* 169, 283–290. doi: 10.1046/j.1365-201x.2000.00742.x

Malomouzh, A. I., Nikolsky, E. E., and Vyskočil, F. (2011). Purine P2Y receptors in ATP-mediated regulation of non-quantal acetylcholine release from motor nerve endings of rat diaphragm. *Neurosci. Res.* 71, 219–225. doi: 10.1016/j.neures.2011.07.1829

Marmiroli, P., and Cavaletti, G. (2012). The glutamatergic neurotransmission in the central nervous system. *Curr. Med. Chem.* 19, 1269–1276. doi: 10.2174/092986712799462711

Minic, J., Molgó, J., Karlsson, E., and Krejci, E. (2002). Regulation of acetylcholine release by muscarinic receptors at the mouse neuromuscular junction depends on the activity of acetylcholinesterase. *Eur. J. Neurosci.* 15, 439–448. doi: 10.1046/j.0953-816x.2001.01875.x

Nadal, L., Garcia, N., Hurtado, E., Simó, A., Tomàs, M., Lanuza, M. A., et al. (2016a). Synergistic action of presynaptic muscarinic acetylcholine receptors and adenosine receptors in developmental axonal competition at the neuromuscular junction. *Dev. Neurosci.* 38, 407–419. doi: 10.1159/000458437

Nadal, L., Garcia, N., Hurtado, E., Simó, A., Tomàs, M., Lanuza, M. A., et al. (2016b). Presynaptic muscarinic acetylcholine autoreceptors (M1, M2 and M4 subtypes), adenosine receptors (A1 and A2A) and tropomyosin-related kinase B receptor (TrkB) modulate the developmental synapse elimination process at the neuromuscular junction. *Mol. Brain* 9, 1–19. doi: 10.1186/s13041-016-0248-9

Nadal, L., Garcia, N., Hurtado, E., Simó, A., Tomàs, M., Lanuza, M. A., et al. (2017). Presynaptic muscarinic acetylcholine receptors and TrkB receptor cooperate in the elimination of redundant motor nerve terminals during development). *Front. Aging Neurosci.* 9:24. doi: 10.3389/fnagi.2017.00024

Nelson, P. G., Lanuza, M. A., Jia, M., Li, M.-X., and Tomas, J. (2003). Phosphorylation reactions in activity-dependent synapse modification at the neuromuscular junction during development. *J. Neurocytol.* 32, 803–816. doi: 10.1023/B:NEUR.0000020625.70284.a6

Nguyen, Q. T., and Lichtman, J. W. (1996). Mechanism of synapse disassembly at the developing neuromuscular junction. *Curr. Opin. Neurobiol.* 6, 104–112. doi: 10.1016/S0959-4388(96)80015-8

Obis, T., Besalduch, N., Hurtado, E., Nadal, L., Santafe, M. M., Garcia, N., et al. (2015). The novel protein kinase C epsilon isoform at the adult neuromuscular synapse: location, regulation by synaptic activity-dependent muscle contraction through TrkB signaling and coupling to ACh release. *Mol. Brain* 8, 1–16. doi: 10.1186/s13041-015-0098-x

Oliveira, L., Timóteo, M. A., and Correia-de-Sá, P. (2009). Negative crosstalk between M1 and M2 muscarinic autoreceptors involves endogenous adenosine activating A1 receptors at the rat motor endplate. *Neurosci. Lett.* 459, 127–131. doi: 10.1016/j.neulet.2009.05.001

Personius, K. E., Slusher, B. S., and Udin, S. B. (2016). Neuromuscular NMDA receptors modulate developmental synapse elimination. *J. Neurosci.* 36, 8783–8789. doi: 10.1523/JNEUROSCI.1181-16.2016

Pitts, E. V., Potluri, S., Hess, D. M., and Balice-Gordon, R. J. (2006). Neurotrophin and Trk-mediated signaling in the neuromuscular system. *Int. Anesthesiol. Clin.* 44, 21–76. doi: 10.1097/00004311-200604420-00004

Pousinha, P. A., Correia, A. M., Sebastiao, A. M., and Ribeiro, J. A. (2010). Predominance of adenosine excitatory over inhibitory effects on transmission at the neuromuscular junction of infant rats. *J. Pharmacol. Exp. Ther.* 332, 153–163. doi: 10.1124/jpet.109.157255

Purves, D., and Lichtman, J. W. (1980). Elimination of synapses in the developing nervous system. *Science* 210, 153–157. doi: 10.1126/science.7414326

Ribchester, R. R., and Barry, J. A. (1994). Spatial versus consumptive competition at polyneuronally innervated neuromuscular junctions. *Exp. Physiol.* 79, 465–494. doi: 10.1113/expphysiol.1994.sp003781

Ribchester, R. R., Thomson, D., Haddow, L. J., and Ushkaryov, Y. A. (1998). Enhancement of spontaneous transmitter release at neonatal mouse neuromuscular junctions by the glial cell line-derived neurotrophic factor (GDNF). *J. Physiol.* 512, 635–641. doi: 10.1111/j.1469-7793.1998.635bd.x

Ribeiro, J. A., Cunha, R. A., Correia-de-Sá, P., and Sebastião, A. M. (1996). Purinergic regulation of acetylcholine release. *Prog. Brain Res.* 109, 231–241. doi: 10.1016/S0079-6123(08)62107-X

Ribeiro, J. A., and Walker, J. (1973). Action of adenosine triphosphate on endplate potentials recorded from muscle fibres of the rat-diaphragm and frog sartorius. *Br. J. Pharmacol.* 49, 724–725. doi: 10.1111/j.1476-5381.1973.tb08555.x

Ribeiro, J. A., and Walker, J. (1975). The effects of adenosine triphosphate and adenosine diphosphate on transmission at the rat and frog neuromuscular junctions. *Br. J. Pharmacol.* 54, 213–218. doi: 10.1111/j.1476-5381.1975.tb06931.x

Roux, P. P., and Barker, P. A. (2002). Neurotrophin signaling through the p75 neurotrophin receptor. *Prog. Neurobiol.* 67, 203–233. doi: 10.1016/S0301-0082(02)00016-3

Salgado, A. I., Cunha, R. A., and Ribeiro, J. (2000). Facilitation by P2 receptor activation of acetylcholine release from rat motor nerve terminals: interaction with presynaptic nicotinic receptors. *Brain Res.* 877, 245–250. doi: 10.1016/S0006-8993(00)02679-2

Sanes, J. R., and Lichtman, J. W. (1999). Developement of the vertebrate neuromuscular junction. *Annu. Rev. Neurosci.* 22, 389–442. doi: 10.1146/annurev.neuro.22.1.389

Santafé, M. M., Garcia, N., Lanuza, M. A., Tomàs, M., and Tomàs, J. (2009). Interaction between protein kinase C and protein kinase A can modulate transmitter release at the rat neuromuscular synapse. *J. Neurosci. Res.* 87, 683–690. doi: 10.1002/jnr.21885

Santafé, M. M., Lanuza, M. A., Garcia, N., Tomàs, M., and Tomàs, J. (2007). Coupling of presynaptic muscarinic autoreceptors to serine kinases in low and high release conditions on the rat motor nerve terminal. *Neuroscience* 148, 432–440. doi: 10.1016/j.neuroscience.2007.06.017

Santafé, M. M., Priego, M., Obis, T., Garcia, N., Tomàs, M., Lanuza, M. A., et al. (2015). Adenosine receptors and muscarinic receptors cooperate in acetylcholine release modulation in the neuromuscular synapse. *Eur. J. Neurosci.* 42, 1775–1787. doi: 10.1111/ejn.12922

Santafé, M. M., Salon, I., Garcia, N., Lanuza, M. A., Uchitel, O. D., and Tomàs, J. (2003). Modulation of ACh release by presynaptic muscarinic autoreceptors in the neuromuscular junction of the newborn and adult rat. *Eur. J. Neurosci.* 17, 119–127. doi: 10.1046/j.1460-9568.2003.02428.x

Santafé, M. M., Salon, I., Garcia, N., Lanuza, M. A., Uchitel, O. D., and Tomàs, J. (2004). Muscarinic autoreceptors related with calcium channels in the strong and weak inputs at polyinnervated developing rat neuromuscular junctions. *Neuroscience* 123, 61–73. doi: 10.1016/j.neuroscience.2003.09.012

Schmidt, N., Akaaboune, M., Gajendran, N., Martinez-Pena, Y., Valenzuela, I., Wakefield, S., et al. (2011). Neuregulin/ErbB regulate neuromuscular junction development by phosphorylation of α-dystrobrevin. *J. Cell Biol.* 195, 1171–1184. doi: 10.1083/jcb.201107083

Searl, T. J., and Silinsky, E. M. (2005). Modulation of Ca(2+)-dependent and Ca(2+)-independent miniature endplate potentials by phorbol ester and adenosine in frog. *Br. J. Pharmacol.* 145, 954–962. doi: 10.1038/sj.bjp.0706248

Shakirzyanova, A. V., Bukharaeva, E. A., Nikolsky, E. E., and Giniatullin, R. A. (2006). Negative cross-talk between presynaptic adenosine and acetylcholine receptors. *Eur. J. Neurosci.* 24, 105–115. doi: 10.1111/j.1460-9568.2006.04884.x

Silinsky, E. M. (2004). Adenosine decreases both presynaptic calcium currents and neurotransmitter release at the mouse neuromuscular junction. *J. Physiol.* 558, 389–401. doi: 10.1113/jphysiol.2004.061457

Silinsky, E. M., Solsona, C., and Hirsh, J. K. (1989). Pertussis toxin prevents the inhibitory effect of adenosine and unmasks adenosine-induced excitation of mammalian motor nerve endings. *Br. J. Pharmacol.* 97, 16–18. doi: 10.1111/j.1476-5381.1989.tb11918.x

Simeone, L., Straubinger, M., Khan, M. A., Nalleweg, N., Cheusova, T., and Hashemolhosseini, S. (2010). Identification of Erbin interlinking MuSK and ErbB2 and its impact on acetylcholine receptor aggregation at the neuromuscular junction. *J. Neurosci.* 30, 6620–6634. doi: 10.1523/JNEUROSCI.5778-09.2010

Singh, Y. N., Dryden, W. F., and Chen, H. (1986). The inhibitory effects of some adenosine analogues on transmitter release at the mammalian neuromuscular junction. *Can. J. Physiol. Pharmacol.* 64, 1446–1450. doi: 10.1139/y86-245

Slater, C. R. (1982a). Neural influence on the postnatal changes in acetylcholine receptor distribution at nerve-muscle junctions in the mouse. *Dev. Biol.* 94, 23–30. doi: 10.1016/0012-1606(82)90064-1

Slater, C. R. (1982b). Postnatal maturation of nerve-muscle junctions in hindlimb muscles of the mouse. *Dev. Biol.* 94, 11–22. doi: 10.1016/0012-1606(82)90063-X

Slutsky, I., Silman, I., Parnas, I., and Parnas, H. (2001). Presynaptic M2 muscarinic receptors are involved in controlling the kinetics of ACh release at the frog neuromuscular junction. *J. Physiol.* 536, 717–725. doi: 10.1111/j.1469-7793.2001.00717.x

Steinbach, J. H. (1981). Developmental changes in acetylcholine receptor aggregates at rat skeletal neuromuscular junctions. *Dev. Biol.* 84, 267–276. doi: 10.1016/0012-1606(81)90394-8

Thomas, U., and Sigrist, S. J. (2012). Glutamate receptors in synaptic assembly and plasticity: case studies on fly NMJs. *Adv. Exp. Med. Biol.* 970, 3–28. doi: 10.1007/978-3-7091-0932-8_1

Todd, K. J., and Robitaille, R. (2006). Purinergic modulation of synaptic signalling at the neuromuscular junction. *Pflügers Arch.* 452, 608–614. doi: 10.1007/s00424-006-0068-3

Tomàs, J., Garcia, N., Lanuza, M. A., Santafé, M. M., Tomàs, M., Nadal, L., et al. (2017). Presynaptic membrane receptors modulate ACh release, axonal competition and synapse elimination during neuromuscular junction development. *Front. Mol. Neurosci.* 10:132. doi: 10.3389/fnmol.2017.00132

Tomàs, J. M., Garcia, N., Lanuza, M. A., Nadal, L., Tomàs, M., Hurtado, E., et al. (2017). Membrane receptor-induced changes of the protein kinases A and C activity may play a leading role in promoting developmental synapse elimination at the neuromuscular junction. *Front. Mol. Neurosci.* 10:255. doi: 10.3389/fnmol.2017.00255

Tomàs, J., Santafé, M. M., Garcia, N., Lanuza, M. A., Tomàs, M., Besalduch, N., et al. (2014). Presynaptic membrane receptors in acetylcholine release modulation in the neuromuscular synapse. *J. Neurosci. Res.* 92, 543–554. doi: 10.1002/jnr.23346

Tomàs, J., Santafé, M. M., Lanuza, M. A., García, N., Besalduch, N., and Tomàs, M. (2011). Silent synapses in neuromuscular junction development. *J. Neurosci. Res.* 89, 3–12. doi: 10.1002/jnr.22494

Tsentsevitsky, A., Nurullin, L., Nikolsky, E., and Malomouzh, A. (2017). Metabotropic and ionotropic glutamate receptors mediate the modulation of acetylcholine release at the frog neuromuscular junction. *J. Neurosci. Res.* 95, 1391–1401. doi: 10.1002/jnr.23977

Tsim, K. W. K., and Barnard, E. A. (2002). The signaling pathways mediated by P2Y nucleotide receptors in the formation and maintenance of the skeletal neuromuscular junction. *Neurosignals* 11, 58–64. doi: 10.1159/000057322

Veggetti, M., Muchnik, S., and Losavio, A. (2008). Effect of purines on calcium-independent acetylcholine release at the mouse neuromuscular junction. *Neuroscience* 154, 1324–1336. doi: 10.1016/j.neuroscience.2008.04.056

Waerhaug, O., and Ottersen, O. P. (1993). Demonstration of glutamate-like immunoreactivity at rat neuromuscular junctions by quantitative electron microscopic immunocytochemistry. *Anat. Embryol.* 188, 501–513. doi: 10.1007/bf00190144

Walder, K. K., Ryan, S. B., Bzdega, T , Olszewski, R. T., Neale, J. H., and Lindgren, C. A. (2013). Immunohistological and electrophysiological evidence that *N*-acetylaspartylglutamate is a co-transmitter at the vertebrate neuromuscular junction. *Eur. J. Neurosci.* 37, 118–129. doi: 10.1111/ejn.12027

Wang, C.-Y., Yang, F., He, X.-P., Je, H.-S., Zhou, J.-Z., Eckermann, K., et al. (2002). Regulation of neuromuscular synapse development by glial cell line-derived neurotrophic factor and neurturin. *J. Biol. Chem.* 277, 10614–10625. doi: 10.1074/jbc.M106116200

Wang, J., Song, F., and Loeb, J. A. (2017). Neuregulin1 fine-tunes pre-, post-, and perisynaptic neuromuscular junction development. *Dev. Dyn.* 246, 368–380. doi: 10.1002/dvdy.24494

Wiese, S., Jablonka, S., Holtmann, B., Orel, N., Rajagopal, R., Chao, M. V., et al. (2007). Adenosine receptor A2A-R contributes to motoneuron survival by transactivating the tyrosine kinase receptor TrkB. *Proc. Natl. Acad. Sci. U.S.A.* 104, 17210–17215. doi: 10.1073/pnas.0705267104

Wright, M. C., Potluri, S., Wang, X., Dentcheva, E., Gautam, D., Tessler, A., et al. (2009). Distinct muscarinic acetylcholine receptor subtypes contribute to stability and growth, but not compensatory plasticity, of neuromuscular synapses. *J. Neurosci.* 29, 14942–14955. doi: 10.1523/JNEUROSCI.2276-09.2009

Wyatt, R. M., and Balice-Gordon, R. J. (2003). Activity-dependent elimination of neuromuscular synapses. *J. Neurocytol.* 32, 777–794. doi: 10.1023/B:NEUR.0000020623.62043.33

13

Nanobody-Based Biologics for Modulating Purinergic Signaling in Inflammation and Immunity

Stephan Menzel, Nicole Schwarz, Friedrich Haag and Friedrich Koch-Nolte*

Institute of Immunology, University Medical Center Hamburg-Eppendorf, Hamburg, Germany

***Correspondence:**
Friedrich Koch-Nolte
nolte@uke.de

Adenosine triphosphate (ATP) and nicotinamide adenine dinucleotide (NAD^+) are released as danger signals from cells during infection and sterile inflammation. In the extracellular compartment ATP is converted by CD39, CD73, and other ecto-enzymes into metabolites that modulate the activity of T cells and macrophages. While ATP mediates pro-inflammatory signals via P2X7 and other P2 receptors, adenosine triggers anti-inflammatory signaling via the adenosine 2a receptor (Adora2a) and other P1 receptors. The latter also plays a role in maintaining an immunosuppressive tumor microenvironment. NAD^+ is converted by CD38, CD203 and other ecto-enzymes to the Ca^{2+} mobilizing messengers cyclic ADP-ribose and ADP-ribose, and to adenosine. Recent findings on the roles of CD38, CD39, CD73, CD203, P2X7, and Adora2a in inflammation and immunity underscore the potential of these proteins as drug targets. However, available small molecule inhibitors often lack specificity and mediate unwanted off-target toxicity. Nanobodies – single domain antibodies derived from heavy chain antibodies that naturally occur in camelids – display a propensity to bind functional epitopes not accessible to conventional antibodies. Like conventional antibodies, nanobodies and nanobody-based biologics are highly specific and have well-understood, tunable *in vivo* pharmacodynamics with little if any toxicity. Nanobodies thus represent attractive alternatives to small molecule inhibitors for modulating purinergic signaling in inflammation and immunity. Here we review recent progress made in developing nanobodies against key targets of purinergic signaling.

Keywords: nanobody, purinergic signaling, biologics, heavy chain antibody, antibody engineering

INTRODUCTION

Purinergic signaling by extracellular ATP, NAD^+ and their metabolites is recognized as an important regulatory mechanism in inflammation and immunity (Junger, 2011; Eltzschig et al., 2012; Idzko et al., 2014; Burnstock, 2016). The intact nucleotides and their common metabolite adenosine play pro- and anti-inflammatory roles, respectively. The ecto-enzymes and receptors that mediate purinergic signaling, therefore, represent promising targets for immunomodulatory drugs (Burnstock, 2017). A number of small molecule inhibitors are available that antagonize

---

Abbreviations: ADCC, antibody-dependent cytotoxicity; ADP, adenosine diphosphate; ADPR, adenosine diphosphate ribose; AMP, adenosine monophosphate; ATP, adenosine triphosphate; BBB, blood brain barrier; CDC, complement-dependent cytotoxicity; GPCR, G-protein coupled receptor; HLE, half-life extended; Ig, immunoglobulin, IL-, interleukin; kD, kilodalton; NAD^+, nicotinamide adenine dinucleotide; NICD, NAD^+ induced cell death.

ionotropic (P2X) and metabotropic (P2Y) ATP-receptors, ATP- and NAD- hydrolyzing enzymes (CD38, CD39, CD73, CD203), and metabotropic (P1) adenosine receptors (Buque et al., 2016; Jacobson and Muller, 2016). Several of these show promising therapeutic benefit in animal models of inflammatory diseases and/or in animal tumor models (Buque et al., 2016; Burnstock, 2016). Recently, antibodies and nanobodies have emerged as a potent alternative class of therapeutics (Wesolowski et al., 2009; Krah et al., 2016; Steeland et al., 2016).

Nanobodies are single domain antibody fragments derived from heavy chain antibodies naturally occurring in dromedaries, llamas, and other camelids (**Figure 1A**) (Hamers-Casterman et al., 1993; Muyldermans, 2013). In these animals, the IgG2 and IgG3 isotypes lack light chains and the CH1 domain. Nanobodies correspond to the variable domain of these heavy chain antibodies (also designated VHH). VHHs carry mutations that render them highly soluble in the absence of a paired light chain. VHHs often have longer CDR3 loops than the VH domain of conventional antibodies. These long CDR3 loops can mediate binding to hidden epitopes on target proteins such as the catalytic cavity of an enzyme, the ligand binding site of an ion channel or of a GPCR (Lauwereys et al., 1998; De Genst et al., 2006; Wesolowski et al., 2009). Because of their small size (15 kD, 3 nm), nanobodies generally show excellent tissue penetration. On the other hand, these small proteins pass the renal filtration barrier, accounting for a much shorter serum half life than that of conventional antibodies. Their robust, soluble single domain format, renders nanobodies amenable for genetic fusion to other protein domains. It is much easier to link two or more nanobodies into bi- or multivalent formats than the corresponding VH+VL domains of conventional antibodies. Linkage to an albumin-specific nanobody, for example, provides a simple strategy to extend the *in vivo* half life (Tijink et al., 2008). Nanobodies, thus represent promising tools to target the key players of purinergic signaling, in particular hidden functional epitopes of these proteins (**Figure 1B**).

NUCLEOTIDE METABOLIZING ECTO-ENZYMES AS TARGET FOR NANOBODIES

Adenosine triphosphate (ATP) and nicotinamide adenine dinucleotide (NAD^+) are released as danger signals from cells during infection and sterile inflammation (Haag et al., 2007; Junger, 2011; Eltzschig et al., 2012; Idzko et al., 2014). In the extracellular compartment ATP is converted by CD39, CD73, CD203 and related enzymes into ADP, AMP, and adenosine, metabolites that modulate the activity of T cells and macrophages. NAD^+ is converted by CD38, CD73, and CD203 into nicotinamide and the Ca^{2+} mobilizing messengers cyclic ADP-ribose (cADPR) and ADP-ribose (ADPR), and finally to adenosine (**Figure 1C**). Extracellular NAD^+ is also a substrate for the CD296 family of toxin-related ecto-enzymes that modify cell surface proteins by ADP-ribosylation.

Nanobodies Targeting CD296/ARTC2.2

In response to NAD^+ released from cells during inflammation, the ARTC2.2 ecto-enzyme ADP-ribosylates the P2X7 ion channel (Adriouch et al., 2008; Laing et al., 2010) and other cell surface proteins. ADP-ribosylation of P2X7 at R125 covalently attaches the weak ligand ADP-ribose close to the ATP binding pocket.

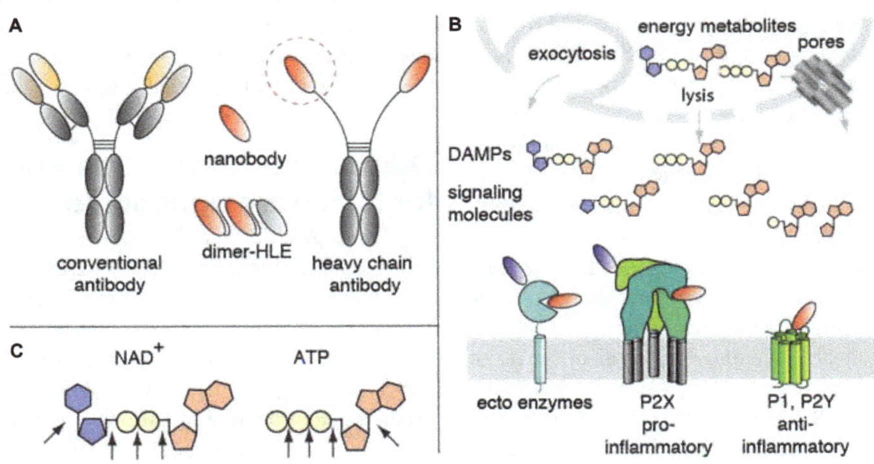

FIGURE 1 | Mediators of purinergic signaling as potential nanobody targets. **(A)** Nanobodies correspond to the variable domain of heavy chain antibodies. These single domain antibodies often contain a long CDR3 that can extend into crevices on proteins that are not accessible to conventional antibodies. Nanobodies are highly soluble and are thus easily linked into bivalent and/or bispecific formats. For example, fusion of a homodimeric nanobody to an albumin-specific nanobody yields a half-life extended dimer (Dimer-HLE). **(B)** The energy metabolites ATP and NAD^+ are released from cells during inflammation. In the extracellular space, these nucleotides function as danger associated molecular patterns (DAMPs) or signaling molecules. Immune cells express ecto-enzymes that convert pro-inflammatory ATP and NAD^+ into anti-inflammatory adenosine. Immune cells also express ionotropic ligand-gated ion channels (P2X) and metabotropic GPCRs (P1, P2Y) that respond to ATP, NAD^+ and their metabolites. These ecto-enzymes and purinergic receptors represent potential targets for immunomodulatory nanobodies. Antagonist nanobodies are illustrated schematically in red, potentiating nanobodies in blue. **(C)** Schematic diagram of NAD^+, ATP and the linkages that are targets for ecto-enzymes.

Chronic activation of P2X7 leads to cell death. This phenomenon is designated NICD (Seman et al., 2003). Regulatory T cells, NKT cells, and tissue resident memory T cells (Trm) are particularly sensitive to NICD (Hubert et al., 2010; Rissiek et al., 2014; Fernandez-Ruiz et al., 2016).

ARTC2 ecto-enzymes are not expressed by human cells because the orthologous gene in humans and other primates is inactivated by premature stop codons (Haag et al., 1994). Notwithstanding, ARTC2.2 is the first immune cell ecto-enzyme for which potent, highly specific, antagonistic nanobodies have been developed (Koch-Nolte et al., 2007). Systemic application of ARTC2.2 -blocking nanobodies in mouse models have yielded important insights that may be relevant also to nanobodies targeting other mediators of purinergic signaling. Nanobodies reach and opsonize ARTC2.2 on the surface of immune cells much faster than conventional antibodies: After intravenous or intraperitoneal injection at moderate dosage (2 mg/kg), the nanobodies completely opsonized ARTC2.2 within 10 min after injection, whereas conventional antibodies achieved this only at 2 h after injection (Koch-Nolte et al., 2007; Hubert et al., 2010; Scheuplein et al., 2010). Conversely, unbound nanobodies were rapidly eliminated via renal infiltration while conventional antibodies and nanobody-based heavy chain antibodies were shown to have a much longer half life (Bannas et al., 2014, 2015). The effective functional blockade of ARTC2.2 enzyme activity by the injected nanobodies and nanobody-based heavy chain antibodies could readily be monitored on T cells recovered from lymphatic tissues of nanobody-injected mice: both formats effectively blocked ARTC2.2-catalyzed ADP-ribosylation of cell surface proteins and ARTC2.2-mediated NICD (Koch-Nolte et al., 2007; Hubert et al., 2010; Scheuplein et al., 2010). By introducing three amino acid substitutions into the Fc domain [LSF previously shown to mediate enhanced binding of IgG to the neonatal Fc-receptor (Ghetie et al., 1997)] blockade of ARTC2.2 *in vivo* could be extended to >1 week, even after injection of only a very low dose (0.2 mg/kg) of the nanobody-based heavy chain antibody LSF mutant (Scheuplein et al., 2010). In the NOD mouse model of genetically determined type 1 diabetes, weekly injections of this ARTC2.2-blocking heavy chain antibody resulted in a significant elevation of iNKT cell numbers in lymph nodes and spleen for at least 4 weeks after injection.

During the preparation of primary lymphocytes from spleen, lymph node, blood or liver, sufficient quantities of NAD^+ are released from the mechanically stressed cells to permit ARTC2.2-catalyzed ADP-ribosylation of P2X7 and induction of NICD of Tregs, NKT, and Trm cells (Hubert et al., 2010; Rissiek et al., 2014; Fernandez-Ruiz et al., 2016). A single systemic injection of ARTC2.2-blocking nanobodies or nanobody-based heavy chain antibodies 30 min before sacrifice effectively prevents NICD of NKT cells and Tregs during cell preparation. Without such treatment ARTC2.2-expressing regulatory immune cells show poor survival during *in vitro* re-stimulation as well in adoptive transfer studies.

Nanobodies Targeting CD38

CD38, the major NAD^+-hydrolyzing ecto-enzyme, plays a decisive role in controlling the local levels of extracellular NAD^+. CD38 is expressed by various hematopoietic cells, in particular by B cells and NK cells. CD38 hydrolyzes NAD^+ to ADPR and cADPR, releasing nicotinamide. ADP-ribose is further hydrolyzed to phosphoriboside and AMP by members of the CD203 family of phosphodiesterases and eventually to adenosine by CD73. Two CD38-specific antibodies (daratumumab, isatuximab) have recently been licensed for the treatment of multiple myeloma, since these tumor cells often upregulate cell surface expression of CD38 to very high levels (van de Donk et al., 2017). The therapeutic benefit of these antibodies is thought to be mediated by their cytotoxic effects on tumor cells rather than by antagonizing the enzymatic activity of CD38. Recent evidence indicates that CD38 is also strongly upregulated by many solid tumors. It has been proposed that CD38 contributes to the immunosuppressive tumor microenvironment by hydrolyzing NAD^+ (Horenstein et al., 2015). In line with this hypothesis, blocking CD38 enzyme activity in the tumor microenvironment may be a therapeutic strategy. Isatuximab was shown to inhibit the enzymatic activity of CD38, even though its binding site is far away from the NAD^+ binding crevice, implying that this antibody acts by an allosteric mechanism (Deckert et al., 2014). Recently, 22 CD38-specific nanobodies were reported, two of which inhibited and two of which enhanced CD38 enzymatic activity (Li et al., 2016; Fumey et al., 2017). The results of epitope mapping and cocrystallization analyses indicate that these functional nanobodies, like isatuximab, act in an allosteric fashion rather than by direct binding to the active site. It is conceivable that the active site cleft of CD38 faces the plasma membrane and therefore is not easily accessible to antibodies or nanobodies. Some of the nanobodies have been shown to effectively target CD38 on human tumor cells in a mouse Xenograft model (Fumey et al., 2017) and some of these nanobodies bind independently of daratumumab and isatuximab and may, therefore, be useful for detecting cell surface CD38 in daratumumab- and isatuximab-treated patients (Oberle et al., 2017).

Other Ecto-Enzymes as Potential Targets for Inhibitory Nanobodies

Similar to ARTC2.2 and CD38, other nucleotide metabolizing ecto-enzymes including CD39, CD73, CD203, and alkaline phosphatase represent promising targets for nanobody-based antagonists and/or agonists (Yegutkin, 2008; Deaglio and Robson, 2011; Horenstein et al., 2013; al-Rashida and Iqbal, 2014) Blocking the hydrolysis of nucleotides to adenosine is predicted to promote inflammatory responses and thus may represent viable therapeutic strategies in chronic infection and oncology. Conversely, promoting the conversion of extracellular nucleotides to adenosine may be beneficial in chronic inflammation. Many of these enzymes display deep active site crevices that are difficult to block with conventional antibodies but may be accessible for nanobodies. CD73 may present an exception from this theme. The crystal structures of CD73 in closed and open conformation revealed that this enzyme undergoes a dramatic conformational rearrangement upon AMP-binding (Knapp et al., 2012). This dramatic conformational shift may facilitate antibody mediated inhibition of CD73 by non-competitive mechanisms, e.g., by sterically blocking the shift in conformation, rather than occluding the active site (Geoghegan et al., 2016).

PURINERGIC P1 AND P2 RECEPTORS AS TARGETS FOR NANOBODIES

ATP, NAD^+ and their metabolites act as ligands for ionotropic (P2X) and metabotropic (P1, P2Y) receptors, many of which are expressed by immune cells (Burnstock and Boeynaems, 2014; Di Virgilio and Vuerich, 2015). Targeting these cell surface receptors with antagonistic and/or agonistic nanobodies thus might also provide novel therapeutic approaches in inflammation and immunity.

Nanobodies Targeting P2X7

The P2X7 ion channel is expressed by monocytes and T cells and is gated upon binding of extracellular ATP, permitting influx of calcium (Ca^{2+}) and sodium (Na^+) and efflux of potassium (K^+) (Bartlett et al., 2014; Di Virgilio et al., 2017). This triggers assembly of the inflammasome, release of the pro-inflammatory cytokine IL-1 β (IL-1β), ectodomain shedding of membrane proteins and externalization of phosphatidylserine (Ferrari et al., 2006; Giuliani et al., 2017). P2X7 is a potential therapeutic target in inflammatory diseases, such as glomerulonephritis, multiple sclerosis, and chronic pain (Bartlett et al., 2014; McInnes et al., 2014).

A set of 21 nanobodies was selected by phage display from llamas immunized with cDNA expression vectors encoding mouse and human P2X7 (Danquah et al., 2016). Six of eighteen nanobody families either blocked or enhanced activation of mouse P2X7 by both ATP and NAD^+-mediated pathways and two of three nanobody families effectively blocked ATP-mediated gating of human P2X7. Dimerization via a flexible G4S linker enhanced the potencies of both, the antagonistic 13A7 nanobody and the potentiating 14D5 nanobody to low nanomolar/high picomolar IC_{50} values. Both nanobodies modulated P2X7 function when added either before or after the ligand ATP. Intriguingly, addition of the 13A7 blocked binding of the 14D5 and vice versa, indicating that these nanobodies either bind to overlapping epitopes or to alternative conformational states of P2X7. Genetic fusion of homodimeric nanobodies to the albumin-binding nanobody Alb8 markedly increased the *in vivo* half-life from hours to days. This trimeric nanobody-format was designated HLE-dimer (half-life extended αP2X7 dimer). A similar extension of the *in vivo* half life was achieved by fusing the nanobody monomers to the hinge and Fc domains of mouse or human IgG, thereby reconstituting a bivalent heavy chain antibody format. In two different mouse models systemic administration of the P2X7-antagonistic 13A7 HLE-dimer at a moderate dosage (1 mg/kg every 3 days) significantly ameliorated inflammation scores. In the model of DNTB-induced allergic contact dermatitis, 13A7 HLE-dimer reduced local inflammation as measured by ear weight and levels of the inflammatory cytokines IL-1ß and IL-6 to a similar extent as the corticosteroid Dexamethasone. Similarly, in the model of antibody-induced glomerulonephritis, the P2X7-antagonistic 13A7 HLE-dimer significantly reduced leukocyte infiltration of glomeruli and proteinuria. In a surrogate human inflammation model with endotoxin-treated blood samples, the human P2X7 antagonistic Dano1 nanobody effectively blocked ATP-induced release of IL-1β with subnanomolar IC_{50} values, i.e., at >1.000 fold higher potency than benchmark small molecule inhibitors of P2X7. Nanobody Dano1 thus is an excellent clinical candidate.

Other Purinergic Receptors as Potential Targets for Inhibitory Nanobodies

Analogous to P2X7, P2X4, and P2X1 are expressed by immune cells and could be targets for nanobody-based antagonists and/or agonists (Burnstock, 2016). The P1 and P2Y receptors are GPCRs that respond to adenosine and purine nucleotides, respectively (Jacobson and Muller, 2016) and Adora2a and P2Y11 receptors are most relevant for inflammation and immunity (Sitkovsky et al., 2014; Young et al., 2016; Kennedy, 2017). Since these GPCRs have much smaller extracellular domains than the P2X receptors, inducing specific antibodies against GPCRs is much more challenging than in case of P2XRs. Notwithstanding, potent antagonistic nanobodies have been developed from llamas immunized with cDNA expression vectors encoding two non-purinergic lymphocyte GPCRs: CXCR4 and ChemR23, receptors for chemotactic proteins (Jahnichen et al., 2010; Claes et al., 2016; Peyrassol et al., 2016). It is thus not farfetched to propose that this strategy may also yield nanobodies targeting P1 and P2Y receptors.

ADVANTAGES AND LIMITATIONS OF NANOBODY-BASED BIOLOGICS IN PURINERGIC PHARMACOLOGY

Nanobodies directed against key players of purinergic signaling are valuable tools for research and diagnosis. Fluorochrome-conjugated nanobodies, for example, are well suited for flow cytometry, microscopy, and molecular imaging applications (Fumey et al., 2017). For example, nanobody JK36 recognizes a non-overlapping epitope on CD38 and can therefore detect cell surface CD38 by flow cytometry even in patients under treatment with daratumumab – where occupancy of CD38 by daratumumab prevents binding of most commercial diagnostic mAbs (Oberle et al., 2017). Owing to their small size, fluorochrome-conjugated nanobodies often provide much higher resolution images in fluorescence microscopy than conventional antibodies (Pleiner et al., 2015). Nanobodies have also proven useful as crystallization chaperones for 3D-structure analyses of GPCRs (Steyaert and Kobilka, 2011). On the other hand, native membrane protein-specific nanobodies usually do not work well in Western-Blot analyses, since their target epitopes are often destroyed by denaturing gel electrophoresis.

Table 1 summarizes advantages and limitations of nanobodies vs. antibodies and small molecule drugs. In contrast to most small molecule drugs, antibodies and nanobodies generally are

TABLE 1 | Advantages and limitations of nanobodies and antibodies vs. small molecule drugs in purinergic pharmacology.

	Antibodies	Nanobodies	Small molecules
Size	150 kD	15 kD	~1 kD
Development costs	High	Moderate	Usually low
Administration	i.v., s.c.	i.v., s.c., aerosol, topical	oral, i.v.
Specificity	High	High	Variable
Off target adverse effects	None	None	P1, P2, kinases, ATPases, dehydrogenases
On target adverse effects	Depends on target	Depends on target	Depends on target
In Vivo half-life	Can be adjusted by Fc-engineering	Can be adjusted by PEGylation or fusion to albumin-specific Nb	Variable (usually short)
Metabolites	Non-toxic, biodegradable	Non-toxic, biodegradable	Potentially toxic
Tissue penetration	Slow	Excellent in periphery	Variable
Tissue specificity	Targetable (bi-specific Abs)	Targetable (bi- specific Nbs)	Variable
Albumin binding	Usually not	Via albumin-specific Nb to extend half life, usually no effect on potency	May reduce potency

not orally available, i.e., they need to be administered by infusion or subcutaneous injection. High costs of clinical development and production still are handicaps of antibodies and nanobodies (Brekke and Sandlie, 2003). On the other hand, antibodies and nanobodies show exquisite specificity to the target molecule and – in contrast to small molecules – show little if any off-target side effects (Steeland et al., 2016). Nanobodies and antibodies are biodegradable and – in contrast to small molecules – do not suffer from conversion to toxic metabolites. While antibodies display uniform pharmacodynamics and a longer *in vivo* or serum half life than small molecules and nanobodies, their large size (150 kD) limits their penetration into solid tumors and other tissues. With a small size (15 kD), excellent tissue penetration and rapid renal filtration of unbound molecules, nanobodies, however, are exceptionally well suited for *in vivo* molecular imaging applications (Chakravarty et al., 2014; Bannas et al., 2015; Rashidian et al., 2015; Beghein and Gettemans, 2017).

Antibodies and nanobodies both show little if any capacity to cross the BBB. This can be an advantage for the therapeutic targeting of purinergic enzymes and receptors in inflammation and oncology outside the nervous system, because this limits on-target side effects in the central nervous system. The BBB, however, presents a limitation for therapeutic targeting inflammation and oncology in the CNS. If desired, passage of antibodies through the BBB can be enhanced by genetic fusion or conjugation to binding modules for the transferrin receptor and other transcytosis receptors (Farrington et al., 2014). Because of their small size and modular nature, nanobodies may be suited better for this strategy than conventional antibodies. The Fc-domain of conventional antibodies can mediate unwanted complement dependent and/or cell-mediated cytotoxicity (CDC, ADCC). Here, lack of an Fc domain can be an advantage for nanobodies. If the deletion of tumor cells or certain immune cell subsets is desired for therapeutic purposes, nanobodies can readily be fused to the Fc domain of conventional antibodies to generate a nanobody-based heavy chain antibody (75 kD). Such heavy chain antibodies are amenable for the full power of Fc-engineering technologies, i.e., substitution of amino acid residues that enhance/reduce *in vivo* half life and/or cytotoxicity (Liu et al., 2017).

Most purine metabolizing ecto-enzymes and purinergic receptors are not restricted to immune cells. Many of these enzymes and receptors are also expressed by cells of the cardiovascular system and the CNS. It will thus be important to monitor potential on-target side effects of the nanobodies that modulate their target on cells of other tissues. Owing to their high solubility and modular format, nanobodies can easily be linked to other nanobodies (Els Conrath et al., 2001; Bannas et al., 2017). This opens the opportunity to generate bi-specific biologics with improved cellular specificity, e.g., by linking a purinergic receptor-specific nanobody to a nanobody directed against a tissue differentiation antigen.

CONCLUSION AND OUTLOOK

Nanobodies display a propensity to bind functional epitopes not accessible to conventional antibodies. Nanobodies that antagonize the purine-metabolizing ecto-enzymes ARTC2.2 and CD38 or the ATP-gated ion channel P2X7 have provided proof of concept for the notion that these small biologics represent attractive alternatives to small molecule inhibitors for modulating purinergic signaling in inflammation and immunity. It is thus not unlikely that caplacizumab, the first nanobody that is bound to reach the clinic next year, will pave the way for nanobody-based therapeutics also in the field of purinergic pharmacology.

AUTHOR CONTRIBUTIONS

FH and FK-N conceived the project. SM, NS, and FK-N wrote the manuscript. All authors reviewed and approved the manuscript.

FUNDING

This work was supported by Grant Nos. 310/11-1, SFB1192 B5, and Ha2369/5-1 to FK-N and FH.

REFERENCES

Adriouch, S., Bannas, P., Schwarz, N., Fliegert, R., Guse, A. H., Seman, M., et al. (2008). ADP-ribosylation at R125 gates the P2X7 ion channel by presenting a covalent ligand to its nucleotide binding site. *FASEB J.* 22, 861–869. doi: 10.1096/fj.07-9294com

al-Rashida, M., and Iqbal, J. (2014). Therapeutic potentials of ecto-nucleoside triphosphate diphosphohydrolase, ecto-nucleotide pyrophosphatase/phosphodiesterase, ecto-5'-nucleotidase, and alkaline phosphatase inhibitors. *Med. Res. Rev.* 34, 703–743. doi: 10.1002/med.21302

Bannas, P., Hambach, J., and Koch-Nolte, F. (2017). Nanobodies and nanobody-based human heavy chain antibodies as antitumor therapeutics. *Front. Immunol.* 8:1603. doi: 10.3389/fimmu.2017.01603

Bannas, P., Lenz, A., Kunick, V., Well, L., Fumey, W., Rissiek, B., et al. (2015). Molecular imaging of tumors with nanobodies and antibodies: timing and dosage are crucial factors for improved in vivo detection. *Contrast Media Mol. Imaging* 10, 367–378. doi: 10.1002/cmmi.1637

Bannas, P., Well, L., Lenz, A., Rissiek, B., Haag, F., Schmid, J., et al. (2014). In vivo near-infrared fluorescence targeting of T cells: comparison of nanobodies and conventional monoclonal antibodies. *Contrast Media Mol. Imaging* 9, 135–142. doi: 10.1002/cmmi.1548

Bartlett, R., Stokes, L., and Sluyter, R. (2014). The P2X7 receptor channel: recent developments and the use of P2X7 antagonists in models of disease. *Pharmacol. Rev.* 66, 638–675. doi: 10.1124/pr.113.008003

Beghein, E., and Gettemans, J. (2017). Nanobody technology: a versatile toolkit for microscopic imaging, protein-protein interaction analysis, and protein function exploration. *Front. Immunol.* 8:771. doi: 10.3389/fimmu.2017.00771

Brekke, O. H., and Sandlie, I. (2003). Therapeutic antibodies for human diseases at the dawn of the twenty-first century. *Nat. Rev. Drug Discov.* 2, 52–62. doi: 10.1038/nrd984

Buque, A., Bloy, N., Aranda, F., Cremer, I., Eggermont, A., Fridman, W. H., et al. (2016). Trial watch-small molecules targeting the immunological tumor microenvironment for cancer therapy. *Oncoimmunology* 5:e1149674. doi: 10.1080/2162402X.2016.1149674

Burnstock, G. (2016). P2X ion channel receptors and inflammation. *Purinergic Signal.* 12, 59–67. doi: 10.1007/s11302-015-9493-0

Burnstock, G. (2017). The therapeutic potential of purinergic signalling. *Biochem. Pharmacol.* doi: 10.1016/j.bcp.2017.07.016 [Epub ahead of print].

Burnstock, G., and Boeynaems, J. M. (2014). Purinergic signalling and immune cells. *Purinergic Signal.* 10, 529–564. doi: 10.1007/s11302-014-9427-2

Chakravarty, R., Goel, S., and Cai, W. (2014). Nanobody: the "magic bullet" for molecular imaging? *Theranostics* 4, 386–398. doi: 10.7150/thno.8006

Claes, K., Vandewalle, K., Laukens, B., Laeremans, T., Vosters, O., Langer, I., et al. (2016). Modular integrated secretory system engineering in pichia pastoris to enhance G-protein coupled receptor expression. *ACS Synth. Biol.* 5, 1070–1075. doi: 10.1021/acssynbio.6b00032

Danquah, W., Meyer-Schwesinger, C., Rissiek, B., Pinto, C., Serracant-Prat, A., Amadi, M., et al. (2016). Nanobodies that block gating of the P2X7 ion channel ameliorate inflammation. *Sci. Transl. Med.* 8:366ra162. doi: 10.1126/scitranslmed.aaf8463

De Genst, E., Silence, K., Decanniere, K., Conrath, K., Loris, R., Kinne, J., et al. (2006). Molecular basis for the preferential cleft recognition by dromedary heavy-chain antibodies. *Proc. Natl. Acad. Sci. U.S.A.* 103, 4586–4591. doi: 10.1073/pnas.0505379103

Deaglio, S., and Robson, S. C. (2011). Ectonucleotidases as regulators of purinergic signaling in thrombosis, inflammation, and immunity. *Adv. Pharmacol.* 61, 301–332. doi: 10.1016/B978-0-12-385526-8.00010-2

Deckert, J., Wetzel, M. C., Bartle, L. M., Skaletskaya, A., Goldmacher, V. S., Vallee, F., et al. (2014). SAR650984, a novel humanized CD38-targeting antibody, demonstrates potent antitumor activity in models of multiple myeloma and other CD38+ hematologic malignancies. *Clin. Cancer Res.* 20, 4574–4583. doi: 10.1158/1078-0432.CCR-14-0695

Di Virgilio, F., Dal Ben, D., Sarti, A. C., Giuliani, A. L., and Falzoni, S. (2017). The P2X7 receptor in infection and inflammation. *Immunity* 47, 15–31. doi: 10.1016/j.immuni.2017.06.020

Di Virgilio, F., and Vuerich, M. (2015). Purinergic signaling in the immune system. *Auton. Neurosci.* 191, 117–123. doi: 10.1016/j.autneu.2015.04.011

Els Conrath, K., Lauwereys, M., Wyns, L., and Muyldermans, S. (2001). Camel single-domain antibodies as modular building units in bispecific and bivalent antibody constructs. *J. Biol. Chem.* 276, 7346–7350. doi: 10.1074/jbc.M007734200

Eltzschig, H. K., Sitkovsky, M. V., and Robson, S. C. (2012). Purinergic signaling during inflammation. *N. Engl. J. Med.* 367, 2322–2333. doi: 10.1056/NEJMra1205750

Farrington, G. K., Caram-Salas, N., Haqqani, A. S., Brunette, E., Eldredge, J., Pepinsky, B., et al. (2014). A novel platform for engineering blood-brain barrier-crossing bispecific biologics. *FASEB J.* 28, 4764–4778. doi: 10.1096/fj.14-253369

Fernandez-Ruiz, D., Ng, W. Y., Holz, L. E., Ma, J. Z., Zaid, A., Wong, Y. C., et al. (2016). Liver-resident memory CD8(+) T cells form a front-line defense against malaria liver-stage infection. *Immunity* 45, 889–902. doi: 10.1016/j.immuni.2016.08.011

Ferrari, D., Pizzirani, C., Adinolfi, E., Lemoli, R. M., Curti, A., Idzko, M., et al. (2006). The P2X7 receptor: a key player in IL-1 processing and release. *J. Immunol.* 176, 3877–3883. doi: 10.4049/jimmunol.176.7.3877

Fumey, W., Koenigsdorf, J., Kunick, V., Menzel, S., Schutze, K., Unger, M., et al. (2017). Nanobodies effectively modulate the enzymatic activity of CD38 and allow specific imaging of CD38(+) tumors in mouse models in vivo. *Sci. Rep.* 7:14289. doi: 10.1038/s41598-017-14112-6

Geoghegan, J. C., Diedrich, G., Lu, X., Rosenthal, K., Sachsenmeier, K. F., Wu, H., et al. (2016). Inhibition of CD73 AMP hydrolysis by a therapeutic antibody with a dual, non-competitive mechanism of action. *mAbs* 8, 454–467. doi: 10.1080/19420862.2016.1143182

Ghetie, V., Popov, S., Borvak, J., Radu, C., Matesoi, D., Medesan, C., et al. (1997). Increasing the serum persistence of an IgG fragment by random mutagenesis. *Nat. Biotechnol.* 15, 637–640. doi: 10.1038/nbt0797-637

Giuliani, A. L., Sarti, A. C., Falzoni, S., and Di Virgilio, F. (2017). The P2X7 Receptor-Interleukin-1 Liaison. *Front. Pharmacol.* 8:123. doi: 10.3389/fphar.2017.00123

Haag, F., Adriouch, S., Brass, A., Jung, C., Moller, S., Scheuplein, F., et al. (2007). Extracellular NAD and ATP: partners in immune cell modulation. *Purinergic Signal.* 3, 71–81. doi: 10.1007/s11302-006-9038-7

Haag, F., Koch-Nolte, F., Kuhl, M., Lorenzen, S., and Thiele, H. G. (1994). Premature stop codons inactivate the RT6 genes of the human and chimpanzee species. *J. Mol. Biol.* 243, 537–546. doi: 10.1006/jmbi.1994.1680

Hamers-Casterman, C., Atarhouch, T., Muyldermans, S., Robinson, G., Hamers, C., Songa, E. B., et al. (1993). Naturally occurring antibodies devoid of light chains. *Nature* 363, 446–448. doi: 10.1038/363446a0

Horenstein, A. L., Chillemi, A., Quarona, V., Zito, A., Roato, I., Morandi, F., et al. (2015). NAD(+)-metabolizing ectoenzymes in remodeling tumor-host interactions: the human myeloma model. *Cells* 4, 520–537. doi: 10.3390/cells4030520

Horenstein, A. L., Chillemi, A., Zaccarello, G., Bruzzone, S., Quarona, V., Zito, A., et al. (2013). A CD38/CD203a/CD73 ectoenzymatic pathway independent of CD39 drives a novel adenosinergic loop in human T lymphocytes. *Oncoimmunology* 2:e26246. doi: 10.4161/onci.26246

Hubert, S., Rissiek, B., Klages, K., Huehn, J., Sparwasser, T., Haag, F., et al. (2010). Extracellular NAD+ shapes the Foxp3+ regulatory T cell compartment through the ART2-P2X7 pathway. *J. Exp. Med.* 207, 2561–2568. doi: 10.1084/jem.20091154

Idzko, M., Ferrari, D., and Eltzschig, H. K. (2014). Nucleotide signalling during inflammation. *Nature* 509, 310–317. doi: 10.1038/nature13085

Jacobson, K. A., and Muller, C. E. (2016). Medicinal chemistry of adenosine, P2Y and P2X receptors. *Neuropharmacology* 104, 31–49. doi: 10.1016/j.neuropharm.2015.12.001

Jahnichen, S., Blanchetot, C., Maussang, D., Gonzalez-Pajuelo, M., Chow, K. Y., Bosch, L., et al. (2010). CXCR4 nanobodies (VHH-based single variable domains) potently inhibit chemotaxis and HIV-1 replication and mobilize stem cells. *Proc. Natl. Acad. Sci. U.S.A.* 107, 20565–20570. doi: 10.1073/pnas.1012865107

Junger, W. G. (2011). Immune cell regulation by autocrine purinergic signalling. *Nat. Rev. Immunol.* 11, 201–212. doi: 10.1038/nri2938

Kennedy, C. (2017). P2Y11 receptors: properties. distribution and functions. *Adv. Exp. Med. Biol.* 1051, 107–122. doi: 10.1007/5584_2017_89

Knapp, K., Zebisch, M., Pippel, J., El-Tayeb, A., Muller, C. E., and Strater, N. (2012). Crystal structure of the human ecto-5'-nucleotidase (CD73): insights into the regulation of purinergic signaling. *Structure* 20, 2161–2173. doi: 10.1016/j.str.2012.10.001

Koch-Nolte, F., Reyelt, J., Schossow, B., Schwarz, N., Scheuplein, F., Rothenburg, S., et al. (2007). Single domain antibodies from llama effectively and specifically block T cell ecto-ADP-ribosyltransferase ART2.2 in vivo. *FASEB J.* 21, 3490–3498. doi: 10.1096/fj.07-8661com

Krah, S., Schroter, C., Zielonka, S., Empting, M., Valldorf, B., and Kolmar, H. (2016). Single-domain antibodies for biomedical applications. *Immunopharmacol. Immunotoxicol.* 38, 21–28. doi: 10.3109/08923973.2015.1102934

Laing, S., Unger, M., Koch-Nolte, F., and Haag, F. (2010). ADP-ribosylation of arginine. *Amino Acids* 41, 257–269. doi: 10.1007/s00726-010-0676-2

Lauwereys, M., Arbabi Ghahroudi, M., Desmyter, A., Kinne, J., Holzer, W., De Genst, E., et al. (1998). Potent enzyme inhibitors derived from dromedary heavy-chain antibodies. *EMBO J.* 17, 3512–3520. doi: 10.1093/emboj/17.13.3512

Li, T., Qi, S., Unger, M., Hou, Y. N., Deng, Q. W., Liu, J., et al. (2016). Immuno-targeting the multifunctional CD38 using nanobody. *Sci. Rep.* 6:27055. doi: 10.1038/srep27055

Liu, H., Saxena, A., Sidhu, S. S., and Wu, D. (2017). Fc engineering for developing therapeutic bispecific antibodies and novel scaffolds. *Front. Immunol.* 8:38. doi: 10.3389/fimmu.2017.00038

McInnes, I. B., Cruwys, S., Bowers, K., and Braddock, M. (2014). Targeting the P2X7 receptor in rheumatoid arthritis: biological rationale for P2X7 antagonism. *Clin. Exp. Rheumatol.* 32, 878–882.

Muyldermans, S. (2013). Nanobodies: natural single-domain antibodies. *Annu. Rev. Biochem.* 82, 775–797. doi: 10.1146/annurev-biochem-063011-092449

Oberle, A., Brandt, A., Alawi, M., Langebrake, C., Janjetovic, S., Wolschke, C., et al. (2017). Long-term CD38 saturation by daratumumab interferes with diagnostic myeloma cell detection. *Haematologica* 102, e368–e370. doi: 10.3324/haematol.2017.169235

Peyrassol, X., Laeremans, T., Gouwy, M., Lahura, V., Debulpaep, M., Van Damme, J., et al. (2016). Development by genetic immunization of monovalent antibodies (nanobodies) behaving as antagonists of the human ChemR23 receptor. *J. Immunol.* 196, 2893–2901. doi: 10.4049/jimmunol.1500888

Pleiner, T., Bates, M., Trakhanov, S., Lee, C. T., Schliep, J. E., Chug, H., et al. (2015). Nanobodies: site-specific labeling for super-resolution imaging, rapid epitope-mapping and native protein complex isolation. *eLife* 4:e11349. doi: 10.7554/eLife.11349

Rashidian, M., Keliher, E. J., Bilate, A. M., Duarte, J. N., Wojtkiewicz, G. R., Jacobsen, J. T., et al. (2015). Noninvasive imaging of immune responses. *Proc. Natl. Acad. Sci. U.S.A.* 112, 6146–6151. doi: 10.1073/pnas.1502609112

Rissiek, B., Danquah, W., Haag, F., and Koch-Nolte, F. (2014). Technical advance: a new cell preparation strategy that greatly improves the yield of vital and functional Tregs and NKT cells. *J. Leukoc. Biol.* 95, 543–549. doi: 10.1189/jlb.0713407

Scheuplein, F., Rissiek, B., Driver, J. P., Chen, Y. G., Koch-Nolte, F., and Serreze, D. V. (2010). A recombinant heavy chain antibody approach blocks ART2 mediated deletion of an iNKT cell population that upon activation inhibits autoimmune diabetes. *J. Autoimmun.* 34, 145–154. doi: 10.1016/j.jaut.2009.08.012

Seman, M., Adriouch, S., Scheuplein, F., Krebs, C., Freese, D., Glowacki, G., et al. (2003). NAD-induced T cell death: ADP-ribosylation of cell surface proteins by ART2 activates the cytolytic P2X7 purinoceptor. *Immunity* 19, 571–582. doi: 10.1016/S1074-7613(03)00266-8

Sitkovsky, M. V., Hatfield, S., Abbott, R., Belikoff, B., Lukashev, D., and Ohta, A. (2014). Hostile, hypoxia-A2-adenosinergic tumor biology as the next barrier to overcome for tumor immunologists. *Cancer Immunol. Res.* 2, 598–605. doi: 10.1158/2326-6066.CIR-14-0075

Steeland, S., Vandenbroucke, R. E., and Libert, C. (2016). Nanobodies as therapeutics: big opportunities for small antibodies. *Drug Discov. Today* 21, 1076–1113. doi: 10.1016/j.drudis.2016.04.003

Steyaert, J., and Kobilka, B. K. (2011). Nanobody stabilization of G protein-coupled receptor conformational states. *Curr. Opin. Struct. Biol.* 21, 567–572. doi: 10.1016/j.sbi.2011.06.011

Tijink, B. M., Laeremans, T., Budde, M., Stigter-van Walsum, M., Dreier, T., de Haard, H. J., et al. (2008). Improved tumor targeting of anti-epidermal growth factor receptor nanobodies through albumin binding: taking advantage of modular Nanobody technology. *Mol. Cancer Ther.* 7, 2288–2297. doi: 10.1158/1535-7163.MCT-07-2384

van de Donk, N., Richardson, P. G., and Malavasi, F. (2017). CD38 antibodies in multiple myeloma: back to the future. *Blood* 131, 13–29. doi: 10.1182/blood-2017-06-740944

Wesolowski, J., Alzogaray, V., Reyelt, J., Unger, M., Juarez, K., Urrutia, M., et al. (2009). Single domain antibodies: promising experimental and therapeutic tools in infection and immunity. *Med. Microbiol. Immunol.* 198, 157–174. doi: 10.1007/s00430-009-0116-7

Yegutkin, G. G. (2008). Nucleotide- and nucleoside-converting ectoenzymes: important modulators of purinergic signalling cascade. *Biochim. Biophys. Acta* 1783, 673–694. doi: 10.1016/j.bbamcr.2008.01.024

Young, A., Ngiow, S. F., Barkauskas, D. S., Sult, E., Hay, C., Blake, S. J., et al. (2016). Co-inhibition of CD73 and A2AR adenosine signaling improves anti-tumor immune responses. *Cancer Cell* 30, 391–403. doi: 10.1016/j.ccell.2016.06.025

14

Purinergic Receptors in Neurological Diseases with Motor Symptoms: Targets for Therapy

*Ágatha Oliveira-Giacomelli[1], Yahaira Naaldijk[1], Laura Sardá-Arroyo[1], Maria C. B. Gonçalves[2], Juliana Corrêa-Velloso[1], Micheli M. Pillat[1], Héllio D. N. de Souza[1] and Henning Ulrich[1]**

[1] Department of Biochemistry, Institute of Chemistry, University of São Paulo, São Paulo, Brazil, [2] Department of Neurology and Neuroscience, Medical School, Federal University of São Paulo, São Paulo, Brazil

***Correspondence:**
Henning Ulrich
henning@iq.usp.br

Since proving adenosine triphosphate (ATP) functions as a neurotransmitter in neuron/glia interactions, the purinergic system has been more intensely studied within the scope of the central nervous system. In neurological disorders with associated motor symptoms, including Parkinson's disease (PD), motor neuron diseases (MND), multiple sclerosis (MS), amyotrophic lateral sclerosis (ALS), Huntington's Disease (HD), restless leg syndrome (RLS), and ataxias, alterations in purinergic receptor expression and activity have been noted, indicating a potential role for this system in disease etiology and progression. In neurodegenerative conditions, neural cell death provokes extensive ATP release and alters calcium signaling through purinergic receptor modulation. Consequently, neuroinflammatory responses, excitotoxicity and apoptosis are directly or indirectly induced. This review analyzes currently available data, which suggests involvement of the purinergic system in neuro-associated motor dysfunctions and underlying mechanisms. Possible targets for pharmacological interventions are also discussed.

Keywords: Parkinson's disease, amyotrophic lateral sclerosis (ALS), multiple sclerosis, neurodegeneration, ataxia, Huntington's disease, restless leg syndrome, purinergic receptors

INTRODUCTION

The unexpected discovery and description of non-adrenergic and non-cholinergic inhibitory nerves working through adenosine triphosphate (ATP) and its metabolites gave rise to the introduction of the purinergic system concept in the early 70's (Burnstock et al., 1970; Burnstock, 1972). Later, purines were also described as important co-transmitters in both central (CNS) and peripheral nervous systems, as they are able to modulate and be modulated by many other neurotransmission systems and signaling pathways (Burnstock, 1997, 2009; Abbracchio et al., 2009).

After proposal of purinergic neurotransmission, the following decades were dedicated to the isolation and characterization of the two families of purinergic receptors, which are distinguished by their main agonists: P1 receptors, a family of protein G-coupled metabotropic adenosine (A_1, $_{2A}A_{2A}$, A_{2B}, A_3) receptors, and P2 receptors. P2 receptors are sub-divided into P2X(1–7) channels, activated by ATP, and G protein-coupled metabotropic P2Y(1–12) receptors, which show sensitivity to ATP, adenosine diphosphate (ADP), uridine di- and triphosphate (UDP and UTP, respectively), or UDP-glucose depending on the receptor subtype. Beyond receptors, membrane nucleotide/nucleoside transporters and channels (e.g., pannexins) as well as ectonucleotidases play important roles in purinergic signaling. These are responsible for the exchange of purines between intracellular and extracellular environments and their enzymatic extracellular conversion, respectively (Zimmermann et al., 1998; Zimmermann, 2006; Scemes et al., 2007; Abbracchio et al., 2009; Lapato and Tiwari-Woodruff, 2017).

P2X receptors are ion channels that promote a non-selective exchange of cations, mainly Ca^{2+}, Na^{+}, Mg^{2+}, and K^{+}. ATP-activation of P2X receptors is especially important for Ca^{2+}-induced intracellular signaling pathways (Surprenant and North, 2009; Puchałowicz et al., 2015). P2Y and adenosine receptors are coupled to Gq/Gi/Gs proteins, depending on the receptor subtype (Puchałowicz et al., 2015). The activation of Gq proteins triggers a signaling cascade through phospholipase C/inositol-1,4,5-triphosphate (PLC/IP3), resulting in the release of Ca^{2+} from the endoplasmic reticulum into the cytoplasm. Gs/Gi protein activation, however, will work through the stimulation/inhibition of adenylate cyclase, respectively, with subsequent up- or down-regulation of cyclic AMP (cAMP) production. Final effects of purinergic receptor-promoted signaling will depend on the cell type and other intra-/inter-cellular conditions, as i.e., in physiological embryonic and adult neurogenesis (Oliveira et al., 2016), and in various pathological scenarios, such as inflammatory (Beamer et al., 2016; Madeira et al., 2017; Przybyła et al., 2018), oncological (Allard et al., 2016; Vijayan et al., 2017; Whiteside, 2017; Kazemi et al., 2018), neurological (Burnstock et al., 2011; Stockwell et al., 2017), metabolic (Lindberg et al., 2015; Csóka et al., 2017; Parpura et al., 2017; Tozzi and Novak, 2017; Labazi et al., 2018), psychiatric (Cunha, 2008; Lindberg et al., 2015; Ortiz et al., 2015; Krügel, 2016; Cheffer et al., 2017; Oliveros et al., 2017), cognitive (Illes and Verkhratsky, 2016), and peripheral neuromuscular and/or neuromotor diseases (Robitaille, 1995; Kalmar, 2005; Burnstock et al., 2013; Jiménez et al., 2014; Bogacheva and Balezina, 2015; Puchałowicz et al., 2015; Safarzadeh et al., 2016).

In the CNS, extracellular nucleotides also participate as messengers for communication between neuronal and non-neuronal cells. As key players in neuron-glia interactions and microglial activation (Fields and Burnstock, 2006; Cunha, 2008, 2016; Färber et al., 2008; Boison et al., 2010; Lecca et al., 2012; Tsuda and Inoue, 2016; Inoue, 2017; Tsuda, 2017), both adenosine and ATP are essential modulators of neuroinflammatory responses, excitotoxicity, oxidative stress and cell death, especially via A_{2A} and P2X7 receptors activity, respectively (Cunha, 2016; Borea et al., 2017; Faas et al., 2017; Faria et al., 2017; He et al., 2017; Lu et al., 2017; Miras-Portugal et al., 2017; Vuorimaa et al., 2017). Differently from other P2X receptors, the P2X7 receptor subtype needs higher ATP concentrations for channel opening and Ca^{2+} influx and remains longer activated, recruiting pannexin pores (Volont et al., 2012; Sun et al., 2013). Through pannexin pores, large amounts of ATP are released into the extracellular environment, stimulating other purinergic receptors, and signaling cascades widely associated with pathological conditions (Bartlett et al., 2014), such as the A_{2A} receptor, which is activated by adenosine released from damaged cells or produced from ATP hydrolysis (Cunha, 2016).

Here, we explore the importance of purinergic signaling in neurological diseases with motor symptoms, including Parkinson's disease (PD), motor neuron diseases (MND), multiple sclerosis (MS), amyotrophic lateral sclerosis (ALS), Huntington's Disease (HD), restless leg syndrome (RLS), and ataxias. We discuss common mechanisms already known to be involved in these conditions (**Table 1**), revise the role of the purinergic system in demyelination processes (**Figure 1**), and discuss new insights for further neural pathologies that might have motor impairments to identify potential targets for pharmacological therapies to decelerate disease progression and improve motor activity.

MOTOR NEURON DISEASES

Motor neurons (MNs) are classified in different categories according to their soma location, electrical speed transmission, and other cellular and physiological characteristics. Regarding the location of their somas, MNs can be classified as upper or lower MNs. Lower MNs have their soma located either in the brainstem—where they control head and neck muscle contraction through cranial nerves—and in the anterior horn of the spinal cord—where their axons innervate and control skeletal muscle contraction through spinal nerves. Upper MNs have somas located in the primary motor cortex and axons that project either to the brainstem or to the spinal cord through corticobulbar and corticospinal tracts, respectively. Upper MNs axons in the brainstem interact with lower MNs, regulating their control of head and neck contraction, while upper MNs project to the spinal cord synapse with lower MNs that innervate skeletal muscles, controlling their contraction (Rezania and Roos, 2013; Verschueren, 2017).

MND are neurodegenerative conditions that affect MNs and result in motor dysfunctions without compromising sensorial neurons. MND are classified according to the damage location in relation to the spinal cord. Diseases affecting lower MNs and upper MNs are known as lower MNDs and upper MNDs, respectively. Lower MNDs include progressive muscular atrophy, spinal muscular atrophy (SMA), spinal and bulbar muscular atrophy, and monomelic amyotrophy (Hirayama disease). However, the most prevalent subtype of MND is ALS,

Abbreviations: 6-OHDA, 6-hydroxydopamine; ALS, amyotrophic lateral sclerosis; ATP, ADP, AMP, adenosine tri-, di-, monophosphate; BBG, Brilliant Blue G; BDNF, brain-derived neurotrophic factor; BzATP, 2′-3′-O-(benzoyl-benzoyl) ATP; cAMP, cyclic AMP; CNS, central nervous system; COX2, cyclooxigenase 2; EAE, encephalomyelitis; HD, Huntington Disease; Htt, huntingtin protein; IL-1β/2/6/17A/23, Interleukin 1β/2/6/17A/23; iPSC, induced pluripotent stem cells; L-DOPA, L-3,4-dihydroxyphenylalanine; LPS, lipopolysaccharide; MAPK/ERK, mitogen activated protein kinases/extracellular signal-regulated kinases signaling induction pathway; MNs, motor neurons; MND, motor neuron diseases; MPP+, 1-methyl-4-phenylpyridinium; MS, multiple sclerosis; NOX2, nicotinamide adenine dinucleotide phosphate-oxidase 2; PBMC, peripheral blood mononuclear cells; PD, Parkinson's disease; QA, quinolinic acid; ROS, Reactive oxygen species; RLS, Restless leg syndrome; SCA, Spinocerebellar ataxia; SMA, spinal muscular atrophy; SNc, substantia nigra pars compacta; SOD1 (G93A), superoxide dismutase 1 (glycin-93 to serine)-mutant mouse; TNF-α, tumor necrosis factor alpha; TrkB, tropomyosin kinase receptor b; UTP, UDP, uridine tri-, diphosphate.

TABLE 1 | Evidence of purinergic receptors involvement in neurological diseases with major motor dysfunctions.

Disease	Purinergic involvement	Model/Sample	Drug	Effects	References
ALS	P2X4 receptor positive activity modulation	MNs culture/SOD1 (G93A) mice	Preincubation with Ivermectin (10 mM); Ivermectin 12 mg per liter of water during 70 days	Neuroprotective against glutamate-induced excitotoxicity; Improves lifespan and increases ventral horn MNs numbers	Andries et al., 2007
	P2X4 receptor	SOD1 (G93A) rats	–	Strong immunoreactivity in the ventral horns	Casanovas et al., 2008
	P2X7 receptor activation	Microglial cells derived from transgenic SOD1 (G93A) mice;	BzATP (10 and 100 μM)	Increase in NCX2 activity and ROS synthesis	Apolloni et al., 2013b
			BzATP (10 μM)	Transition from microglial M2 to M1 activated phenotype, increased TNF-α production and COX2 activation	D'Ambrosi et al., 2009
		Microglia/Neuron co-culture	BzATP (10 μM)	Cell death due to ROS and NOS production	Skaper et al., 2006; D'Ambrosi et al., 2009
		Cultured rat spinal cord MNs	ATP (1–100 μM)	MNs cell death through peroxinitrite/Fas death pathway	Gandelman et al., 2013
		MNs co-cultured with SOD1G93 astrocytes	ATP (100 μM, 5 days) or BzATP (10 μM, 48 h)	Astrocytes become neurotoxic for MNs through increased oxidative stress	Gandelman et al., 2010
	P2X7 receptor deletion	$P2X7^{(-/-)}$/SOD1-G93A mice	–	Accelerates disease onset and progression, increased pro-inflammatory markers as well as astrogliosis, microgliosis, and MNs cell death	Apolloni et al., 2013a
	A_{2A} receptor antagonism	SOD1 (G93A) mice	Caffeine, 1.5 mg/day for 70 days, in drinking water	Shortened mice survival	Potenza et al., 2013
		Rat spinal cord cells culture	Chronic enprofylline treatment	Decreased MNs susceptibility to excitotoxic environment through inhibition of BDNF-promoted death pathway	Mojsilovic-Petrovic et al., 2006
	A_{2A} receptor expression or levels	SOD1 G93A mice	–	Decreased expression in spinal cord	Potenza et al., 2013
		SOD1 G93A mice and end-stage humans with ALS	–	Increased expression in spinal cord of symptomatic mice and patients	Ng et al., 2015
		ALS patient lymphocytes	–	Increased density in lymphocytes, positively related with clinical status of patients	Vincenzi et al., 2013
	A_{2A} receptor activation	SOD1 G93A mice	CGS21680, 5 mg/kg, i.p., during 4 weeks	Delays ALS onset possibly by stimulating non-truncated forms of the TrkB receptor	Yanpallewar et al., 2012
		NSC34 cells	T1–11 (30 μM)	Normalized abnormal cellular redistribution of human antigen R, found in MNs of ALS patients	Liu et al., 2015
	A_1 and A_{2A} receptors	SOD1 G93A mice presymptomatic (4–6 weeks old) symptomatic (12–14 weeks old)	N(6)-cyclopentyladenosine (50 nM); CGS 21680 (5 nM)	Impaired cross-talk between receptors in presymptomatic mice, increased A_1 receptor activation in symptomatic mice	Nascimento et al., 2015

(Continued)

TABLE 1 | Continued

Disease	Purinergic involvement	Model/Sample	Drug	Effects	References
Spinal muscular atrophy	ATP response	iPSC-derived astrocyte culture from SMA patients	ATP (10 μM)	Increased basal intracellular calcium levels accompanied by a reduced calcium response to ATP application	McGivern et al., 2013
Multiple sclerosis	P2X7 receptor expression and protein levels	Cultured PBMC from MS patients	Glatiramer acetate (50 μg/ml, 48 h) BzATP (300 μM, 30 min)	Glatiramer acetate, used to treat MS patients, reduced P2X7 receptor expression in BzATP-stimulated cells	Caragnano et al., 2012
		MS patients' spinal cords	–	Increased P2X7 receptor protein levels in microglia	Yiangou et al., 2006
		EAE rat brains	–	Increased P2X7 receptor expression related to synaptosomal fraction in the symptomatic phase and to the glial fraction in recovered rat brains	Grygorowicz et al., 2011
	P2X7 receptor polymorphisms	MS patients	–	Patients with T allele of rs17525809 polymorphism present a more prominent activity, which may contribute to MS development	Oyanguren-Desez et al., 2011
	P2X7 receptor deletion	P2X7R$^{-/-}$ EAE mice model	–	Enhanced mouse susceptibility to EAE	Chen and Brosnan, 2006
				Suppressed clinical symptoms in EAE mice	Sharp et al., 2008
	P2X7 receptor antagonism	EAE mouse model	BBG (10 mg/kg daily, delivered from pellets, during 20 days)	Antagonism improved symptoms and promoted remyelination	Matute et al., 2007
	P2Y12 receptor levels	MS patients cortical tissue	–	Reduced protein levels near demyelination areas	Amadio et al., 2010
	P2Y12 receptor deletion	P2Y12 knockout EAE mice	–	Mice developed more severe EAE related to higher release of IL-23 cytokines and imbalanced Th-cell subtype frequencies	Zhang et al., 2017
	A_{2A} receptor antagonism	MS patients	Coffee consumption exceeding 900 mL daily	Reduced MS risk in comparison to control group	Hedström et al., 2016
	A_1 receptor deletion	A1AR$^{-/-}$ EAE mice		Induced severe EAE, with more prominent demyelination, axonal injury, and microglia activation	Tsutsui et al., 2004
	A_1 receptor activation	A1AR$^{-/-}$ EAE mice	Caffeine (2 mg/kg) + adenosine amine congener (10 μg/kg), subcutaneous pump, during 25 days	Reduced EAE severity induced by A_1 receptor expression deletion	Tsutsui et al., 2004
		Cultured PBMC from MS patients	R-phenylisopropyl-adenosine (1 mM)	Inhibited IL-6 production	Mayne et al., 1999
Parkinson's disease	P2X1 receptor antagonism	H4 cells overexpressing α-synuclein	Pre-treatment with NF449 (1–5 μM) followed by 48 h treatment with ATP (3 mM, every hour)	Prevented ATP-induced α-synuclein aggregation in a dose dependent manner	Gan et al., 2015
	P2X7 receptor antagonism	6-OHDA lesioned rats	A-438079 (30 mg/kg, i.p., before lesion establishment)	Prevented depletion of dopamine in striatum without reducing dopaminergic neuron cell death	Marcellino et al., 2010

(Continued)

TABLE 1 | Continued

Disease	Purinergic involvement	Model/Sample	Drug	Effects	References
			BBG (45 mg/kg, i.p., every 48 h during 2 weeks, before lesion establishment)	Prevented loss of tyrosine-hydroxylase immunoreactivity and attenuated rotational behavior and memory deficit	Carmo et al., 2014
			BBG (50 mg/kg, i.p., daily, during 1 week, after lesion establishment)	Reverted dopaminergic neurons loss in substantia nigra and rotational behavior	Ferrazoli et al., 2017
		BV2 microglia cells	Pretreatment with BBG (1 μM)	Antagonism and/or deletion of P2X7 receptor blocked the interaction between α-synuclein and P2X7 receptors and decreased ROS production induced by α-synuclein	Jiang et al., 2015
		SH-SY5Y cells	Pretreatment with PPADS (100 μM) or AZ 11645373 (10 μM)	Prevented abnormal calcium influx induced by α-synuclein	Wilkaniec et al., 2017
	P2X7 receptor polymorphism	PBMC from PD patients	–	1513A>C (rs3751143) polymorphism increased PD risk by facilitating pore formation and cell death	Liu et al., 2013
	P2Y6 receptor antagonism	SH-SY5Y cells	Pretreatment with MRS2578 (1.0 μM)	Decreased ROS production and other inflammatory markers induced by MPP+	Qian et al., 2017
	A_{2A} receptor antagonism	6-OHDA lesioned rats	8-ethoxy-9-ethyladenine (8 mg/kg, daily, during 28 days, minipumps)	Enhanced effect of low doses of L-DOPA without increased dyskinesia	Fuzzati-Armentero et al., 2015
		MPTP treated monkeys	KW-6002 (10.0 mg/kg, orally)	Increased effect of D2 receptor agonist quinpirole, D1 receptor agonist SKF80723 and low doses of L-DOPA without increased dyskinesia	Kanda et al., 2000
		PD patients with PD gene risk variant *LRRK2* R1628P	Caffeine intake through coffee and tea consumption	Decreased PD risk in subjects with LRRK2 variant R1628P	Kumar et al., 2015
		PD patients with GRIN2A variant rs4998386-T allele	Caffeine intake through coffee consumption	Increased protective effect of GRIN2A variant rs4998386-T allele	Hamza et al., 2011; Yamada-Fowler et al., 2014
		A_{2A} receptor knockout mice, SH-SY5Y cells	SCH 58261, ZM 241385	Decreased α-synuclein aggregation, prevent neuronal death induced by extracellular α-synuclein and restrain overactivation of NMDA receptors	Ferreira et al., 2015
		Brain slices from mice treated with MPTP	Preladenant (5 μM)	Facilitated beneficial microglial responses to injury	Gyoneva et al., 2014
		Rats treated with LPS	Caffeine 10 and 20 mg/kg; KW6002 1.5 and 3 mg/kg; i.p. for 6 days	Prevented striatal dopaminergic deficit and hydroxyl radicals release	Gołembiowska et al., 2013
	A_{2A} receptor number	Mice injected with α-Syn fibrils	–	Hippocampal A_{2A} receptors number increased after injections of α-synuclein in mice	Hu et al., 2016
	A_{2A} receptor polymorphisms	PD patients	–	rs3032740 and rs5996696 polymorphisms are inversely linked to PD risk	Popat et al., 2011

(Continued)

TABLE 1 | Continued

Disease	Purinergic involvement	Model/Sample	Drug	Effects	References
Huntington's disease	P2X7 receptor antagonist	Tet/HD94 and R6/1	BBG (45.5 mg/kg, i.p., every 48 h during 28 days)	Reduce body weight loss, improve motor functions, and prevent neuronal loss	Diaz-Hernandez et al., 2009
	A_1 receptor agonist	3-NPA mouse and rat model	Pre-treatment of R-PIA (1.75 mg/kg, i.p.) 15 min prior 3-NPA application	Reduction of seizure but not prevention of neuronal loss	Zuchora and Urbañska, 2001
		3-NPA rat model	ADAC (100 μg/kg, i.p., daily for 2 days) 3 days after 3-NPA	Reduction in striatal lesion and degeneration, improvement of motor functions	Blum et al., 2002
	A_1 receptor antagonist	Intracraneal application malonate 6 μmol in Swiss-Webster mice and 3 μmol Sprague Dawley rats	Pre-treatment with CPX 1 mg/kg, i.p.	Stimulate DAergic and GABAergic neuron death	Alfinito et al., 2003
	A_{2A} receptor polymorphisms	1876 C/T		Silent mutation in A_{2A} receptor	Dhaenens et al., 2009
		1876 T/T		Accelerates HD onset by 3.5 years	
		rs2298383		Early onset of HD	Taherzadeh-Fard et al., 2010
	A_{2A} receptor antagonist	Intracranial application malonate 6 μmol in Swiss-Webster mice and 3 μmol Sprague Dawley rats	Pre-treatment with DMPX 5 mg/kg, i.p.	Provided protection to DAergic and GABAergic cells against malonate	Alfinito et al., 2003
		Human	<190 mg/day caffeine	Accelerates HD onset.	Simonin et al., 2013
		3-NPA mouse model	8-(3-chlorostyryl) caffeine (5 mg/kg and 20 mg/kg, i.p.) 2x day for 5 days prior 3-NPA application	Reduction in striatal damage	Fink et al., 2004
		R6/2 mice	SCH58261 (0.01 mg/kg, i.p.)	Reduction in striatal BDNF levels at earlier HD stage	Potenza et al., 2007
			SCH58261 (50 nM): microdialysis application in striatum)	Reduction of glutamate and adenosine level	Gianfriddo et al., 2004
			Application of SCH58261 (0.01 mg/kg, i.p.) daily for 7 days at age of 5 weeks	Reduced NMDA-induced toxicity and emotional responses	Domenici et al., 2007
		Corticostriatal slices from R6/2 mice	ZM241385 (100 nM)	Prevention of BDNF positive effect on NMDA toxicity	Martire et al., 2010
		ST14/SQ120 cells			
		Primary rat striatal culture	Pre-treatment with SCH 58261 (30 nM) prior bath application QA 900 μM	Enhanced QA-induced increase in intracellular calcium concentration	Popoli et al., 2002
		QA rat model	Pre-treatment with SCH 58261 (0.01 mg/kg, i.p.) prior to QA application	Blocked the effect of QA on striatal gliosis, EEG changes, motor activity and glutamate levels	Popoli et al., 2002
			DMPX (0.2 μg, i.p.) application 5 min after QA application	Blocked QA-induced EEG abnormalities in frontal cortex	Reggio et al., 1999

(Continued)

TABLE 1 | Continued

Disease	Purinergic involvement	Model/Sample	Drug	Effects	References
			Pre-treatment with SCH58261 (0.01 mg/kg, i.p.) 20 min before QA application	Reduction in rearing behavior and anxiety levels	Scattoni et al., 2007
			SCH58261 (0.01 and 1 mg/kg, i.p.) daily for 1 or 3 weeks	Reduction in striatal BDNF levels	Potenza et al., 2007
		Transgenic HD rat model	KW-6002 (1 and 3 mg/kg, i.p.)	No beneficial locomotor activity at 6 and 12 month age	Orrú et al., 2011
			SCH 442416 (0.3 and 1 mg/kg, i.p.)	No significant effect in reducing electromyography responses	
	A_{2A} receptor agonist	Primary rat striatal culture	Pre-treatment with CGS21680 (100 nM.) prior bath application QA 900 μM	Reduced QA-induced increase in intracellular calcium concentration	Popoli et al., 2002
		Corticostriatal slices from R6/2 mice	CGS21680 (30 nM)	Beneficial effect against NDMA-induced toxicity	Ferrante et al., 2010
		R6/2 mice	CGS21680 (5 μg/kg, i.p.) daily for 2 weeks	Delay decline in motor performance and inhibit reduction in brain weight	Chou et al., 2005
			CGS21680 (0.5 mg/kg, i.p.) daily for 3 weeks	Brain region dependent alteration in NMDA glutamate receptor subunits density	Ferrante et al., 2010
			CGS21680 (0.5 mg/kg, i.p.)	No changes in behavior compared to wild type	Martire et al., 2007
		Corticostriatal slices from R6/2 mice	CGS21680 (5 μg/kg, i.p.) daily for 2 weeks	Brain region dependent alteration in NMDA subunits	Ferrante et al., 2010
	A_{2A} receptor knockout	N171-82Q mouse model	–	Aggravate survival and motor functions and decrease in specific markers for sub-population medium spiny neurons	Mievis et al., 2011
		3-NPA mouse model	A_{2A} receptor knockout mice treated with 3-NPA	Reduction in striatal damage	Fink et al., 2004
Ataxia	A_{2A} receptor antagonism	SCA3 mice model	Caffeine (1 g/L, drinking water during 2 weeks)	Decreased synaptotoxicity and reactive gliosis	Gonçalves et al., 2013
		(TgMJD) mice	Caffeine (1 g/L, drinking water during 2 weeks)	Prevented motor symptoms and cognitive impairment	Gonçalves et al., 2013
	P2X receptors	CHO-K1 cells with mutant PKCγ	ATP (1 mM)	Increased damaging aggregation of mutant PKCγ	Seki et al., 2005
Restless leg syndrome	A_{2A} receptor	Iron deficient mice	–	Increased in striatal presynaptic neurons	Gulyani et al., 2009
	A_1 and A_{2A} receptors	Iron deficient mice	–	Decreased A_1 and D2 receptor density in animals with mild, moderate and severe deficiency; increased pre-synaptic A_{2A} receptor density in the latter	Quiroz et al., 2016

in which both upper and lower MNs are affected and where non-neuronal cells as microglia and astrocytes play a central role in its pathogenesis and progression (Rezania and Roos, 2013; Verschueren, 2017).

Amyotrophic Lateral Sclerosis

ALS is the main motor disorder in adulthood. It is characterized by a progressive loss of MNs from the motor cortex, brainstem, and spinal cord (Kiernan et al., 2011). As a result of this neuronal

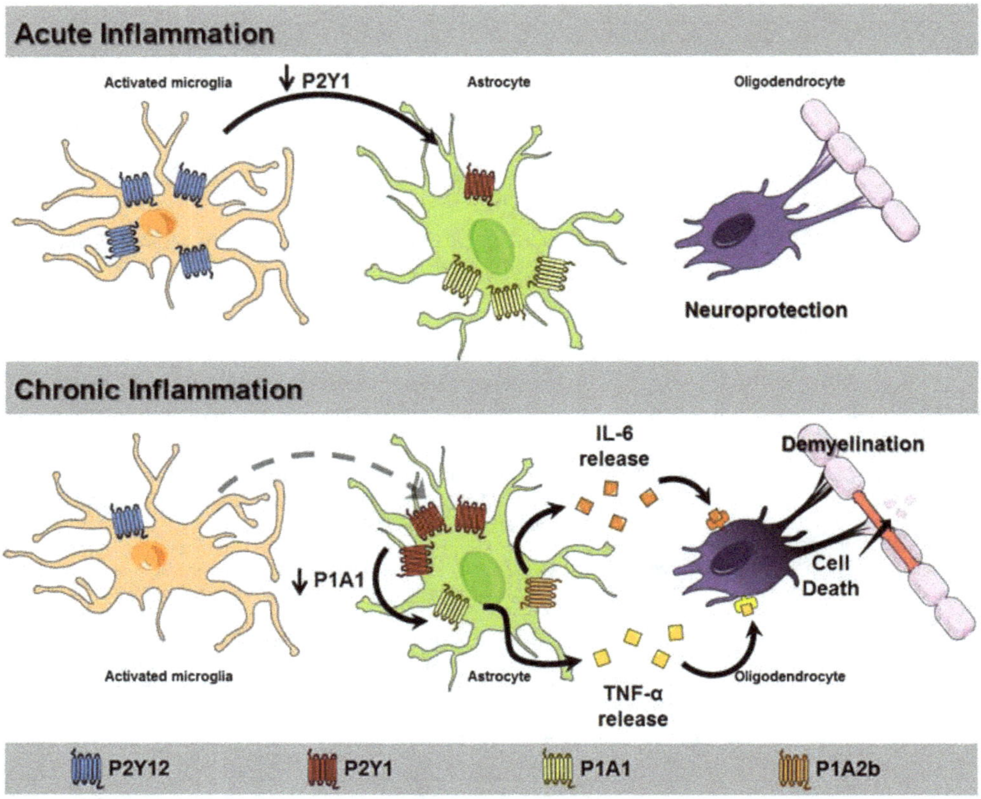

FIGURE 1 | Proposed mechanism for glial purinergic dysfunction leading to loss of myelination and cell death. In acute inflammation scenarios, microglial activation upregulates P2Y12 receptor expression and activity (blue), stimulating microglial motility to the injury site. The activation of these receptors reduces P2Y1 receptor (red) expression in astrocytes, increasing reactive astrogliosis and promoting neuroprotection. Chronic inflammation, as observed in motor neuron diseases (MND), unable of upregulating microglial P2Y12 receptor expression results in constant astrocytic P2Y1 receptor activation and reduction of A_1 receptor expression (yellow). These events result in stimulating tumor necrosis factor α (TNF-α) release, which in turn induces A_{2B} receptor activation (orange) and release of IL-6. These detrimental factors induce oligodendrocyte death and neuron demyelination, aggravating the pathological scenario.

loss, muscle weakness, spasticity, and muscle atrophy occur, inducing progressive paralysis. ALS is a very aggressive pathology that usually evolves in a fast-progressive way. Patients have a lifespan of 2–5 years after diagnosis. Death is frequently due to breathing failure. Most of ALS cases (90%) are sporadic, while a small proportion (10%) is linked to genetic mutations that usually follow an autosomal dominant transmission (Harms and Baloh, 2013; Renton et al., 2013). Cognitive impairment is also associated with ALS. In fact, 30% of ALS cases develop frontotemporal dementia (Lomen-Hoerth, 2011). The C9ORF72 mutation is responsible for the main part of ALS and frontotemporal dementia inherited cases (DeJesus-Hernandez et al., 2011).

The cause of and reasons for MNs death are still unknown. Particularly, it is still not known why this specific neuronal population is affected. However, intense research performed throughout the last two decades has uncovered several hallmarks and molecular mechanisms involved in ALS neurodegeneration. Among them, neuroinflammation, which is understood to be a maintained immune system response in the CNS, plays a central role in the pathogenesis of ALS. This response includes astrocytic and microglial activation and lymphocyte infiltration (Barbeito et al., 2010). There is strong evidence for a compromised energetic metabolism in ALS. Several genes involved in the mitochondrial electron transport chain are altered in their mRNA expression levels (Ferraiuolo et al., 2007, 2011; Lederer et al., 2007; Raman et al., 2015). Further, numerous studies reported structural and functional abnormalities in mitochondria, resulting in increased reactive oxygen species (ROS) and decreased ATP production (Jung et al., 2002; Mattiazzi et al., 2002; Menzies et al., 2002; Wiedemann et al., 2002; Browne et al., 2006), with supposed impacts on purinergic signaling. Here, we will discuss the contribution of purinergic signaling in ALS etiology.

Purinergic Involvement in ALS

P2X receptors

ATP mediates intercellular communication by acting as a messenger between neurons and glia via activation of several purinergic P2 receptors. The involvement of purinergic receptors in ALS has been documented, such as the P2X4 receptor subtype, which is implicated in neuroprotection (Andries et al., 2007) and microglial activation (Tsuda et al., 2003). Positive allosteric modulation of P2X4 receptor activity with Ivermectin and pre-incubation with low ATP concentration has shown to induce neuroprotection against glutamate-induced excitotoxicity in MNs cultures, a phenotype observed in several ALS models. Allosteric P2X4 receptor activation also improved the lifespan of superoxide dismutase 1 (SOD1) transgenic mice harboring the G92A mutation (Gly-93 to Ala)—a conventional animal model of ALS—by 10% and increased the number of ventral horn MNs in the spinal cord (Andries et al., 2007). Ventral horns are the main neurodegenerative regions affected in ALS. These findings indicate that purinergic receptors modulate excitability, exerting neuroprotection in ALS (Miles et al., 2002). However, it has been described that the allosteric P2X4 receptor activator Ivermectin acts on AMPA receptors inhibiting glutamate excitotoxicity, which could be also responsible for these observed beneficial effects.

Interestingly, the P2X4 receptor has been suggested as a novel marker for non-typical apoptotic and degenerating MNs both in the spinal cord and in other degenerated areas, which had not been previously linked to ALS. P2X4 receptor-immunoreactivity was enhanced in the ventral horns of SOD1 (G93A) transgenic rats. These P2X4 receptor-positive cells were surrounded by microglia with a neuronophagic phenotype (Casanovas et al., 2008). Moreover, Tsuda et al. proved that the P2X4 receptor is expressed selectively in activated microglia after neural injury in the spinal cord and that this expression is required for neuropathic pain (Tsuda et al., 2003). The same study showed that pharmacological inhibition of P2X4 receptors induced a reduction in neuropathic pain, indicating a direct relationship between P2X4 receptor activation and microglial reactivity (Tsuda et al., 2003). Further studies regarding the role of P2X4 receptors in activated and resting microglia are needed for elucidating the participation of the P2X4 receptor in ALS etiology and progression.

The P2X7 receptor is expressed in microglia (Ferrari et al., 1996), spinal cord neurons (Deuchars et al., 2001; Wang et al., 2004), astrocytes (Ballerini et al., 1996), and oligodendrocytes (Matute et al., 2007). Activated microglia from the dorsolateral white matter in the spinal cord of sporadic ALS patients presented increased P2X7 receptor immunoreactivity (Yiangou et al., 2006). This receptor has been tightly linked to neuroinflammation. *In vitro* studies also showed increased densities of P2X7 and P2X4 receptors, upregulation of P2Y6 receptor expression, and decreased ectonucleotidase CD39 hydrolytic activity in transgenic mice SOD1 (G93A)-derived microglia, all indicating a potentiation of the purinergic system in ALS. In fact, SOD1 (G93A) microglia treated with ATP or 2′-3′-O-(benzoyl-benzoyl) ATP (BzATP), a potent P2X7 receptor agonist, presented a prominent transition from the microglial M2 to the M1 activated phenotype, accompanied by augmented production of tumor necrosis factor alpha (TNF-α) and cycloxygenase 2 (COX2) (D'Ambrosi et al., 2009). BzATP treatment of SOD1 (G93A) microglia also increased the presence of inflammatory markers, such as nicotinamide adenine dinucleotide phosphate-oxidase 2 (NOX2) activity and ROS production, indicating damaging effects resulting from P2X7 receptor activation (Apolloni et al., 2013b). As expected, P2X7 receptor activation in microglia-neuronal co-culture induced cell death by ROS and reactive nitrogen species generation (Skaper et al., 2006; D'Ambrosi et al., 2009). Complementary to the involvement of P2X7 receptors, Parisi et al. (2013, 2016) reported an overproduction of several microRNAs in neuroinflammation. In agreement, expression rates of these microRNAs were upregulated in ALS models upon P2X7 receptor stimulation (Parisi et al., 2016).

Astrocytes, the most abundant cell type in the CNS, show low expression of P2X7 receptor under physiological conditions. However, this potential cytotoxic receptor presents upregulated expression and increased activity following injury or under pro-inflammatory conditions (Franke et al., 2004; Narcisse et al., 2005; Lovatt et al., 2007). SOD1 (G93A) mice-derived astrocytes showed increased extracellular ATP-induced signaling as well as increased ATP hydrolysis (Gandelman et al., 2010). As previously reported for microglia, P2X7 receptor activation resulted in astrocyte cytotoxicity accompanied by production of reactive oxygen and nitrogen species that are harmful to MNs (D'Ambrosi et al., 2009).

In vitro studies presented consistent data regarding P2X7 receptor function in inflammation through microglia and astrocytes, which are detrimental for MNs survival. Low doses of ATP or BzATP induced spinal MNs death through the peroxinitrite/Fas pathway (Gandelman et al., 2013). However, *in vitro* studies fail to mimic the biological interplay between neuronal and glial cell types. Activation of the Fas pathway, or "Fas-death pathway," is required for inducing death of MNs in trophic factor deprivation environment (Raoul et al., 1999; Barthélémy et al., 2004). Fas can trigger two different signaling pathways: (1) activation of Fas-associated death domain (FADD) and caspase 8, inducing mitochondrial cytochrome c release, or (2) activation of FADD-associated protein 6 (Daxx), activating Ask1 and p38, ultimately increasing production of nitric oxide and peroxynitrite through NOS1 (Estévez et al., 1998, 2000; Raoul et al., 1999, 2002). Although the latter pathway has been described in MNs, it is not restricted to this neuronal population alone.

Though studies have linked the P2X7 receptor to neuroinflammation, surprising results have been found in ALS murine models lacking P2X7 receptor. The genetic deletion of P2X7 receptor expression ($P2X7^{-/-}$) accelerated disease onset and progression, induced neuroinflammatory responses, and produced MNs depletion at end stages of the disease in comparison with $P2X7^{+/+}$/SOD1 (G93A) animals (Apolloni et al., 2013a). The heterozygous SOD1 (G93A) P2X7 receptor$^{+/-}$ animal model did not present any significant differences in body weight, disease onset or motor performance.

While the heterozygous SOD1 (G93A) P2X7 receptor$^{+/-}$ animal model did not present any significant differences in body weight, disease onset, or motor performance, the genetic deletion of P2X7 receptor expression ($P2X7^{-/-}$), instead of improving ALS disease conditions, accelerated disease onset and progression, induced neuroinflammatory responses, and produced MNs depletion at end stages of the disease in comparison with $P2X7^{+/+}$/SOD1 (G93A) animals (Apolloni et al., 2013a). These detrimental effects on P2X7 receptor-knockout SOD1 (G93A) mice shed light on possible dual effects of the P2X7 receptor in maintaining normal glial activation/trophic phenotypes at early stages of ALS and promoting a pronounced immunoinflammatory response in advanced stages of the disease. Moreover, P2X7 as well as P2X4 receptor expression levels were upregulated in neurons of asymptomatic SOD1 (G93A) mouse peripheral nervous system; however, more information about the mechanisms of action of these receptors in ALS is required (Volont et al., 2016).

The P2X7 receptor has been implicated in detrimental processes other than neuroinflammation. For instance, heat shock proteins that are elements involved in the unfolded protein response are also a neuroprotective mechanism against unfolded proteins that accumulate in the endoplasmic reticulum in response to stress, a phenotype associated with several ALS models. Specifically, the heat shock protein 90 (Hsp90) expression is upregulated in SOD1 (G93A) animal models as well as in ALS patients. However, it is not clear whether this upregulation is beneficial or prejudicial as *in vitro* studies reported that Hsp90 is able to induce MNs cell death through P2X7 receptor and FAS signaling (Franco et al., 2013). On the other hand, two chaperones, HSP90α and HSP70-1A, interact with A_{2A} purinergic receptors. By this interaction, they retain the receptor in the endoplasmic reticulum prior to exportation, ensuring its correct folding and acting as a protein quality control system (Bergmayr et al., 2013).

P2Y receptors

The metabotropic P2Y12 receptor has been proposed as a marker for ALS progression. It is co-expressed with CD11b in microglia and is also functional in oligodendrocytes. Its immunoreactivity is gradually lost in the dorsal and ventral horns of the spinal cord during ALS disease in the SOD1 (G93A) model, while CD68 immunoreactivity increases, indicating that P2Y12 receptor expression as marker for M2 microglia (Amadio et al., 2014). However, no specific function of this receptor has yet been described in association with either microglia or oligodendrocytes.

Adenosine receptors

Among the four adenosine receptors, the A_{2A} receptor subtype has been mostly described to be involved in ALS. *In vivo* and *in vitro* studies suggest a role of A_{2A} receptor associated with both improvement and attenuation of ALS progression, which could suggest a stage-dependent role of this receptor.

The A_{2A} receptor has been reported as the main target for caffeine, a non-selective adenosine antagonist (Fredholm et al., 1999; Karcz-Kubicha et al., 2003). The first investigation of the possible neuroprotective effect of caffeine intake and ALS development was performed in an epidemiological study, showing a reduced ALS risk in 377 European patients (Beghi et al., 2011). However, a longitudinal analysis based on over one million individuals from five cohort studies failed to demonstrate this association (Fondell et al., 2015). Similarly, an Italian case-control study found no association with caffeine intake (Pupillo et al., 2017). In the SOD1 (G93A) ALS mouse model, A_{2A} receptor blockade by chronic consumption of caffeine shortened survival and decreased motor performance (Potenza et al., 2013). An interesting finding of this study was the decrease in A_{2A} receptor protein levels only in the spinal cord from the SOD1 (G93A) control group and not in caffeine-treated animals. Whether this downregulation of receptor protein expression is due to the heterogeneity of analyzed cell types (MNs, astrocytes and microglia) or a true outcome of the disease must be determined. In fact, another study showed an increased expression of A_{2A}, but not A_1 receptors, in the spinal cords of symptomatic SOD1 (G93A) mice and in spinal cords of human end-stage ALS patients (Ng et al., 2015).

In the pathophysiology of ALS, one described mechanism that is associated with susceptibility of MNs to excitotoxic insults is activation of the receptor tropomyosin kinase receptor B (TrkB) by brain-derived neurotrophic factor (BDNF) (Fryer et al., 2001; Hu and Kalb, 2003). In this pro-death pathway, BDNF (Koh et al., 1995; Ishikawa et al., 2000; Kim, 2003) agonist stimulation of A_{2A} receptors leads to the damaging transactivation of TrkB (Lee and Chao, 2001; Rajagopal et al., 2004). This neurotoxic pathway is diminished by blockade of A_{2A} receptor in rat MNs *in vitro* injured by the levels of ALS-related mutated proteins, such as SOD1 (G85R) and p150glued (G59S) (Mojsilovic-Petrovic et al., 2006). A physical interaction between TrkB and A_{2A} receptor was demonstrated, in which their disruption by cholesterol depletion blocks the detrimental effect of BDNF to render MNs vulnerable to insult in a similar way observed by *in vitro* A_{2A} receptor blockade (Mojsilovic-Petrovic et al., 2006). In addition to pharmacological inhibition, partial genetic ablation of A_{2A} receptors in SOD1 (G93A) mice protected MNs from astrocyte-induced cell death and delayed disease progression in the mouse model (Ng et al., 2015).

During neuromuscular transmission, adenosine is an important modulator of acetylcholine release by acting on both inhibitory A_1 and excitatory A_{2A} receptors (Correia-de-Sá et al., 1991). In pre-symptomatic SOD1 (G93A) mice, a loss of functional cross-talk between A_1 and A_{2A} receptors was reported, suggesting adenosine signaling dysfunction prior to ALS onset (Nascimento et al., 2015). In the early asymptomatic ALS phase, activation of A_{2A} receptors by the agonist CGS21680 enhanced acetylcholine-evoked release, whereas this excitatory effect was no longer observed during the symptomatic phase (Nascimento et al., 2015). Intracellular Ca^{2+} homeostasis was also dysfunctional in MNs from SOD1 (G93A) mice (Fuchs et al., 2013). A_{2A} receptor activation increased the levels of cytosolic Ca^{2+} (Kobayashi et al., 1998; Palma et al., 2011), while the opposite effect was observed after A_{2A} receptor blockade (Li and Wong, 2000; Correia-de-Sá et al., 2002) and after A_1 receptor activation (De Lorenzo et al., 2004). The described loss of a functional equilibrium between A_1 and A_{2A} receptor actions in presymptomatic ALS mice could induce a hyperexcitable adenosinergic tonus in neuromuscular transmission, contributing to the Ca^{2+}-mediated excitotoxicity at initial stages of the disease (Nascimento et al., 2015). According to this hypothesis, A_{2A} receptors could act in an excitatory context during the pre-symptomatic phase, whereas A_{2A} receptor excitatory action disappears during the symptomatic phase (Nascimento et al., 2015). This stage-dependent effect of A_{2A} receptors could explain the different effects on modulation of this receptor in ALS models. Nevertheless, further investigation of this receptor through ALS progression is needed.

Outside the neuromuscular context, only A_{2A} receptor density was up-regulated in lymphocytes from ALS patients, while A_1, A_{2B}, and A_3 receptors densities and affinities did not change compared to age-matched healthy subjects. Surprisingly, A_{2A} receptor density was positively correlated with improved clinical and functional status according to the revised ALS Functional Rating Scale (Vincenzi et al., 2013). Furthermore, cAMP production in ALS lymphocytes was increased by pharmacological stimulation of the A_{2A} receptor by its agonist CGS21680. Within the immune system, higher levels of cAMP reduce the production of pro-inflammatory mediators and increase the production of anti-inflammatory factors (Raker et al., 2016). Therefore, in addition to its described anti-inflammatory function (Sitkovsky, 2003; Haskó, 2004), these findings indicate a possible protective role for the A_{2A} receptor, specifically in the peripheral immune system.

In MNs, aberrant RNA metabolism—due to mislocalization and/or dysfunction of RNA-binding proteins—has been implicated in ALS (Strong, 2010). Human antigen R, a RNA-binding protein that translocates from nucleus to the cytoplasm, could be associated with pathogenic pathways of ALS (Liu et al., 2015). Stimulation of A_{2A} receptors with the agonist T1-11 normalized the cellular redistribution of human antigen R in the MNs cell line NSC-34, providing potential therapeutic interventions for improving the sustainability of MNs against stress and delaying ALS progression.

Conclusion

ALS is a multifactorial disease with a marked loss of MNs and an important contribution of non-neuronal cells to its pathogenesis and progression. Several works reported the involvement of diverse elements from the purinergic system in ALS, with a critical contribution to neuroinflammation through microglia and astrocyte activation. Two elements play a crucial role in ALS pathogenesis regarding the purinergic system. P2X4 and P2X7 receptors participate in microglia reactivity and astrogliosis, which both produce detrimental effects on MNs maintenance and survival. However, their involvement in ALS progression is more complex as shown *in vivo* models. There is a specific time window, at late pre-symptomatic stages of the disease, where antagonism of the purinergic P2X7 receptor may be beneficial. However, P2X7 receptor inhibition after this point produces negative effects on cell survival. During the early phase of ALS, the A_{2A} receptor mediates excitotoxicity effects on neuromuscular junction, whereas this effect is no longer observed with the progression of the disease, at the symptomatic phase. These observations indicate a possible change of function of this receptor depending on disease state. In terms of the variety of extracellular nucleotide-degrading enzymes and purinergic receptors, which assemble as homo- or heterocomplexes and vary in composition in different CNS cell types, more intense research has to be performed to clarify short- and long-term implications of purinergic signaling in ALS.

Other Motor Neuron Diseases

Spinal Muscular Atrophy (SMA) is a MND that affects MNs in the spinal cord and brainstem. Patients share manifestations similar to ALS, such as weakness, muscle atrophy/paralysis, and respiratory impairment that can lead to death (Crawford and Pardo, 1996; Lefebvre et al., 1997). The most frequent type of SMA is caused by deletions in the survival motor neuron 1 (SMN1) gene, which is involved in biosynthesis of RNA and proteins (Burghes et al., 1994; Lefebvre et al., 1995; Jablonka et al., 2000; Gabanella et al., 2007; Bebee et al., 2010; Lotti et al., 2012). High SMN1 expression in neurons and glia in a SMA transgenic mice model rescued MNs survival, indicating a non-autonomous cellular contribution in SMA (Gavrilina et al., 2008).

Currently, the only study shedding light on the involvement of the purinergic system in SMA used human induced pluripotent stem cell (iPSC)-derived astrocytes (McGivern et al., 2013). Authors reported that this population presented increased basal cytosolic Ca^{2+} concentrations and reduced responses to ATP application, suggesting a possible impairment of the purinergic system in the disease. For instance, P2Y2 receptor activation triggered intracellular Ca^{2+} mobilization in control cells, which was not observed in iPSC-derived astrocytes (Zhu and Kimelberg, 2001; Verkhratsky et al., 2012). The cause for this dysfunction, either because of altered kinetics or compromise of downstream signaling elements, still needs to be clarified. Further, this work was restricted to P2Y2 receptors, while other purinergic receptor subtypes may be involved in the same pathology. The role of the purinergic system in SMA disease should also be studied in microglia and neurons for postulating mechanisms of purinergic signaling in this MNs disorder.

Although no direct experimental evidence links the purinergic system to other previously mentioned MND, the participation of P2 and A_{2A} receptors in the physiology of peripheral nervous system is well-established. Schwann cells—peripheral glial cells responsible for myelin maintenance and injury—destroy their own myelin after peripheral nerve injury and remove myelin and cell debris (Band et al., 1986). Since demyelination is a secondary process present in MND pathophysiology, Schwann cell activity may contribute to disease progression. In fact, injured sciatic nerve induces Schwann cell proliferation via ATP activation of P2X7 receptor while A_{2A} receptors activation inhibits it, both through MAPK/ERK pathways (Stevens and Fields, 2000; Song et al., 2015).

Schwann cells located near the amphibian neuromuscular junction are activated by synaptic ATP release (Robitaille, 1998), and purinergic signaling has key roles in presynaptic modulation (Todd and Robitaille, 2006). However, as suggested by the use of suramin (a non-selective P2 receptor antagonist), activation of Schwann cells by local applications of ATP did not depend on P2 receptors, indicating a possible involvement of A_1 receptor activation by ATP metabolites (Rochon et al., 2001). An *in vitro* model of neuromuscular junction injury showed that ATP was an activating signal for Schwann cells in response to nerve function impairment, triggering purinergic signaling (Rodella et al., 2017). Xu et al. (2013) brought evidence for the involvement of purinergic signaling pathway in glia-derived neurotrophic factor (GDNF) release by Schwann cells in nerve injure. ALS patients presented increased GDNF levels in the cerebrospinal fluid in comparison to control groups as a protective response to nerve injury (Grundström et al., 2000). Moreover, ATP and ADP released by injured nerves activated purinergic receptors that stimulate protein kinase-C and -D pathways (Xu et al., 2013). Furthermore, purinergic receptors promoted myelination processes in oligodendrocytes and inhibited them in Schwann cells. The importance of the purinergic system involvement in demyelination process in MND is clear, but a better understanding of the degenerative process is necessary for developing therapies (Xu et al., 2013).

MULTIPLE SCLEROSIS

MS is an autoimmune disease of the CNS. It is estimated to affect ~2.5 million people worldwide and is highly incapacitating; 50% of patients will need to use a wheelchair in the years following disease onset between 25 and 45 years of age. The symptomatology of MS is heterogeneous and includes motor impairment, cognitive, visual, and sensory deficits, fatigue, and pain (Compston and Coles, 2008). The etiology of MS is unknown. However, it is speculated that environmental and genetic factors play a role in disease development (Dendrou et al., 2015).

The pathophysiology of MS is characterized by chronic inflammation, in which T cells become responsive for different myelin epitopes, triggering a cascade of events resulting in axonal demyelination and neuronal transmission impairment (Sun et al., 1991; Koehler et al., 2002). The hallmarks of MS are axonal loss, astrogliosis/microgliosis, oligodendrocytes damage, inflammatory focal lesions and T-cell activation (Goldenberg, 2012; Luo et al., 2017). There is a range of immune modulatory drugs used to alleviate MS symptoms. However, these drugs induce troubling side effects including development of other autoimmune disorders and fatal opportunistic infections (Dendrou et al., 2015). Thus, better understanding of the disease in order to develop more effective and safe treatments is needed.

Purinergic Involvement in MS

The first report of the involvement of purinergic signaling in MS came from Mayne et al. (1999), when it was found increased plasma and serum TNF-α levels in MS patients correlated with low levels of adenosine. The induced experimental autoimmune encephalomyelitis (EAE) mouse model, established by myelin oligodendrocyte glycoprotein or myelin basic protein peptide inoculation and immunization, provides some clues on the mechanical role of purinergic signaling in early-stage MS. The EAE model shows similar features as seen in the CNS of MS patients, such as infiltrating T-cells and presence of IgG antibodies as well as hind limb paralysis (Lassmann, 1983; Miller and Karpus, 1994; Eng et al., 1996; Constantinescu et al., 2011). The four purinergic receptors especially known to be involved in MS are P2X7, P2Y12, A_1, and A_{2A} receptors.

P2X receptors

The participation of P2X receptors in MS has been proposed, since they modulate astrocytes and axon-oligodendrocyte communication, which is necessary for myelination formation and repair (Butt, 2006). *Post-mortem* tissue from MS patients exhibited increased P2X7 receptor expression in microglia from spinal cord and brain white matter (Yiangou et al., 2006) in astrocytes localized in active brain lesions (Narcisse et al., 2005) and in oligodendrocytes from optic nerve samples (Matute et al., 2007). Immunohistochemistry analysis of brain sections from the frontal cortex of MS patients showed immunostaining for P2X1, P2X2, P2X3, P2X4, and P2X7 receptors, while P2X6 receptor subunits could not be detected (Amadio et al., 2010). Analysis of blood monocytes from MS patients did not show any differences in P2X7 receptor expression in comparison to healthy controls (Caragnano et al., 2012). However, monocytes from MS patients undergoing treatment with glatiramer acetate—which acts displacing myelin basic protein from the binding site on MHC-II molecules, preventing the activation of myelin-specific T cells—exhibit reduced P2X7 receptor and interleukin (IL)-1β expression, indicating that this treatment may act by decreasing P2X7 receptor pro-inflammatory effects (Caragnano et al., 2012).

Alterations in the P2X7 receptor gene have been identified in MS, leading to gain-of-function of this protein (Oyanguren-Desez et al., 2011). A polymorphism in P2X7 receptor T-allele, resulting in an Ala-76 to Val transition (A76V), induced an increase in Ca^{2+} permeability, ethidium bromide uptake, and electrophysiological responses. Also, P2X7 receptor A-allele substitution of His-155 to Tyr-382, increased Ca^{2+} influx (Oyanguren-Desez et al., 2011). Similar findings in P2X7 receptor gain-of-function due to His-155 to Tyr substitution (H155T) was previously described for leukemic lymphocytes (Cabrini et al., 2005) and suggested to be essential for ATP-dependent P2X7 receptor activation, since the residue 155 is important for P2X7 receptor protein folding (Bradley et al., 2011). On the other hand, a genetic study demonstrated that the presence of P2X7 receptor loss-of-function due to an Arg-307 to Gln (N307Q) polymorphism provided a two-fold protective effect against MS outcome (Gu et al., 2015). Thus, human P2X7 receptor variants are associated with a reduced or increased risk of MS development (Oyanguren-Desez et al., 2011; Gu et al., 2015).

In vivo studies with the EAE mouse model demonstrated that absence of P2X7 receptors resulted in a severe disease phenotype. In addition, microglia and invading brain macrophages were positive for P2X7 receptor immunostaining (Witting et al., 2006). P2X7 receptor knockout mice ($P2X7^{-/-}$), where EAE was experimentally induced, showed lower number of apoptotic lymphocytes in the CNS and increased expression of interferon γ in the spinal cord, with no alterations in TNF-α and IL-2 protein levels (Chen and Brosnan, 2006). Furthermore, P2X7 $receptor^{-/-}$ EAE mice have lower production of endocannabinoids and reduced axonal damage in comparison to wild type animals (Witting et al., 2006). The administration of a P2X7 receptor antagonist during the chronic phase of EAE in mice attenuated symptoms and tissue damage, including remyelination, by improving axonal conductivity and neurological latency (Matute et al., 2007). These results suggest that the P2X7 receptor plays a detrimental role in the development and chronic phase of MS.

A study by Sharp et al. (2008) demonstrated that the absence of P2X7 receptor results in lower frequency of EAE development, including reduced astrocyte activation with no changes in microglia, antigen responsive T-cell population, or cytokine production by splenic-T cells. These results differ from previous available data on P2X7 receptor $^{-/-}$ and EAE mice. In the former two studies, deletion of exon 5 in P2X7 receptor was used to derive the knockout mice (Chen and Brosnan, 2006; Witting et al., 2006), while in Sharp et al. (2008) exon 1 was deleted, resulting in macrophages inability to produce IL-1β. Based on these data, regulation of P2X7 receptor activation status can provide beneficial advantages for MS.

Activation of P2X7 receptors in astrocytes induces the release of purines (Ballerini et al., 1996) and limits glutamate removal from the extracellular compartment (Lo et al., 2008), eventually culminating in neuronal/oligodendrocyte excitotoxicity (Pitt et al., 2000; Matute, 2011). Upon stimulation with IL-1β, astrocytes showed P2X7 receptor expression upregulation, indicating that the P2X7 receptor expression depends on the presence of pro-inflammatory cytokines (Narcisse et al., 2005). Furthermore, a hyperactivation of P2X7 receptors in oligodendrocytes causes excitotoxicity by cytosolic Ca^{2+} overload and consequent tissue damage (Matute et al., 2007).

Yiangou et al. (2006) proposed a mechanism for the involvement of P2X7 receptor in MS: increased extracellular ATP levels caused by cell death activate P2X7 receptors in microglia and macrophages, consequently stimulate IL-1β production and release. IL-1β will induce COX2, an enzyme known to be detrimental during inflammation (Minghetti, 2004). This induction will intensify cell death and production of pro-inflammatory cytokines. In addition, in the EAE rat model, protein levels of P2X7 receptor were analyzed at symptomatic manifestation and after recovery (Grygorowicz et al., 2011). During symptom onset, P2X7 receptor was found to be overproduced in synaptosomes and in glial cells homogenates. The elevated protein level of P2X7 receptor was stable at the recovery phase mainly in the glial fraction, suggesting sustained astrogliosis. The use of P2X7 receptor antagonists, such as periodate-oxidized ATP and Brilliant Blue G (BBG), for the treatment of the neurodegenerative phase of MS has been patented (EP1655032 B1), providing novel tools for clinical and research purposes.

P2Y receptors

During inflammatory responses, P2Y receptors are up regulated in microglia to promote phagocytosis and migration, preventing oxidative stress followed by apoptosis and controlling the expression of pro-inflammatory cytokines (Förster and Reiser, 2015). In MS, the P2Y12 receptor was found in oligodendrocytes from *post-mortem* brain samples and its expression was decreased in areas corresponding to demyelination in gray and subcortical white matter (Amadio et al., 2010). Immunohistochemistry studies revealed expression of P2Y12, P2Y11, and P2Y14 receptors in the frontal cortex of MS patients (Amadio et al., 2010). However, the functions of P2Y11 and P2Y14 receptors are not known. Therefore, we will further focus on the P2Y12 receptor.

Microglia, macrophages and neuronal cells did not show any expression of P2Y12 receptors, while receptor-positive staining was found to be co-localized with myelin-binding proteins and astrocytes. In the white matter of MS patients, microglia expressing the major histocompatibility complex class II, revealed immunostaining for P2Y12 receptors, indicating that microglia possibly phagocytized myelin-bearing P2Y12 receptors (Amadio et al., 2010). Presence of P2Y12 receptors in astrocytes and oligodendrocytes suggests that signaling of this receptor is involved in remyelination.

To determine the effect of P2Y12 receptor in MS, knockout models of this receptor resulted in an enhanced EAE phenotype in mice (Zhang et al., 2017). The EAE pathology was characterized by an increase in IL-17A cytokine levels in serum, higher number of T-helper cell subset (Th17) in spleen and CNS, as well as the presence of granulocyte-macrophage colony-stimulating factor (Zhang et al., 2017). Bone marrow-derived dendritic cells from P2Y12$^{-/-}$ mice challenged to model EAE have increased release of IL-23, which is an essential factor to promote differentiation of CD4+ T cells toward the Th17 cell subtype (Zhang et al., 2017). The authors concluded that P2Y12 receptors are important for balancing Th-cell populations, and receptor function dysregulation leads to altered cytokine profiles, contributing to EAE.

Adenosine receptors

Analysis of peripheral blood mononuclear cells (PBMC) from MS patients showed that A_1 receptor protein level was significantly reduced (Mayne et al., 1999; Johnston et al., 2001), but gene expression was unaltered (Mayne et al., 1999). In healthy controls, activation of A_1 receptors in PBMCs resulted in inhibition of TNF-α while in MS patients IL-6 was inhibited and had no effect on TNF-α protein level (Mayne et al., 1999). It has been previously demonstrated that constant presence of high TNF-α levels can induce demyelination in a similar way as observed in MS patients, indicating that dysregulation of TNF-α by A_1 receptors can be an initiating factor for MS pathology (Probert et al., 1995).

Histological analyses of *post-mortem* brain tissues showed lower expression of A_1 receptor in the glial population, specifically the A_1-β receptor spliced variant (Johnston et al., 2001). Induction of the EAE model in $A_1^{-/-}$ mice caused a severe progressive-relapsing form of MS with myelin and axonal loss (Tsutsui et al., 2004). Macrophages produced IL-1β and metalloproteinase 12, as well as soluble factors that damaged oligodendrocytes. Analysis of spinal cord of $A_1^{-/-}$ EAE mice showed increased release of pro-inflammatory cytokines. In contrast, $A_1^{+/+}$ EAE mice had diminished A_1 receptor expression in microglia, corresponding to inflammation. Chronic caffeine administration upregulated A_1 receptor expression in microglia, and when treated concomitantly with A_1 receptor agonist alleviated EAE pathology in the $A_1^{+/+}$ EAE mice model (Tsutsui et al., 2004). Furthermore, coffee consumption and MS risk were recently investigated. In individuals, who reported high coffee consumption and in animal models of MS, caffeine decreased the risk of developing neuroinflammation and had neuroprotective and anti-inflammatory properties (Hedström et al., 2016; Olsson et al., 2017).

Current therapeutic recommendations in MS include interferon-β and *glatiramer* (Wiendl et al., 2008). Worthwhile of mentioning, interferon-β treatment increases expression of CD73, responsible for the conversion of AMP into adenosine, in endothelial cells (Airas et al., 2007). Similarly, in an induced-demyelinated rat model, interferon-β treatment also enhanced CD73 activity in synaptosomes from cerebral cortex (Spanevello et al., 2006). CD73 activity is also required for lymphocyte infiltration into the CNS during EAE development (Mills et al., 2008). Thus, interference with levels of purines could be an additional factor, by which interferon-β benefits MS patients.

While the A_1 receptor subtype is an unequivocal negative modulator of MS and EAE (Tsutsui et al., 2004), the A_{2A} receptor subtype presents a complex role in this disease. Interestingly, A_{2A} receptor expression is increased in the brain of patients with secondary progressive MS, evidenced by positron emission tomography (PET) imaging of radioligand binding to the A_{2A} receptor (Rissanen et al., 2013). This receptor is both highly expressed by lymphocytes and the main mediator of anti-inflammatory effects of adenosine (Blackburn et al., 2009). In the EAE model, A_{2A} receptor-selective antagonist SCH58261 treatment protected mice from EAE induction and CNS lymphocyte infiltration (Mills et al., 2008, 2012). On the other hand, A_{2A} receptor-deficient ($A_{2A}^{-/-}$) mice developed a more severe paralysis after EAE induction, characterized by increased numbers of lymphocytes and activated macrophages/microglia in the CNS (Mills et al., 2012), severe demyelinated phenotype, axonal injury in spinal cord and cerebral cortex and pro-inflammatory cytokine profile in the CNS, blood, and spleen (Yao et al., 2012). Mechanisms of these opposite effects following genetic (knockout animal) or pharmacological (antagonists) blockade of A_{2A} receptors were revealed by assays with bone marrow chimeric mice (subjected to radiation and replacement of immune cells by bone marrow from donor animals) (Mills et al., 2012). This model also reveals the contribution of A_{2A} receptor signaling in immune and non-immune cells during EAE. In fact, $A_{2A}^{-/-}$ donor hematopoietic cells induced severe EAE, whereas the absence of A_{2A} receptor in non-immune cells protected mice from disease development. Taken together, these data demonstrate that expression of A_{2A} receptors in lymphocytes is crucial for limiting the severity of inflammation, while the A_{2A} receptor on nonimmune cells is necessary for disease development. Moreover, without A_{2A} receptor expression by blood brain barrier cells (and other non-immune cells), immune cells fail to infiltrate the CNS, protecting mice from disease development (Mills et al., 2012), similarly to the effects of pharmacological blockade of A_{2A} receptors (Mills et al., 2008, 2012).

A_3 receptor signaling is associated with degranulation of mast cells. Activation of A_3 receptor inhibits adenylate cyclase, stimulates phospholipase C and B, and induces calcium release from intracellular stores. It has been suggested that A_3 receptors may also inhibit binding of neutrophils to endothelial cells. A_3 receptor is expressed in whole brain (Safarzadeh et al., 2016). Though it is still unclear whether the A_3 receptor is involved in MS, this receptor has been demonstrated to mediate the inhibition of TNF-α production by adenosine (Lee et al., 2006; Levy et al., 2006). Therefore, this receptor may play important roles in the pathophysiology of MS and, such as for the A_{2A} receptor, A_3 receptor inhibition may be a potential therapeutic approach.

A_{2B} receptor signaling also modulates the pathogenesis of EAE phenotype. This receptor is upregulated in peripheral leukocytes of MS patients and in the mouse model. Activity inhibition of A_{2B} receptor with the selective antagonist CVT-6883 or its genetic deletion attenuated adenosine-mediated IL-6 production, infiltration of peripheral leukocytes and clinical symptoms in the EAE model (Wei et al., 2013). The presented studies suggest that adenosinergic activation of A_1 receptor regulating inflammatory cytokine TNF-α and IL-6 production is altered in MS, probably due to alterations at transcriptional levels of A_1 receptor and/or to adenosine availability (Mayne et al., 1999; Johnston et al., 2001).

Conclusion

Since current therapeutic recommendations for MS have partial efficacy on clinical outcomes and disease progression, the search for new therapeutic tools is necessary. In this context, *post-mortem* analysis of brain tissue from both MS patients and EAE mouse/rat models elicited potential therapeutic targets through: (1) blockade of P2X7 receptor and stimulation of A_1 receptor, inhibiting inflammation; (2) P2Y12 receptor stimulation, favoring remyelination; and (3) blockade of A_{2B} receptors and CD73, inhibiting the infiltration of leukocytes into the CNS.

PARKINSON'S DISEASE

Parkinson's Disease (PD) is the second most common neurodegenerative disease. Its incidence increases with age reaching over 4% of the population over 80 years old (de Lau and Breteler, 2006). PD is considered a motor disease as a reflex of its clinical symptoms, as resting tremors of extremities, muscular rigidity, postural imbalance, and bradykinesia (Braak et al., 2013). The pathology of PD is characterized by progressive loss of dopaminergic neurons in the *substantia nigra pars compacta* (SNc) and their projections to the striatum, structures associated to voluntary motor movements' control. Besides dopaminergic neuronal degeneration, the presence of protein aggregates (known as Lewy bodies) due to misfolding of α-synuclein occurs in the SNc, *locus ceruleus*, amygdala, and the CA2 area of the hippocampus (Jellinger, 2011). The mechanisms underlying these events have yet to be clarified, although a genetic predisposition associated with insults as traumatic brain injury and ischemia seems to induce α-synuclein aggregation (Shahaduzzaman et al., 2013; Kim and Vemuganti, 2017). The majority of genes linked to familial PD development, such as α-synuclein and leucine-rich repeat kinase-2 (LRRK2) apparently follow a non-Mendelian genetic inheritance pattern. Even so, people who have first-degree relatives affected by sporadic PD have increased chances of developing PD (Elbaz et al., 1999).

Mitochondrial dysfunction and purinergic receptor signaling are also involved in the mechanism of the disorder (Takenouchi et al., 2010; Hoang, 2014).

Currently, dopamine agonists as L-3,4-dihydroxyphenylalanine (L-DOPA) are the most common agents used in therapy. L-DOPA is a precursor of catecholamines such as dopamine and is able to cross the blood-brain barrier. However, long term use of L-DOPA loses efficacy and dose adjustments are needed, triggering side effects such as dyskinesias in 50% of patients after 5 years of continuous treatments (Lang, 2009; Olanow et al., 2009). Present studies on molecular aspects of PD, together with the development of new drugs and tests for improving diagnosis accuracy, will bring new therapeutics perspectives for the disease.

Purinergic Involvement in PD

P2X receptors

Although immunohistochemistry analysis did not reveal any difference between intact and lesioned striatum and SNc (Amadio et al., 2007) for P2X7 receptors, antagonism of this receptor has been shown to prevent or reverse hemiparkinsonian behavior in animals lesioned with 6-hydroxydopamine (6-OHDA), a neurotoxin that mimics PD's pathology. Acute SNc injections of the P2X7 receptor antagonist A-438059, 60 min before and 60 min after rat 6-OHDA lesion, prevented dopamine striatal deficit in comparison to the intact hemisphere, with the P2X7 receptor localized in glial cells (Marcellino et al., 2010). BBG administered in a dose of 45 mg/kg daily after 6-OHDA lesion prevented hemiparkinsonian behavior, short-term memory impairment and dopamine deficit in the striatum and SNc (Carmo et al., 2014). While these studies showed only a preventive effect of P2X7 receptor antagonism, BBG at a dose of 50 mg/kg reversed 6-OHDA lesion in striatum and SNc. In this work, BBG treatment started 1 week after 6-OHDA injection, a period of time sufficient for the lesion to settle, thus proving the reversal effect (Ferrazoli et al., 2017).

Neuronal death seems to aggravate protein aggregation observed in PD. Intense ATP release and consequent purinergic receptors activation were considered to be a key trigger. In fact, P2X1 receptor antagonism or genetic deletion reduced α-synuclein aggregation induced by ATP released by dying cells *in vitro* (Gan et al., 2015). Moreover, P2X1 receptor activation induced lysosomal dysfunction that seems to be involved in α-synuclein aggregation, since it delayed protein turnover and led to its accumulation (Gan et al., 2015). Although P2X7 receptor blockade did not result in reduction of α-synuclein aggregation in this study, ATP release triggered by α-synuclein *in vitro* activated the P2X7 receptor and mobilized the release of intracellular Ca^{2+}, showing that P2X7 receptor activation is a consequence of α-synuclein aggregation (Wilkaniec et al., 2017). Additionally, another study showed that microglial cells challenged with α-synuclein presented increased ROS production through P2X7 receptor activation, which was prevented in the presence of a receptor antagonist (Jiang et al., 2015). Thus, it seems that P2X1 receptor activation contributes to α-synuclein aggregation, which in turn modulates P2X7 receptor activity, ROS production and, finally, ATP release.

Taking into account that few studies directly link purinergic receptors with genetic predisposition to PD, the P2X7R 1513A>C polymorphism that facilitates pore formation by P2X7 receptor activation and leads to cell death (Gu et al., 2001) was shown to be a risk factor in sporadic PD in a Han Chinese population (Liu et al., 2013)

P2Y receptors

There is little data directly connecting P2Y receptors to PD. Recent studies are drawing attention to the role of P2Y6 receptors in PD development and progression. An *in vitro* study showed that P2Y6 receptor gene expression is increased in SH-SY5Y cells—a human neuroblastoma lineage that when differentiated presents markers for dopaminergic neurons—when challenged with neurotoxin 1-methyl-4-phenylpyridinium (MPP^+) (Qian et al., 2017). Thus, its antagonism or deletion decreased MPP^+ effects in cell death through reduced ROS production (Yang et al., 2017). In the CNS, UDP released by damaged cells induces expression of cytokines CCL2 and CCL3 in microglia and phagocytic activity through activation of P2Y6 receptors, indicating that this receptor subtype may be involved in inflammatory response in neurodegenerative diseases (Kim et al., 2011).

Recently, P2Y6 receptor levels were found to be increased in PBMC of PD patients younger than 80 years. To elucidate the involvement of P2Y6 receptor in these patients, the authors used an *in vitro* model of microglia challenged with lipopolysaccharide (LPS) and found increased P2Y6 receptor expression, supporting the hypothesized neuroinflammatory effect of microglia (Yang et al., 2017). Taking into account that P2Y6 receptor selective inhibition by MRS2578 is able to prevent microglial phagoptosis in a mixed neuronal/glial culture in inflammatory conditions (Neher et al., 2014), P2Y6 receptor antagonism seems to be a promising tool to attenuate neuronal death in PD by preventing lesion worsening due to phagocytosis of viable neurons.

Adenosine receptors

It is known that A_{2A} receptors are enriched in dopaminergic brain areas and that their activity modulation affects dopamine receptors (Burnstock et al., 2011). In fact, A_{2A} receptors form heterodimers with dopaminergic D2 and A_1 receptors in glutamatergic synapses, modulating the balance between excitatory and inhibitory impulses that may aggravate PD symptomatology (reviewed by Schiffmann et al., 2007). In animals, a range of A_{2A} receptor antagonists have being shown to potentiate therapeutic effect of low doses of L-DOPA in MPP^+ lesioned monkeys and marmosets and in 6-OHDA lesioned rodents (Kanda et al., 2000; Fuzzati-Armentero et al., 2015) In fact *istradefylline,* a A_{2A} receptor antagonist, was recently approved in Japan to be used concomitantly with L-DOPA treatment, once the compound enhances antiparkinsonian effect of L-DOPA and allow the usage of lower doses of L-DOPA with less long-term side effects (Zhu et al., 2014).

A_{2A} receptors are supposedly involved in synucleinopathy process. A_{2A} receptor-knock out mice presented resistance in preventing dopaminergic deficits upon α-synuclein-induced insults (Kachroo and Schwarzschild, 2012). Attempting to clarify involved mechanisms, Ferreira et al. found that A_{2A} receptor antagonism decreased α-synuclein aggregation, prevented neuronal death induced by extracellular α-synuclein and restrained hyperactivation of NMDA-glutamate receptors (Ferreira et al., 2015). A_{2A} receptor protein expression levels are increased upon hippocampal injections of α-synuclein in mice and closely co-localized with aggregates, suggesting a pathogenic role of this receptor in synucleinopathy (Hu et al., 2016).

Moreover, A_{2A} receptor antagonism may facilitate microglial response to injury. Microglial delayed containment of debris resulted from cell death can be associated with expansion of the lesion (Gyoneva et al., 2014). Further, both caffeine and selective A_{2A} receptor antagonist KW60002 prevented rat striatal dopaminergic deficit and hydroxyl radical release in LPS-induced inflammation (Gołembiowska et al., 2013). These data suggest inflammatory modulation by A_{2A} receptor antagonism in PD models.

Two polymorphisms of A_{2A} receptor (rs71651683 or rs5996696) were inversely associated with genetic PD risk, wherein caffeine intake intensified the inverse association. Moreover, two polymorphisms in CYP1A2a (rs762551 or rs2470890), an enzyme responsible for caffeine metabolism, in homozygous caffeine consumers showed a prominent reduction in the risk of developing PD (Popat et al., 2011).

Caffeine intake interferes with other genetic risk factors for PD. Subjects with LRRK2 risk variant R1628P showed 15 times increased risk of developing PD than not caffeine consumers (Kumar et al., 2015). GRIN2A rs4998386-T allele encodes a subtype of NMDA receptor, whose activity is enhanced by A_{2A} receptor activation and leads to glutamatergic excitotoxicity. A polymorphism in the GRIN2A rs4998386-T is considered protective for PD development *per se,* but in association with caffeine consumption, it can beneficially impact PD risk in a greater magnitude (Hamza et al., 2011; Yamada-Fowler et al., 2014). However, creatine consumption that increases ATP storage accelerated PD progression in GRIN2A caffeine consumers, possibly due to ATP conversion to adenosine and later A_{2A} receptor activation (Simon et al., 2017).

Conclusion

Taken together, evidence indicates that modulation of purinergic receptor expression and activity could be useful in PD treatment in several ways: (1) reducing microglia activation by damaged cells and α-synuclein aggregation through P2X7 and P2Y6 receptors antagonism; (2) preventing α-synuclein aggregation through P2X1 and A_{2A} receptors antagonism; (3) modulating inflammatory scenario through A_{2A} receptors antagonism; or (4) preventing dyskinesia induced by L-DOPA long-term use through combined treatment with A_{2A} receptor antagonists.

OTHER NEUROLOGICAL CONDITIONS WITH MOTOR DYSFUNCTIONS

Huntington's Disease

HD is an inherited neurological disorder caused by a mutation in IT15 gene that encodes huntingtin protein (Htt) predominantly found in neurons. This mutation results in abnormal (CAG)n repeats localized in 5′ coding sequence. HD is characterized by neurodegeneration of neuronal cells located in striatum and cerebral cortex, ultimately causing neuronal dysfunction and striatal death (Vonsattel and DiFiglia, 1998; Ross and Tabrizi, 2011).

Purinergic Involvement in HD

Adenosine receptor

Adenosinergic pathway plays an essential role in HD etiology and progression, especially through the A_{2A} receptor, as observed in patients and animal models (Popoli et al., 2007). The A_{2A} receptor is highly expressed in striatum (Schiffmann et al., 1991; Fink et al., 1992) especially in GABAergic/enkephalinergic neurons (Taherzadeh-Fard et al., 2010) and in post-synaptic striatopallidal GABAergic neurons (Martinez-Mir et al., 1991; Hettinger et al., 2001), antagonizing dopamine D2 receptors (Schiffmann et al., 2007), while presynaptic A_{2A} receptor activity promotes glutamate release (Shen et al., 2013). Further, presynaptic A_{2A} receptors in glutamatergic terminals impinging into medium spiny neurons play an essential role in the initial maladaptive plasticity in animal models of HD (Li et al., 2015), suggesting its involvement in the degeneration of striatal neurons. Reduction of A_{2A} receptor expression is based on the overexpression of mutant Htt protein showing expanded poly (Q), which affects CREB binding to its promoter region in the A_{2A} receptor gene. Under stimulation, A_{2A} receptor is able to promote its own gene expression via activation of PKC/CREB signaling as well as reduce Htt aggregations (Chiang et al., 2005). Striatal cells expressing mutant Htt showed increased A_{2A} receptor density and cAMP activity due to A_{2A} receptor activation (Varani et al., 2001). As expected, transgenic HD mice showed reduced A_{2A} receptor expression (Cha et al., 1999; Glass et al., 2000; Luthi-Carter et al., 2000), while exhibiting transient increases in A_{2A} receptor density and A_{2A} receptor-dependent activation of cAMP signaling at the earlier pre-symptomatic stage (Tarditi et al., 2006).

It has been proposed that modulation of A_{2A} receptor activity either by agonists or antagonists may prove to be beneficial for HD treatment. However, available data indicate that the beneficial effect observed after stimulation or inhibition of A_{2A} receptor activity depends on the disease stage. At earlier stages of HD, the use of SCH58261 (an A_{2A} receptor antagonist) in quinolinic acid (QA)-induced HD rats and R6/2 transgenic mice reduced striatal BDNF expression, precluding BDNF control of NMDA toxicity (Potenza et al., 2007; Tebano et al., 2010). In later stages, no effect on BDNF expression was observed (Martire et al., 2010; Tebano et al., 2010). QA-induced rats reproduced neurochemical changes of NMDA receptor from HD, e.g., increased glutamate outflow, reduced adenosine levels and degeneration of A_{2A} and dopamine receptors (Beal et al., 1991; Ishiwata et al., 2002; Gianfriddo et al., 2003). Treatment with SCH58261 2-3 weeks after QA injection increased striatal glutamate release, acting as damaging factor (Gianfriddo et al., 2003).

Preventive treatment with SCH58261 before QA induction in rats minimizes the effect of QA on motor activity, striatal gliosis, electroencephalographic (EEG) changes, and glutamate levels

(Popoli et al., 2002). However, cyclooxygenase-2 (COX-2) is inhibited in microglia but increased in cortical neurons, probably as a consequence of NMDA receptors activation, leading to neurotoxicity (Minghetti, 2004). Pretreated QA-induced rats also showed less rearing behavior and no changes in baseline motor activity after 2 weeks of induction; 6 months later, rats showed reduced anxiety but no changes in learning task when compared to QA-induced rats not pre-treated with SCH58261 (Scattoni et al., 2007). These findings suggest that SCH58261 acts on damaged striatum and not on damaged hippocampus, and that different populations of striatal neurons are responsive to SCH58261 (Scattoni et al., 2007). As reviewed by Cunha (Cunha, 2016), the blockage of A_{2A} receptor improves memory and motor functions indicating hippocampal activity, contradicting the findings of Scattoni et al.

On the other hand, in primary striatal cultures treated with QA, an increase in intracellular calcium concentration was observed which enhanced in presence of SCH58261, but reduced in presence of A_{2A} receptor agonist CGS21680 (Popoli et al., 2002). Another A_{2A} receptor antagonist, 3,7-dimethyl-1-propargylxanthine (DMPX), completely blocked encephalographic changes in prefrontal cortex in QA-induced rats (Reggio et al., 1999). The beneficial effect can be due to dopamine receptor activation that provides neuroprotection as a result of abolishment of A_{2A} receptor function, since D2 dopaminergic receptors are downregulated by A_{2A} receptors in D2/A_{2A} receptor heteromers (Reggio et al., 1999).

In a transgenic rat model of HD showing 51 repeated CAG sequences, the presence of post-synaptic A_{2A} receptor antagonist KW-6002, a known stimulant of locomotion, didn't alter the locomotion pattern between 3 and 6 months old. This indicated that the animals become indifferent to A_{2A} receptor modulation during that period (Orr,ú et al., 2011). Furthermore, the presynaptic A_{2A} receptor antagonist SCH-442416 did not reduce electromyography responses (Orr,ú et al., 2011).

The function of A_{2A} receptors has been studied in HD transgenic mouse models (R6/1 with later symptoms and R6/2 with earlier symptoms), which contain the first exon of human Htt gene and 115-150 CAG repeats (Li et al., 2005). During R6/2 mouse development, A_{2A} receptor protein density and A_{2A} receptor-dependent production of cAMP slightly increased at post-natal days 7–14, before the onset of motor symptoms (Tarditi et al., 2006). On the 21st day, changes are normalized to control (Tarditi et al., 2006). A_{2A} receptor expression, but not protein density, starts decreasing, indicating that protein turnover is altered in HD (Cha et al., 1999; Tarditi et al., 2006). Reduction of A_{2A} receptor coding mRNA can be explained by regulation of A_{2A} receptor gene methylation patterns, once R6/1 mice has less hydroxymethylcytosine and higher methylcytosine levels in 5′-UTR regions of the A_{2A} receptor gene (Villar-Menéndez et al., 2013).

Since turnover of A_{2A} receptor protein is altered in HD, inhibition of this receptor function is an advisable therapeutic approach. Starting at 5 weeks, the use of the A_{2A} receptor antagonist SCH58261 in R6/2 mice ameliorated NMDA-induced toxicity and emotional/anxiety response (Domenici et al., 2007). After week 8, administration of SCH58261 leads to NMDA receptors remodeling (NR_1 and NR_{2A} receptor /NR_{2B} ratio) in striatum (Martire et al., 2010). R6/2 mice at age of 10–11 weeks old showed increased adenosine levels correlated with the presence of p38 MAPK in striatal neurons, resulting in striatal damage (Gianfriddo et al., 2004). The usage of SCH58261 greatly reduced striatal adenosine levels and glutamate outflow, suggesting that SCH58261 was acting on A_{2A} receptors located in corticostriatal glutamatergic terminals (Gianfriddo et al., 2004). When treated with SCH58261, rearing and grooming behaviors were reduced in R6/2 mice, but increased in wild type mice, suggesting that A_{2A} receptor antagonism effects on behavior depended on the presence of mutant Htt (Domenici et al., 2007). However, there are contradictory findings regarding the effect of SCH58261. While this compound has shown beneficial effect by reducing NMDA toxicity in striatum *in vivo*, it did not prevent NMDA toxicity from *in vitro* culture of corticostriatal slices obtained from R6/2 mice (Martire et al., 2010).

In order to determine whether the A_{2A} receptor is involved in HD etiology, A_{2A} receptor knockout mice were induced with mitochondrial toxin 3-nitropropionic acid (3-NPA) which blocks succinate dehydrogenase, inducing HD phenotype. Only 1 out of 8 showed striatal lesion after 3-NPA induction, indicating that the absence of A_{2A} receptor has protective effect against HD development (Fink et al., 2004). To confirm this finding, wild type mice were pre-treated with the A_{2A} receptor antagonist 8-(3-chlorostypyl)-caffeine. The animals did not show any striatal lesions after 3-NPA treatment (Fink et al., 2004). On the other hand, ablation of A_{2A} receptors in HD N171-82Q transgenic mouse model completely aggravated motor performance and survival, reducing the expression of striatal encephalin (Mievis et al., 2011). This observation suggests that early and chronic blockade of A_{2A} receptor is not favorable for HD development (Mievis et al., 2011), but memory improvement was observed in R6/2 mice with complete genetic A_{2A} receptor ablation (Li et al., 2015).

In symptomatic R6/2 mice, activation of A_{2A} receptors by CGS21680 delayed the deterioration of motor conditions, prevented reduction in brain weight, diminished the levels of choline, normalized glucose levels, and altered NMDA receptor subunit composition and basal synaptic transmission, without changing its expression (Chou et al., 2005; Martire et al., 2007; Potenza et al., 2007; Ferrante et al., 2010; Tebano et al., 2010). Cultivation of corticostriatal slices from R6/2 mice in presence of CGS21680 also showed reduced NMDA toxicity, suggesting a crosstalk between A_{2A} receptor and BDNF (Tebano et al., 2010). Treatment of striatum slices from R6/2 with CGS21680 resulted in an increase in extracellular field potential, while the opposite effect was observed in wild type slices, where the use of an A_{2A} receptor agonist potentiated toxicity via NMDA receptor activation (Martire et al., 2007).

Single nucleotide polymorphisms (SNPs) in the ADORA$_{2A}$ gene have been identified in HD patients. A C>T genotype (1876 C/T; rs5751876) SNP results in a silent mutation with unknown function and influences the age of onset of HD, while the T/T genotype increases the age of onset of HD by 3.8 years when compared to the C/C genotype (Dhaenens et al., 2009). A SNP in intron 1 (rs2298383) is linked to early onset of HD

(Taherzadeh-Fard et al., 2010). Analysis of HD patient peripheral blood cells led to increased aberrant A_{2A} receptor signaling, which correlates with the age of the patient, numbers of expanded CAG repeats and number of A_{2A} receptor ligand-binding sites (Maglione et al., 2005a,b). The linear correlation is more evident in patients suffering from chorea—an early disruption of the striatum in HD. Neutrophils from HD patients have higher A_{2A} receptor dysfunction in homozygous vs. heterozygous HD patients while no changes in A_1 or A_3 receptors are observed in peripheral blood cells (Varani et al., 2003). A_{2A}-cannabinoid CB1 receptor heterodimers exert crucial function by controlling neuronal excitability (Moreno et al., 2017), while activation of striatal A_{2A} receptors may inhibit CB1 function independent from heterodimer formation (Ferreira et al., 2015). Patients harboring high-grade HD do not possess A_{2A}-CB1 receptor heterodimers in the caudate-putamen region due to the lack of CB1 receptors (Moreno et al., 2017). Recent evidence suggests that consuming more than 190 mg/day of caffeine may accelerate HD onset (Simonin et al., 2013), contradicting findings in animal models that point toward beneficial effects of A_{2A} receptor antagonism in HD.

HD is also characterized by oxidative stress resulting from mitochondrial dysfunction, leading to GABAergic neuronal loss and proneness to DNA damage (Chiu et al., 2015). GABAergic neurons derived from HD-iPSC showed an increase in DNA damage and oxidative stress, which can be dramatically reduced by A_{2A} receptor activation (Chiu et al., 2015). Stimulation of A_{2A} receptors minimizes oxidative stress-induced apoptosis by activation of the cAMP/PKA signaling pathway (Chiu et al., 2015), which is essential for reversing the effect of reduced A_{2A} receptor activity via CREB transcription factor activation (Chiang et al., 2005). However, findings *in vivo* contradict the beneficial effect of A_{2A} receptor agonism on PKA signaling. In R6/1 mice, dopamine D1 and A_{2A} receptors are hyperactive showing greater cAMP/PKA signaling (Tyebji et al., 2015). Chronic administration of antagonists of dopamine D1 and A_{2A} receptors normalized PKA levels and improved cognitive dysfunction and synaptic plasticity. Pre-treatment of rats and mice with either 8-cyclopentyl-1,3-dipropylxanthine (CPX; A_1 receptor antagonist) or DMPX prior application of manolate (an inhibitor of mitochondria acting in striatum) showed that DMPX prevented GABAergic cell loss while CPX promotes cell death (Alfinito et al., 2003). The A_1 receptor agonist R-PIA prevented seizures but not neurodegeneration in the 3-nitropropionic acid (3-NPA) model of neurotoxicity (Zuchora and Urbańska, 2001), while the A_1 receptor agonist adenosine amine congener (ADAC) protects against excitotoxicity, delays degeneration and improves motor functions in the same model (Blum et al., 2002). In view of that, the effect of A_1 receptors depended on the respective used antagonist.

P2 receptors

The role of P2X signaling in HD has not yet been studied in detail. Evidence exists that signaling via ATP induced cell death in HD models while blockade of ATP production reduces cell loss (Varma et al., 2007). At the present, the only evidence available is the role of P2X7 receptor in HD pathogenesis. In two HD mice model, Tet/HD94 and R6/1, P2X7 receptor expression is increased, as well as P2X7 receptor-induced Ca^{2+} permeability (Diaz-Hernandez et al., 2009). Treatment with the P2X7 receptor antagonist BBG ameliorates motor coordination deficits and body weight loss while inhibiting neuronal loss. *In vitro*, neurons expressing mutant Htt are prone to cell death induction by apoptosis after P2X7 receptor stimulation (Diaz-Hernandez et al., 2009).

Conclusion

The available data on the involvement of A_{2A} receptors in HD progression is evident, suggesting that the prevention of its activation could delay disease progression. Taken together, it can be proposed that a combination of A_1 receptor agonist and A_{2A} receptor antagonist might be a good therapeutic approach for HD. It must be taken in consideration that the effect of A_{2A} receptor antagonism depends on age, doses, and length of treatment. Although antagonism of P2X7 receptor may be promising, the involvement of other P2 receptors remains unclear and needs to be investigated.

Ataxias

Ataxia, or dysfunction in motor coordination, is a major consequence of cerebellar and spinocerebellar tract dysfunction that can be induced by several factors, including genetic and sporadic forms, commonly related to immune system mechanisms (Mariotti et al., 2005). Spinocerebellar ataxia (SCA), a genetic-related form of progressive ataxia resulted by cerebellar degeneration, is classified according to mode of inheritance and gene/chromosome locus affected (Matilla-Dueñas et al., 2012). The most prevalent and severe forms of SCA are caused by an increase in CAG sequence repeats in genes that encode proteins related to disease development (Paulson et al., 2017). For example, the expansion in polyglutamine affecting ataxin-2 protein can be observed in SCA type 2, while ataxin-3 related expansion occurs in SCA type 3. Other forms of SCA can be characterized by other genetic mutations, such as the type 14, in which mutations in the protein kinase C-γ gene induce cerebellar degeneration (Seki et al., 2005).

Purinergic Involvement in Ataxias

Attempting to identify survival characteristics of some cell in SCA type 2, wild type ataxin-2 positive neurons showed resistance in cell-death induced by axotomy (Viscomi et al., 2005) and, although this lesion up-regulated P2X1 and P2X2 receptors in precerebellar nuclei (Florenzano et al., 2002) and induced P2X1 receptor in ataxin-2 positive neurons, the percentage of cells expressing P2X1 receptor was not altered (Viscomi et al., 2005). Viscomi and co-workers suggested that these purinergic receptors could influence resistance against cell death without being essential for cell survival, since there are several pathways involved in neuronal death. The elucidation of purinergic receptor involvement in SCA type 3 is focused on adenosine receptors. The blockade of A_{2A} receptors through caffeine ingestion reduced damaging morphological changes induced by mutant ataxin-3 injection. Moreover, these damaging effects were abolished in knockout mice for A_{2A} receptors (Gonçalves et al., 2013). Behavioral improvements were also observed in transgenic c57Bl6 mice expressing truncated polyglutamine ataxin-3 with severe ataxia, reinforcing the protective effect of A_{2A} receptor antagonism in the SCA type 3 (Gonçalves et al., 2017). In the SCA type 14 *in vitro* model, stimulation of purinergic receptors with ATP transiently increased translocation of mutant protein kinase C-γ to the plasma membrane and subsequent increased damaging aggregation in the cytoplasm (Seki et al., 2005).

Restless Leg Syndrome

Restless leg syndrome (RLS) is a neurological condition characterized by an urge to move legs during rest, following a circadian cycle with worsening during night and even during sleep (named periodic limb movements of sleep). Pathophysiological mechanisms have not been fully elucidated, and conflicting results are reported in the literature. Dopaminergic transmission seems to be involved, since the use of dopaminergic-inducing drugs improved symptoms (Garcia-Borreguero and Cano-Pumarega, 2017). Due to the high affinity of the agonists with best responsiveness to RLS for D3 dopaminergic receptors, it is postulated that the D3 receptor subtype has major responsibility for RLS improvement (Ferré et al., 2018). However, the risk of symptoms worsening after long-term use of these drugs stimulated the search for alternative therapies, based on glutamatergic ligands and reversal of iron deficiency (Ferré et al., 2017). Striatal glutamatergic terminals are found to be hypersensitive in an animal model of RLS with increased glutamate and dopamine release. It is known that, besides increased dopamine release, there is a decreased synaptic D2 receptor density in this animal model (Ferré et al., 2018).

Purinergic Involvement in RLS

Recently, Ferré's group pointed at a relation between adenosine receptors and brain iron deficiency in RLS. Using an animal model for RLS, in which mice and rats adhered to an iron deficient diet, striatal presynaptic A_{2A} receptor density was upregulated (Gulyani et al., 2009). In the same animal model, A_1 receptor density was found decreased in animals with mild, moderate and severe deficiency accompanied by dopaminergic D2 receptor downregulation, and increased pre-synaptic A_{2A} receptor density in animals submitted to a more iron deficient diet (Quiroz et al., 2016). Thus, the post-synaptic A_1 receptor, which can be found as heteromers with D1 dopaminergic receptors and antagonizes their activity, as well as presynaptic A_{2A} receptors forming heteromers with D2 receptors whose activation decreases D2 receptor affinity for agonists, could be targets to improve movement impairment (Ferré et al., 1994; Ferre et al., 1996; Ferré et al., 2007, 2018). Finally, A_1/A_{2A} receptor heteromers found in the striatal glutamatergic terminals, activated by different adenosine concentrations, decreased glutamate release, a condition found in brain iron deficiency animals (Ciruela et al., 2006; Ferré, 2010).

OUTCOMES FOR HYPOTHESES ON P2 PURINERGIC SIGNALING

Although P2X7 receptor expression and levels in neurons is controversial, the involvement of this receptor in neurodegeneration is well-stated (Illes et al., 2017). Of all purinergic receptors, the P2X7 receptor has the lowest affinity for ATP, and only high concentrations of this nucleotide induce channel formation (North, 2002; Khakh and Alan North, 2006). Of the neurological diseases presented here, immune system responses and neural cell death correspond with the release of elevated levels of ATP into the extracellular space. In these scenarios, ATP in excess acts as a toxin that can directly induce oligodendrocyte death by activating P2X7 receptors, resulting in progressive neural damage (Matute et al., 2007; Domercq et al., 2009). Corroborating this idea, it is well-known that the P2X7 receptor triggers pro-inflammatory effects (Lister et al., 2007), and its antagonism can counteract chronic inflammation observed in these diseases (**Figure 2**). Thus, beneficial effects of P2X7 receptor antagonism are of interest for future therapeutic approaches.

As further investigations are necessary to better understand the real role of purinergic signaling in the diseases here presented, we also propose a novel mechanistic perspective, in which purinergic receptors from glial cells are key initiators of motor dysfunction in PD, MS, ALS and other MND. Although there is no data regarding P2Y1 receptor functions in these pathological conditions, it is known that this receptor plays a crucial role in astrocyte responses accompanied by P2Y12 and adenosine receptor activity modulation (Mamedova et al., 2006).

During an initial inflammatory response, microglial activation induces P2Y12 receptor expression level and/or activity upregulation, stimulating motility toward the injury site and resulting in reduced P2Y1 receptor expression in astrocytes. This downregulation in P2Y1 receptor expression stimulates an increase in reactive astrogliosis and a phenotypical change in order to promote neuroprotection (Haynes et al., 2006; Mamedova et al., 2006; Shinozaki et al., 2017). However, constant inflammatory responses disable microglia of stimulating P2Y12 receptor expression and activity, resulting in a permanent activation of P2Y1 receptors in astrocytes and extended ROS production (Rodrigues et al., 2015). This condition will lead to a downregulation of A_1 receptor expression, stimulating TNF-α production and release, thereby promoting IL-6 secretion through A_{2B} receptor activation. As a result, TNF-α and IL-6 accumulation damages oligodendrocytes and provoke demyelination. A scheme of this mechanism is proposed in **Figure 1**.

OVERALL CONCLUSION

The purinergic signaling system has risen in the past years as a meaningful research object for understanding and treating several pathologies, as reviewed by Burnstock (2017). Purinergic receptors and enzymes are in the spotlight for new therapeutic interventions as key regulators of neuron-glia communication, as well as modulators of many signaling pathways associated to neuroprotection, neurodegeneration, and neuroregeneration (Burnstock, 2016; Ribeiro et al., 2016). In this review, we highlighted available data linking purinergic signaling pathways to neurological diseases, such as PD, MS, ALS, and other MND, putting together published knowledge with novel hypotheses for overcoming motor dysfunctions. The evidence is summarized in **Table 1**. A common mechanism supporting P2X7 receptor

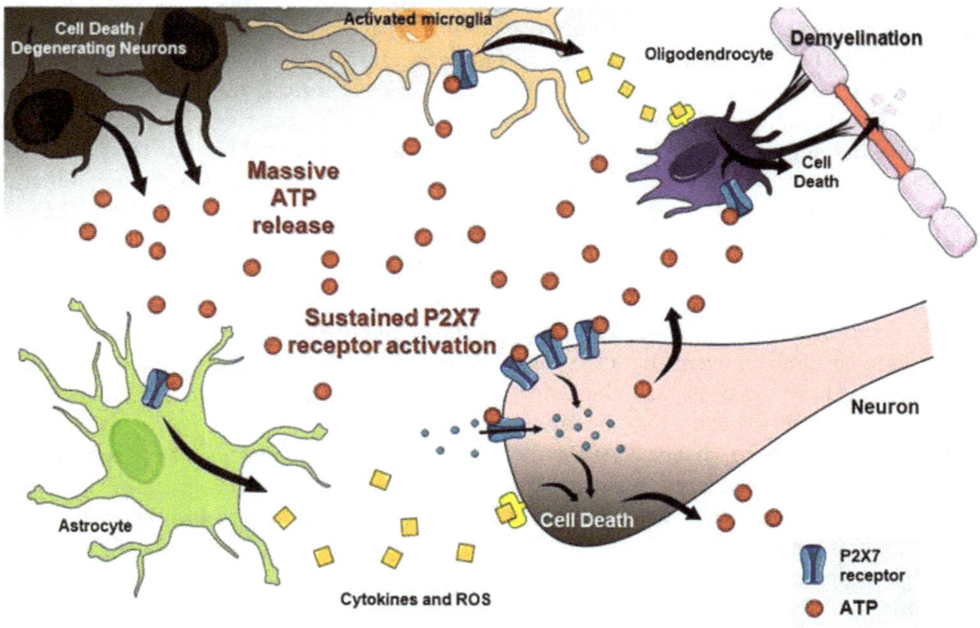

FIGURE 2 | Common mechanism involving P2X7 receptor-mediated cell death in the central nervous system under neurological diseases affecting motor functions. Degenerating neurons release large amounts of ATP, leading to sustained P2X7 receptor activation in: a. Astrocytes, inducing the release of cytokines and reactive oxygen species (ROS); b. Microglia, inducing an activated state and release of cytokines and ROS; c. Oligodendrocytes, inducing cell death and neuron demyelination; d. Neurons (in spite of the controversial discussion on expression of P2X7 receptors in this cell type), inducing pore formation, ion influx and cell death, releasing more ATP into the extracellular space. Moreover, cytokines and ROS released by astrocytes and microglia act on other neural cells, culminating in apoptotic pathway activation.

hyperactivation through high levels of ATP release during disease development is illustrated in **Figure 2**. Moreover, a novel mechanism based on purinergic modulation of glial cells is proposed in **Figure 1**. These approaches suggest novel possible research targets to understand the here presented motor dysfunctions and other factors associated to neurological impairment that have not been studied yet. Applied research will need to be conducted for the development of novel pharmacological treatments to improve patients' lifespan and quality.

AUTHOR CONTRIBUTIONS

ÁO-G: Contribution to idea proposal, organization of sections, writing PD, other MND, RLS, and Ataxia sections, figures, table. YN: Writing MS, HD, and mechanism hypothesis sections. LS-A: Writing ALS and SMA sections. MG: Writing introduction, HD, and conclusion sections. JC-V: Writing ALS section. MP: Writing MS section. HdS: Writing PD section. HU: Conceptualization of the manuscript, supervision of manuscript elaboration, editing and revision, and critical overview.

ACKNOWLEDGMENTS

HU is grateful for grant support by the São Paulo State Foundation FAPESP (Project No. 2012/50880-4) and the National Research Council CNPq (Project No. 306429/2013-6), Brazil. ÁO-G (Project No. 141979/2014-3) and MG (Project No. 870458/1997-3) are grateful for a doctorate fellowship granted by CNPq; Fellowships were granted by FAPESP to HdS (doctorate; Project No. 2012/20685-5), LS-A (doctorate, Project No. 2013/25338-4), MP (pos-doctorate, Project No. 2015/19478-3) and YN (pos-doctorate, Project No. 2015/14343-2). We thank ME Caitlyn A. Moore for English editing and comments on the manuscript.

REFERENCES

Abbracchio, M. P., Burnstock, G., Verkhratsky, A., and Zimmermann, H. (2009). Purinergic signalling in the nervous system: an overview. *Trends Neurosci.* 32, 19–29. doi: 10.1016/j.tins.2008.10.001

Airas, L., Niemela, J., Yegutkin, G., and Jalkanen, S. (2007). Mechanism of action of IFN-beta in the treatment of multiple sclerosis: a special reference to CD73 and adenosine. *Ann. N. Y. Acad. Sci.* 1110, 641–648. doi: 10.1196/annals.1423.067

Alfinito, P. D., Wang, S.-P., Manzino, L., Rijhsinghani, S., Zeevalk, G. D., and Sonsalla, P. K. (2003). Adenosinergic protection of dopaminergic and GABAergic neurons against mitochondrial inhibition through receptors located in the substantia nigra and striatum, respectively. *J. Neurosci.* 23, 10982–10987.

Allard, B., Beavis, P. A., Darcy, P. K., and Stagg, J. (2016). Immunosuppressive activities of adenosine in cancer. *Curr. Opin. Pharmacol.* 29, 7–16. doi: 10.1016/j.coph.2016.04.001

Amadio, S., Montilli, C., Magliozzi, R., Bernardi, G., Reynolds, R., and Volonté, C. (2010). P2Y12 receptor protein in cortical gray matter lesions in multiple sclerosis. *Cereb. Cortex* 20, 1263–1273. doi: 10.1093/cercor/bhp193

Amadio, S., Montilli, C., Picconi, B., Calabresi, P., and Volonté, C. (2007). Mapping P2X and P2Y receptor proteins in striatum and substantia nigra: an immunohistological study. *Purinergic Signal.* 3, 389–398. doi: 10.1007/s11302-007-9069-8

Amadio, S., Parisi, C., Montilli, C., Carrubba, A. S., Apolloni, S., and Volonté, C. (2014). P2Y 12 receptor on the verge of a neuroinflammatory breakdown. *Mediators Inflamm.* 2014:975849. doi: 10.1155/2014/975849

Andries, M., Van Damme, P., Robberecht, W., and Van Den Bosch, L. (2007). Ivermectin inhibits AMPA receptor-mediated excitotoxicity in cultured motor neurons and extends the life span of a transgenic mouse model of amyotrophic lateral sclerosis. *Neurobiol. Dis.* 25, 8–16. doi: 10.1016/j.nbd.2006.08.018

Apolloni, S., Amadio, S., Montilli, C., Volonté, C., and D'Ambrosi, N. (2013a). Ablation of P2X7 receptor exacerbates gliosis and motoneuron death in the SOD1-G93A mouse model of amyotrophic lateral sclerosis. *Hum. Mol. Genet.* 22, 4102–4116. doi: 10.1093/hmg/ddt259

Apolloni, S., Parisi, C., Pesaresi, M. G., Rossi, S., Carrì, M. T., Cozzolino, M., et al. (2013b). The NADPH oxidase pathway is dysregulated by the P2X7 receptor in the SOD1-G93A microglia model of amyotrophic lateral sclerosis. *J. Immunol.* 190, 5187–5195. doi: 10.4049/jimmunol.1203262

Ballerini, P., Rathbone, M. P., Di Iorio, P., Renzetti, A., Giuliani, P., D'Alimonte, I., et al. (1996). Rat astroglial P2Z (P2X7) receptors regulate intracellular calcium and purine release. *Neuroreport* 7, 2533–2537.

Band, H., Bhattacharya, A., and Talwar, G. P. (1986). Mechanism of phagocytosis by Schwann cells. *J. Neurol. Sci.* 75, 113–119. doi: 10.1016/0022-510X(86)90054-7

Barbeito, A. G., Mesci, P., and Boillée, S. (2010). Motor neuron–immune interactions: the vicious circle of ALS. *J. Neural Transm.* 117, 981–1000. doi: 10.1007/s00702-010-0429-0

Barthélémy, C., Henderson, C. E., and Pettmann, B. (2004). Foxo3a induces motoneuron death through the Fas pathway in cooperation with JNK. *BMC Neurosci.* 5:48. doi: 10.1186/1471-2202-5-48

Bartlett, R., Stokes, L., and Sluyter, R. (2014). The P2X7 receptor channel: recent developments and the use of P2X7 antagonists in models of disease. *Pharmacol. Rev.* 66, 638–675. doi: 10.1124/pr.113.008003

Beal, M. F., Ferrante, R. J., Swartz, K. J., and Kowall, N. W. (1991). Chronic quinolinic acid lesions in rats closely resemble Huntington's disease. *J. Neurosci.* 11, 1649–659.

Beamer, E., Gölöncsér, F., Horváth, G., Beko, K., Otrokocsi, L., Koványi, B., et al. (2016). Purinergic mechanisms in neuroinflammation: an update from molecules to behavior. *Neuropharmacology* 104, 94–104. doi: 10.1016/j.neuropharm.2015.09.019

Bebee, T. W., Gladman, J. T., and Chandler, D. S. (2010). Splicing of the survival motor neuron genes and implications for treatment of SMA. *Front. Biosci. (Landmark Ed).* 15, 1191–1204. doi: 10.2741/3670

Beghi, E., Pupillo, E., Messina, P., Giussani, G., Chiò, A., Zoccolella, S., et al. (2011). Coffee and amyotrophic lateral sclerosis: a possible preventive role. *Am. J. Epidemiol.* 174, 1002–1008. doi: 10.1093/aje/kwr229

Bergmayr, C., Thurner, P., Keuerleber, S., Kudlacek, O., Nanoff, C., Freissmuth, M., et al. (2013). Recruitment of a cytoplasmic chaperone relay by the A $_{2A}$ adenosine receptor. *J. Biol. Chem.* 288, 28831–28844. doi: 10.1074/jbc.M113.464776

Blackburn, M. R., Vance, C. O., Morschl, E., and Wilson, C. N. (2009). Adenosine receptors and inflammation. *Handb. Exp. Pharmacol.* 193, 215–269. doi: 10.1007/978-3-540-89615-9_8

Blum, D., Gall, D., Galas, M.-C., D'alcantara, P., Bantubungi, K., and Schiffmann, S. N. (2002). The adenosine A 1 receptor agonist adenosine amine congener exerts a neuroprotective effect against the development of striatal lesions and motor impairments in the 3-nitropropionic acid model of neurotoxicity. *J. Neurosci.* 22, 9122–9133.

Bogacheva, P. O., and Balezina, O. P. (2015). Postsynaptic potentiation in mouse motor synapses induced by ATP accumulation in synaptic cleft. *Bull. Exp. Biol. Med.* 159, 583–587. doi: 10.1007/s10517-015-3018-2

Boison, D., Chen, J.-F., and Fredholm, B. B. (2010). Adenosine signaling and function in glial cells. *Cell Death Differ.* 17, 1071–1082. doi: 10.1038/cdd.2009.131

Borea, P. A., Gessi, S., Merighi, S., Vincenzi, F., and Varani, K. (2017). Pathological overproduction: the bad side of adenosine. *Br. J. Pharmacol.* 174, 1945–1960. doi: 10.1111/bph.13763

Braak, H., Del Tredici, K., Rüb, U., de Vos, R. A., Jansen Steur, E. N., and Braak, E. (2013). Staging of brain pathology related to sporadic Parkinson's disease. *Neurobiol. Aging* 24, 197–211. doi: 10.1016/S0197-4580(02)00065-9

Bradley, H. J., Baldwin, J. M., Goli, G. R., Johnson, B., Zou, J., Sivaprasadarao, A., et al. (2011). Residues 155 and 348 contribute to the determination of P2X7 receptor function via distinct mechanisms revealed by single-nucleotide polymorphisms. *J. Biol. Chem.* 286, 8176–8187. doi: 10.1074/jbc.M110.211284

Browne, S. E., Yang, L., DiMauro, J.-P., Fuller, S. W., Licata, S. C., and Beal, M. F. (2006). Bioenergetic abnormalities in discrete cerebral motor pathways presage spinal cord pathology in the G93A SOD1 mouse model of ALS. *Neurobiol. Dis.* 22, 599–610. doi: 10.1016/j.nbd.2006.01.001

Burghes, A. H., Ingraham, S. E., Kóte-Jarai, Z., Rosenfeld, S., Herta, N., Nadkarni, N., et al. (1994). Linkage mapping of the spinal muscular atrophy gene. *Hum. Genet.* 93, 305–312. doi: 10.1007/BF00212028

Burnstock, G. (1972). Purinergic nerves. *Pharmacol. Rev.* 24, 509–581.

Burnstock, G. (1997). The past, present and future of purine nucleotides as signalling molecules. *Neuropharmacology* 36, 1127–1139. doi: 10.1016/S0028-3908(97)00125-1

Burnstock, G. (2009). Purinergic cotransmission. *Exp. Physiol.* 94, 20–24. doi: 10.1113/expphysiol.2008.043620

Burnstock, G. (2016). An introduction to the roles of purinergic signalling in neurodegeneration, neuroprotection and neuroregeneration. *Neuropharmacology* 104, 4–17. doi: 10.1016/j.neuropharm.2015.05.031

Burnstock, G. (2017). The therapeutic potential of purinergic signalling. *Biochem. Pharmacol.* doi: 10.1016/j.bcp.2017.07.016. [Epub ahead of print].

Burnstock, G., Arnett, T. R., and Orriss, I. R. (2013). Purinergic signalling in the musculoskeletal system. *Purinergic Signal.* 9, 541–572. doi: 10.1007/s11302-013-9381-4

Burnstock, G., Fredholm, B. B., and Verkhratsky, A. (2011). Adenosine and ATP receptors in the brain. *Curr. Top. Med. Chem.* 11, 973–1011. doi: 10.2174/156802611795347627

Burnstock, G., Campbell, G., Satchell, D., and Smythe, A. (1970). Evidence that adenosine triphosphate or a related nucleotide is the transmitter substance released by non-adrenergic inhibitory nerves in the gut. *Br. J. Pharmacol.* 40, 668–688. doi: 10.1111/j.1476-5381.1970.tb10646.x

Butt, A. M. (2006). Neurotransmitter-mediated calcium signalling in oligodendrocyte physiology and pathology. *Glia* 54, 666–675. doi: 10.1002/glia.20424

Cabrini, G., Falzoni, S., Forchap, S. L., Pellegatti, P., Balboni, A., Agostini, P., et al. (2005). A His-155 to Tyr polymorphism confers gain-of-function to the human P2X7 receptor of human leukemic lymphocytes. *J. Immunol.* 175, 82–89. doi: 10.4049/jimmunol.175.1.82

Caragnano, M., Tortorella, P., Bergami, A., Ruggieri, M., Livrea, P., Specchio, L. M., et al. (2012). Monocytes P2X7 purinergic receptor is modulated by glatiramer acetate in multiple sclerosis. *J. Neuroimmunol.* 245, 93–97. doi: 10.1016/j.jneuroim.2012.02.002

Carmo, M. R., Menezes, A. P., Nunes, A. C., Pliássova, A., Rolo, A. P., Palmeira, C. M., et al. (2014). The P2X7 receptor antagonist Brilliant Blue G attenuates contralateral rotations in a rat model of Parkinsonism through a combined control of synaptotoxicity, neurotoxicity and gliosis. *Neuropharmacology* 81, 142–152. doi: 10.1016/j.neuropharm.2014.01.045

Casanovas, A., Hernández, S., Tarabal, O., Rosselló, J., and Esquerda, J. E. (2008). Strong P2X4 purinergic receptor-like immunoreactivity is selectively associated with degenerating neurons in transgenic rodent models of amyotrophic lateral sclerosis. *J. Comp. Neurol.* 506, 75–92. doi: 10.1002/cne.21527

Cha, J. H., Frey, A. S., Alsdorf, S. A., Kerner, J. A., Kosinski, C. M., Mangiarini, L., et al. (1999). Altered neurotransmitter receptor expression in transgenic mouse models of Huntington's disease. *Philos. Trans. R. Soc. Lond. B Biol. Sci.* 354, 981–989.

Cheffer, A., Castillo, A. R., Corrêa-Velloso, J. C., Gonçalves, M. C. B., Naaldijk, Y., Nascimento, I. C., et al. (2017). Purinergic system in psychiatric diseases. *Mol. Psychiatry* 23, 94–106. doi: 10.1038/mp.2017.188

Chen, L., and Brosnan, C. F. (2006). Exacerbation of experimental autoimmune encephalomyelitis in P2X7R-/- mice: evidence for loss of apoptotic activity in lymphocytes. *J. Immunol.* 176, 3115–3126. doi: 10.4049/jimmunol.176.5.3115

Chiang, M. C., Lee, Y. C., Huang, C. L., and Chern, Y. (2005). cAMP-response element-binding protein contributes to suppression of the A2A adenosine receptor promoter by mutant huntingtin with expanded polyglutamine residues. *J. Biol. Chem.* 280, 14331–14340. doi: 10.1074/jbc.M413279200

Chiu, F. L., Lin, J. T., Chuang, C. Y., Chien, T., Chen, C. M., Chen, K. H., et al. (2015). Elucidating the role of the A2Aadenosine receptor in neurodegeneration using neurons derived from Huntington's disease iPSCs. *Hum. Mol. Genet.* 24, 6066–6079. doi: 10.1093/hmg/ddv318

Chou, S.-Y., Lee, Y.-C., Chen, H.-M., Chiang, M.-C., Lai, H.-L., Chang, H.-H., et al. (2005). CGS21680 attenuates symptoms of Huntington's disease in a transgenic mouse model. *J. Neurochem.* 93, 310–320. doi: 10.1111/j.1471-4159.2005.03029.x

Ciruela, F., Casadó, V., Rodrigues, R. J., Luján, R., Burgueño, J., Canals, M., et al. (2006). Presynaptic control of striatal glutamatergic neurotransmission by adenosine A1-A2A receptor heteromers. *J. Neurosci.* 26, 2080–2087. doi: 10.1523/JNEUROSCI.3574-05.2006

Compston, A., and Coles, A. (2008). Multiple sclerosis. *Lancet* 372, 1502–1517. doi: 10.1016/S0140-6736(08)61620-7

Constantinescu, C. S., Farooqi, N., O'Brien, K., and Gran, B. (2011). Experimental autoimmune encephalomyelitis (EAE) as a model for multiple sclerosis (MS). *Br. J. Pharmacol.* 164, 1079–1106. doi: 10.1111/j.1476-5381.2011.01302.x

Correia-de-Sá, P., Sebastião, A. M., and Ribeiro, J. A. (1991). Inhibitory and excitatory effects of adenosine receptor agonists on evoked transmitter release from phrenic nerve endings of the rat. *Br. J. Pharmacol.* 103, 1614–1620. doi: 10.1111/j.1476-5381.1991.tb09836.x

Correia-de-Sá, P., Timóteo, M. A., and Ribeiro, J. A. (2002). A2A adenosine receptor facilitation of neuromuscular transmission. *J. Neurochem.* 74, 2462–2469. doi: 10.1046/j.1471-4159.2000.0742462.x

Crawford, T. O., and Pardo, C. A. (1996). The neurobiology of childhood spinal muscular atrophy. *Neurobiol. Dis.* 3, 97–110. doi: 10.1006/nbdi.1996.0010

Csóka, B., Töro, G., Vindeirinho, J., Varga, Z. V., Koscsó, B., Németh, Z. H., et al. (2017). A2A adenosine receptors control pancreatic dysfunction in high-fat-diet-induced obesity. *FASEB J.* 31, 4985–4997. doi: 10.1096/fj.201700398R

Cunha, R. A. (2008). Different cellular sources and different roles of adenosine: A1 receptor-mediated inhibition through astrocytic-driven volume transmission and synapse-restricted A2A receptor-mediated facilitation of plasticity. *Neurochem. Int.* 52, 65–72. doi: 10.1016/j.neuint.2007.06.026

Cunha, R. A. (2016). How does adenosine control neuronal dysfunction and neurodegeneration? *J. Neurochem.* 139, 1019–1055. doi: 10.1111/jnc.13724

D'Ambrosi, N., Finocchi, P., Apolloni, S., Cozzolino, M., Ferri, A., Padovano, V., et al. (2009). The proinflammatory action of microglial P2 receptors is enhanced in SOD1 models for amyotrophic lateral sclerosis. *J. Immunol.* 183, 4648–4656. doi: 10.4049/jimmunol.0901212

DeJesus-Hernandez, M., Mackenzie, I. R., Boeve, B. F., Boxer, A. L., Baker, M., Rutherford, N. J., et al. (2011). Expanded GGGGCC hexanucleotide repeat in noncoding region of C9ORF72 causes chromosome 9p-linked FTD and ALS. *Neuron* 72, 245–256. doi: 10.1016/j.neuron.2011.09.011

de Lau, L. M., and Breteler, M. M. (2006). Epidemiology of Parkinson's disease. *Lancet Neurol.* 5, 525–535. doi: 10.1016/S1474-4422(06)70471-9

Dendrou, C. A., Fugger, L., and Friese, M. A. (2015). Immunopathology of multiple sclerosis. *Nat. Rev. Immunol.* 15, 545–558. doi: 10.1038/nri3871

De Lorenzo, S., Veggetti, M., Muchnik, S., and Losavio, A. (2004). Presynaptic inhibition of spontaneous acetylcholine release induced by adenosine at the mouse neuromuscular junction. *Br. J. Pharmacol.* 142, 113–124. doi: 10.1038/sj.bjp.0705656

Deuchars, S. A., Atkinson, L., Brooke, R. E., Musa, H., Milligan, C. J., Batten, T. F., et al. (2001). Neuronal P2X7 receptors are targeted to presynaptic terminals in the central and peripheral nervous systems. *J. Neurosci.* 21, 7143–7152.

Dhaenens, C. M., Burnouf, S., Simonin, C., Van Brussel, E., Duhamel, A., Defebvre, L., et al. (2009). A genetic variation in the ADORA2A gene modifies age at onset in Huntington's disease. *Neurobiol. Dis.* 35, 474–476. doi: 10.1016/j.nbd.2009.06.009

Díaz-Hernández, M., Díez-Zaera, M., Sánchez-Nogueiro, J., Gómez-Villafuertes, R., Canals, J. M., Alberch, J., et al. (2009). Altered P2X7-receptor level and function in mouse models of Huntington's disease and therapeutic efficacy of antagonist administration. *FASEB J.* 23, 1893–906. doi: 10.1096/fj.08-122275

Domenici, M. R., Scattoni, M. L., Martire, A., Lastoria, G., Potenza, R. L., Borioni, A., et al. (2007). Behavioral and electrophysiological effects of the adenosine A 2A receptor antagonist SCH 58261 in R6/2 Huntington's disease mice. *Neurobiol. Dis.* 28, 197–205. doi: 10.1016/j.nbd.2007.07.009

Domercq, M., Perez-Samartin, A., Aparicio, D., Alberdi, E., Pampliega, O., and Matute, C. (2009). P2X7 receptors mediate ischemic damage to oligodendrocytes. *Glia* 58, 730–740. doi: 10.1002/glia.20958

Elbaz, A., Grigoletto, F., Baldereschi, M., Breteler, M. M., Manubens-Bertran, J. M., Lopez-Pousa, S., et al. (1999). Familial aggregation of Parkinson's disease: a population-based case-control study in Europe. EUROPARKINSON study group. *Neurology* 52, 1876–1882.

Eng, L. F., Ghirnikar, R. S., and Lee, Y. L. (1996). Inflammation in EAE: role of chemokine/cytokine expression by resident and infiltrating cells. *Neurochem. Res.* 21, 511–525. doi: 10.1007/BF02527717

Estévez, A. G., Sampson, J. B., Zhuang, Y. X., Spear, N., Richardson, G. J., Crow, J. P., et al. (2000). Liposome-delivered superoxide dismutase prevents nitric oxide-dependent motor neuron death induced by trophic factor withdrawal. *Free Radic. Biol. Med.* 28, 437–446. doi: 10.1016/S0891-5849(99)00261-0

Estévez, A. G., Spear, N., Manuel, S. M., Barbeito, L., Radi, R., and Beckman, J. S. (1998). Role of endogenous nitric oxide and peroxynitrite formation in the survival and death of motor neurons in culture. *Prog. Brain Res.* 118, 269–280. doi: 10.1016/S0079-6123(08)63214-8

Faas, M. M., Sáez, T., and de Vos, P. (2017). Extracellular ATP and adenosine: the Yin and Yang in immune responses? *Mol. Aspects Med.* 55, 9–19. doi: 10.1016/j.mam.2017.01.002

Färber, K., Markworth, S., Pannasch, U., Nolte, C., Prinz, V., Kronenberg, G., et al. (2008). The ectonucleotidase *cd39* /ENTPDase1 modulates purinergic-mediated microglial migration. *Glia* 56, 331–341. doi: 10.1002/glia.20606

Faria, R. X., Freitas, H. R., and Reis, R. A. M. (2017). P2X7 receptor large pore signaling in avian Müller glial cells. *J. Bioenerg. Biomembr.* 49, 215–229. doi: 10.1007/s10863-017-9717-9

Ferré, S. (2010). Role of the central ascending neurotransmitter systems in the psychostimulant effects of caffeine. *J. Alzheimers Dis.* 20, S35–S49. doi: 10.3233/JAD-2010-1400

Ferré, S., Agnati, L. F., Ciruela, F., Lluis, C., Woods, A. S., Fuxe, K., et al. (2007). Neurotransmitter receptor heteromers and their integrative role in "local modules": the striatal spine module. *Brain Res. Rev.* 55, 55–67. doi: 10.1016/j.brainresrev.2007.01.007

Ferré, S., Earley, C., Gulyani, S., and Garcia-Borreguero, D. (2017). In search of alternatives to dopaminergic ligands for the treatment of restless legs syndrome: iron, glutamate, and adenosine. *Sleep Med.* 31, 86–92. doi: 10.1016/j.sleep.2016.08.019

Ferré, S., O'Connor, W. T., Snaprud, P., Ungerstedt, U., and Fuxe, K. (1994). Antagonistic interaction between adenosine A2A receptors and dopamine D2 receptors in the ventral striopallidal system. Implications for the treatment of schizophrenia. *Neuroscience* 63, 765–773.

Ferre, S., O'Connor, W. T., Svenningsson, P., Bjorklund, L., Lindberg, J., Tinner, B., et al. (1996). Dopamine D1 receptor-mediated facilitation of GABAergic neurotransmission in the rat strioentopenduncular pathway and its modulation by adenosine A1 receptor-mediated mechanisms. *Eur. J. Neurosci.* 8, 1545–1553.

Ferré, S., Quiroz, C., Guitart, X., Rea, W., Seyedian, A., Moreno, E., et al. (2018). Pivotal role of adenosine neurotransmission in restless legs syndrome. *Front. Neurosci.* 11:722. doi: 10.3389/fnins.2017.00722

Ferraiuolo, L., Heath, P. R., Holden, H., Kasher, P., Kirby, J., and Shaw, P. J. (2007). Microarray analysis of the cellular pathways involved in the adaptation to and progression of motor neuron injury in the SOD1 G93A mouse model of familial ALS. *J. Neurosci.* 27, 9201–9219. doi: 10.1523/JNEUROSCI.1470-07.2007

Ferraiuolo, L., Higginbottom, A., Heath, P. R., Barber, S., Greenald, D., Kirby, J., et al. (2011). Dysregulation of astrocyte-motoneuron cross-talk in mutant superoxide dismutase 1-related amyotrophic lateral sclerosis. *Brain* 134, 2627–2641. doi: 10.1093/brain/awr193

Ferrante, A., Martire, A., Armida, M., Chiodi, V., Pézzola, A., Potenza, R. L., et al. (2010). Influence of CGS 21680, a selective adenosine A 2A receptor agonist, on NMDA receptor function and expression in the brain of Huntington's disease mice. *Brain Res.* 1323, 184–191. doi: 10.1016/j.brainres.2010.01.080

Ferrari, D., Villalba, M., Chiozzi, P., Falzoni, S., Ricciardi-Castagnoli, P., and Di Virgilio, F. (1996). Mouse microglial cells express a plasma membrane pore gated by extracellular ATP. *J. Immunol.* 156, 1531–1539.

Ferrazoli, E. G., de Souza, H. D. N., Nascimento, I. C., Oliveira-Giacomelli, Á., Schwindt, T. T., Britto, L. R., et al. (2017). Brilliant blue G, but not fenofibrate, treatment reverts hemiparkinsonian behavior and restores dopamine levels in an animal model of Parkinson's disease. *Cell Transplant.* 26, 669–677. doi: 10.3727/096368917X695227

Ferreira, D. G., Batalha, V. L., Vicente Miranda, H., Coelho, J. E., Gomes, R., Gonçalves, F. Q., et al. (2015). Adenosine A $_{2A}$ receptors modulate α-synuclein aggregation and toxicity. *Cereb. Cortex* 27:bhv268. doi: 10.1093/cercor/bhv268

Fields, R. D., and Burnstock, G. (2006). Purinergic signalling in neuron-glia interactions. *Nat. Rev. Neurosci.* 7, 423–436. doi: 10.1038/nrn1928

Fink, J. S., Kalda, A., Ryu, H., Stack, E. C., Schwarzschild, M. A., Chen, J. F., et al. (2004). Genetic and pharmacological inactivation of the adenosine A2Areceptor attenuates 3-nitropropionic acid-induced striatal damage. *J. Neurochem.* 88, 538–544. doi: 10.1046/j.1471-4159.2003.02145.x

Fink, J. S., Weaver, D. R., Rivkees, S. A., Peterfreund, R. A., Pollack, A. E., Adler, E. M., et al. (1992). Molecular cloning of the rat A2 adenosine receptor: selective co-expression with D2 dopamine receptors in rat striatum. *Brain Res. Mol. Brain Res.* 14, 186–195. doi: 10.1016/0169-328X(92)90173-9

Florenzano, F., Viscomi, M. T., Cavaliere, F., Volonté, C., and Molinari, M. (2002). Cerebellar lesion up-regulates P2X1 and P2X2 purinergic receptors in precerebellar nuclei. *Neuroscience* 115, 425–434. doi: 10.1016/S0306-4522(02)00397-4

Fondell, E., O'Reilly, É. I., Fitzgerald, K. C., Falcone, G. J., Kolonel, L. N., Park, Y., et al. (2015). Intakes of caffeine, coffee and tea and risk of amyotrophic lateral sclerosis: Results from five cohort studies. *Amyotroph. Lateral Scler. Front. Degener.* 16, 366–371. doi: 10.3109/21678421.2015.1020813

Förster, D., and Reiser, G. (2015). Supportive or detrimental roles of P2Y receptors in brain pathology?-The two faces of P2Y receptors in stroke and neurodegeneration detected in neural cell and in animal model studies. *Purinergic Signal.* 11, 441–454. doi: 10.1007/s11302-015-9471-6

Franco, M. C., Ye, Y., Refakis, C. A., Feldman, J. L., Stokes, A. L., Basso, M., et al. (2013). Nitration of Hsp90 induces cell death. *Proc. Natl. Acad. Sci. U.S.A.* 110, E1102–E1111. doi: 10.1073/pnas.1215177110

Franke, H., Günther, A., Grosche, J., Schmidt, R., Rossner, S., Reinhardt, R., et al. (2004). P2X7 receptor expression after ischemia in the cerebral cortex of rats. *J. Neuropathol. Exp. Neurol.* 63, 686–699. doi: 10.1093/jnen/63.7.686

Fredholm, B. B., Bättig, K., Holmén, J., Nehlig, A., and Zvartau, E. E. (1999). Actions of caffeine in the brain with special reference to factors that contribute to its widespread use. *Pharmacol. Rev.* 51, 83–133.

Fryer, H. J., Wolf, D. H., Knox, R. J., Strittmatter, S. M., Pennica, D., O'Leary, R. M., et al. (2001). Brain-derived neurotrophic factor induces excitotoxic sensitivity in cultured embryonic rat spinal motor neurons through activation of the phosphatidylinositol 3-kinase pathway. *J. Neurochem.* 74, 582–595. doi: 10.1046/j.1471-4159.2000.740582.x

Fuchs, A., Kutterer, S., Mühling, T., Duda, J., Schütz, B., Liss, B., et al. (2013). Selective mitochondrial Ca $^{2+}$ uptake deficit in disease endstage vulnerable motoneurons of the SOD1 ^{G93A} mouse model of amyotrophic lateral sclerosis. *J. Physiol. (Lond).* 591, 2723–2745. doi: 10.1113/jphysiol.2012.247981

Fuzzati-Armentero, M.-T., Cerri, S., Levandis, G., Ambrosi, G., Montepeloso, E., Antoninetti, G., et al. (2015). Dual target strategy: combining distinct non-dopaminergic treatments reduces neuronal cell loss and synergistically modulates l -DOPA-induced rotational behavior in a rodent model of Parkinson's disease. *J. Neurochem.* 134, 740–747. doi: 10.1111/jnc.13162

Gabanella, F., Butchbach, M. E., Saieva, L., Carissimi, C., Burghes, A. H., and Pellizzoni, L. (2007). Ribonucleoprotein assembly defects correlate with spinal muscular atrophy severity and preferentially affect a subset of spliceosomal snRNPs. *PLoS ONE* 2:e921. doi: 10.1371/journal.pone.0000921

Gan, M., Moussaud, S., Jiang, P., and McLean, P. J. (2015). Extracellular ATP induces intracellular alpha-synuclein accumulation via P2X1 receptor-mediated lysosomal dysfunction. *Neurobiol. Aging* 36, 1209–1220. doi: 10.1016/j.neurobiolaging.2014.10.037

Gandelman, M., Levy, M., Cassina, P., Barbeito, L., and Beckman, J. S. (2013). P2X7 receptor-induced death of motor neurons by a peroxynitrite/FAS-dependent pathway. *J. Neurochem.* 126, 382–388. doi: 10.1111/jnc.12286

Gandelman, M., Peluffo, H., Beckman, J. S., Cassina, P., and Barbeito, L. (2010). Extracellular ATP and the P2X7 receptor in astrocyte-mediated motor neuron death: implications for amyotrophic lateral sclerosis. *J. Neuroinflammation* 7:33. doi: 10.1186/1742-2094-7-33

Garcia-Borreguero, D., and Cano-Pumarega, I. (2017). New concepts in the management of restless legs syndrome. *BMJ* 356:j104. doi: 10.1136/bmj.j104

Gavrilina, T. O., McGovern, V. L., Workman, E., Crawford, T. O., Gogliotti, R. G., DiDonato, C. J., et al. (2008). Neuronal SMN expression corrects spinal muscular atrophy in severe SMA mice while muscle-specific SMN expression has no phenotypic effect. *Hum. Mol. Genet.* 17, 1063–1075. doi: 10.1093/hmg/ddm379

Gianfriddo, M., Corsi, C., Melani, A., Pèzzola, A., Reggio, R., Popoli, P., et al. (2003). A denosine A antagonism increases striatal glutamate outflow in the 2A quinolinic acid rat model of Huntington's disease. *Brain Res.* 979, 225–229. doi: 10.1016/S0006-8993(03)02942-1

Gianfriddo, M., Melani, A., Turchi, D., Giovannini, M. G., and Pedata, F. (2004). Adenosine and glutamate extracellular concentrations and mitogen-activated protein kinases in the striatum of Huntington transgenic mice. Selective antagonism of adenosine A_{2A} receptors reduces transmitter outflow. *Neurobiol. Dis.* 17, 77–88. doi: 10.1016/j.nbd.2004.05.008

Glass, M., Dragunow, M., and Faull, R. L. (2000). The pattern of neurodegeneration in Huntington's disease: a comparative study of cannabinoid, dopamine, adenosine and GABA(A) receptor alterations in the human basal ganglia in Huntington's disease. *Neuroscience* 97, 505–519. doi: 10.1016/S0306-4522(00)00008-7

Goldenberg, M. M. (2012). Multiple sclerosis review. *P T* 37, 175–184.

Gołembiowska, K., Wardas, J., Noworyta-Sokołowska, K., Kaminska, K., and Górska, A. (2013). Effects of adenosine receptor antagonists on the *in vivo* LPS-induced inflammation model of Parkinson's disease. *Neurotox. Res.* 24, 29–40. doi: 10.1007/s12640-012-9372-1

Gonçalves, N., Simões, A. T., Cunha, R. A., and de Almeida, L. P. (2013). Caffeine and adenosine A_{2A} receptor inactivation decrease striatal neuropathology in a lentiviral-based model of Machado-Joseph disease. *Ann. Neurol.* 73, 655–666. doi: 10.1002/ana.23866

Gonçalves, N., Simões, A. T., Prediger, R. D., Hirai, H., Cunha, R. A., and Pereira de Almeida, L. (2017). Caffeine alleviates progressive motor deficits in a transgenic mouse model of spinocerebellar ataxia. *Ann. Neurol.* 81, 407–418. doi: 10.1002/ana.24867

Grundström, E., Lindholm, D., Johansson, A., Blennow, K., and Askmark, H. (2000). GDNF but not BDNF is increased in cerebrospinal fluid in amyotrophic lateral sclerosis. *Neuroreport* 11, 1781–1783. doi: 10.1097/00001756-200006050-00037

Grygorowicz, T., Sulejczak, D., and Struzynska, L. (2011). Expression of purinergic P2X7 receptor in rat brain during the symptomatic phase of experimental autoimmune encephalomyelitis and after recovery of neurological deficits. *Acta Neurobiol. Exp.* 71, 65–73.

Gu, B. J., Field, J., Dutertre, S., Ou, A., Kilpatrick, T. J., Lechner-Scott, J., et al. (2015). A rare P2X7 variant Arg307Gln with absent pore formation function protects against neuroinflammation in multiple sclerosis. *Hum. Mol. Genet.* 24, 5644–5654. doi: 10.1093/hmg/ddv278

Gu, B. J., Zhang, W., Worthington, R. A., Sluyter, R., Dao-Ung, P., Petrou, S., et al. (2001). A Glu-496 to Ala polymorphism leads to loss of function of the human P2X7 receptor. *J. Biol. Chem.* 276, 11135–11142. doi: 10.1074/jbc.M010353200

Gulyani, S., Earley, C. J., Camandola, S., Maudsley, S., Ferré, S., Mughal, M. R., et al. (2009). Diminished iron concentrations increase adenosine A_{2A} receptor levels in mouse striatum and cultured human neuroblastoma cells. *Exp. Neurol.* 215, 236–242. doi: 10.1016/j.expneurol.2008.10.007

Gyoneva, S., Shapiro, L., Lazo, C., Garnier-Amblard, E., Smith, Y., Miller, G. W., et al. (2014). Adenosine A_{2A} receptor antagonism reverses inflammation-induced impairment of microglial process extension in a model of Parkinson's disease. *Neurobiol. Dis.* 67, 191–202. doi: 10.1016/j.nbd.2014.03.004

Hamza, T. H., Chen, H., Hill-Burns, E. M., Rhodes, S. L., Montimurro, J., Kay, D. M., et al. (2011). Genome-wide gene-environment study identifies glutamate receptor gene GRIN2A as a Parkinson's disease modifier gene via interaction with coffee. *PLoS Genet.* 7:e1002237. doi: 10.1371/journal.pgen.1002237

Harms, M. B., and Baloh, R. H. (2013). Clinical neurogenetics: amyotrophic lateral sclerosis. *Neurol. Clin.* 31, 929–950. doi: 10.1016/j.ncl.2013.05.003

Haskó, G. (2004). Adenosine: an endogenous regulator of innate immunity. *Trends Immunol.* 25, 33–39. doi: 10.1016/j.it.2003.11.003

Haynes, S. E., Hollopeter, G., Yang, G., Kurpius, D., Dailey, M. E., Gan, W.-B., et al. (2006). The P2Y12 receptor regulates microglial activation by extracellular nucleotides. *Nat. Neurosci.* 9, 1512–1519. doi: 10.1038/nn1805

He, Y., Taylor, N., Fourgeaud, L., and Bhattacharya, A. (2017). The role of microglial P2X7: modulation of cell death and cytokine release. *J. Neuroinflammation* 14:135. doi: 10.1186/s12974-017-0904-8

Hedström, A. K., Mowry, E. M., Gianfrancesco, M. A., Shao, X., Schaefer, C. A., Shen, L., et al. (2016). High consumption of coffee is associated with decreased multiple sclerosis risk; results from two independent studies. *J. Neurol. Neurosurg. Psychiatry* 87, 454–460. doi: 10.1136/jnnp-2015-312176

Hettinger, B. D., Lee, A., Linden, J., and Rosin, D. L. (2001). Ultrastructural localization of adenosine A2A receptors suggests multiple cellular sites for modulation of GABAergic neurons in rat striatum. *J. Comp. Neurol.* 431, 331–346. doi: 10.1002/1096-9861(20010312)431:3<331::AID-CNE1074>3.0.CO;2-W

Hoang, Q. Q. (2014). Pathway for Parkinson disease. *Proc. Natl. Acad. Sci. U.S.A.* 111, 2402–2403. doi: 10.1073/pnas.1324284111

Hu, P., and Kalb, R. G. (2003). BDNF heightens the sensitivity of motor neurons to excitotoxic insults through activation of TrkB. *J. Neurochem.* 84, 1421–1430. doi: 10.1046/j.1471-4159.2003.01599.x

Hu, Q., Ren, X., Liu, Y., Li, Z., Zhang, L., Chen, X., et al. (2016). Aberrant adenosine A2A receptor signaling contributes to neurodegeneration and cognitive impairments in a mouse model of synucleinopathy. *Exp. Neurol.* 283, 213–223. doi: 10.1016/j.expneurol.2016.05.040

Illes, P., Khan, T. M., and Rubini, P. (2017). Neuronal P2X7 receptors revisited: do they really exist? *J. Neurosci.* 37, 7049–7062. doi: 10.1523/JNEUROSCI.3103-16.2017

Illes, P., and Verkhratsky, A. (2016). Purinergic neurone-glia signalling in cognitive-related pathologies. *Neuropharmacology* 104, 62–75. doi: 10.1016/j.neuropharm.2015.08.005

Inoue, K. (2017). Purinergic signaling in microglia in the pathogenesis of neuropathic pain. *Proc. Japan Acad. Ser. B* 93, 174–182. doi: 10.2183/pjab.93.011

Ishikawa, Y., Ikeuchi, T., and Hatanaka, H. (2000). Brain-derived neurotrophic factor accelerates nitric oxide donor-induced apoptosis of cultured cortical neurons. *J. Neurochem.* 75, 494–502. doi: 10.1046/j.1471-4159.2000.0750494.x

Ishiwata, K., Ogi, N., Hayakawa, N., Oda, K., Nagaoka, T., Toyama, H., et al. (2002). Adenosine A_{2A} receptor imaging with $[^{11}C]$KF18446 PET in the rat brain after quinolinic acid lesion: comparison with the dopamine receptor imaging. *Ann. Nucl. Med.* 16, 467–475. doi: 10.1007/BF02988643

Jablonka, S., Rossoll, W., Schrank, B., and Sendtner, M. (2000). The role of SMN in spinal muscular atrophy. *J. Neurol.* 247(Suppl. 1), I37–I42. doi: 10.1007/s004150050555

Jellinger, K. A. (2011). "Parkinson's disease," in *Neurodegeneration : The Molecular Pathology of Dementia and Movement Disorders*, eds D. W. Dickson and R. O. Welle (Bassel: Wiley-Blackwell), 477.

Jiang, T., Hoekstra, J., Heng, X., Kang, W., Ding, J., Liu, J., et al. (2015). P2X7 receptor is critical in α-synuclein–mediated microglial NADPH oxidase activation. *Neurobiol. Aging* 36, 2304–2318. doi: 10.1016/j.neurobiolaging.2015.03.015

Jiménez, M., Clavé, P., Accarino, A., and Gallego, D. (2014). Purinergic neuromuscular transmission in the gastrointestinal tract; functional basis for future clinical and pharmacological studies. *Br. J. Pharmacol.* 171, 4360–4375. doi: 10.1111/bph.12802

Johnston, J. B., Silva, C., Gonzalez, G., Holden, J., Warren, K. G., Metz, L. M., et al. (2001). Diminished adenosine A1 receptor expression on macrophages in brain and blood of patients with multiple sclerosis. *Ann. Neurol.* 49, 650–658. doi: 10.1002/ana.1007

Jung, C., Higgins, C. M., and Xu, Z. (2002). Mitochondrial electron transport chain complex dysfunction in a transgenic mouse model for amyotrophic lateral sclerosis. *J. Neurochem.* 83, 535–545. doi: 10.1046/j.1471-4159.2002.01112.x

Kachroo, A., and Schwarzschild, M. A. (2012). Adenosine A_{2A} receptor gene disruption protects in an α-synuclein model of Parkinson's disease. *Ann. Neurol.* 71, 278–282. doi: 10.1002/ana.22630

Kalmar, J. M. (2005). The influence of caffeine on voluntary muscle activation. *Med. Sci. Sports Exerc.* 37, 2113–2119. doi: 10.1249/01.mss.0000178219.18086.9e

Kanda, T., Jackson, M. J., Smith, L. A., Pearce, R. K., Nakamura, J., Kase, H., et al. (2000). Combined use of the adenosine A2A antagonist KW-6002 with l-DOPA or with selective D1 or D2 dopamine agonists increases antiparkinsonian activity but not dyskinesia in MPTP-treated monkeys. *Exp. Neurol.* 162, 321–327. doi: 10.1006/exnr.2000.7350

Karcz-Kubicha, M., Antoniou, K., Terasmaa, A., Quarta, D., Solinas, M., Justinova, Z., et al. (2003). Involvement of adenosine A1 and A2A receptors in the motor effects of caffeine after its acute and chronic administration. *Neuropsychopharmacology* 28, 1281–1291. doi: 10.1038/sj.npp.1300167

Kazemi, M. H., Raoofi Mohseni, S., Hojjat-Farsangi, M., Anvari, E., Ghalamfarsa, G., Mohammadi, H., et al. (2018). Adenosine and adenosine receptors in the immunopathogenesis and treatment of cancer. *J. Cell. Physiol.* 233, 2032–2057. doi: 10.1002/jcp.25873

Khakh, B. S., and Alan North, R. (2006). P2X receptors as cell-surface ATP sensors in health and disease. *Nature* 442, 527–532. doi: 10.1038/nature04886

Kiernan, M. C., Vucic, S., Cheah, B. C., Turner, M. R., Eisen, A., Hardiman, O., et al. (2011). Amyotrophic lateral sclerosis. *Lancet* 377, 942–955. doi: 10.1016/S0140-6736(10)61156-7

Kim, B., Jeong, H. K., Kim, J. H., Lee, S. Y., Jou, I., and Joe, E. H. (2011). Uridine 5′-diphosphate induces chemokine expression in microglia and astrocytes through activation of the P2Y6 receptor. *J. Immunol.* 186, 3701–3709. doi: 10.4049/jimmunol.1000212

Kim, H. (2003). TrkB mediates BDNF-induced potentiation of neuronal necrosis in cortical culture. *Neurobiol. Dis.* 14, 110–119. doi: 10.1016/S0969-9961(03)00103-7

Kim, T., and Vemuganti, R. (2017). Mechanisms of Parkinson's disease-related proteins in mediating secondary brain damage after cerebral ischemia. *J. Cereb. Blood Flow Metab.* 37, 1910–1926. doi: 10.1177/0271678X17694186

Kobayashi, S., Conforti, L., Pun, R. Y. K., and Millhorn, D. E. (1998). Adenosine modulates hypoxia-induced responses in rat PC12 cells via the A_{2A} receptor. *J. Physiol.* 508, 95–107. doi: 10.1111/j.1469-7793.1998.095br.x

Koehler, N. K., Genain, C. P., Giesser, B., and Hauser, S. L. (2002). The human T cell response to myelin oligodendrocyte glycoprotein: a multiple sclerosis family-based study. *J. Immunol.* 168, 5920–5927. doi: 10.4049/jimmunol.168.11.5920

Koh, J., Gwag, B. J., Lobner, D., and Choi, D. W. (1995). Potentiated necrosis of cultured cortical neurons by neurotrophins. *Science* 268, 573–575. doi: 10.1126/science.7725105

Krügel, U. (2016). Purinergic receptors in psychiatric disorders. *Neuropharmacology* 104, 212–225. doi: 10.1016/j.neuropharm.2015.10.032

Kumar, P. M., Paing, S. S., Li, H., Pavanni, R., Yuen, Y., Zhao, Y., et al. (2015). Differential effect of caffeine intake in subjects with genetic susceptibility to Parkinson's Disease. *Sci. Rep.* 5:15492. doi: 10.1038/srep15492

Labazi, H., Teng, B., and Mustafa, S. J. (2018). Functional changes in vascular reactivity to adenosine receptor activation in type I diabetic mice. *Eur. J. Pharmacol.* 820, 191–197. doi: 10.1016/j.ejphar.2017.12.034

Lang, A. E. (2009). When and how should treatment be started in Parkinson disease? *Neurology* 72, S39–S43. doi: 10.1212/WNL.0b013e318198e177

Lapato, A. S., and Tiwari-Woodruff, S. K. (2017). Connexins and pannexins: At the junction of neuro-glial homeostasis & disease. *J. Neurosci. Res.* 96, 31–44. doi: 10.1002/jnr.24088

Lassmann, H. (1983). Chronic relapsing experimental allergic encephalomyelitis: its value as an experimental model for multiple sclerosis. *J. Neurol.* 229, 207–220. doi: 10.1007/BF00313549

Lecca, D., Ceruti, S., Fumagalli, M., and Abbracchio, M. P. (2012). Purinergic trophic signalling in glial cells: functional effects and modulation of cell proliferation, differentiation, and death. *Purinergic Signal.* 8, 539–557. doi: 10.1007/s11302-012-9310-y

Lederer, C. W., Torrisi, A., Pantelidou, M., Santama, N., and Cavallaro, S. (2007). Pathways and genes differentially expressed in the motor cortex of patients with sporadic amyotrophic lateral sclerosis. *BMC Genomics* 8:26. doi: 10.1186/1471-2164-8-26

Lee, F. S., and Chao, M. V. (2001). Activation of Trk neurotrophin receptors in the absence of neurotrophins. *Proc. Natl. Acad. Sci. U.S.A.* 98, 3555–3560. doi: 10.1073/pnas.061020198

Lee, J. Y., Jhun, B. S., Oh, Y. T., Lee, J. H., Choe, W., Baik, H. H., et al. (2006). Activation of adenosine A3 receptor suppresses lipopolysaccharide-induced TNF-alpha production through inhibition of PI 3-kinase/Akt and NF-kappaB activation in murine BV2 microglial cells. *Neurosci. Lett.* 396, 1–6. doi: 10.1016/j.neulet.2005.11.004

Lefebvre, S., Bürglen, L., Reboullet, S., Clermont, O., Burlet, P., Viollet, L., et al. (1995). Identification and characterization of a spinal muscular atrophy-determining gene. *Cell* 80, 155–165. doi: 10.1016/0092-8674(95)90460-3

Lefebvre, S., Burlet, P., Liu, Q., Bertrandy, S., Clermont, O., Munnich, A., et al. (1997). Correlation between severity and SMN protein level in spinal muscular atrophy. *Nat. Genet.* 16, 265–269. doi: 10.1038/ng0797-265

Levy, O., Coughlin, M., Cronstein, B. N., Roy, R. M., Desai, A., and Wessels, M. R. (2006). The adenosine system selectively inhibits TLR-mediated TNF-alpha production in the human newborn. *J. Immunol.* 177, 1956–1966. doi: 10.4049/jimmunol.177.3.1956

Li, J. Y., Popovic, N., and Brundin, P. (2005). The use of the R6 transgenic mouse models of Huntington's disease in attempts to develop novel therapeutic strategies. *NeuroRx* 2, 447–464. doi: 10.1602/neurorx.2.3.447

Li, S. N., and Wong, P. T. (2000). The adenosine receptor agonist, APNEA, increases calcium influx into rat cortical synaptosomes through N-type channels associated with A2a receptors. *Neurochem. Res.* 25, 457–459. doi: 10.1023/A:1007503907823

Li, W., Silva, H. B., Real, J., Wang, Y.-M., Rial, D., Li, P., et al. (2015). Inactivation of adenosine A2A receptors reverses working memory deficits at early stages of Huntington's disease models. *Neurobiol. Dis.* 79, 70–80. doi: 10.1016/j.nbd.2015.03.030

Lindberg, D., Shan, D., Ayers-Ringler, J., Oliveros, A., Benitez, J., Prieto, M., et al. (2015). Purinergic signaling and energy homeostasis in psychiatric disorders. *Curr. Mol. Med.* 15, 275–295. doi: 10.2174/156652401566615033016 3724

Lister, M. F., Sharkey, J., Sawatzky, D. A., Hodgkiss, J. P., Davidson, D. J., Rossi, A. G., et al. (2007). The role of the purinergic P2X7 receptor in inflammation. *J. Inflamm. (Lond).* 4:5. doi: 10.1186/1476-9255-4-5

Liu, H., Han, X., Li, Y., Zou, H., and Xie, A. (2013). Association of P2X7 receptor gene polymorphisms with sporadic Parkinson's disease in a Han Chinese population. *Neurosci. Lett.* 546, 42–45. doi: 10.1016/j.neulet.2013.04.049

Liu, Y.-J., Lee, L.-M., Lai, H.-L., and Chern, Y. (2015). Aberrant activation of AMP-activated protein kinase contributes to the abnormal distribution of HuR in amyotrophic lateral sclerosis. *FEBS Lett.* 589, 432–439. doi: 10.1016/j.febslet.2014.12.029

Lo, J.-C., Huang, W.-C., Chou, Y.-C., Tseng, C.-H., Lee, W.-L., and Sun, S. H. (2008). Activation of P2X$_7$ receptors decreases glutamate uptake and glutamine synthetase activity in RBA-2 astrocytes via distinct mechanisms. *J. Neurochem.* 105, 151–164. doi: 10.1111/j.1471-4159.2007.05119.x

Lomen-Hoerth, C. (2011). Clinical phenomenology and neuroimaging correlates in ALS-FTD. *J. Mol. Neurosci.* 45, 656–662. doi: 10.1007/s12031-011-9636-x

Lotti, F., Imlach, W. L., Saieva, L., Beck, E. S., Hao, L. T., Li, D. K., et al. (2012). An SMN-dependent U12 splicing event essential for motor circuit function. *Cell* 151, 440–454. doi: 10.1016/j.cell.2012.09.012

Lovatt, D., Sonnewald, U., Waagepetersen, H. S., Schousboe, A., He, W., Lin, J. H.-C., et al. (2007). The transcriptome and metabolic gene signature of protoplasmic astrocytes in the adult murine cortex. *J. Neurosci.* 27, 12255–12266. doi: 10.1523/JNEUROSCI.3404-07.2007

Lu, W., Albalawi, F., Beckel, J. M., Lim, J. C., Laties, A. M., and Mitchell, C. H. (2017). The P2X7 receptor links mechanical strain to cytokine IL-6 up-regulation and release in neurons and astrocytes. *J. Neurochem.* 141, 436–448. doi: 10.1111/jnc.13998

Luo, C., Jian, C., Liao, Y., Huang, Q., Wu, Y., Liu, X., et al. (2017). The role of microglia in multiple sclerosis. *Neuropsychiatr. Dis. Treat.* 13, 1661–1667. doi: 10.2147/NDT.S140634

Luthi-Carter, R., Strand, A., Peters, N. L., Solano, S. M., Hollingsworth, Z. R., Menon, A. S., et al. (2000). Decreased expression of striatal signaling genes in a mouse model of Huntington's disease. *Hum. Mol. Genet.* 9, 1259–1271. doi: 10.1093/hmg/9.9.1259

Madeira, M. H., Boia, R., Ambrósio, A. F., and Santiago, A. R. (2017). Having a coffee break: the impact of caffeine consumption on microglia-mediated inflammation in neurodegenerative diseases. *Mediators Inflamm.* 2017, 1–12. doi: 10.1155/2017/4761081

Maglione, V., Cannella, M., Martino, T., De Blasi, A., Frati, L., and Squitieri, F. (2005a). The platelet maximum number of A2A-receptor binding sites (Bmax) linearly correlates with age at onset and CAG repeat expansion in Huntington's disease patients with predominant chorea. *Neurosci. Lett.* 393, 27–30. doi: 10.1016/j.neulet.2005.09.037

Maglione, V., Giallonardo, P., Cannella, M., Martino, T., Frati, L., and Squitieri, F. (2005b). Adenosine A_{2A} receptor dysfunction correlates with age at onset anticipation in blood platelets of subjects with Huntington's disease. *Am. J. Med. Genet.* 139B, 101–105. doi: 10.1002/ajmg.b.30223

Mamedova, L. K., Gao, Z.-G., and Jacobson, K. A. (2006). Regulation of death and survival in astrocytes by ADP activating P2Y1 and P2Y12 receptors. *Biochem. Pharmacol.* 72, 1031–1041. doi: 10.1016/j.bcp.2006.07.017

Marcellino, D., Suárez-Boomgaard, D., Sánchez-Reina, M. D., Aguirre, J. A., Yoshitake, T., Yoshitake, S., et al. (2010). On the role of P2X7 receptors in dopamine nerve cell degeneration in a rat model of Parkinson's disease: studies with the P2X7 receptor antagonist A-438079. *J. Neural Transm.* 117, 681–687. doi: 10.1007/s00702-010-0400-0

Mariotti, C., Fancellu, R., and Donato, S. (2005). An overview of the patient with ataxia. *J. Neurol.* 252, 511–518. doi: 10.1007/s00415-005-0814-z

Martinez-Mir, M. I., Probst, A., and Palacios, J. M. (1991). Adenosine A2 receptors: Selective localization in the human basal ganglia and alterations with disease. *Neuroscience* 42, 697–706. doi: 10.1016/0306-4522(91)90038-P

Martire, A., Calamandrei, G., Felici, F., Scattoni, M. L., Lastoria, G., Domenici, M. R., et al. (2007). Opposite effects of the A_{2A} receptor agonist CGS21680 in the striatum of Huntington's disease versus wild-type mice.*Neurosci. Lett.* 417, 78–83. doi: 10.1016/j.neulet.2007.02.034

Martire, A., Ferrante, A., Potenza, R. L., Armida, M., Ferretti, R., Pézzola, A., et al. (2010). Remodeling of striatal NMDA receptors by chronic A2A receptor blockade in Huntington's disease mice. *Neurobiol. Dis.* 37, 99–105. doi: 10.1016/j.nbd.2009.09.012

Matilla-Dueñas, A., Corral-Juan, M., Volpini, V., and Sanchez, I. (2012). *The Spinocerebellar Ataxias: Clinical Aspects And Molecular Genetics.* New York, NY: Springer.

Mattiazzi, M., D'Aurelio, M., Gajewski, C. D., Martushova, K., Kiaei, M., Beal, M. F., et al. (2002). Mutated human SOD1 causes dysfunction of oxidative phosphorylation in mitochondria of transgenic mice. *J. Biol. Chem.* 277, 29626–29633. doi: 10.1074/jbc.M203065200

Matute, C. (2011). Glutamate and ATP signalling in white matter pathology. *J. Anat.* 219, 53–64. doi: 10.1111/j.1469-7580.2010.01339.x

Matute, C., Torre, I., Perez-Cerda, F., Perez-Samartin, A., Alberdi, E., Etxebarria, E., et al. (2007). P2X7 Receptor blockade prevents ATP excitotoxicity in oligodendrocytes and ameliorates experimental autoimmune encephalomyelitis. *J. Neurosci.* 27, 9525–9533. doi: 10.1523/JNEUROSCI.0579-07.2007

Mayne, M., Shepel, P. N., Jiang, Y., Geiger, J. D., and Power, C. (1999). Dysregulation of Adenosine A 1 Receptor– Mediated Cytokine Expression in Peripheral Blood Mononuclear Cells from Multiple Sclerosis Patients. *Ann. Neurol.* 45, 633–639. doi: 10.1002/1531-8249(199905)45:5<633::AID-ANA12>3.0.CO;2-X

McGivern, J. V., Patitucci, T. N., Nord, J. A., Barabas, M. A., Stucky, C. L., and Ebert, A. D. (2013). Spinal muscular atrophy astrocytes exhibit abnormal calcium regulation and reduced growth factor production. *Glia* 61, 1418–1428. doi: 10.1002/glia.22522

Menzies, F. M., Cookson, M. R., Taylor, R. W., Turnbull, D. M., Chrzanowska-Lightowlers, Z. M., Dong, L., et al. (2002). Mitochondrial dysfunction in a cell culture model of familial amyotrophic lateral sclerosis. *Brain* 125, 1522–1533. doi: 10.1093/brain/awf167

Mievis, S., Blum, D., and Ledent, C. (2011). A_{2A} receptor knockout worsens survival and motor behaviour in a transgenic mouse model of Huntington's disease. *Neurobiol. Dis.* 41, 570–576. doi: 10.1016/j.nbd.2010.09.021

Miles, G. B., Parkis, M. A., Lipski, J., and Funk, G. D. (2002). Modulation of phrenic motoneuron excitability by ATP: consequences for respiratory-related output *in vitro. J. Appl. Physiol.* 92, 1899–1910. doi: 10.1152/japplphysiol. 00475.2001

Miller, S. D., and Karpus, W. J. (1994). The immunopathogenesis and regulation of T-cell-mediated demyelinating diseases. *Immunol. Today* 15, 356–361. doi: 10.1016/0167-5699(94)90173-2

Mills, J. H., Kim, D.-G., Krenz, A., Chen, J.-F., and Bynoe, M. S. (2012). A2A adenosine receptor signaling in lymphocytes and the central nervous system regulates inflammation during experimental autoimmune encephalomyelitis. *J. Immunol.* 188, 5713–5722. doi: 10.4049/jimmunol.1200545

Mills, J. H., Thompson, L. F., Mueller, C., Waickman, A. T., Jalkanen, S., Niemela, J., et al. (2008). CD73 is required for efficient entry of lymphocytes into the central nervous system during experimental autoimmune encephalomyelitis. *Proc. Natl. Acad. Sci. U.S.A.* 105, 9325–9330. doi: 10.1073/pnas.0711175105

Minghetti, L. (2004). Cyclooxygenase-2 (COX-2) in inflammatory and degenerative brain diseases. *J. Neuropathol. Exp. Neurol.* 63, 901–910. doi: 10.1093/jnen/63.9.901

Miras-Portugal, M. T., Sebastián-Serrano, Á., de Diego García, L., and Díaz-Hernández, M. (2017). Neuronal P2X7 Receptor: Involvement in Neuronal Physiology and Pathology. *J. Neurosci.* 37, 7063–7072. doi: 10.1523/JNEUROSCI.3104-16.2017

Mojsilovic-Petrovic, J., Jeong, G.-B., Crocker, A., Arneja, A., David, S., Russell, D., et al. (2006). protecting motor neurons from toxic insult by antagonism of adenosine A2a and Trk receptors. *J. Neurosci.* 26, 9250–9263. doi: 10.1523/JNEUROSCI.1856-06.2006

Moreno, E., Chiarlone, A., Medrano, M., Puigdellívol, M., Bibic, L., Howell, L. A., et al. (2017). Singular location and signaling profile of adenosine A 2A-Cannabinoid CB 1 receptor heteromers in the dorsal striatum. *Neuropsychopharmacology* 43, 964–977. doi: 10.1038/npp.2017.12

Narcisse, L., Scemes, E., Zhao, Y., Lee, S. C., and Brosnan, C. F. (2005). The cytokine IL-1beta transiently enhances P2X7 receptor expression and function in human astrocytes. *Glia* 49, 245–258. doi: 10.1002/glia.20110

Nascimento, F., Sebastião, A. M., and Ribeiro, J. A. (2015). Presymptomatic and symptomatic ALS SOD1(G93A) mice differ in adenosine A1 and A2A receptor-mediated tonic modulation of neuromuscular transmission. *Purinergic Signal.* 11, 471–480. doi: 10.1007/s11302-015-9465-4

Neher, J. J., Neniskyte, U., Hornik, T., and Brown, G. C. (2014). Inhibition of UDP/P2Y $_6$ purinergic signaling prevents phagocytosis of viable neurons by activated microglia *in vitro* and *in vivo*. *Glia* 62, 1463–1475. doi: 10.1002/glia.22693

Ng, S. K., kah, Higashimori, H., Tolman, M., and Yang, Y. (2015). Suppression of adenosine 2a receptor (A2aR)-mediated adenosine signaling improves disease phenotypes in a mouse model of amyotrophic lateral sclerosis. *Exp. Neurol.* 267, 115–122. doi: 10.1016/j.expneurol.2015.03.004

North, R. A. (2002). Molecular Physiology of P2X Receptors. *Physiol. Rev.* 82, 1013–1067. doi: 10.1152/physrev.00015.2002

Olanow, C. W., Stern, M. B., and Sethi, K. (2009). The scientific and clinical basis for the treatment of Parkinson disease (2009). *Neurology* 72, S1–S136. doi: 10.1212/WNL.0b013e3181a1d44c

Oliveira, A., Illes, P., and Ulrich, H. (2016). Purinergic receptors in embryonic and adult neurogenesis. *Neuropharmacology* 104, 272–281. doi: 10.1016/j.neuropharm.2015.10.008

Oliveros, A., Cho, C. H., Cui, A., Choi, S., Lindberg, D., Hinton, D., et al. (2017). Adenosine A2A receptor and ERK-driven impulsivity potentiates hippocampal neuroblast proliferation. *Transl. Psychiatry* 7, e1095. doi: 10.1038/tp.2017.64

Olsson, T., Barcellos, L. F., and Alfredsson, L. (2017). Interactions between genetic, lifestyle and environmental risk factors for multiple sclerosis. *Nat. Rev. Neurol.* 13, 25–36. doi: 10.1038/nrneurol.2016.187

Orr,ú, M., Zanoveli, J., Quiroz, C., Nguyen, H. P., Guitart, X., and Ferr,é, S. (2011). Functional changes in postsynaptic adenosine A 2A receptors during early stages of a rat model of Huntington disease. *Exp. Neurol.* 232, 76–80. doi: 10.1016/j.expneurol.2011.08.005

Ortiz, R., Ulrich, H., Zarate, C. A., and Machado-Vieira, R. (2015). Purinergic system dysfunction in mood disorders: a key target for developing improved therapeutics. *Prog. Neuro-Psychopharmacology Biol. Psychiatry* 57, 117–131. doi: 10.1016/j.pnpbp.2014.10.016

Oyanguren-Desez, O., Rodríguez-Antigüedad, A., Villoslada, P., Domercq, M., Alberdi, E., and Matute, C. (2011). Gain-of-function of P2X7 receptor gene variants in multiple sclerosis. *Cell Calcium* 50, 468–472. doi: 10.1016/j.ceca.2011.08.002

Palma, A. G., Muchnik, S., and Losavio, A. S. (2011). Excitatory effect of the A2A adenosine receptor agonist CGS-21680 on spontaneous and K+-evoked acetylcholine release at the mouse neuromuscular junction. *Neuroscience* 172, 164–176. doi: 10.1016/j.neuroscience.2010.10.015

Parisi, C., Arisi, I., D'Ambrosi, N., Storti, A. E., Brandi, R., D'Onofrio, M., et al. (2013). Dysregulated microRNAs in amyotrophic lateral sclerosis microglia modulate genes linked to neuroinflammation. *Cell Death Dis.* 4:e959. doi: 10.1038/cddis.2013.491

Parisi, C., Napoli, G., Amadio, S., Spalloni, A., Apolloni, S., Longone, P., et al. (2016). MicroRNA-125b regulates microglia activation and motor neuron death in ALS. *Cell Death Differ.* 23, 531–541. doi: 10.1038/cdd.2015.153

Parpura, V., Fisher, E. S., Lechleiter, J. D., Schousboe, A., Waagepetersen, H. S., Brunet, S., et al. (2017). Glutamate and ATP at the Interface Between Signaling and Metabolism in Astroglia: Examples from Pathology. *Neurochem. Res.* 42, 19–34. doi: 10.1007/s11064-016-1848-6

Paulson, H. L., Shakkottai, V. G., Clark, H. B., and Orr, H. T. (2017). Polyglutamine spinocerebellar ataxias — from genes to potential treatments. *Nat. Rev. Neurosci.* 18, 613–626. doi: 10.1038/nrn.2017.92

Pitt, D., Werner, P., and Rain, C. S. (2000). Glutamate excitotoxicity in a model of multiple sclerosis. *Nat. Med.* 6, 67–70. doi: 10.1038/71555

Popat, R. A., Van Den Eeden, S. K., Tanner, C. M., Kamel, F., Umbach, D. M., Marder, K., et al. (2011). Coffee, ADORA2A, and CYP1A2: the caffeine connection in Parkinson's disease. *Eur. J. Neurol.* 18, 756–765. doi: 10.1111/j.1468-1331.2011.03353.x

Popoli, P., Blum, D., Martire, A., Ledent, C., Ceruti, S., and Abbracchio, M. P. (2007). Functions, dysfunctions and possible therapeutic relevance of adenosine A2A receptors in Huntington's disease. *Prog. Neurobiol.* 81, 331–348. doi: 10.1016/j.pneurobio.2006.12.005

Popoli, P., Pintor, A., Domenici, M. R., Frank, C., Tebano, M. T., P.è, Zzola, A., et al. (2002). Blockade of Striatal Adenosine A 2A Receptor Reduces, through a Presynaptic Mechanism, Quinolinic Acid-Induced Excitotoxicity: Possible Relevance to Neuroprotective Interventions in Neurodegenerative Diseases of the Striatum. *J. Neurosci.* 22, 1967–1975.

Potenza, R. L., Armida, M., Ferrante, A., Pèzzola, A., Matteucci, A., Puopolo, M., et al. (2013). Effects of chronic caffeine intake in a mouse model of amyotrophic lateral sclerosis. *J. Neurosci. Res.* 91, 585–592. doi: 10.1002/jnr.23185

Potenza, R. L., Tebano, M. T., Martire, A., Domenici, M. R., Pepponi, R., Armida, M., et al. (2007). Adenosine A2A receptors modulate BDNF both in normal conditions and in experimental models of Huntington's disease. *Purinergic Signal.* 3, 333–338. doi: 10.1007/s11302-007-9066-y

Probert, L., Akassoglou, K., Pasparakis, M., Kontogeorgost, G., Kollias, G., and Levi-Montalcini, R. (1995). Spontaneous inflammatory demyelinating disease in transgenic mice showing central nervous system-specific expression of tumor necrosis factor a. *Neurobiology* 92, 11294–11298. doi: 10.1073/pnas.92.24.11294

Przybyła, T., Sakowicz-Burkiewicz, M., and Pawełczyk, T. (2018). Purinergic signaling in B cells. *Acta Biochim. Pol.* 65, 1–7. doi: 10.18388/abp.2017_1588

Puchałowicz, K., Baranowska-Bosiacka, I., Dziedziejko, V., and Chlubek, D. (2015). Purinergic signaling and the functioning of the nervous system cells. *Cell. Mol. Biol. Lett.* 20, 867–918. doi: 10.1515/cmble-2015-0050

Pupillo, E., Bianchi, E., Chi,ò, A., Casale, F., Zecca, C., Tortelli, R., et al. (2017). Amyotrophic lateral sclerosis and food intake. *Amyotroph. Lateral Scler. Front. Degener.* 19, 267–274. doi: 10.1080/21678421.2017.1418002

Qian, Y., Xu, S., Yang, X., and Xiao, Q. (2017). Purinergic receptor P2Y6 contributes to 1-methyl-4-phenylpyridinium-induced oxidative stress and cell death in neuronal SH-SY5Y cells. *J. Neurosci. Res.* 96, 253–264. doi: 10.1002/jnr.24119

Quiroz, C., Gulyani, S., Ruiqian, W., Bonaventura, J., Cutler, R., Pearson, V., et al. (2016). Adenosine receptors as markers of brain iron deficiency: Implications for Restless Legs Syndrome. *Neuropharmacology* 111, 160–168. doi: 10.1016/j.neuropharm.2016.09.002

Rajagopal, R., Chen, Z.-Y., Lee, F. S., and Chao, M. V. (2004). Transactivation of Trk neurotrophin receptors by G-protein-coupled receptor ligands occurs on intracellular membranes. *J. Neurosci.* 24, 6650–6658. doi: 10.1523/JNEUROSCI.0010-04.2004

Raker, V. K., Becker, C., and Steinbrink, K. (2016). The cAMP pathway as therapeutic target in autoimmune and inflammatory diseases. *Front. Immunol.* 7:123. doi: 10.3389/fimmu.2016.00123

Raman, R., Allen, S. P., Goodall, E. F., Kramer, S., Ponger, L.-L., Heath, P. R., et al. (2015). Gene expression signatures in motor neurone disease fibroblasts reveal dysregulation of metabolism, hypoxia-response and RNA processing functions. *Neuropathol. Appl. Neurobiol.* 41, 201–226. doi: 10.1111/nan.12147

Raoul, C., Estévez, A. G., Nishimune, H., Cleveland, D. W., deLapeyrière, O., Henderson, C. E., et al. (2002). Motoneuron death triggered by a specific pathway downstream of Fas. potentiation by ALS-linked SOD1 mutations. *Neuron* 35, 1067–1083. doi: 10.1016/S0896-6273(02)00905-4

Raoul, C., Henderson, C. E., and Pettmann, B. (1999). Programmed cell death of embryonic motoneurons triggered through the Fas death receptor. *J. Cell Biol.* 147, 1049–1062. doi: 10.1083/jcb.147.5.1049

Reggio, R., Pèzzola, A., and Popoli, P. (1999). The intrastratial injection of an adenosine A2 receptor antagonist prevents frontal cortex EEG abnormalities in a rat model of Huntington's disease. *Brain Res.* 83, 315–318. doi: 10.1016/S0006-8993(99)01489-4

Renton, A. E., Chi,ò, A., and Traynor, B. J. (2013). State of play in amyotrophic lateral sclerosis genetics. *Nat. Neurosci.* 17, 17–23. doi: 10.1038/nn.3584

Rezania, K., and Roos, R. P. (2013). Spinal Cord. *Neurol. Clin.* 31, 219–239. doi: 10.1016/j.ncl.2012.09.014

Ribeiro, F. F., Xapelli, S., Miranda-Lourenço, C., Tanqueiro, S. R., Fonseca-Gomes, J., Diógenes, M. J., et al. (2016). Purine nucleosides in neuroregeneration and neuroprotection. *Neuropharmacology* 104, 226–242. doi: 10.1016/j.neuropharm.2015.11.006

Rissanen, E., Virta, J. R., Paavilainen, T., Tuisku, J., Helin, S., Luoto, P., et al. (2013). Adenosine A2A receptors in secondary progressive multiple sclerosis: a [(11)C]TMSX brain PET study. *J. Cereb. Blood Flow Metab.* 33, 1394–1401. doi: 10.1038/jcbfm.2013.85

Robitaille, R. (1995). Purinergic receptors and their activation by endogenous purines at perisynaptic glial cells of the frog neuromuscular junction. *J. Neurosci.* 15, 7121–7131.

Robitaille, R. (1998). Modulation of synaptic efficacy and synaptic depression by glial cells at the frog neuromuscular junction. *Neuron* 21, 847–855. doi: 10.1016/S0896-6273(00)80600-5

Rochon, D., Rousse, I., and Robitaille, R. (2001). Synapse-glia interactions at the mammalian neuromuscular junction. *J. Neurosci.* 21, 3819–3829.

Rodella, U., Negro, S., Scorzeto, M., Bergamin, E., Jalink, K., Montecucco, C., et al. (2017). Schwann cells are activated by ATP released from neurons in an *in vitro* cellular model of Miller Fisher syndrome. *Dis. Model. Mech.* 10, 597–603. doi: 10.1242/dmm.027870

Rodrigues, R. J., Tomé, A. R., and Cunha, R. A. (2015). ATP as a multi-target danger signal in the brain. *Front. Neurosci.* 9:148. doi: 10.3389/fnins.2015.00148

Ross, C. A., and Tabrizi, S. J. (2011). Huntington's disease: from molecular pathogenesis to clinical treatment. *Lancet Neurol.* 10, 83–98. doi: 10.1016/S1474-4422(10)70245-3

Safarzadeh, E., Jadidi-Niaragh, F., Motallebnezhad, M., and Yousefi, M. (2016). The role of adenosine and adenosine receptors in the immunopathogenesis of multiple sclerosis. *Inflamm. Res.* 65, 511–520. doi: 10.1007/s00011-016-0936-z

Scattoni, M. L., Valanzano, A., Pezzola, A., March, Z. D., De Fusco, F. R., Popoli, P., et al. (2007). Adenosine A2A receptor blockade before striatal excitotoxic lesions prevents long term behavioural disturbances in the quinolinic rat model of Huntington's disease. *Behav. Brain Res.* 176, 216–221. doi: 10.1016/j.bbr.2006.10.004

Scemes, E., Suadicani, S. O., Dahl, G., and Spray, D. C. (2007). Connexin and pannexin mediated cell-cell communication. *Neuron Glia Biol.* 3, 199–208. doi: 10.1017/S1740925X08000069

Schiffmann, S. N., Fisone, G., Moresco, R., Cunha, R. A., and Ferré, S. (2007). Adenosine A2Areceptors and basal ganglia physiology. *Prog. Neurobiol.* 83, 277–292. doi: 10.1016/j.pneurobio.2007.05.001

Schiffmann, S. N., Jacobs, O., and Vanderhaeghen, J. J. (1991). Striatal restricted adenosine A2 receptor (RDC8) is expressed by enkephalin but not by substance P neurons: an *in situ* hybridization histochemistry study. *J. Neurochem.* 57, 1062–1067. doi: 10.1111/j.1471-4159.1991.tb08257.x

Seki, T., Adachi, N., Ono, Y., Mochizuki, H., Hiramoto, K., Amano, T., et al. (2005). Mutant protein kinase Cγ found in spinocerebellar ataxia type 14 is susceptible to aggregation and causes cell death. *J. Biol. Chem.* 280, 29096–29106. doi: 10.1074/jbc.M501716200

Shahaduzzaman, M., Acosta, S., Bickford, P. C., and Borlongan, C. V. (2013). α-Synuclein is a pathological link and therapeutic target for Parkinson's disease and traumatic brain injury. *Med. Hypotheses* 81, 675–680. doi: 10.1016/j.mehy.2013.07.025

Sharp, A. J., Polak, P. E., Simonini, V., Lin, S. X., Richardson, J. C., Bongarzone, E. R., et al. (2008). P2x7 deficiency suppresses development of experimental autoimmune encephalomyelitis. *J. Neuroinflammation* 5:33. doi: 10.1186/1742-2094-5-33

Shen, H.-Y., Canas, P. M., Garcia-Sanz, P., Lan, J.-Q., Boison, D., Moratalla, R., et al. (2013). Adenosine A2A receptors in striatal glutamatergic terminals and GABAergic neurons oppositely modulate psychostimulant action and DARPP-32 phosphorylation. *PLoS ONE* 8:e80902. doi: 10.1371/journal.pone.0080902

Shinozaki, Y., Shibata, K., Yoshida, K., Ikenaka, K., Tanaka, K. F., Correspondence, S. K., et al. (2017). Transformation of Astrocytes to a neuroprotective phenotype by microglia via P2Y 1 receptor downregulation. *Cell Rep.* 19, 1151–1164. doi: 10.1016/j.celrep.2017.04.047

Simon, D. K., Wu, C., Tilley, B. C., Lohmann, K., Klein, C., Payami, H., et al. (2017). Caffeine, creatine, GRIN2A and Parkinson's disease progression. *J. Neurol. Sci.* 375, 355–359. doi: 10.1016/j.jns.2017.02.032

Simonin, C., Duru, C., Salleron, J., Hincker, P., Charles, P., Delval, A., et al. (2013). Association between caffeine intake and age at onset in huntington's disease. *Neurobiol. Dis.* 58, 179–182. doi: 10.1016/j.nbd.2013.05.013

Sitkovsky, M., V (2003). Use of the A2A adenosine receptor as a physiological immunosuppressor and to engineer inflammation *in vivo*. *Biochem. Pharmacol.* 65, 493–501. doi: 10.1016/S0006-2952(02)01548-4

Skaper, S. D., Facci, L., Culbert, A. A., Evans, N. A., Chessell, I., Davis, J. B., et al. (2006). P2X7 receptors on microglial cells mediate injury to cortical neurons *in vitro*. *Glia* 54, 234–242. doi: 10.1002/glia.20379

Song, X. M., Xu, X. H., Zhu, J., Guo, Z., Li, J., He, C., et al. (2015). Up-regulation of P2X7 receptors mediating proliferation of Schwann cells after sciatic nerve injury. *Purinergic Signal.* 11, 203–213. doi: 10.1007/s11302-015-9445-8

Spanevello, R. M., Mazzanti, C. M., Kaizer, R., Zanin, R., Cargnelutti, D., Hannel, L., et al. (2006). Apyrase and 5'-nucleotidase activities in synaptosomes from the cerebral cortex of rats experimentally demyelinated with ethidium bromide and treated with interferon-beta. *Neurochem. Res.* 31, 455–462. doi: 10.1007/s11064-006-9039-5

Stevens, B., and Fields, R. D. (2000). Response of Schwann cells to action potentials in development. *Science* 287, 2267–2271. doi: 10.1126/science.287.5461.2267

Stockwell, J., Jakova, E., and Cayabyab, F. S. (2017). Adenosine A1 and A2A receptors in the brain: current research and their role in neurodegeneration. *Molecules* 22:676. doi: 10.3390/molecules22040676

Strong, M. J. (2010). The evidence for altered RNA metabolism in amyotrophic lateral sclerosis (ALS). *J. Neurol. Sci.* 288, 1–12. doi: 10.1016/j.jns.2009.09.029

Sun, C., Heid, M. E., Keyel, P. A., and Salter, R. D. (2013). The second transmembrane domain of P2X7 contributes to dilated pore formation. *PLoS ONE* 8:e61886. doi: 10.1371/journal.pone.0061886

Sun, J., Link, H., Olsson, T., Xiao, B. G., Andersson, G., Ekre, H. P., et al. (1991). T and B cell responses to myelin-oligodendrocyte glycoprotein in multiple sclerosis. *J. Immunol.* 146, 1490–1495.

Surprenant, A., and North, R. A. (2009). Signaling at Purinergic P2X Receptors. *Annu. Rev. Physiol.* 71, 333–359. doi: 10.1146/annurev.physiol.70.113006.100630

Taherzadeh-Fard, E., Saft, C., Wieczorek, S., Epplen, J. T., and Arning, L. (2010). Age at onset in Huntington's disease: replication study on the associations of ADORA2A, HAP1 and OGG1. *Neurogenetics* 11, 435–439. doi: 10.1007/s10048-010-0248-3

Takenouchi, T., Sekiyama, K, Sekigawa, A., Fujita, M., Waragai, M., Sugama, S., et al. (2010). P2X7 receptor signaling pathway as a therapeutic target for neurodegenerative diseases. *Arch. Immunol. Ther. Exp. (Warsz).* 58, 91–96. doi: 10.1007/s00005-010-0069-y

Tarditi, A., Camurri, A., Varani, K., Borea, P. A., Woodman, B., Bates, G., et al. (2006). Early and transient alteration of adenosine A2A receptor signaling in a mouse model of Huntington disease. *Neurobiol. Dis.* 23, 44–53. doi: 10.1016/j.nbd.2006.01.014

Tebano, M. T., Martire, A., Chiodi, V., Ferrante, A., and Popoli, P. (2010). Role of adenosine A 2A receptors in modulating synaptic functions and brain levels of BDNF: a possible key mechanism in the pathophysiology of Huntington's disease. *Rev. ScientificWorldJournal.* 10, 1768–1782. doi: 10.1100/tsw.2010.164

Todd, K. J., and Robitaille, R. (2006). Purinergic modulation of synaptic signalling at the neuromuscular junction. *Pflügers Arch. Eur. J. Physiol.* 452, 608–614. doi: 10.1007/s00424-006-0068-3

Tozzi, M., and Novak, I. (2017). Purinergic receptors in adipose tissue as potential targets in metabolic disorders. *Front. Pharmacol.* 8:878. doi: 10.3389/fphar.2017.00878

Tsuda, M. (2017). P2 receptors, microglial cytokines and chemokines, and neuropathic pain. *J. Neurosci. Res.* 95, 1319–1329. doi: 10.1002/jnr.23816

Tsuda, M., and Inoue, K. (2016). Neuron–microglia interaction by purinergic signaling in neuropathic pain following neurodegeneration. *Neuropharmacology* 104, 76–81. doi: 10.1016/j.neuropharm.2015.08.042

Tsuda, M., Shigemoto-Mogami, Y., Koizumi, S., Mizokoshi, A., Kohsaka, S., Salter, M. W., et al. (2003). P2X4 receptors induced in spinal microglia gate tactile allodynia after nerve injury. *Nature* 424, 778–783. doi: 10.1038/nature01786

Tsutsui, S., Schnermann, J., Noorbakhsh, F., Henry, S., Yong, V. W., Winston, B. W., et al. (2004). Neurobiology of disease A1 adenosine receptor upregulation and activation attenuates neuroinflammation and demyelination in a model of multiple sclerosis. *J. Neurosci.* 24, 1521–1529. doi: 10.1523/JNEUROSCI.4271-03.2004

Tyebji, S., Saavedra, A., Canas, P. M., Pliassova, A., Delgado-García, J. M., Alberch, J., et al. (2015). Hyperactivation of D1 and A 2A receptors contributes to cognitive dysfunction in Huntington's disease. *Neurobiol. Dis.* 74, 41–57. doi: 10.1016/j.nbd.2014.11.004

Varani, K., Abbracchio, M. P., Cannella, M., Cislaghi, G., Giallonardo, P., Mariotti, C., et al. (2003). Aberrant A_{2A} receptor function in peripheral blood cells in Huntington's disease. *FASEB J.* 17, 2148–2150. doi: 10.1096/fj.03-0079fje

Varani, K., Rigamonti, D., Sipione, S., Camurri, A., Borea, P. A., Cattabeni, F., et al. (2001). Aberrant amplification of A 2A receptor signaling in striatal cells expressing mutant huntingtin. *FASEB J.* 15, 1245–1247. doi: 10.1096/fj.00-0730fje

Varma, H., Cheng, R., Voisine, C., Hart, A. C., and Stockwell, B. R. (2007). Inhibitors of metabolism rescue cell death in Huntington's disease models. *Proc. Natl. Acad. Sci. U.S.A.* 104, 14525–14530. doi: 10.1073/pnas.0704482104

Verkhratsky, A., Rodríguez, J. J., and Parpura, V. (2012). Calcium signalling in astroglia. *Mol. Cell. Endocrinol.* 353, 45–56. doi: 10.1016/j.mce.2011.08.039

Verschueren, A. (2017). Motor neuropathies and lower motor neuron syndromes. *Rev. Neurol. (Paris).* 173, 320–325. doi: 10.1016/j.neurol.2017.03.018

Vijayan, D., Young, A., Teng, M. W. L., and Smyth, M. J. (2017). Targeting immunosuppressive adenosine in cancer. *Nat. Rev. Cancer* 17, 709–724. doi: 10.1038/nrc.2017.86

Villar-Menéndez, I., Blanch, M., Tyebji, S., Pereira-Veiga, T., Albasanz, J. L., Martín, M., et al. (2013). Increased 5-methylcytosine and decreased 5-hydroxymethylcytosine levels are associated with reduced striatal A2AR levels in Huntington's disease. *NeuroMolecular Med.* 15, 295–309. doi: 10.1007/s12017-013-8219-0

Vincenzi, F., Corciulo, C., Targa, M., Casetta, I., Gentile, M., Granieri, E., et al. (2013). A_{2A} adenosine receptors are up-regulated in lymphocytes from amyotrophic lateral sclerosis patients. *Amyotroph. Lateral Scler. Front. Degener.* 14, 406–413. doi: 10.3109/21678421.2013.793358

Viscomi, M. T., Florenzano, F., Amadio, S., Bernardi, G., and Molinari, M. (2005). Partial resistance of ataxin-2-containing olivary and pontine neurons to axotomy-induced degeneration. *Brain Res. Bull.* 66, 212–221. doi: 10.1016/j.brainresbull.2005.04.016

Volont,é, C., Apolloni, S., Parisi, C., and Amadio, S. (2016). Purinergic contribution to amyotrophic lateral sclerosis. *Neuropharmacology* 104, 180–193. doi: 10.1016/j.neuropharm.2015.10.026

Volont,é, C., Apolloni, S., Skaper, S. D., and Burnstock, G. (2012). P2X7 receptors: channels, pores and more. *CNS Neurol. Disord. Drug Targets* 11, 705–721. doi: 10.2174/187152712803581137

Vonsattel, J. P., and DiFiglia, M. (1998). Huntington disease. *J. Neuropathol. Exp. Neurol.* 57, 369–384. doi: 10.1097/00005072-199805000-00001

Vuorimaa, A., Rissanen, E., and Airas, L. (2017). *In vivo* PET Imaging of adenosine 2A receptors in neuroinflammatory and neurodegenerative disease. *Contrast Media Mol. Imaging* 2017:6975841. doi: 10.1155/2017/6975841

Wang, X., Arcuino, G., Takano, T., Lin, J., Peng, W. G., Wan, P., et al. (2004). P2X7 receptor inhibition improves recovery after spinal cord injury. *Nat. Med.* 10, 821–827. doi: 10.1038/nm1082

Wei, W., Du, C., Lv, J., Zhao, G., Li, Z., Wu, Z., et al. (2013). Blocking A2B adenosine receptor alleviates pathogenesis of experimental autoimmune encephalomyelitis via inhibition of IL-6 production and Th17 differentiation. *J. Immunol.* 190, 138–146. doi: 10.4049/jimmunol.1103721

Whiteside, T. L. (2017). Targeting adenosine in cancer immunotherapy: a review of recent progress. *Expert Rev. Anticancer Ther.* 17, 527–535. doi: 10.1080/14737140.2017.1316197

Wiendl, H., Toyka, K. V., Rieckmann, P., Gold, R., Hartung, H.-P., Hohlfeld, R., et al. (2008). Basic and escalating immunomodulatory treatments in multiple sclerosis: Current therapeutic recommendations. *J. Neurol.* 255, 1449–1463. doi: 10.1007/s00415-008-0061-1

Wiedemann, F. R., Manfredi, G., Mawrin, C., Beal, M. F., and Schon, E. A. (2002). Mitochondrial DNA and respiratory chain function in spinal cords of ALS patients. *J. Neurochem.* 80, 616–625. doi: 10.1046/j.0022-3042.2001.00731.x

Wilkaniec, A., Gassowska, M., Czapski, G. A., Cieślik, M., Sulkowski, G., and Adamczyk, A. (2017). P2X7 receptor-pannexin 1 interaction mediates extracellular alpha-synuclein-induced ATP release in neuroblastoma SH-SY5Y cells. *Purinergic Signal.* 13, 347–361. doi: 10.1007/s11302-017-9567-2

Witting, A., Chen, L., Cudaback, E., Straiker, A., Walter, L., Rickman, B., et al. (2006). Experimental autoimmune encephalomyelitis disrupts endocannabinoid-mediated neuroprotection. *Proc. Natl. Acad. Sci. U.S.A.* 103, 6362–6367. doi: 10.1073/pnas.0510418103

Xu, P., Rosen, K. M., Hedstrom, K., Rey, O., Guha, S., Hart, C., et al. (2013). Nerve injury induces glial cell line-derived neurotrophic factor (GDNF) expression in Schwann cells through purinergic signaling and the PKC-PKD pathway. *Glia* 61, 1029–1040. doi: 10.1002/glia.22491

Yamada-Fowler, N., Fredrikson, M., and Söderkvist, P. (2014). Caffeine interaction with glutamate receptor gene GRIN2A: Parkinson's disease in Swedish population. *PLoS ONE* 9:e99294. doi: 10.1371/journal.pone.00 99294

Yang, X., Lou, Y., Liu, G., Wang, X., Qian, Y., Ding, J., et al. (2017). Microglia P2Y6 receptor is related to Parkinson's disease through neuroinflammatory process. *J. Neuroinflammation* 14:38. doi: 10.1186/s12974-017-0795-8

Yanpallewar, S. U., Barrick, C. A., Buckley, H., Becker, J., and Tessarollo, L. (2012). Deletion of the BDNF truncated receptor TrkB.T1 delays disease onset in a mouse model of amyotrophic lateral sclerosis. *PLoS ONE* 7:e39946. doi: 10.1371/journal.pone.0039946

Yao, S.-Q., Li, Z.-Z., Huang, Q.-Y., Li, F., Wang, Z.-W., Augusto, E., et al. (2012). Genetic inactivation of the adenosine A(2A) receptor exacerbates brain damage in mice with experimental autoimmune encephalomyelitis. *J. Neurochem.* 123, 100–112. doi: 10.1111/j.1471-4159.2012.07807.x

Yiangou, Y., Facer, P., Durrenberger, P., Chessell, I. P., Naylor, A., Bountra, C., et al. (2006). COX-2, CB2 and P2X7-immunoreactivities are increased in activated microglial cells/macrophages of multiple sclerosis and amyotrophic lateral sclerosis spinal cord. *BMC Neurol.* 6:12. doi: 10.1186/1471-2377-6-12

Zhang, J., Li, Z., Hu, X., Su, Q., He, C., Liu, J., et al. (2017). Knockout of P2Y 12 aggravates experimental autoimmune encephalomyelitis in mice via increasing of IL-23 production and Th17 cell differentiation by dendritic cells. *Brain Behav Immun.* 62, 245–255. doi: 10.1016/j.bbi.2016.12.001

Zhu, C., Wang, G., Li, J., Chen, L., Wang, C., Wang, Y., et al. (2014). Adenosine A2A receptor antagonist istradefylline 20 versus 40 mg/day as augmentation for Parkinson's disease: a meta-analysis. *Neurol. Res.* 36, 1028–1034. doi: 10.1179/1743132814Y.0000000375

Zhu, Y., and Kimelberg, H. K. (2001). Developmental expression of metabotropic P2Y1 and P2Y2 receptors in freshly isolated astrocytes from rat hippocampus. *J. Neurochem.* 77, 530–541. doi: 10.1046/j.1471-4159.2001.00241.x

Zimmermann, H. (2006). Ectonucleotidases in the nervous system. *Novartis Found. Symp.* 276, 113–128; discussion 128–130, 233–237, 275–281. doi: 10.1002/9780470032244.ch10

Zimmermann, H., Braun, N., Kegel, B., and Heine, P. (1998). New insights into molecular structure and function of ectonucleotidases in the nervous system. *Neurochem. Int.* 32, 421–425. doi: 10.1016/S0197-0186(97)00126-5

Zuchora, B., and Urbañska, E. M. (2001). Effect of adenosine receptor agonists on neurodegenerative and convulsive activity of mitochondrial toxin, 3-nitropropionic acid. *Polish J. Pharmacol. Pol. J. Pharmacol* 53, 69–71.

15

Adenosine A_{2A} Receptors Control Glutamatergic Synaptic Plasticity in Fast Spiking Interneurons of the Prefrontal Cortex

*Amber Kerkhofs[1,2], Paula M. Canas[2], A. J. Timmerman[1], Tim S. Heistek[1], Joana I. Real[2], Carolina Xavier[2], Rodrigo A. Cunha[2,3], Huibert D. Mansvelder[1] and Samira G. Ferreira[2]**

[1] Department of Integrative Neurophysiology, Center for Neurogenomics and Cognitive Research, VU University, Amsterdam, Netherlands, [2] Center for Neuroscience and Cell Biology, University of Coimbra, Coimbra, Portugal, [3] Faculty of Medicine, University of Coimbra, Coimbra, Portugal

***Correspondence:**
Samira G. Ferreira
carsamira@gmail.com

Adenosine A_{2A} receptors ($A_{2A}R$) are activated upon increased synaptic activity to assist in the implementation of long-term plastic changes at synapses. While it is reported that $A_{2A}R$ are involved in the control of prefrontal cortex (PFC)-dependent behavior such as working memory, reversal learning and effort-based decision making, it is not known whether $A_{2A}R$ control glutamatergic synapse plasticity within the medial PFC (mPFC). To elucidate that, we tested whether $A_{2A}R$ blockade affects long-term plasticity (LTP) of excitatory post-synaptic potentials in pyramidal neurons and fast spiking (FS) interneurons in layer 5 of the mPFC and of population spikes. Our results show that $A_{2A}R$ are enriched at mPFC synapses, where their blockade reversed the direction of plasticity at excitatory synapses onto layer 5 FS interneurons from LTP to long-term depression, while their blockade had no effect on the induction of LTP at excitatory synapses onto layer 5 pyramidal neurons. At the network level, extracellularly induced LTP of population spikes was reduced by $A_{2A}R$ blockade. The interneuron-specificity of $A_{2A}R$ in controlling glutamatergic synapse LTP may ensure that during periods of high synaptic activity, a proper excitation/inhibition balance is maintained within the mPFC.

Keywords: A_{2A} receptor, prefrontal cortex (PFC), synaptic plasticity, fast-spiking interneurons, adenosine, LTP and LTD, electrophysiology

INTRODUCTION

The prefrontal cortex (PFC) is involved in the control of cognitive and executive functions, such as decision making, working memory, inhibitory control, attention, and behavioral flexibility (Dalley et al., 2004; Euston et al., 2013). The flexible regulation of these types of behavior makes it possible to properly respond to a changing environment (Arnsten, 2009). Such flexibility is thought to require plastic changes in the strength of synaptic connections (Kandel, 1976; Mayford et al., 2012), which is heavily dependent on the action of several neuromodulators (Pawlak et al., 2010; Bloem et al., 2014; Dembrow and Johnston, 2014).

One of the neuromodulators that can impact synaptic plasticity is adenosine, which is released in an activity-dependent fashion at synapses (Cunha et al., 1996; Wall and Dale, 2013). Its actions are mediated by a balanced activation of the inhibitory A_1 receptors (A_1R) and the facilitatory A_{2A} receptors ($A_{2A}R$) (Cunha, 2008), which act predominantly on glutamatergic but also on

GABAergic signaling (Shen et al., 2008; Rombo et al., 2015; Qi et al., 2017). While A_1R control basal synaptic transmission, $A_{2A}R$ are selectively engaged in events where long-term potentiation (LTP) is induced (d'Alcantara et al., 2001; Rebola et al., 2008; Simões et al., 2016).

$A_{2A}R$ are present in the PFC (Van Dort et al., 2009; Pandolfo et al., 2013; van Aerde et al., 2013) and affect PFC-dependent behavior. Indeed, genetic elimination of $A_{2A}R$ decreases effort-based decision-making (Pardo et al., 2012), while enhancing working memory (Zhou et al., 2009; Wei et al., 2011) and reversal learning (Wei et al., 2011). Their possible pathophysiological relevance is highlighted by the ability of selective $A_{2A}R$ antagonists to attenuate working memory deficits (Horita et al., 2013; Li et al., 2015), and by the ability of caffeine, which antagonizes both adenosine receptors, to counteract cognitive behavioral deficits both in human subjects suffering from attention deficit hyperactivity disorder (ADHD; Leon, 2000) as well as in a rat model of ADHD (Pandolfo et al., 2013).

Despite the effects of $A_{2A}R$ on PFC-dependent behavior, it is not known how $A_{2A}R$ control the information flow and whether $A_{2A}R$ affect glutamatergic synaptic plasticity of information within the local PFC circuit. Therefore, we studied the impact of $A_{2A}R$ on synaptic transmission and plasticity at excitatory synapses onto pyramidal neurons and interneurons and at the network level in the medial PFC (mPFC). We found that $A_{2A}R$ are enriched at mPFC synapses, where $A_{2A}R$ blockade shifts the direction of plasticity at excitatory synapses onto layer 5 fast spiking (FS) interneurons from LTP to LTD, while it is ineffective at excitatory synapses onto layer 5 pyramidal neurons and reduces plasticity at the network level.

MATERIALS AND METHODS

Animals

All studies were conducted in accordance with the principles and procedures outlined as "3Rs" in the guidelines of EU (210/63), FELASA, and the National Centre for the 3Rs (the ARRIVE; Kilkenny et al., 2010), and were approved by the Animal Care Committee of the Center for Neuroscience and Cell Biology (ORBEA 78/2013) or by the VU University's Animal Experimentation Ethics Committee (DEC) and were in accordance with institutional and Dutch license procedures. Rats were housed in a temperature and humidity-controlled environment with 12 h light on/off cycles and *ad libitum* access to food and water.

Membrane-Binding Assay

The density of $A_{2A}R$ in total membranes or synaptosomal membranes from the PFC was estimated by a radioligand-binding assay using a supramaximal concentration of the $A_{2A}R$ antagonist ^{3}H-SCH58261 (6 nM; provided by E. Ongini, Schering-Plough, Milan, Italy), as described previously (Kaster et al., 2015; Viana da Silva et al., 2016). Specific binding was determined by the subtraction of non-specific binding measured in the presence of 3 μM XAC (Tocris).

Subsynaptic Fractionation of mPFC Synaptosomes and Western Blot Analysis

To separate the extra-synaptic (non-active) zone, presynaptic active zone and post-synaptic fractions from synaptosomes, we used a fractionation method previously described in detail (Rebola et al., 2005; Canas and Cunha, 2016). The efficiency of separation is based on the segregation of different markers in the several fractions: SNAP-25 in the presynaptic active zone, PSD-95 in the post-synaptic density (PSD) and synaptophysin outside the active zone (extra-synaptic fraction). Western blot analysis was performed with an anti-$A_{2A}R$ antibody (1:500; sc-32261 from Santa Cruz Biotechnology; Santa Cruz, CA, United States), of which selectivity was confirmed by the lack of signal in $A_{2A}R$ knockout mice (Rebola et al., 2005).

Whole-Cell-Recordings

Male Wistar rats (5–6.5 week-old) purchased from Charles River (Harlan) were decapitated, their brain was carefully removed and the mPFC was sliced in carbogen buffered (pH 7.4) ice-cold choline-based slicing solution containing (in mM): choline chloride 110, sodium ascorbate 11.6, KCl 2.5, NaH_2PO_4 1.3, $MgCl_2$ 7, $CaCl_2$ 0.5, $NaHCO_3$ 26, and glucose 10. Slices (350 μm) were kept at room temperature in aCSF oxygenated with carbogen in a holding chamber. Following recovery for at least 1 h, recordings from cells in L5 of the mPFC were made in oxygenated aCSF (flow rate of 2–3 ml/min, 32°C). Whole-cell patch-clamp recordings were made with borosilicate glass pipettes (3–6 MΩ) filled with an intracellular solution containing (in mM): K-gluconate 111, KCl 8, HEPES 10, Mg-ATP 4, K_2 phosphocreatine 10, GTP 0.4, EGTA 0.2. Biocytin (0.2–0.5%) was added to all solutions for *post hoc* cell identification, and osmolarity was adjusted to 290–295 mOsm. Pyramidal L5 cells were visualized with differential interference contrast microscopy, selected on their large and pyramidal shape and further identified by their spike profile. FS interneurons were selected based on their small, round shape and further identified by their spike profile. During recordings, neurons were kept at a holding potential close to −70 mV. Recordings were made using MultiClamp 700 A/B amplifiers (Axon Instruments, Sunnyvale, CA, United States), with sampling at 10 kHz and low-pass filtering at 3–4 kHz. Recordings were digitized with an Axon Digidata 1440A and acquired using pClamp software (Axon). After experiments were completed, slices were stored in 4% paraformaldehyde for subsequent neuronal visualization and reconstruction as previously described (Mohan et al., 2015).

Spontaneous EPSCs

Spontaneous excitatory post-synaptic currents (sEPSCs) were recorded 5–10 min before and 25–30 min after drug incubation. Acquired data were stored for off-line analysis and events were detected using MiniAnalysis software. EPSC amplitude and frequency were determined and averaged over a 5-min time-course in each condition.

Evoked EPSCs

Excitatory post-synaptic currents (EPSCs) were evoked (eEPSCs) every 3.5 s using bipolar stimulating electrodes in glass pipettes filled with aCSF positioned 100–150 μm along the cell's apical dendrite. Duration (0.5 ms) and amplitude (100–350 mA) of extracellular stimulation were controlled by Isoflex stimulators (A.M.P.I., Jerusalem, Israel) to generate a monosynaptic response. After recording a baseline for 5–10 min, drugs were added and the eEPSC response was recorded for another 20 min. In pyramidal neurons, 15 datapoints were determined and averaged in each condition (baseline, 5 min after incubation and 15 min after incubation). In FS cells, EPSC amplitude was averaged over a 5-min time-course in all conditions (baseline, 5 min after incubation and 15 min after incubation).

Long-Term Potentiation

Excitatory post-synaptic potentials (EPSPs) were evoked every 7 s (0.14 Hz) using bipolar stimulating electrodes in glass pipettes filled with aCSF positioned 100–150 μm along the cell's apical dendrite. The duration (0.5 ms) and amplitude (100–350 μA) of extracellular stimulation were controlled by Isoflex stimulators (A.M.P.I., Jerusalem, Israel) to generate a monosynaptic response. Baseline EPSP was defined with an input/output curve, stimulating at below half maximum response. After obtaining a stable baseline of 3–5 min (30–43 EPSPs), LTP was induced within 15 min of whole-cell configuration with an unpaired theta burst stimulation (TBS) protocol (10 bursts of five pulses each at 100 Hz, repeated three times). This protocol triggered an optimal potentiated response in the cells, which was more reliable than other tested protocols such as spike timing dependent potentiation (STDP), although it was still highly variable especially in pyramidal neurons. Timing of EPSPs and the induction protocol was controlled by a Master-8 stimulator (A.M.P.I.). The slope of the initial 2 ms of the EPSP was taken as a measure of EPSP strength. The change in synaptic strength was defined as the percent change in EPSP slope 20–30 min after the TBS relative to baseline. Cell input resistance was monitored by applying a hyperpolarizing pulse at the end of each sweep (−30 pA). After LTP induction, membrane potential was returned to approximate baseline value by modest current injection. Criteria for inclusion of recordings were: (1) baseline resting membrane potential < -60 mV, (2) smooth rise of EPSP and clear separation from stimulation artifact, (3) stable baseline EPSP slope, (4) less than 30% change in input resistance, (5) no AP-firing evoked by extracellular stimulation in post-pairing period. In total, five cases of extreme EPSP rundown (slope $< 20\%$ of baseline) were excluded from analysis.

Extracellular Recordings

Male Wistar rats (6–8 week-old) were purchased from Charles River Laboratories (Barcelona, Spain). Rats were anesthetized under halothane atmosphere, decapitated and the brain rapidly removed from the skull and submerged in ice-cold artificial cerebrospinal fluid (aCSF) solution of the following composition, in mM: NaCl 125, KCl 3, $MgSO_4$ 1, $CaCl_2$ 2, Na_2HPO_4 1.25 $NaHCO_3$ 25–26 and glucose 11, pH 7.4 (osmolality, ~300 mOsmol.kg^{-1}), oxygenated with carbogen (95% O_2 + 5% CO_2). Coronal slices (300 μm-thick) containing the medial prefrontal cortex (mPFC) were cut with a Vibratome 1500 sectioning system (Vibratome, Germany). The slices were then transferred to a pre-chamber containing aCSF under continuous oxygenation to recover at 32°C for at least 1 h. Slices were then transferred to a submerged recording chamber where they were continuously superfused at a rate of 2–3 ml/min with oxygenated aCSF at 30–32°C. A bipolar concentric stimulation electrode SNE-100 (Kopf, Germany) was placed on the layer II/III of the mPFC delivering rectangular pulses (80–160 μA) of 0.1 ms duration applied with a Digitimer DS3 stimulator (Digitimer, Ltd., United Kingdom) once every 20 s. The evoked population spikes were recorded through an extracellular borosilicate microelectrode (filled with 4 M NaCl, 2–4 MΩ resistance) placed in the layer V of the mPFC, using an Axopatch 200B amplifier (Axon Instruments, Inc., United States), coupled to an analog/digital acquisition board (Digidata 1322A; Axon Instruments, Inc., United States). Responses were digitized at 10 kHz and continuously monitored on a personal computer via WinLTP 1.1 software (Anderson and Collingridge, 2007). Responses were quantified as the amplitude of the population spike recordings. After stabilizing the response, the input/output curve was obtained. Then the intensity of the stimulus was regulated to obtain 40–50% of the maximum response before induction of LTP. LTP was induced by delivering a train of 100 Hz (50 pulses, 0.5 s duration) for a priming effect, which was 15 min later followed by four trains of 100 Hz (50 pulses, 0.5 s duration, 1 every 10 s). Due to difficulties in inducing LTP in rat PFC slices, LTP protocols were extensively tested and this protocol, which has been used by Gemperle et al. (2003), was the most reliable one in our hands.

Experimental Design and Statistics

For membrane binding assays, PFC from five adult male Wistar rats were used, and the density of $A_{2A}R$ in synaptosomal membranes was compared to that in total membranes using unpaired t-test. For Western blotting of sub-synaptic fractions, we pooled together mPFC tissue from 22 rats (30–45 days-old). This was due to the requirement of 1 g of tissue for the sub-synaptic fractionation step. For pharmacology in electrophysiology experiments, all the drugs used were dissolved in aCSF at the desired concentration and bath applied during the experiments. The drugs were diluted from stock solutions made in dimethylsulfoxide (DMSO) to their final concentrations: SCH58261 (50–100 nM from 5 mM stock solution, Tocris). All experiments were performed without application of synaptic blockers. In extracellular recordings, due to high variability in LTP magnitude, whenever SCH58261 was tested, a control slice was also done in parallel. In the end, data from 25 slices per group (from 25 different rats) were pooled together for statistical comparison using an unpaired t-test. For plasticity in whole-cell patch-clamp experiments, due to cellular variability, strict exclusion criteria (see above), long duration of the experiment and high quality of slices needed, more animals were needed than are presented in our figures. When relevant and possible, we recorded one cell in control and one cell in drug condition from every animal. For the pyramidal-TBS experiment, 51 animals were used. For the FS interneuron-TBS experiment, 27 animals were used. Raw data was analyzed using Clampfit 10.4 and custom Matlab scripts. For all LTP experiments, we used the percentage of increase in EPSP slope (whole-cell recordings) or population spike amplitude (extracellular recordings) induced by the LTP protocol per cell (whole-cell recordings) or per slice (extracellular recordings) as input for statistical tests. An unpaired *t*-test was used to compare two groups consisting of multiple such experiments, comparing the percentage of LTP induction in control experiments *versus* the percentage of LTP induction in $A_{2A}R$ antagonist-treated experiments. This method for comparing differences in LTP induction in control *versus* drug treated slices is adopted from our previous research on LTP induction (Mansvelder and McGehee, 2000; Couey et al., 2007; Meredith et al., 2007; Rebola et al., 2008; Verhoog et al., 2013, 2016; Simões et al., 2016). For whole-cell spontaneous recordings, 12 slices from 10 different animals were used in sEPSC on pyramidal neurons; 2 recordings were excluded for rundown reasons (>20% change in resistance). For sEPSC on FS interneurons, 32 recordings of interneurons were made from slices of 21 different animals. Of these, 13 cells were actual FS interneurons; 1 was excluded for rundown. For eEPCS experiments on pyramidal neurons, 14 slices were used from four different animals. For eEPSC experiments on FS interneurons, eight slices from three animals were used, four animals were used in total for these experiments. All recorded sEPSCs were analyzed with MiniAnalysis software (Synaptosoft, version 6.0.7). All the statistical analysis was performed using Prism 6 (GraphPad software). Data was analyzed by using the appropriate parametric statistical test as mentioned in the text and $p < 0.05$ was taken as statistically significant.

RESULTS

$A_{2A}R$ Are Enriched in Synaptosomal Membranes and Present in All Sub-synaptic Fractions

To investigate the density and synaptic distribution of $A_{2A}R$, we compared the binding of ^{3}H-SCH58261 in total and synaptosomal membranes from the PFC. The binding density of ^{3}H-SCH58261 was higher ($n = 5$; $t_8 = 4.56$; $p = 0.0018$; unpaired *t*-test) in the synaptosomal membrane fraction (39.0 ± 3.6 fmol/mg protein) compared to the total membrane fraction (19.4 ± 2.4 fmol/mg protein; $n = 5$) from the PFC (**Figure 1A**). Given this enrichment of $A_{2A}R$ in synaptosomal membranes, we used mPFC synaptosomes (pooled from 22 rats) to separate the different subsynaptic fractions, and probed for the subsynaptic distribution of $A_{2A}R$. $A_{2A}R$ were present in all the subsynaptic fractions, inside and outside the presynaptic active zone and PSD, with a higher $A_{2A}R$ density observed outside the presynaptic active zone and PSD (**Figure 1B**). The presence of $A_{2A}R$ in all PFC sub-synaptic fractions suggests a role for $A_{2A}R$ in the control of synaptic communication in the mPFC.

$A_{2A}R$ Do Not Control Spontaneous and Evoked Excitatory Synaptic Transmission

To determine whether sEPSCs or eEPSCs are affected by $A_{2A}R$, we recorded sEPSCs and eEPSCs onto both pyramidal neurons and FS interneurons, the two largest groups of neurons in the PFC (Markram et al., 2004) and tested the effect of the selective $A_{2A}R$ antagonist SCH58261. After recording a baseline in ACSF, SCH58261 (100 nM) was incubated into the bath and cells were recorded for another 20–30 min. Spontaneous events onto pyramidal neurons were unaffected by incubation of SCH58261 (100 nM; **Figures 2A–E**) in both frequency (**Figures 2B,C**; Frequency mean control: 1.22 ± 1.2 Hz, $n = 10$; 5 min after SCH58261: 1.12 ± 0.83 Hz, $n = 10$; 25 min after SCH58261: 0.78 ± 0.46 Hz, $n = 10$; difference: $F_{2,9} = 6.05$, $p = 0.21$, ANOVA) and amplitude (**Figures 2D,E**; Amplitude

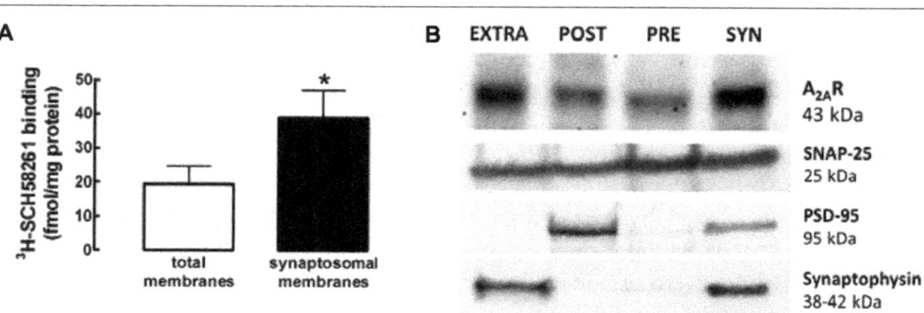

FIGURE 1 | $A_{2A}R$ are enriched in synaptosomal membranes and present in all subsynaptic fractions. **(A)** The binding density of a supra-maximal concentration of a selective $A_{2A}R$ antagonist ^{3}H-SCH58261 (6 nM) was higher in synaptosomal when compared to total membranes from Wistar rat PFC. Data are mean ± SEM of five rats; *$p < 0.05$, unpaired Student's *t*-test. **(B)** Western blots of subsynaptic fractions showing the subsynaptic distribution of $A_{2A}R$ in the mPFC (pooled from 22 rats due to the requirement of large sample size – 1 g of tissue – at the start of the subsynaptic fractionation procedure). The efficiency of separation is based on the segregation of different markers in the several fractions: SNAP-25 in the presynaptic active zone, PSD-95 in the post-synaptic density (PSD) and synaptophysin outside the active zone (extrasynaptic fraction). $A_{2A}R$ are present in all the subsynaptic fractions, inside and outside the presynaptic active zone and PSD. However, there is an enrichment outside the presynaptic active zone and PSD.

mean control: 36.38 ± 6.2 pA, $n = 10$; 5 min after SCH58261: 38.18 ± 8.9 pA, $n = 10$; 25 min after SCH58261: 37.50 ± 6.5 pA, $n = 10$; difference: $F_{2,9} = 0.95$, $p = 0.39$, ANOVA). Similarly, spontaneous events onto FS interneurons were unaffected by incubation of SCH58261 (100 nM; **Figures 2H–L**) in both frequency (**Figures 2I,J**; Frequency mean control: 3.25 ± 2.7 Hz, $n = 12$; 5 min after SCH58261: 3.50 ± 2.64 Hz, $n = 12$; 25 min after SCH58261: 3.72 ± 2.7 Hz, $n = 12$; difference: $F_{2,11} = 1.52$, $p = 0.24$, ANOVA) and amplitude (**Figures 2K,L**; Amplitude mean control: 40.34 ± 9.3 pA, $n = 12$; 5 min after SCH58261: 41.83 ± 11.5 pA, $n = 12$; 25 min after SCH58261: 41.34 ± 10.5 pA, $n = 12$; difference: $F_{2,11} = 0.32$, $p = 0.65$, ANOVA). Also, eEPSCs onto both pyramidal neurons (**Figures 2F,G**) and interneurons (**Figures 2M,N**) were unaffected by incubation of SCH58261. Specifically, the amplitude of eEPSCs onto pyramidal neurons did not differ between baseline and incubation conditions (**Figures 2F,G**; Amplitude mean control: 522.6 ± 160.4 pA, $n = 14$; 5 min after SCH58261: 574.7 ± 218.9 pA, $n = 14$; 15 min after SCH58261: 554.1 ± 239.1 pA, $n = 14$; difference: $F_{2,13} = 0.67$, $p = 0.46$, ANOVA) and likewise, the amplitude of eEPSCs onto FS interneurons did not differ between baseline and incubation conditions (**Figures 2M,N**; Amplitude mean control: 242.5 ± 107.3 pA, $n = 8$; 5 min after SCH58261: 246.5 ± 115.4 pA, $n = 8$; 15 min after SCH58261: 237.9 ± 116.1 pA, $n = 8$; difference: $F_{2,7} = 0.14$, $p = 0.79$, ANOVA). Thus, $A_{2A}R$ do not seem necessary for excitatory synaptic transmission in the mPFC as their blockade does not affect either sEPSCs or eEPSCs in pyramidal neurons and FS interneurons.

$A_{2A}R$ Blockade Does Not Affect Glutamatergic Synapse LTP in Layer 5 Pyramidal Neurons

Under endogenous levels of adenosine, $A_{2A}R$ mainly act as a modulator of processes in which plasticity is engaged (d'Alcantara et al., 2001; Rebola et al., 2008; Costenla et al., 2011). Therefore, we tested whether $A_{2A}R$ blockade affected the induction of glutamatergic synaptic plasticity in mPFC pyramidal neurons. We made whole-cell recordings from L5 pyramidal neurons (**Figures 3A,B**) and glutamatergic EPSPs were evoked by extracellular stimulation. To induce LTP, a TBS protocol was applied (Larson and Munkácsy, 2015). After recording a stable baseline of EPSPs, 10 bursts of five pulses each were given at 100 Hz (**Figure 3C**), and this was repeated three times within 30 s. Following this induction protocol, the slope of EPSPs was increased in a sustained manner, 20–30 min after the induction protocol (128.2 ± 46.6%, $n = 32$; **Figures 3D–F,H**). When slices were pre-incubated with SCH58261 (100 nM), the increase in EPSP slope (122.8 ± 59.8%, $n = 17$; **Figures 3D–F,H**) was not significantly different from control experiments without SCH58261 ($t_{47} = 0.35$, $p = 0.731$, unpaired t-test). Indeed, in the absence of SCH58261, 53% of cells showed TBS-induced LTP (17 out of 32), 28% did not show a change in EPSP slope (9 out of 32) and 19% showed a reduction in EPSP slope (6 out of 32), while in the presence of SCH58261 (100 nM), 47% of the pyramidal cells showed TBS-induced LTP (8 out of 17), 29% showed no change (5 out of 17), and 24% showed a reduction in EPSP slope (4 out of 17). These distributions were not significantly different between control and SCH58261 conditions (**Figure 3G**, chi-square test, $p = 0.52$). In both conditions - control and presence of SCH58261 - cells had on average similar resting membrane potential and input resistance (mean RMP of control: −67.6 ± 0.4 mV; mean RMP with SCH58261: −69.1 ± 0.7 mV, $t_{49} = 1.82$, $p = 0.07$, unpaired t-test; mean R input of control: 52.3 ± 4.7 mΩ; mean R input with SCH58261: 54.4 ± 7.6 mΩ, $t_{49} = 0.26$, $p = 0.80$, unpaired t-test). Thus, blockade of $A_{2A}R$ has no significant effect on the induction of glutamatergic synaptic plasticity in L5 pyramidal neurons in mPFC slices.

$A_{2A}R$ Blockade Shifts the Direction of Plasticity From LTP Into LTD at Excitatory Synapses Onto Layer 5 Fast Spiking (FS) Interneurons

Next, we tested the effects of $A_{2A}R$ blockade on glutamatergic synaptic plasticity in FS interneurons. Glutamatergic synapses on FS interneurons can undergo LTP, albeit through different mechanisms than pyramidal neurons (Lamsa et al., 2007; Lu et al., 2007; Sarihi et al., 2008; Nissen et al., 2010; Sambandan et al., 2010; Huang et al., 2013). To test whether $A_{2A}R$ are involved in this type of plasticity, we made whole-cell recordings from mPFC L5 FS interneurons (**Figure 4A**). These neurons had FS patterns, short action potential half widths, showed no inter-spike interval adaptation, and displayed fast hyperpolarization time constants and minimal hyperpolarization amplitude (**Figure 4B**). To induce LTP, we applied the same TBS protocol as in the pyramidal neuron recordings (**Figure 4C**). This induced a robust potentiation of EPSP slope in FS interneurons (159.4 ± 44.9%, $n = 10$; **Figures 4D–G,H**). When slices were pre-incubated with SCH58261 (100 nM), stimulation with the TBS protocol induced long-term depression (LTD), rather than potentiation (64.4 ± 25.2%, $n = 10$; **Figures 4D–G,H**), which was significantly different from control ($t_{18} = 5.84$, $p < 0.0001$, unpaired t-test). In the two conditions - absence or presence of SCH58261 - the resting membrane potential and input resistance were similar (mean RMP of control: −71.2 ± 0.9 mV; mean RMP with SCH58261: −69.6 ± 1.9 mV, $t_{18} = 0.75$, $p = 0.46$, unpaired t-test; mean R input of control: 164.3 ± 17.8 mΩ; mean R input with SCH58261: 160.2 ± 19.2 mΩ, $t_{18} = 0.15$, $p = 0.88$, unpaired t-test). In the absence of SCH58261, 70% of all cells displayed LTP, compared to 0% in the SCH58261 group. Conversely, 70% of all cells displayed LTD in the SCH58261 group, whereas none of the cells in the control condition displayed LTD (**Figure 4G**). This shows that $A_{2A}R$ control the direction of plasticity at glutamatergic synapses onto FS interneurons in the mPFC.

$A_{2A}R$ Control LTP of Population Spikes in the Layer V mPFC (mPFC)

Since population spikes represent the integrated responses of all local cells, i.e., responses from both pyramidal cells and interneurons, we next recorded population spikes to determine

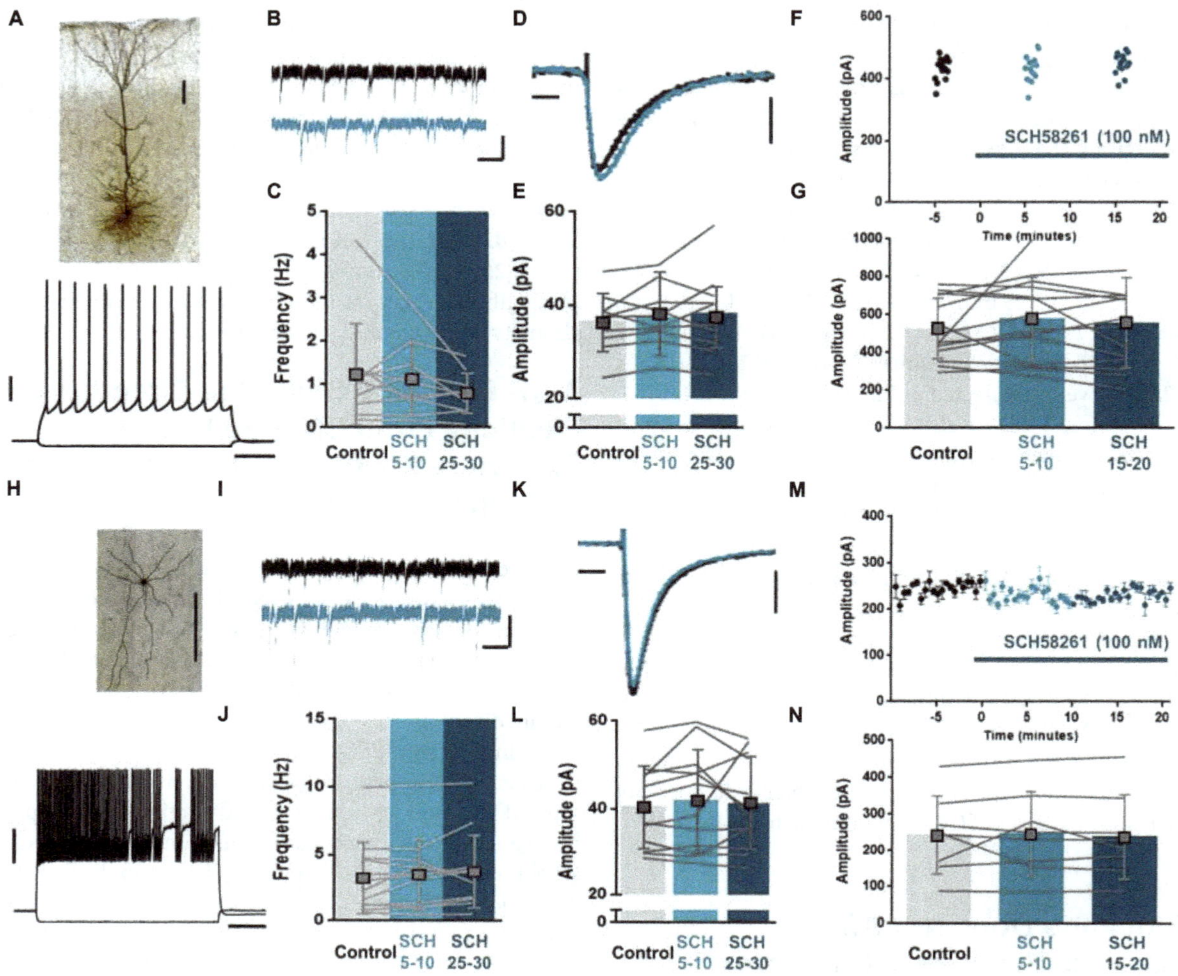

FIGURE 2 | $A_{2A}R$ do not affect spontaneous or evoked excitatory synaptic transmission in the mPFC. Biocytin staining of layer 5 pyramidal neuron (**A**, top) and fast spiking (FS) interneuron (**H**, top) from coronal slice of rat prelimbic mPFC. Scale bars: 100 μm. Voltage responses to hyperpolarizing (–50 pA) and depolarizing (+225 pA) somatic current injections to the soma of a L5 pyramidal neuron (**A**, bottom) and to hyperpolarizing (–60 pA) and depolarizing (+400 pA) somatic current injections to the soma of a FS interneuron (**H**, bottom). Scale bars: 20 mV, 200 ms. **(B,C)** Bath application of the selective $A_{2A}R$ antagonist, SCH58261 (100 nM, blue) did not affect the frequency of sEPSCs onto pyramidal neurons. A representative trace is depicted in control (black) and prolonged SCH58261 (100 nM, blue) wash-in condition **(B)**. The frequency over 5 min does not change after SCH58261 (100 nM, blue) wash-in; data are mean ± SD of $n = 10$, individual lines show the average of one cell over the course of 5 min per condition **(C)**. Scale bars: 30 pA, 50 ms. **(D,E)** Bath application of SCH58261 (100 nM, blue) did not affect the amplitude of sEPSCs onto pyramidal neurons. The average sEPSC amplitude of a representative cell is depicted in control (black) and prolonged SCH58261 (100 nM, blue) wash-in condition **(D)**. The average amplitude over 5 min does not change after SCH58261 (100 nM, blue) wash-in; data are mean ± SD of $n = 10$ **(E)**. Scale bars: 10 pA, 1 ms. **(F,G)** Bath application of SCH58261 (100 nM, blue) did not affect the amplitude of eEPSCs onto pyramidal neurons. The eEPSC amplitude of a representative cell is depicted during 15 sweeps in all three conditions; control (black), short- (light blue) and prolonged SCH58261 (100 nM, blue) wash-in conditions are shown **(F)**. The average amplitude does not change after SCH58261 (100 nM, blue) wash-in; data are mean ± SD of $n = 14$ **(G)**. **(I,J)** Bath application of SCH58261 (100 nM, blue) did not affect the frequency of sEPSCs onto interneurons. A representative trace is depicted in control (black) and prolonged SCH58261 (100 nM, blue) wash-in condition **(I)**. The frequency over 5 min does not change after SCH58261 (100 nM, blue) wash-in; data are mean ± SD of $n = 12$, individual lines show the average of one cell over the course of 5 min per condition **(J)**. Scale bars: 30 pA, 50 ms. **(K,L)** Bath application of SCH58261 (100 nM, blue) did not affect the amplitude of sEPSCs onto interneurons. The average sEPSC amplitude of a representative cell is depicted in control (black) and prolonged SCH58261 (100 nM, blue) wash-in condition **(K)**. The average amplitude over 5 min does not change after SCH58261 (100 nM, blue) wash-in; data are mean ± SD of $n = 12$ **(L)**. Scale bars: 10 pA, 1 ms. **(M,N)** Bath application of SCH58261 (100 nM, blue) did not affect the amplitude of eEPSCs onto pyramidal neurons. The average eEPSC amplitude of a representative cell is depicted over a time-course of 30 min, in which control (black), short- and prolonged SCH58261 (100 nM, blue) wash-in conditions are shown **(M)**. The average amplitude over 5 min does not change after SCH58261 (100 nM, blue) wash-in; data are mean ± SD of $n = 8$ **(N)**. Paired one-way ANOVA; all data are non-significant ($p > 0.05$).

whether $A_{2A}R$ affect plasticity on the neuronal network level. To that end, we recorded extracellularly evoked AMPA receptor-mediated population spikes in mPFC layer 5 (L5) in acute brain slices, upon stimulation of L2/3 (**Figures 5A,B**). Bath application of SCH58261 (50 nM) affected the stimulus–response relationship of the network by increasing the maximum amplitude of population spikes (1.86 ± 0.03 mV in SCH58261, $n = 23$; 1.58 ± 0.04 mV in control, $n = 26$; $t_{47} = 5.34$,

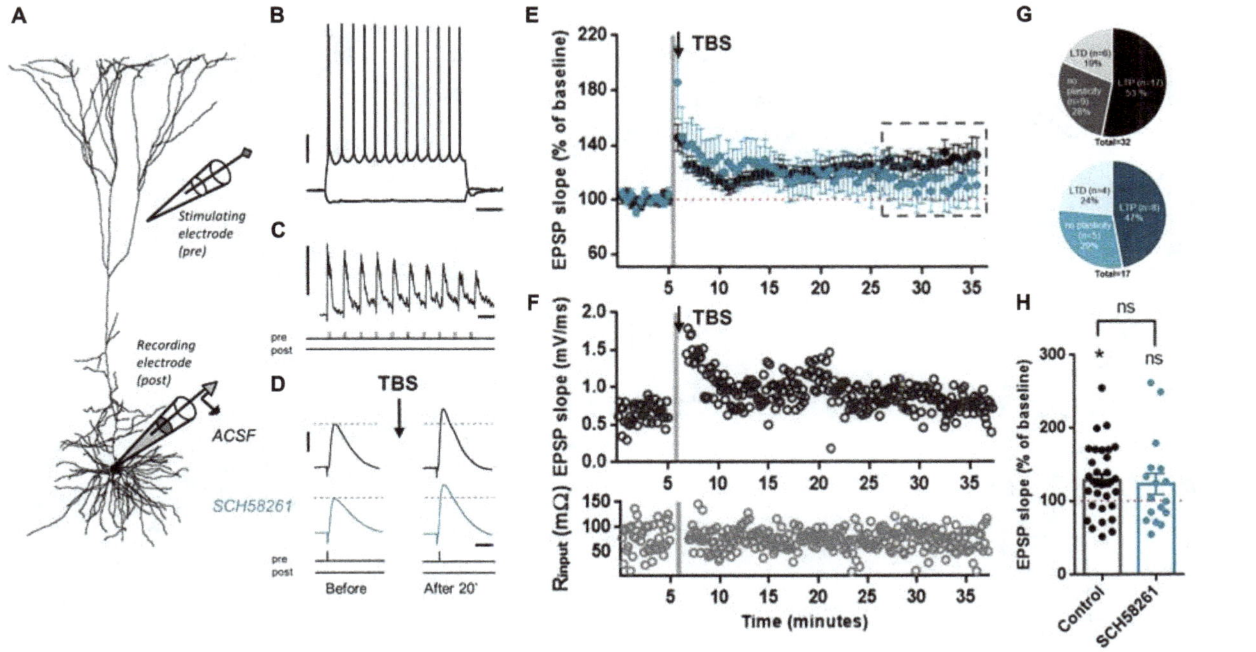

FIGURE 3 | $A_{2A}R$ blockade does not affect glutamatergic synapse LTP in layer 5 pyramidal neurons. **(A)** Biocytin reconstruction of layer 5 pyramidal neuron from coronal slice of rat prelimbic mPFC showing relative positions of recording and stimulating electrodes. **(B)** Voltage responses to hyperpolarizing (–60 pA) and depolarizing (+380 pA) somatic current injections to the soma of a L5 pyramidal neuron. Scale bars: 20 mV, 200 ms. **(C)** Plasticity induction protocol. Theta burst stimulation (TBS) was induced by stimulation of 10 bursts of five pulses each at 100 Hz, repeated three times. Scale bars: 20 mV, 200 ms. **(D)** After obtaining a baseline measure of EPSPs, TBS-LTP was induced. EPSPs were then recorded for up to 30 min to observe changes in EPSP slope. Slices were pre-incubated in either control ACSF or in ACSF with added SCH58261 (100 nM). Scale bars: 2 mV, 20 ms. **(E)** Summary time-course plot of control (black symbols) and SCH58261 (100 nM; blue symbols) experiments, showing a robust LTP in control condition, and a highly variable LTP in SCH58261 pre-incubated cells. **(F)** Example of a TBS-LTP experiment in control conditions showing slope and input resistance (top and bottom panels, respectively) *versus* time. Gray shading indicates time of TBS induction. **(G)** The fraction of cells that display LTP is slightly higher in the control condition than in the presence of SCH58261; however, fraction differences were not significant (Chi-square test, $p = 0.52$). **(H)** Summary bar chart of control and SCH58261 (100 nM) TBS-LTP experiments, showing percentage change of EPSP slope for both conditions (mean ± SEM; control: $n = 32$, SCH58261: $n = 17$). Unpaired t-test $p = 0.73$; $^*p < 0.05$ compared to baseline value of 100%, one-sample t-test.

$p < 0.0001$, unpaired t-test; **Figure 5C**). LTP of the population spike was induced by applying a single train of high-frequency stimulation (HFS), followed 15 min later by four HFS trains (50 pulses at 100 Hz, 0.5 s duration, delivered every 10 s). This induction protocol was run in the absence or presence of SCH58261, and for each experiment a naïve mPFC slice was used. Blockade of $A_{2A}R$ by SCH58261 decreased the magnitude of population spike LTP (120.7 ± 2.9% in SCH58261, $n = 25$; 130.9 ± 3.4% in control slices, $n = 25$; $t_{48} = 2.28$, $p = 0.027$, unpaired t-test; **Figures 5D–F**). These findings show that $A_{2A}R$ control plasticity at a neuronal network level in mPFC.

DISCUSSION

In the present study, we show that in the mPFC, $A_{2A}R$ control LTP at excitatory synapses onto fast-spiking interneurons rather than onto pyramidal neurons. $A_{2A}R$ did not affect spontaneous or evoked synaptic transmission in either cell type. A similar predominant role of $A_{2A}R$ on plasticity has been observed in other brain areas, including hippocampus (Rebola et al., 2008), amygdala (Simões et al., 2016), and striatum (d'Alcantara et al., 2001; Shen et al., 2008; Li et al., 2015). As in the hippocampus (Rebola et al., 2005), $A_{2A}R$ in the mPFC are enriched at synapses. However, mPFC $A_{2A}R$ are enriched outside the presynaptic active zone and PSD, whereas most of the hippocampal $A_{2A}R$ are located inside the presynaptic active zone and PSD (Rebola et al., 2005). It is conceivable that this different sub-synaptic distribution could translate into $A_{2A}R$ playing by different rules to control information flow within the mPFC. Indeed, our results show an effect of $A_{2A}R$ antagonism on the induction of LTP at excitatory synapses specifically in FS interneurons, while the antagonist was ineffective at excitatory synapses onto pyramidal neurons. At excitatory connections to FS interneurons, the blockade of $A_{2A}R$ led to LTD of their excitatory synapses, meaning that without active $A_{2A}R$, LTD would occur at these glutamatergic synapses onto FS interneurons. Thus, $A_{2A}R$ activation would be particularly important for the induction of synaptic potentiation of glutamatergic synapses in FS interneurons, while not affecting glutamatergic synapses in mPFC pyramidal neurons. At the mPFC neuronal network level, blockade of $A_{2A}R$ reduced LTP induction, suggesting a role for $A_{2A}R$ at the network level.

Target cell specificity of $A_{2A}R$ modulation has also been found in the hippocampus, although with the difference that activation

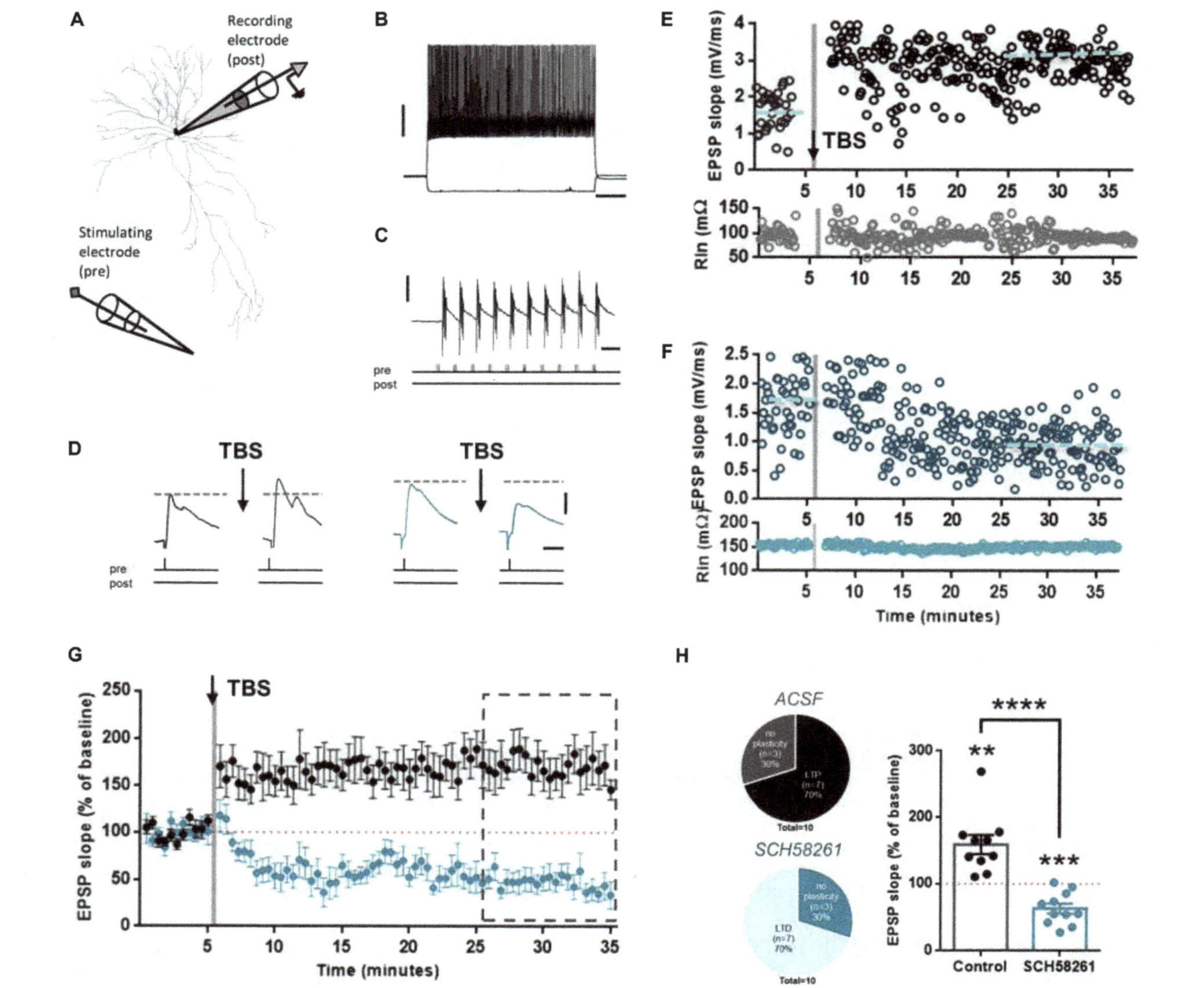

FIGURE 4 | $A_{2A}R$ blockade shifts reverses LTP to LTD at excitatory synapses in layer 5 FS interneurons. **(A)** Biocytin reconstruction of a FS interneuron from coronal slice of rat mPFC showing relative positions of recording and stimulating electrodes. **(B)** Voltage responses to hyperpolarizing (–80 pA) and depolarizing (+360 pA) somatic current injections to the soma of a FS interneuron. Scale bars: 20 mV, 200 ms. **(C)** Plasticity induction protocol. TBS was induced by stimulation of 10 bursts of five pulses each at 100 Hz, repeated three times. Scale bars: 10 mV, 200 ms. **(D)** After obtaining a baseline measure of EPSPs, TBS-LTP was induced. EPSPs were then recorded for up to 30 min to observe changes in EPSP slope. Slices were pre-incubated in either control ACSF (black traces) or in ACSF with added SCH58261 (100 nM; blue traces). Scale bars: 2 mV, 20 ms. Representative TBS-LTP experiments in control **(E)** and 100 nM SCH58261 **(F)** conditions showing slope and input resistance (top and bottom panels, respectively) *versus* time. Gray shading indicates time of TBS induction. **(G)** Summary plot of control (black symbols) and SCH58261 (100 nM; blue symbols) experiments, showing a robust LTP in control condition, and a strong LTD in SCH58261 pre-incubated cells. (**H**, left panel) The fraction of cells that obtain plasticity is reversed in control *versus* SCH58261 conditions. In control, 70% of cells display LTP, whereas in SCH58261, 70% of cells display LTD. (**H**, right panel) Summary bar chart of control and SCH58261 (100 nM) TBS-LTP experiments, showing percentage change in EPSP slope for both conditions (mean ± SEM; control: $n = 10$; SCH58261: $n = 10$). ****$p < 0.0001$ compared to the respective control (*black dots*), unpaired Student's *t*-test. **$p < 0.01$ compared to the hypothetical value of 100, one-sample *t*-test. ***$p < 0.001$ compared to the hypothetical value of 100, one-sample *t*-test.

of hippocampal $A_{2A}R$ increased excitatory transmission to CA1 pyramidal cells but not to inhibitory interneurons (Rombo et al., 2015). The PFC is unique in the magnitude and variety of interneurons, where FS interneurons represent the largest group (Markram et al., 2004). FS interneurons are activated by feedback and feedforward excitation, and they target perisomatic regions of pyramidal neurons (Tremblay et al., 2016) to control the output of pyramidal neurons by exerting fast, powerful and uniform inhibition of their firing (Kvitsiani et al., 2013; Sparta et al., 2014). Both LTP and LTD can be generated in FS interneurons, although LTP seems to be the dominant form of plasticity expressed in this neuron subtype (Lamsa et al., 2007; Lu et al., 2007; Sarihi et al., 2008; Nissen et al., 2010; Sambandan et al., 2010). In contrast to long-term plasticity (LTP) of excitatory synapses onto pyramidal neurons, LTP at glutamatergic synapses in FS neurons is predominantly independent of NMDA receptors

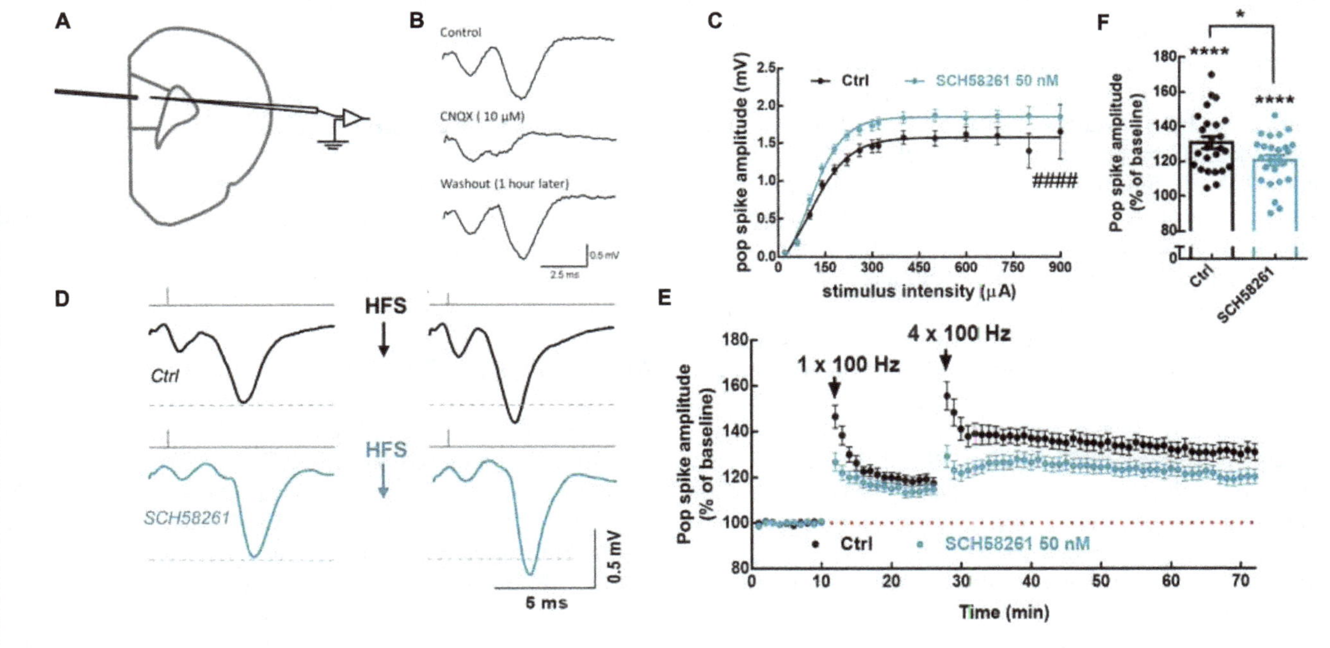

FIGURE 5 | $A_{2A}R$ facilitate LTP of population spikes in mPFC layer 5. **(A)** Positioning of the stimulating (layer 2/3 mPFC) and recording electrodes (layer 5 mPFC). **(B)** The recorded population spikes were abolished by the AMPA/kainate receptor antagonist, CNQX 10 μM. **(C)** Bath application of the selective $A_{2A}R$ antagonist, SCH58261 (50 nM; blue dots) increased the number and synchrony of cells discharging action potentials as indicated by the increase in the maximum response when the input/output response was assessed 20 min after SCH58261 superfusion. **(D)** Representative averaged traces at baseline and 30 min after the induction of LTP, in the absence and presence of SCH58261 (50 nM); SCH58261 decreased LTP magnitude. **(E)** Time course showing that SCH58261 decreased the magnitude of LTP of the population spike responses triggered by a priming train of high-frequency stimulation (HFS), followed 15 min later by four HFS trains (50 pulses at 100 Hz, 0.5 s duration, delivered every 10 s). **(F)** Summary plot displaying the variability of LTP magnitude, estimated 30 min after the induction of LTP, in the absence and presence of SCH58261 (50 nM). Data are mean ± SEM of 25 slices (from 25 rats) per group. $^{\#\#\#\#}p < 0.0001$ comparing the estimated maximum response in the presence of SCH58261 to control (*black bar/dots*), unpaired Student's *t*-test. $^{*}p < 0.05$ comparing SCH58261 to control (*black bar/dots*), unpaired Student's *t*-test. $^{****}p < 0.0001$ compared to the hypothetical value of 100%, one-sample *t*-test.

(Lamsa et al., 2007; Sarihi et al., 2008; Nissen et al., 2010; Sambandan et al., 2010; Huang et al., 2013). In most cases, an essential role for group I metabotropic glutamate receptors (mGluRs) has been demonstrated in LTP and LTD induction in these FS interneurons (Perez et al., 2001; Lu et al., 2007; Sarihi et al., 2008; Huang et al., 2013). Whether LTP or LTD can be induced in these synapses is dependent on post-synaptic calcium fluctuations during LTP induction (Alle et al., 2001; Sambandan et al., 2010; Huang et al., 2013). $A_{2A}R$ control both NMDA receptors and voltage-sensitive calcium channels, thus potentially contributing to modulate the pattern of plasticity (Mogul et al., 1993; Gonçalves et al., 1997; Rebola et al., 2008; Azdad et al., 2009; Higley and Sabatini, 2010). Furthermore, $A_{2A}R$ heteromerize with mGluR5 (Ferré et al., 2002) and tightly interact with mGluR5 receptor function in the hippocampus, changing the efficiency of NMDA receptors (Tebano et al., 2005; Sarantis et al., 2015; Viana da Silva et al., 2016). Whether either of these mechanisms is responsible for the observed effects, should be subject to further investigation.

We here show the role of $A_{2A}R$ in normal, non-pathological, conditions by targeting the endogenous pool of adenosine acting at the $A_{2A}R$ with the $A_{2A}R$ antagonist SCH58261. In these conditions, $A_{2A}R$ act mainly as modulators of synaptic plasticity (d'Alcantara et al., 2001; Rebola et al., 2008; Simões et al., 2016). $A_{2A}R$ have an additional role in pathological conditions, where they can control microglia and astrocytes (Rebola et al., 2011; Matos et al., 2015; Orr et al., 2015; Cunha, 2016). Targeting $A_{2A}R$ with an $A_{2A}R$ agonist would mimic the situation of an additional load onto these microglia- and astrocytic located $A_{2A}R$, thereby recruiting $A_{2A}R$ that are only active in pathological conditions (Matos et al., 2012; Orr et al., 2015). As we are specifically interested in the role of the $A_{2A}R$ in non-pathological conditions, we only evaluated plastic changes under influence of the $A_{2A}R$ antagonist.

The alteration in glutamatergic synapse strength in FS interneurons by $A_{2A}R$ can have a major impact on cortical function. A decreased synaptic strength at FS interneurons has been linked to a loss of temporal fidelity of pyramidal-to-pyramidal signaling (Lamsa et al., 2005), leading to a loss of information processing (Pouille and Scanziani, 2001). Also, the selective control by $A_{2A}R$ of plasticity at glutamatergic synapses onto FS interneurons might have important implications for the excitation–inhibition balance. Indeed, if the activity of interneurons is experimentally reduced in mPFC, LTP of excitatory to pyramidal neurons is impaired (Konstantoudaki et al., 2016). Adenosine, by acting at $A_{2A}R$ at synapses of FS interneurons, could therefore provide a homeostatic mechanism by which inhibition is ensured, thereby maintaining a proper excitation–inhibition balance (Zhang et al., 2015). FS interneurons, in particular the parvalbumin-positive FS cells, have been shown to support working memory and cognitive flexibility (Murray et al., 2015), and to be central for the control of attention (Kim et al., 2016). Therefore, abnormal $A_{2A}R$ function might lead to impaired behavioral functioning through changes in plasticity at FS interneuron synapses. An overexpression of $A_{2A}R$ specifically in the PFC is indeed related to cognitive and attentional deficits in a rat model of attention deficit and hyperactivity disorder (Pandolfo et al., 2013). Furthermore, genetic elimination of $A_{2A}R$ also interferes with behaviors that involve information processing in the PFC, including working memory (Zhou et al., 2009; Wei et al., 2011) and reversal learning (Wei et al., 2011). Future research targeting selectively $A_{2A}R$ in PFC FS interneurons will be needed to elucidate whether specifically $A_{2A}R$ located on glutamatergic synapses in FS interneurons control PFC-related behavior.

In short, we present here a first characterization of the role of endogenous adenosine acting at $A_{2A}R$ to affect synaptic plasticity in the mPFC, showing that $A_{2A}R$ specifically affect plasticity of glutamatergic synapses in cortical FS interneurons. An effect of $A_{2A}R$ manipulation on plasticity at these synapses was never shown before, therefore, further explorations into synaptic plasticity of FS interneurons in the PFC should be considered to reveal the underlying mechanism of $A_{2A}R$ manipulation.

AUTHOR CONTRIBUTIONS

AK, HM, RC, and SF designed the research. AK, SF, AT, TH, JR, CX, PC, and RC performed the experiments. AK, SF, RC, and HM analyzed the data. AK and SF wrote the first draft of the manuscript. All authors commented on the manuscript text.

ACKNOWLEDGMENTS

Supported by Maratona da Saúde, Santa Casa da Misericórdia, GAI-FMUC and Banco Santander-Totta, NARSAD, Erasmus Mundus Joint Doctorate grant (ENC-Network) and ERDF, through Centro 2020 (project no. CENTRO-01-0145-FEDER-000008:BrainHealth 2020), and through FCT (project nos. POCI-01-0145-FEDER-007440 and PTDC/NEU-NMC/4154/2016) to RC. HM received funding for this work from the Netherlands Organization for Scientific Research (NWO; VICI grant), ERC StG "BrainSignals," EU H2020 Framework Program (agreement no. 604102 "Human Brain Project") and the EU 7th Framework Program (no. EU MSCA-ITN CognitionNet FP7-PEOPLE-2013-ITN 607508).

REFERENCES

Alle, H., Jonas, P., and Geiger, J. R. P. (2001). PTP and LTP at a hippocampal mossy fiber-interneuron synapse. *Proc. Natl. Acad. Sci. U.S.A.* 98, 14708–14713. doi: 10.1073/pnas.251610898

Anderson, W. W., and Collingridge, G. L. (2007). Capabilities of the WinLTP data acquisition program extending beyond basic LTP experimental functions. *J. Neurosci. Methods* 162, 346–356. doi: 10.1016/j.jneumeth.2006.12.018

Arnsten, A. F. T. (2009). Stress signalling pathways that impair prefrontal cortex structure and function. *Nat. Rev. Neurosci.* 10, 410–422. doi: 10.1038/nrn2648

Azdad, K., Gall, D., Woods, A. S., Ledent, C., Ferrié, S., and Schiffmann, S. N. (2009). Dopamine D_2 and adenosine A_{2A} receptors regulate NMDA-mediated excitation in accumbens neurons through A_{2A}–D_2 receptor heteromerization. *Neuropsychopharmacology* 34, 972–986. doi: 10.1038/npp.2008.144

Bloem, B., Poorthuis, R. B., and Mansvelder, H. D. (2014). Cholinergic modulation of the medial prefrontal cortex: the role of nicotinic receptors in attention and regulation of neuronal activity. *Front. Neural Circuits* 8:17. doi: 10.3389/fncir.2014.00017

Canas, P. M., and Cunha, R. A. (2016). Subsynaptic membrane fractionation. *Neuromethods* 110, 31–37. doi: 10.1007/978-1-4939-3064-7_3

Costenla, A. R., Diógenes, M. J., Canas, P. M., Rodrigues, R. J., Nogueira, C., Maroco, J., et al. (2011). Enhanced role of adenosine A_{2A} receptors in the modulation of LTP in the rat hippocampus upon ageing. *Eur. J. Neurosci.* 34, 12–21. doi: 10.1111/j.1460-9568.2011.07719.x

Couey, J. J., Meredith, R. M., Spijker, S., Poorthuis, R. B., Smit, A. B., Brussaard, A. B., et al. (2007). Distributed network actions by nicotine increase the threshold for spike-timing-dependent plasticity in prefrontal cortex. *Neuron* 54, 73–87. doi: 10.1016/j.neuron.2007.03.006

Cunha, R. A. (2008). Different cellular sources and different roles of adenosine: A1 receptor-mediated inhibition through astrocytic-driven volume transmission and synapse-restricted A_{2A} receptor-mediated facilitation of plasticity. *Neurochem. Int.* 52, 65–72. doi: 10.1016/j.neuint.2007.06.026

Cunha, R. A. (2016). How does adenosine control neuronal dysfunction and neurodegeneration? *J. Neurochem.* 139, 1019–1055. doi: 10.1111/jnc.13724

Cunha, R. A., Vizi, E. S., Ribeiro, J. A., and Sebastião, A. M. (1996). Preferential release of ATP and its extracellular catabolism as a source of adenosine upon high- but not low-frequency stimulation of rat hippocampal slices. *J. Neurochem.* 67, 2180–2187. doi: 10.1046/j.1471-4159.1996.67052180.x

d'Alcantara, P. D., Ledent, C., Swillens, S., and Schiffmann, S. N. (2001). Inactivation of adenosine A_{2A} receptor impairs long term potentiation in the accumbens nucleus without altering basal synaptic transmission. *Neuroscience* 107, 455–464. doi: 10.1016/S0306-4522(01)00372-4

Dalley, J. W., Cardinal, R. N., and Robbins, T. W. (2004). Prefrontal executive and cognitive functions in rodents: neural and neurochemical substrates. *Neurosci. Biobehav. Rev.* 28, 771–784. doi: 10.1016/j.neubiorev.2004.09.006

Dembrow, N., and Johnston, D. (2014). Subcircuit-specific neuromodulation in the prefrontal cortex. *Front. Neural Circuits* 8:54. doi: 10.3389/fncir.2014.00054

Euston, D. R., Gruber, A. J., and Mcnaughton, B. L. (2013). The role of medial prefrontal cortex in memory and decision making. *Neuron* 76, 1057–1070. doi: 10.1016/j.neuron.2012.12.002

Ferré, S., Karcz-Kubicha, M., Hope, B. T., Popoli, P., Burgueño, J., Gutiérrez, M. A., et al. (2002). Synergistic interaction between adenosine A2A and glutamate mGlu5 receptors: implications for striatal neuronal function. *Proc. Natl. Acad. Sci. U.S.A.* 99, 11940–11945. doi: 10.1073/pnas.172393799

Gemperle, A. Y., Enz, A., Pozza, M. F., Lüthi, A., and Olpe, H. R. (2003). Effects of clozapine, haloperidol and iloperidone on neurotransmission and synaptic plasticity in prefrontal cortex and their accumulation in brain tissue: an in vitro study. *Neuroscience* 117, 681–695. doi: 10.1016/S0306-4522(02)00769-8

Gonçalves, M. L., Cunha, R. A., and Ribeiro, J. A. (1997). Adenosine A_{2A} receptors facilitate $^{45}Ca^{2+}$ uptake through class A calcium channels in rat hippocampal CA3 but not CA1 synaptosomes. *Neurosci. Lett.* 238, 73–77. doi: 10.1016/S0304-3940(97)00803-3

Higley, M. J., and Sabatini, B. L. (2010). Competitive regulation of synaptic Ca^{2+} influx by D2 dopamine and A_{2A} adenosine receptors. *Nat. Neurosci.* 13, 958–966. doi: 10.1038/nn.2592

Horita, T. K., Kobayashi, M., Mori, A., Jenner, P., and Kanda, T. (2013). Effects of the adenosine A_{2A} antagonist istradefylline on cognitive performance in rats with a 6-OHDA lesion in prefrontal cortex. *Psychopharmacology* 230, 345–352. doi: 10.1007/s00213-013-3158-x

Huang, S., Huganir, R. L., and Kirkwood, A. (2013). Adrenergic gating of Hebbian spike-timing-dependent plasticity in cortical interneurons. *J. Neurosci.* 33, 13171–13178. doi: 10.1523/JNEUROSCI.5741-12.2013

Kandel, E. R. (1976). *Cellular Basis of Behavior: An Introduction to Behavioral Neurobiology*. San Francisco, CA: W.H. Freeman.

Kaster, M. P., Machado, N. J., Silva, H. B., Nunes, A., Ardais, A. P., Santana, M., et al. (2015). Caffeine acts through neuronal adenosine A_{2A} receptors to prevent mood and memory dysfunction triggered by chronic stress. *Proc. Natl. Acad. Sci. U.S.A.* 112, 7833–7838. doi: 10.1073/pnas.1423088112

Kilkenny, C., Browne, W. J., Cuthill, I. C., Emerson, M., and Altman, D. G. (2010). Improving bioscience research reporting: the ARRIVE guidelines for reporting animal research. *PLOS Biol.* 8:e1000412. doi: 10.1371/journal.pbio.1000412

Kim, H., Ährlund-Richter, S., Wang, X., Deisseroth, K., and Carlén, M. (2016). Prefrontal parvalbumin neurons in control of attention. *Cell* 164, 208–218. doi: 10.1016/j.cell.2015.11.038

Konstantoudaki, X., Chalkiadaki, K., Tivodar, S., Karagogeos, D., and Sidiropoulou, K. (2016). Impaired synaptic plasticity in the prefrontal cortex of mice with developmentally decreased number of interneurons. *Neuroscience* 322, 333–345. doi: 10.1016/j.neuroscience.2016.02.048

Kvitsiani, D., Ranade, S., Hangya, B., Taniguchi, H., Huang, J., and Kepecs, A. (2013). Distinct behavioural and network correlates of two interneuron types in prefrontal cortex. *Nature* 498, 363–366. doi: 10.1038/nature12176

Lamsa, K., Heeroma, J. H., and Kullmann, D. M. (2005). Hebbian LTP in feed-forward inhibitory interneurons and the temporal fidelity of input discrimination. *Nat. Neurosci.* 8, 916–924. doi: 10.1038/nn1486

Lamsa, K. P., Heeroma, J. H., Somogyi, P., Rusakov, D. A., and Kullmann, D. M. (2007). Anti-Hebbian long-term potentiation in the hippocampal feedback inhibitory circuit. *Science* 315, 1262–1266. doi: 10.1126/science.1137450

Larson, J., and Munkácsy, E. (2015). Theta-burst LTP. *Brain Res.* 1621, 38–50. doi: 10.1016/j.brainres.2014.10.034

Leon, M. R. (2000). Effects of caffeine on cognitive, psychomotor, and affective performance of children with Attention-Deficit/Hyperactivity Disorder. *J. Atten. Disord.* 4, 27–47. doi: 10.1177/108705470000400103

Li, W., Silva, H. B., Real, J., Wang, Y.-M., Rial, D., Li, P., et al. (2015). Inactivation of adenosine A_{2A} receptors reverses working memory deficits at early stages of Huntington's disease models. *Neurobiol. Dis.* 79, 70–80. doi: 10.1016/j.nbd.2015.03.030

Lu, J., Li, C., Zhao, J.-P., Poo, M., and Zhang, X. (2007). Spike-timing-dependent plasticity of neocortical excitatory synapses on inhibitory interneurons depends on target cell type. *J. Neurosci.* 27, 9711–9720. doi: 10.1523/JNEUROSCI.2513-07.2007

Mansvelder, H. D., and McGehee, D. S. (2000). Long-term potentiation of excitatory inputs to brain reward areas by nicotine. *Neuron* 27, 349–357. doi: 10.1016/S0896-6273(00)00042-8

Markram, H., Toledo-Rodriguez, M., Wang, Y., Gupta, A., Silberberg, G., and Wu, C. (2004). Interneurons of the neocortical inhibitory system. *Nat. Rev. Neurosci.* 5, 793–807. doi: 10.1038/nrn1519

Matos, M., Augusto, E., Machado, N. J., dos Santos-Rodrigues, A., Cunha, R. A., and Agostinho, P. (2012). Astrocytic adenosine A2A receptors control the amyloid-β peptide-induced decrease of glutamate uptake. *J. Alzheimers Dis.* 31, 555–567. doi: 10.3233/JAD-2012-120469

Matos, M., Shen, H.-Y., Augusto, E., Wang, Y., Wei, C. J., Wang, Y. T., et al. (2015). Deletion of adenosine A_{2A} receptors from astrocytes disrupts glutamate homeostasis leading to psychomotor and cognitive impairment: relevance to schizophrenia. *Biol. Psychiatry* 78, 763–774. doi: 10.1016/j.biopsych.2015.02.026

Mayford, M., Siegelbaum, S. A., Kandel, E. R., Long-term, N. R., Lüscher, C., Malenka, R. C., et al. (2012). Synapses and memory storage. *Cold Spring Harb. Perspect. Biol.* 4:a005751. doi: 10.1101/cshperspect.a005751

Meredith, R. M., Holmgren, C. D., Weidum, M., Burnashev, N., and Mansvelder, H. D. (2007). Increased threshold for spike-timing-dependent plasticity is caused by unreliable calcium signaling in mice lacking fragile X gene fmr1. *Neuron* 54, 627–638. doi: 10.1016/j.neuron.2007.04.028

Mogul, D. J., Adams, M. E., and Fox, A. P. (1993). Differential activation of adenosine receptors decreases N-type but potentiates P-type Ca^{2+} current in hippocampal CA3 neurons. *Neuron* 10, 327–334. doi: 10.1016/0896-6273(93)90322-I

Mohan, H., Verhoog, M. B., Doreswamy, K. K., Eyal, G., Aardse, R., Lodder, B. N., et al. (2015). Dendritic and axonal architecture of individual pyramidal neurons across layers of adult human neocortex. *Cereb. Cortex* 25, 4839–4853. doi: 10.1093/cercor/bhv188

Murray, A. J., Woloszynowska-Fraser, M. U., Ansel-Bollepalli, L., Cole, K. L. H., Foggetti, A., Crouch, B., et al. (2015). Parvalbumin-positive interneurons of the prefrontal cortex support working memory and cognitive flexibility. *Sci. Rep.* 5:16778. doi: 10.1038/srep16778

Nissen, W., Szabo, A., Somogyi, J., Somogyi, P., and Lamsa, K. P. (2010). Cell type-specific long-term plasticity at glutamatergic synapses onto hippocampal interneurons expressing either parvalbumin or CB1 cannabinoid receptor. *J. Neurosci.* 30, 1337–1347. doi: 10.1523/JNEUROSCI.3481-09.2010

Orr, A. G., Hsiao, E. C., Wang, M. M., Ho, K., Kim, D. H., Wang, X., et al. (2015). Astrocytic adenosine receptor A_{2A} and G_s-coupled signaling regulate memory. *Nat. Neurosci.* 18, 423–434. doi: 10.1038/nn.3930

Pandolfo, P., Machado, N. J., Köfalvi, A., Takahashia, R. N., and Cunha, R. A. (2013). Caffeine regulates frontocorticostriatal dopamine transporter density and improves attention and cognitive deficits in an animal model of attention deficit hyperactivity disorder. *Eur. Neuropsychopharmacol.* 23, 317–328. doi: 10.1016/j.euroneuro.2012.04.011

Pardo, M., Lopez-Cruz, L., Valverde, O., Ledent, C., Baqi, Y., Müller, C. E., et al. (2012). Adenosine A_{2A} receptor antagonism and genetic deletion attenuate the effects of dopamine D_2 antagonism on effort-based decision making in mice. *Neuropharmacology* 62, 2068–2077. doi: 10.1016/j.neuropharm.2011.12.033

Pawlak, V., Wickens, J. R., Kirkwood, A., and Kerr, J. N. D. (2010). Timing is not everything: neuromodulation opens the STDP gate. *Front. Synaptic Neurosci.* 2:146. doi: 10.3389/fnsyn.2010.00146

Perez, Y., Morin, F., and Lacaille, J. (2001). A Hebbian form of long-term potentiation dependent on mGluR1a in hippocampal inhibitory interneurons. *Proc. Natl. Acad. Sci. U.S.A.* 98, 9401–9406. doi: 10.1073/pnas.161493498

Pouille, F., and Scanziani, M. (2001). Enforcement of temporal fidelity in pyramidal cells by somatic feed-forward inhibition. *Science* 293, 1159–1163. doi: 10.1126/science.1060342

Qi, G., van Aerde, K., Abel, T., and Feldmeyer, D. (2017). Adenosine differentially modulates synaptic transmission of excitatory and inhibitory microcircuits in layer 4 of rat barrel cortex. *Cereb. Cortex* 27, 4411–4422. doi: 10.1093/cercor/bhw243

Rebola, N., Canas, P. M., Oliveira, C. R., and Cunha, R. A. (2005). Different synaptic and subsynaptic localization of adenosine A_{2A} receptors in the hippocampus and striatum of the rat. *Neuroscience* 132, 893–903. doi: 10.1016/j.neuroscience.2005.01.014

Rebola, N., Lujan, R., Cunha, R. A., and Mulle, C. (2008). Adenosine A_{2A} receptors are essential for long-term potentiation of NMDA-EPSCs at hippocampal mossy fiber synapses. *Neuron* 57, 121–134. doi: 10.1016/j.neuron.2007.11.023

Rebola, N., Simões, A. P., Canas, P. M., Tomé, A. R., Andrade, G. M., Barry, C. E., et al. (2011). Adenosine A_{2A} receptors control neuroinflammation and consequent hippocampal neuronal dysfunction. *J. Neurochem.* 117, 100–111. doi: 10.1111/j.1471-4159.2011.07178.x

Rombo, D. M., Newton, K., Nissen, W., Badurek, S., Horn, J. M., Minichiello, L., et al. (2015). Synaptic mechanisms of adenosine A_{2A} receptor-mediated hyperexcitability in the hippocampus. *Hippocampus* 25, 566–580. doi: 10.1002/hipo.22392

Sambandan, S., Sauer, J.-F., Vida, I., and Bartos, M. (2010). Associative plasticity at excitatory synapses facilitates recruitment of fast-spiking interneurons in the dentate gyrus. *J. Neurosci.* 30, 11826–11837. doi: 10.1523/JNEUROSCI.2012-10.2010

Sarantis, K., Tsiamaki, E., Kouvaros, S., Papatheodoropoulos, C., and Angelatou, F. (2015). Adenosine A_{2A} receptors permit mGluR5-evoked tyrosine phosphorylation of NR2B (Tyr1472) in rat hippocampus: a possible key mechanism in NMDA receptor modulation. *J. Neurochem.* 135, 714–726. doi: 10.1111/jnc.13291

Sarihi, A., Jiang, B., Komaki, A., Sohya, K., Yanagawa, Y., and Tsumoto, T. (2008). Metabotropic glutamate receptor type 5-dependent long-term potentiation of excitatory synapses on fast-spiking GABAergic neurons in mouse visual cortex. *J. Neurosci.* 28, 1224–1235. doi: 10.1523/JNEUROSCI.4928-07.2008

Shen, H. Y., Coelho, J. E., Ohtsuka, N., Canas, P. M., Day, Y. J., Huang, Q. Y., et al. (2008). A critical role of the adenosine A_{2A} receptor in extrastriatal neurons in modulating psychomotor activity as revealed by opposite phenotypes of striatum and forebrain A_{2A} receptor knock-outs. *J. Neurosci.* 28, 2970–2975. doi: 10.1523/JNEUROSCI.5255-07.2008

Simões, A. P., Machado, N. J., Gonçalves, N., Kaster, M. P., Simões, A. T., Nunes, A., et al. (2016). Adenosine A_{2A} receptors in the amygdala control synaptic plasticity and contextual fear memory. *Neuropsychopharmacology* 41, 2862–2871. doi: 10.1038/npp.2016.98

Sparta, D. R., Hovelsø, N., Mason, A. O., Kantak, P. A., Ung, R. L., Decot, H. K., et al. (2014). Activation of prefrontal cortical parvalbumin interneurons facilitates extinction of reward-seeking behavior. *J. Neurosci.* 34, 3699–3705. doi: 10.1523/JNEUROSCI.0235-13.2014

Tebano, M. T., Martire, A., Rebola, N., Pepponi, R., Domenici, M. R., Grò, M. C., et al. (2005). Adenosine A_{2A} receptors and metabotropic glutamate 5 receptors are co-localized and functionally interact in the hippocampus: a possible key mechanism in the modulation of N-methyl-d-aspartate effects. *J. Neurochem.* 95, 1188–1200.

Tremblay, R., Lee, S., and Rudy, B. (2016). GABAergic interneurons in the neocortex: from cellular properties to circuits. *Neuron* 91, 260–292. doi: 10.1016/j.neuron.2016.06.033

van Aerde, K. I., Qi, G., and Feldmeyer, D. (2013). Cell type-specific effects of adenosine on cortical neurons. *Cereb. Cortex* 25, 772–787. doi: 10.1093/cercor/bht274

Van Dort, C. J., Baghdoyan, H. A., and Lydic, R. (2009). Adenosine A_1 and A_{2A} receptors in mouse prefrontal cortex modulate acetylcholine release and behavioral arousal. *J. Neurosci.* 29, 871–881.

Verhoog, M. B., Goriounova, N. A., Obermayer, J., Stroeder, J., Hjorth, J. J. J., Testa-Silva, G., et al. (2013). Mechanisms underlying the rules for associative plasticity at adult human neocortical synapses. *J. Neurosci.* 33, 17197–17208. doi: 10.1523/JNEUROSCI.3158-13.2013

Verhoog, M. B., Obermayer, J., Kortleven, C. A., Wilbers, R., Wester, J., Baayen, J. C., et al. (2016). Layer-specific cholinergic control of human and mouse cortical synaptic plasticity. *Nat. Commun.* 7:12826. doi: 10.1038/ncomms12826

Viana da Silva, S., Haberl, M. G., Zhang, P., Bethge, P., Lemos, C., Gonçalves, N., et al. (2016). Early synaptic deficits in the APP/PS1 mouse model of Alzheimer's disease involve neuronal adenosine A_{2A} receptors. *Nat. Commun.* 7:11915. doi: 10.1038/ncomms11915

Wall, M. J., and Dale, N. (2013). Neuronal transporter and astrocytic ATP exocytosis underlie activity-dependent adenosine release in the hippocampus. *J. Physiol.* 591, 3853–3871. doi: 10.1113/jphysiol.2013.253450

Wei, C. J., Singer, P., Coelho, J., Boison, D., Feldon, J., Yee, B. K., et al. (2011). Selective inactivation of adenosine A_{2A} receptors in striatal neurons enhances working memory and reversal learning. *Learn. Mem.* 18, 459–474.

Zhang, P., Bannon, N. M., Ilin, V., Volgushev, M., and Chistiakova, M. (2015). Adenosine effects on inhibitory synaptic transmission and excitation–inhibition balance in the rat neocortex. *J. Physiol.* 593, 825–841. doi: 10.1113/jphysiol.2014.279901

Zhou, S.-J., Zhu, M.-E., Shu, D., Du, X.-P., Song, X.-H., Wang, X.-T., et al. (2009). Preferential enhancement of working memory in mice lacking adenosine A_{2A} receptors. *Brain Res.* 1303, 74–83. doi: 10.1016/j.brainres.2009.09.082

16

Essential Control of the Function of the Striatopallidal Neuron by Pre-coupled Complexes of Adenosine A_{2A}-Dopamine D_2 Receptor Heterotetramers and Adenylyl Cyclase

Sergi Ferré[1], Jordi Bonaventura[1], Wendy Zhu[2], Candice Hatcher-Solis[1], Jaume Taura[3,4], César Quiroz[1], Ning-Sheng Cai[1], Estefanía Moreno[5], Verónica Casadó-Anguera[5], Alexxai V. Kravitz[6], Kimberly R. Thompson[2], Dardo G. Tomasi[7], Gemma Navarro[8], Arnau Cordomí[9], Leonardo Pardo[9], Carme Lluís[5], Carmen W. Dessauer[10], Nora D. Volkow[7], Vicent Casadó[5], Francisco Ciruela[3,4], Diomedes E. Logothetis[11] and Daniel Zwilling[2]*

[1] Integrative Neurobiology Section, National Institute on Drug Abuse, Intramural Research Program, National Institutes of Health, Baltimore, MD, United States, [2] Circuit Therapeutics, Inc., Menlo Park, CA, United States, [3] Unitat de Farmacologia, Departament de Patologia i Terapèutica Experimental, Facultat de Medicina i Ciències de la Salut, IDIBELL, Universitat de Barcelona, Barcelona, Spain, [4] Institut de Neurociències, Universitat de Barcelona, Barcelona, Spain, [5] Center for Biomedical Research in Neurodegenerative Diseases Network, Department of Biochemistry and Molecular Biomedicine, Faculty of Biology, Institute of Biomedicine of the University of Barcelona, University of Barcelona, Barcelona, Spain, [6] Eating and Addiction Section, Diabetes, Endocrinology and Obesity Branch, National Institute of Diabetes and Digestive and Kidney Diseases, Intramural Research Program, National Institutes of Health, Bethesda, MD, United States, [7] Laboratory of Neuroimaging, National Institute on Alcohol Abuse and Alcoholism, Intramural Research Program, National Institutes of Health, Rockville, MD, United States, [8] Department of Biochemistry and Physiology, Faculty of Pharmacy, University of Barcelona, Barcelona, Spain, [9] Laboratory of Computational Medicine, School of Medicine, Autonomous University of Barcelona, Bellaterra, Spain, [10] Department of Integrative Biology and Pharmacology, McGovern Medical School, University of Texas Health Science Center at Houston, Houston, TX, United States, [11] Department of Pharmaceutical Sciences, Bouvé College of Health Sciences, Northeastern University, Boston, MA, United States

***Correspondence:**
Sergi Ferré
sferre@intra.nida.nih.gov

The central adenosine system and adenosine receptors play a fundamental role in the modulation of dopaminergic neurotransmission. This is mostly achieved by the strategic co-localization of different adenosine and dopamine receptor subtypes in the two populations of striatal efferent neurons, striatonigral and striatopallidal, that give rise to the direct and indirect striatal efferent pathways, respectively. With optogenetic techniques it has been possible to dissect a differential role of the direct and indirect pathways in mediating "Go" responses upon exposure to reward-related stimuli and "NoGo" responses upon exposure to non-rewarded or aversive-related stimuli, respectively, which depends on their different connecting output structures and their differential expression of dopamine and adenosine receptor subtypes. The striatopallidal neuron selectively expresses dopamine D_2 receptors (D2R) and adenosine A_{2A} receptors (A2AR), and numerous experiments using multiple genetic and pharmacological *in vitro*, *in situ* and *in vivo* approaches, demonstrate they can form A2AR-D2R heteromers. It was initially assumed that different pharmacological interactions between dopamine and adenosine receptor ligands indicated the existence of different subpopulations of A2AR and D2R in the striatopallidal neuron. However, as elaborated in the present essay, most evidence now indicates that all interactions can be explained with a predominant population of striatal A2AR-D2R heteromers forming complexes with adenylyl cyclase subtype 5 (AC5). The A2AR-D2R heteromer has a tetrameric structure, with two homodimers, which allows not only multiple allosteric interactions between different orthosteric ligands, agonists, and antagonists, but also the canonical Gs-Gi antagonistic interaction at the level of AC5. We present a model of the function of the A2AR-D2R heterotetramer-AC5 complex, which acts as an integrative device of adenosine and dopamine signals that determine the excitability and gene expression of the striatopallidal neurons. The model can explain most behavioral effects of A2AR and D2R ligands, including the psychostimulant effects of caffeine. The model is also discussed in the context of different functional striatal compartments, mainly the dorsal and the ventral striatum. The current accumulated knowledge of the biochemical properties of the A2AR-D2R heterotetramer-AC5 complex offers new therapeutic possibilities for Parkinson's disease, schizophrenia, SUD and other neuropsychiatric disorders with dysfunction of dorsal or ventral striatopallidal neurons.

Keywords: striatopallidal neuron, adenosine A_{2A} receptor, dopamine D_2 receptor, GPCR heteromers, adenylyl cyclase, caffeine, akinesia, apathy

INTRODUCTION

One of the most noticeable functions of adenosine in the brain is the ability to impose a brake on the central dopaminergic system. This inhibitory role of adenosine is largely mediated by the activation of one subtype of adenosine receptor, the A_{2A} receptor (A2AR), particularly expressed by one type of neuron localized in the striatum, the striatopallidal neuron. The striatum is the brain area with the highest innervation of dopamine and the highest expression of dopamine receptors in the brain (Gerfen, 2004), and the striatopallidal neuron expresses the highest density of A2AR and dopamine receptors of the D_2 subtype (D2R) than any other neuron in the central nervous system (Gerfen, 2004; Schiffmann et al., 2007). It is now well accepted that adenosine controls the function of the striatopallidal neuron through intermolecular interactions between A2AR and D2R, with the formation of receptor heteromers.

Since its initial discovery, now more than 25 years ago (Ferré et al., 1991b), A2AR-D2R interactions have become a model for the study of allosteric interactions within G protein-coupled receptor (GPCR) heteromers, with the emergence of a new concept: allosteric interactions between orthosteric ligands (reviewed in Ferré et al., 2014). But recent findings indicate that the A2AR-D2R heteromer will also become a model for receptor-receptor interactions previously thought to take place downstream, on converging signaling molecules, which were often labeled as "interactions at the second messenger level." The antagonistic canonical interaction at the level of adenylyl cyclase (AC), between a Gs/olf-coupled receptor, such as the A2AR, and a Gi/o-coupled receptor, such as the D2R, represents a classical example. Thus, a recent study demonstrates that this canonical interaction is dependent on the oligomerization of A2AR and D2R and the AC subtype AC5 (Navarro et al., 2018). This discovery implies that the striatal A2AR-D2R heteromer could explain most pharmacological effects of A2AR and D2R ligands, with implications for various neuropsychiatric disorders.

The understanding of the role of striatal adenosine and A2AR-D2R heteromers in striatal function and dysfunction will be here revisited within the framework of, not only the new developments on A2AR-D2R heteromers, but also most recent developments on the function of different striatal compartments and striatal dopamine, particularly on the function of the striatopallidal neuron. First, we summarize the current knowledge of the role of dopamine in the different striatal compartments. Next, we analyze the role of adenosine-dopamine interactions in the modulation of the function of the striatopallidal neuron. We then propose a functional model for the A2AR-D2R heterotetramer-AC5 complex in the striatopallidal neuron, a complex formed by one A2AR homodimer coupled to a Golf protein, a D2R homodimer coupled to a Gi protein and its signaling molecule AC5. The model is then used to reevaluate the pharmacological effects of adenosine receptor ligands, including caffeine. Finally, it is proposed that A2AR-D2R heterotetramer-AC5 complexes localized in striatopallidal neurons can be used as targets for the treatment of neuropsychiatric symptoms, such as akinesia and apathy. We also present new results of the effect of the A2AR antagonist SCH 442416 in radioligand binding, locomotor activation and optogenetic experiments in mice, which reconcile previous studies with the same compound that were apparently incompatible with our hypothesis of a predominant population of striatal A2AR-D2R heteromers that modulate striatopallidal neuronal function.

FUNCTIONAL DISTINCTION OF STRIATAL COMPARTMENTS

The striatum is the main input structure of the basal ganglia. Although in humans and non-human primates it has been classically subdivided into nucleus accumbens (NAc), caudate and putamen, it can be functionally subdivided in three different compartments: ventral, rostral-dorsal and caudal-dorsal striata (**Figure 1A**). The ventral striatum concept has expanded from its initial inclusion of areas innervated by the dopaminergic cells of the ventral tegmental area (VTA), mostly the NAc with its two compartments core and shell and the olfactory tubercle, to the striatal areas receiving glutamatergic inputs from the ventromedial prefrontal cortex, orbitofrontal cortex and anterior cingulate cortex (Haber and Behrens, 2014) (**Figure 1A**). In fact, the orbitofrontal cortex and the anterior cingulate cortex, respectively, receive partial and predominant dopaminergic innervation from the substantia nigra pars compacta (SNpc; Haber and Behrens, 2014). Furthermore, the ventral striatum receives afferent glutamatergic projections from the insular cortex, amygdala and hippocampus (Haber and Behrens, 2014). The rostral-dorsal striatum receives glutamatergic input from frontal and parietal association areas and the caudal-dorsal striatum from the primary motor and somatosensory cortices (**Figure 1A**). Both rostral-dorsal and caudal-dorsal striata receive their dopaminergic input from the SNpc (Haber, 2014; Haber and Behrens, 2014).

The ventral striatum forms part of decision-making brain circuits involved in reward valuation tasks, which determine and store reward values (often named as "subjective values of rewards") and constantly choose the reward to be obtained by a process of maximizing utilities associated with different options, the highest benefit/cost ratio (Kable and Glimcher, 2009). 'Delay discounting' (DD), 'effort discounting' (ED), and 'low-probability discounting' (LPD) refer to the empirical finding that both humans and animals value immediate, low-effort and high probability rewards more than delayed, high-effort and low probability rewards. A large number of behavioral and clinical studies indicate that DD, ED, and LPD are independent variables possibly involving corticostriatal circuits with different ventral striatal compartments differentially connected to different prefrontal cortical areas (Prévost et al., 2010; Stopper and Floresco, 2011). A main role of the ventral striatum, classically labeled as an interface between motivation and action (Mogenson et al., 1980), can be synthesized as determining "whether to respond" while that of the dorsal striatum is "how to respond" to reward-associated stimuli (Ferré, 2017). All reward-related, dopamine-dependent functions, including the facilitation of reward-oriented behavior and learning of stimulus-reward and reward-response associations (positive reinforcement; Wise, 2004), are simultaneously processed by the rostral-dorsal and caudal-dorsal striata. In relation to positive reinforcement, the rostral-dorsal striatum is predominantly involved in an initial, more controlled (contingent on the outcome) and less permanent learning, while the caudal-dorsal striatum is involved in a slower, less controlled (non-contingent on the outcome) but long-lasting learning (Kim and Hikosaka, 2015). The same functional dichotomy, "volitional" and "automatic" learning, but with a medial-lateral distribution, can also be demonstrated in the rodent striatum (Voorn et al., 2004; Yin and Knowlton, 2006; Balleine and O'Doherty, 2010). However, it is becoming increasingly evident that dopaminergic mesencephalic cells also process aversive-related and non-rewarded stimuli and are involved in negative reinforcement. Most dopamine cells respond by decreasing their activity upon exposure to aversive stimuli and to omission of expected rewards. Dopaminergic cells, therefore, code for positive and negative reward prediction errors, increasing their firing upon presentation of reward-related stimuli or better than expected rewards or with the termination of aversive-related stimuli and decreasing their firing upon omission of reward-related stimuli or presentation of a worse than expected reward (Steinberg et al., 2013; Chang et al., 2016).

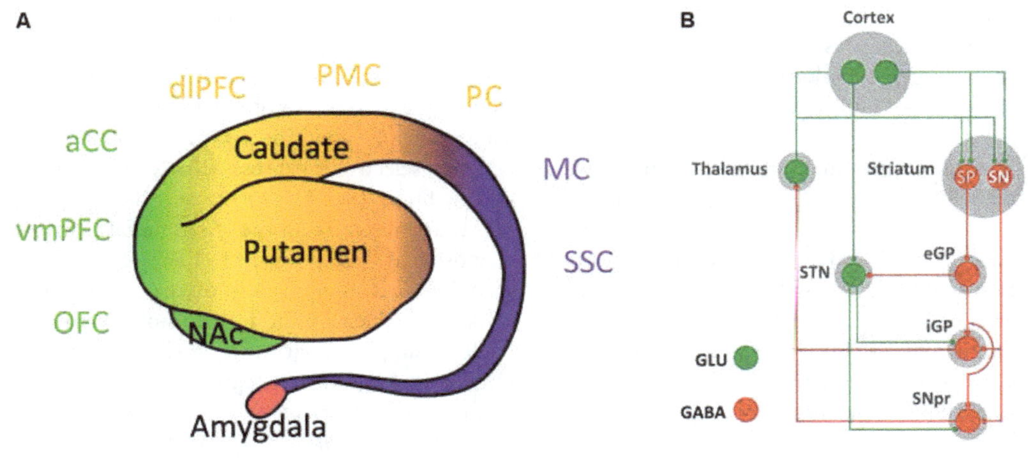

FIGURE 1 | Inputs and outputs of the striatum. **(A)** Lateral view of the striatum and amygdala (of human and non-human primates). The classical morphological subdivision of striatal compartments in nucleus accumbens (NAc), caudate and putamen nuclei can be functionally classified according to the cortical inputs in: ventral striatum (in green), which receives inputs from the ventromedial prefrontal cortex (vmPFC), orbitofrontal cortex (OFC), and anterior cingulate cortex (aCC); rostral-dorsal striatum (in orange), which receives inputs from frontal and parietal association areas, such as the dorsolateral prefrontal cortex (dlPFC), premotor cortex (PMC), and parietal cortex (PC); and caudal-rostral striatum (in purple), which receives inputs from the primary motor cortex (MC) and the somatosensory cortex (SSC). **(B)** Basal ganglia circuitry. The striatonigral neuron (SN) directly connects the striatum with the output structures of the basal ganglia: the internal segment of the globus pallidus (iGP) and the substantia nigra pars reticulata (SNpr). The striatopallidal neuron (SP) connects with the output structures by relays in the external segment of the globus pallidus (eGP) and the subthalamic nucleus (STN); GLU, glutamate.

THE A2AR-D2R-EXPRESSING STRIATOPALLIDAL NEURON

In the striatum, glutamatergic and dopaminergic inputs converge in the dendritic spines of the GABAergic medium-sized spiny neurons, which constitute more than 95% of the striatal neuronal population (Gerfen, 2004). There are two types of medium-sized spiny neurons, which define the two striatal efferent pathways that connect the striatum with the output structures of the basal ganglia, substantia nigra pars reticulata (SNpr) and internal segment of the globus pallidus (**Figure 1B**). The striatonigral neuron constitutes the *direct efferent pathway* since it connects directly with the output structures (Gerfen, 2004). The striatopallidal neuron gives rise to the *indirect efferent pathway* and connects with the pallidal complex (the external segment of the globus pallidus and the ventral pallidum), which connects with the output structures directly and through a relay in the subthalamic nucleus (Gerfen, 2004) (**Figure 1B**). While there are no apparent qualitative or quantitative differences between the glutamatergic inputs impinging on the striatonigral and striatopallidal neurons, there is a clear distinction with the receptors that process the dopaminergic signals. Thus, the striatonigral neuron expresses dopamine D_1 receptors (D1R), a prototypical Gs/olf-coupled stimulatory receptor (Golf in the striatum), while the striatopallidal neuron expresses D2R, a prototypical Gi/o-coupled inhibitory receptor (Gerfen, 2004; Bertran-Gonzalez et al., 2008). This established scheme breaks down in the most ventral striatal compartment, the shell of the NAc. The most ventral striatopallidal neurons project to the ventromedial and ventrolateral parts of the ventral pallidum, which does not connect with the output structures or relay in the subthalamic nucleus (Root et al., 2015). Instead, these regions of the ventral pallidum represent output structures of the basal ganglia themselves, since they project to the medio-dorsal thalamus, lateral hypothalamus and lateral habenula (Root et al., 2015). Furthermore, some ventral striatopallidal neurons also express D1R, with some degree of co-localization but still largely segregated from D2R (Bertran-Gonzalez et al., 2008; Frederick et al., 2015).

A mechanism by which dopamine is directly involved with positive and negative reinforcement is emerging from the study of the functional role of the direct and indirect striatal efferent pathways. Using recently developed optogenetic techniques, it has been possible to dissect a differential role of the direct and indirect pathways in mediating "Go" responses upon exposure to reward-related stimuli and "NoGo" responses upon exposure to non-rewarded or aversive-related stimuli, respectively, which depends on their different connecting output structures and their differential expression of dopamine receptor subtypes (Hikida et al., 2010, 2013; Kravitz et al., 2010, 2012; Freeze et al., 2013; Danjo et al., 2014). The differential connectivity entails that activation of striatonigral and striatopallidal neurons lead to qualitatively different behavioral responses, with the most obvious being the respective facilitation and inhibition of psychomotor activity. At this point, following Wise and Bozarth (1987), we should make the distinction between "psychomotor" and simply "motor" responses. Psychomotor responses, which include forward locomotion or withdraw, have a characteristic dependence on external stimuli; increases or decreases of dopamine enhance or diminish the responsiveness to those stimuli, respectively. The differential affinities of D1R and D2R for endogenous dopamine and their respective predominant expression in striatonigral and striatopallidal neurons provide a fine-tuning device by which bursts and pauses of dopamine neurons can differentially influence their activity (Roitman et al., 2008; Bromberg-Martin et al., 2010; Macpherson et al., 2014). Dopamine has significantly higher affinity for D2R than for D1R. Therefore, D2R are more activated than D1R by basal dopamine levels and are more sensitive to the effects of dopamine pauses, while D1R are more sensitive to dopamine bursts, to conditions of larger dopamine release. Bursts of dopamine neurons result in large dopamine release, which predominantly increases the activation of stimulatory D1R and causes the direct pathway to promote high-value reward-associated movements, whereas the lower basal dopamine levels predominantly activate D2R, which are inhibitory and remove activation of the indirect pathway, thus suppressing low-value reward-associated or high-value punishment-associated movements (Frank, 2005; Hikosaka, 2007; Dreyer et al., 2010; Hikida et al., 2010, 2013; Kravitz et al., 2012; Danjo et al., 2014). Nevertheless, we should not ignore the fact that D2R are not completely occupied by endogenous dopamine and that bursts of dopamine are also able to enhance D2R signaling, therefore participating to the psychomotor activation guided by the stimuli associated with the concomitant increase in dopaminergic cell firing. However, strong dopamine receptor activation basically promotes potentiation of corticostriatal synapses onto the direct pathway and learning from positive outcomes (positive reinforcement), while weak dopamine receptor activation promotes potentiation of corticostriatal synapses onto the indirect pathway and learning from negative outcomes (negative reinforcement) (Frank et al., 2004; Nakamura and Hikosaka, 2006; Shen et al., 2008; Voon et al., 2010).

Another important phenotypical difference between the striatopallidal and striatonigral neurons is their differential expression of adenosine receptor subtypes. The striatopallidal neurons selectively express A2AR, in fact, the highest density in the brain (Schiffmann et al., 2007). On the other hand, A2AR are absent from the striatonigral neurons, which express adenosine A_1 receptors (A1R) (Ferré et al., 1997). A2AR can then be used as a marker of the striatopallidal neuron. For instance, to identify the function of the striatopallidal neuron, studies using Bacterial Artificial Chromosome (BAC) transgenic mice have targeted the regulatory elements of either the D2R or the A2AR (Durieux et al., 2009; Valjent et al., 2009; Freeze et al., 2013). We used BAC transgenic mouse lines that express Cre recombinase under the control of regulatory elements of the D2R (D2R-Cre mice) or the A2AR (A2AR-Cre mice), allowing the selective expression of channelrhodopsin 2 (ChR2) by striatopallidal neurons (Kravitz et al., 2010; Freeze et al., 2013; Zwilling et al., 2014). This was achieved by bilateral injection of an adeno-associated virus (AAV) containing a Cre-sensitive vector with a double-floxed inverted open reading frame encoding a fusion of ChR2 and enhanced yellow fluorescence protein into the dorsomedial striatum. Then, fiber-optic cannulas implanted immediately above the injection site allowed the local delivery of light with the concomitant selective optogenetic activation of a large fraction of dorsal striatopallidal neurons. Unilateral optogenetic stimulation led to significant ipsilateral rotational behavior, while bilateral optogenetic stimulation led to a significant decrease in locomotor activity (Kravitz et al., 2010; Freeze et al., 2013; Zwilling et al., 2014) (**Figure 2A**). These results were opposite to those obtained by the selective ablation of a large proportion of dorsal and ventral striatopallidal neurons in BAC transgenic A2AR-Cre mice by Cre-mediated expression of a diphtheria toxin receptor and diphtheria toxin injection, which led to hyperlocomotion (Durieux et al., 2009).

Altogether, these optogenetic and genetic targeting experiments agree with the increase and decrease of "NoGo" responses upon the respective activation or inactivation of striatopallidal neurons. Hypo- or hyperlocomotion represents an outcome of the respective sustained activation or deactivation of a large number of striatopallidal neurons, which more discretely should represent the respective facilitation and inhibition of withdrawal behavior from low-value reward-associated or high-value punishment-associated movements. We addressed more directly this assumption in optogenetic experiments with A2AR-Cre mice, by selectively inducing the expression of ChR2 in dorsal striatopallidal neurons and by using more discrete parameters of stimulation (Zwilling et al., 2014). **Figure 2B** shows the comparison of two different parameters of bilateral optogenetic stimulation in the dorso-medial striatum on locomotor activity. Continuous light for 1 min induced freezing and therefore an impairment of motor activity that

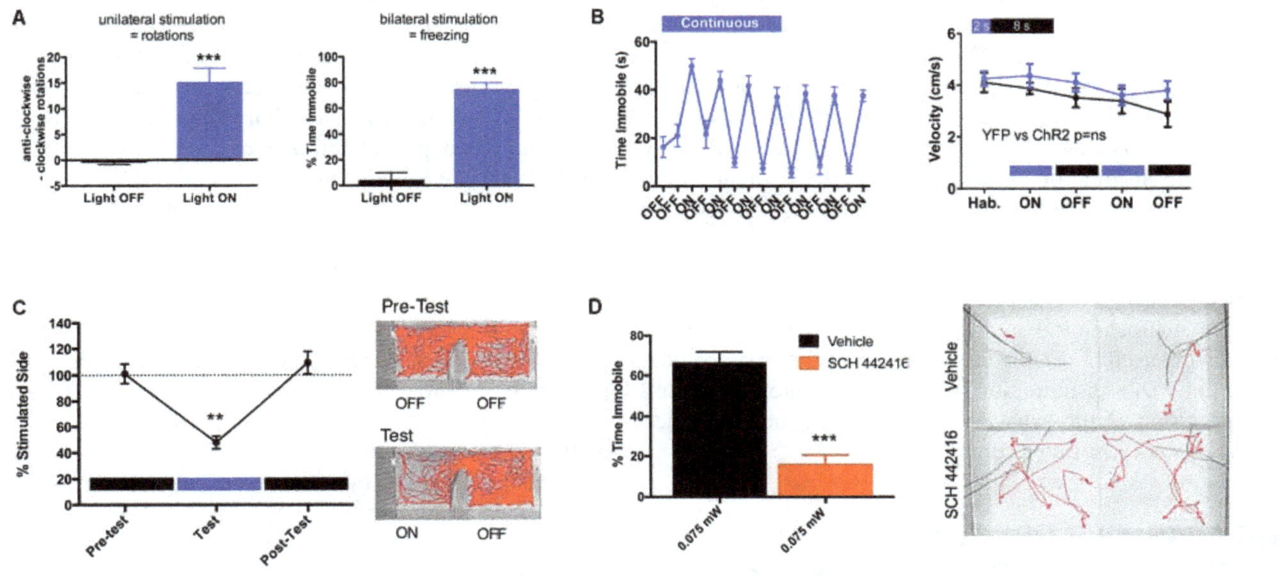

FIGURE 2 | Behavioral effects of the optogenetic stimulation of the striatopallidal neuron in mice. The adeno-associated virus (AAV) containing the Cre-sensitive pAAV5-EF1a-DIO-hChR2(H134R)-YFP virus was bilaterally injected into the dorsal-medial striatum (1 μl at coordinates M-L ± 1.5, A-P + 0.8 and D-V –3.5, relative to bregma) of a BAC transgenic A2AR-Cre mouse (C57BL/6 background). Fiber-optic cannulas were implanted 0.5 μm above the injection site and the virus was allowed to incubate for 4 weeks before the start of behavioral testing. **(A)** At high intensity of stimulation, unilateral illumination results in rotational behavior and bilateral illumination results in freezing. In **(A)** left graph, mice were unilaterally illuminated (left side) with constant light at 1 mW (measured at the fiber tip) and anti-clockwise vs. clockwise (ipsilateral vs. contralateral) rotations were recorded for a duration of 5 min; results are expressed as mean ± SEM; Student's paired *t*-test showed significant differences in the number of rotations in the illuminated condition (light ON) compared to control (light OFF) (***$p < 0.001$, $n = 4$). In **(A)** right graph, mice were illuminated bilaterally with constant light at equal intensity (1 mW per side) and time spent immobile over a period of 1 min was determined; results are expressed as mean ± SEM; Student's paired *t*-test showed significant differences between the illuminated condition (light ON) compared to control (light OFF) (***$p < 0.001$, $n = 11$). **(B)** Comparison of different light illumination paradigms; bilateral circuit activation produced different effects on motor behavior depending on the pattern of light stimulation; continuous light for 1 min induced freezing and motor impairment. In **(B)** left graph, mice were bilaterally stimulated alternating 1-min light ON/OFF blocks, while freezing (expressed as time immobile) was scored through several cycles over 15 min (results are expressed as mean ± SEM, $n = 11$). In **(B)** right graph, mice were pulse stimulated using a 2-s ON/8-s OFF illumination paradigm and did not exhibit ambulatory impairment; velocity of ambulation was monitored over 3-min bins; blue and black plots represent ambulation (in mean ± SEM) of mice injected with the virus expressing ChR-YFP ($n = 20$) or YFP (control, $n = 10$), respectively; two-way ANOVA, did not show significant differences between both groups ($p > 0.05$). **(C)** Aversive behavior driven by striatopallidal neuron activation using stimulation parameters that did not produce motor impairment; in a real-time place-preference assay pulsed light illumination (2-s ON/8 s-OFF) was triggered automatically upon entry into the predesignated 'stimulation side' of the chamber; the amount of time spent in the light-paired chamber was quantified over 20-min blocks recorded before, during and immediately after light stimulation. In **(C)** left graph, mice demonstrated a significant light-mediated aversion, a reduction in the percentage of time (in mean ± SEM) spent in the stimulated side; analyzed statistically by one-way repeated measures ANOVA and Tukey *post hoc* test (**$p < 0.01$; $n = 8$). In **(C)** right panel, example tracks show robust aversion to the left stimulation chamber during the test session. **(D)** A2AR antagonist reduces freezing phenotype. In **(D)** left graph, a 5-min pre-test injection of the A2AR antagonist SCH 442416 (3 mg/kg, i.p.) significantly reduced the percent time freezing (in mean ± SEM) at light power levels of 0.075 mW; Student's paired *t*-test showed significant difference between the groups treated with and without SCH 442416 (***$p < 0.001$; $n = 11$). In **(D)** right panel, example tracks showing SCH-mediated counteraction of optogenetically induced freezing. All behaviors were performed in custom-built arenas and activity monitored and automatically scored using a Noldus Ethovision video tracking system.

would interfere with the analysis of behavior in a real-time place-preference study. On the other hand, mice that were pulse-stimulated using a 2-s ON/8-s OFF illumination paradigm did not demonstrate ambulatory impairment (**Figure 2B**). When this pulse-stimulation was triggered when the mouse entered one of the chambers of a place-preference box, the animal showed a very significant aversion-like behavior to that side (**Figure 2C**) (Zwilling et al., 2014). These results also complement those obtained by Hikida et al. (2010, 2013) in experiments with selective bilateral inactivation of the dorsal or ventral striatopallidal neuron by means of doxycycline-dependent, pathway-specific expression of tetanus toxin (driven by the promoter of the gene coding the neuropeptide enkephalin, selectively expressed by striatopallidal neurons). A counteraction of the expression in addition to the acquisition of aversion-like behavior was also demonstrated by using an asymmetric design, with targeted unilateral inactivation of the ventral striatopallidal neurons with tetanus toxin and the contralateral infusion of a D2R agonist (but not a D2R antagonist or D1R agonists or antagonists) or an A2AR antagonist (Hikida et al., 2013). Similarly, we could demonstrate that the systemic administration of the A2AR antagonist SCH 442416 (3 mg/kg i.p.) significantly decreases the locomotor depression induced by low-intensity optogenetic stimulation of the dorsal-medial striatopallidal neurons (**Figure 2D**). These results would imply a significant role of an endogenous adenosinergic tone in the facilitation of the striatopallidal neuronal function mediated by A2AR. In fact, numerous neurochemical studies imply that A2AR signaling is especially involved in driving the activation of the striatopallidal neuron upon D2R disinhibition (see below), therefore in driving the suppression of the behavior associated with non-rewarded and punishment-associated stimuli.

THE A2AR-D2R RECEPTOR HETEROTETRAMER-AC5 COMPLEX

There is a large amount of experimental evidence indicating the existence of a predominant striatal population of A2AR and D2R that control striatopallidal neuronal function (Ferré et al., 1993, 2016; Azdad et al., 2009; Bonaventura et al., 2015). Recent studies suggested that A2AR-D2R heteromers assemble into a heterotetrameric structure, with A2AR and D2R homodimers coupled to their respective cognate Gs (more precisely the Golf isoform) and Gi proteins (Bonaventura et al., 2015). The heterotetrameric structure would provide the frame for multiple adenosine-dopamine interactions and for interactions between exogenous A2AR and D2R ligands (Navarro et al., 2014; Ferré et al., 2016). One of the most prominent interactions is the allosteric negative effect of A2AR ligands on the affinity and efficacy of D2R ligands (*allosteric interaction*) (Ferré et al., 1991b; Azdad et al., 2009; Bonaventura et al., 2015), which has been demonstrated to depend on A2AR-D2R heteromerization by the use of synthetic peptides that selectively interfere with the heteromeric interface, both in mammalian transfected cells and in striatal tissue (Azdad et al., 2009; Bonaventura et al., 2015).

In addition to the allosteric interaction, a strong reciprocal antagonistic interaction, with the ability of D2R agonists to inhibit A2AR agonist-mediated activation of AC, was first identified in mammalian transfected cells (Kull et al., 1999; Hillion et al., 2002) and more recently characterized in striatal cells in culture (Navarro et al., 2014). This represents an antagonistic Gs-Gi *canonical interaction*, the ability of an activated Gi-coupled receptor to inhibit a Gs-coupled receptor-mediated activation of AC. The A2AR-D2R canonical interaction was first observed *in situ*, in the striatum. The evidence came initially from experiments that demonstrated that the increase in the expression of the immediate-early gene *c-fos* in the striatopallidal neurons upon treatment with D2R antagonists or acute dopamine depletion could be counteracted by blocking A2AR signaling (Boegman and Vincent, 1996; Svenningsson et al., 1999). This A2AR signaling is initiated by the second messenger cyclic-AMP (cAMP), the product of AC activation. The cascade includes protein kinase A (PKA) activation, with phosphorylation of the cAMP-response element binding protein (CREB), a mechanism which is amplified by the PKA-dependent phosphorylation of 'dopamine- and cAMP-regulated phosphoprotein of molecular weight 32,000' (DARPP-32) (Svenningsson et al., 1998; Kull et al., 1999) (**Figure 3A**). A2AR-mediated activation of PKA also promotes phosphorylation of voltage dependent Ca^{2+} channels (VDCC), NMDA, and AMPA receptors (Håkansson et al., 2006; Azdad et al., 2009; Higley and Sabatini, 2010), which determines their degree of activation and, therefore, the degree of excitability of the striatopallidal neurons, which determines the degree of psychomotor depression (**Figure 3A**).

Activation of the D2R, when uninterrupted by co-activation of the A2AR (allosteric interaction), can also signal through phospholipase C (PLC) by a Gßγ subunit-dependent mechanism, which induces the release of inositol (1,4,5)-triphosphate (IP3), a second messenger that causes the release of intracellular Ca^{2+}. This, in turn results in the subsequent activation of the Ca^{2+}/calmodulin-dependent protein phosphatase calcineurin (also called protein phosphatase 2B or PP2B) (Hernandez-Lopez et al., 2000; Azdad et al., 2009) (**Figure 3A**). Phosphorylated forms of VDCC, NMDA, and AMPA receptors and DARPP-32 are main targets of PP2B. Therefore, activation of PP2B leads to a decreased neuronal excitability and represents a downstream additional mechanism of D2R-mediated inhibition of A2AR signaling (Lindskog et al., 1999) (**Figure 3A**). In addition, A2AR and D2R activation can modify gene expression through respective G protein-dependent and independent mechanisms of MAPK activation, which plays a predominant role in the mailing of signals from the synapse to the nucleus by directly activating the constitutive transcription factor Elk-1 (Besnard et al., 2011) (**Figure 3A**). Our previous work indicates that the outcome of co-activation of striatal A2AR and D2R on MAPK activation depends on the intracellular levels of Ca^{2+}, which determines the binding of two different neuronal Ca^{2+}-binding proteins, NCS-1 and calneuron-1 (Navarro et al., 2014). NCS-1 and calneuron bind to the A2AR-D2R heteromer upon low and high concentrations of Ca^{2+}, respectively. Binding of calneuron specifically alters the ability of A2AR ligands

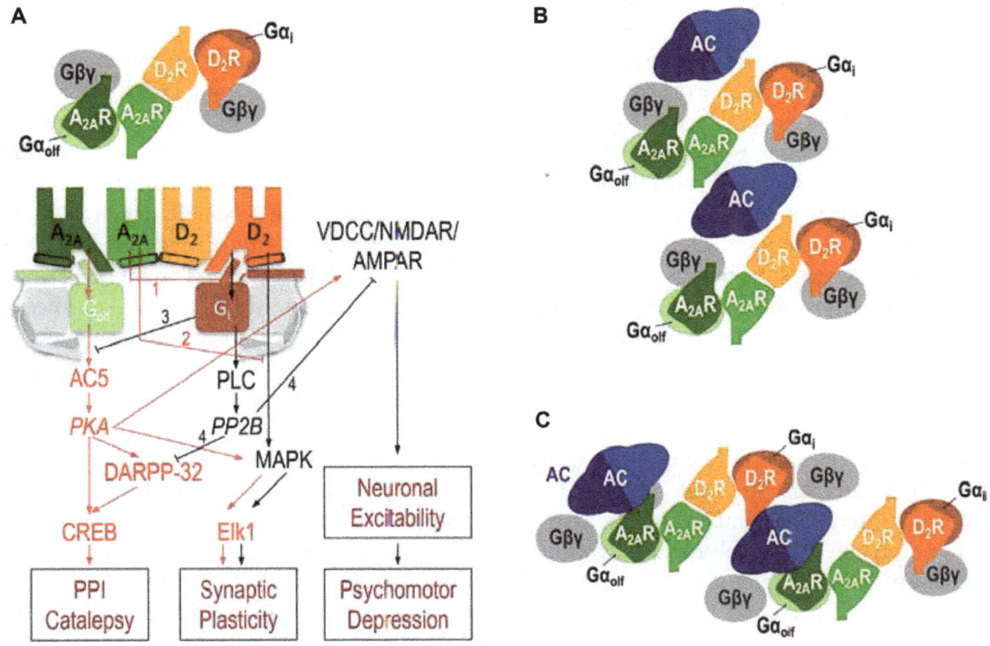

FIGURE 3 | The A2AR-D2R heterotetramer. **(A)** Model representing the striatal A2AR-D2R heteromer-dependent mechanisms that modulate different biochemical and behavioral outputs. The heterotetrameric structure of the A2AR-D2R heteromer allows multiple simultaneous and reciprocal interactions between adenosine and dopamine and exogenous A2AR and D2R ligands. Mainly, the ability of adenosine or exogenous A2AR ligands to decrease G protein-dependent (1) or G protein-independent (2) signaling by dopamine or exogenous D2R ligands (allosteric interactions) and a reciprocal antagonistic interaction, the ability of D2R agonists to inhibit the A2AR agonist-mediated activation of AC5, by means of the antagonistic Gs-Gi canonical interaction at the AC5 level (3). When uninterrupted by the canonical interaction, A2AR signals through activation of AC5 and protein kinase A (PKA) with phosphorylation of 'dopamine- and cAMP-regulated phosphoprotein of molecular weight 32,000' (DARPP-32), which facilitates PPI and catalepsy, and voltage-dependent Ca^{2+} channels (VDCC), NMDA and AMPA receptors, resulting in an increase in the excitability of the striatopallidal neuron. When uninterrupted by the allosteric interaction, D2R signals through PLC, which leads to activation of calcineurin (PP2B). PP2B dephosphorylates PKA substrates, DARPP-32, VDCC, NMDA and AMPA receptors, providing a downstream additional mechanism of D2R-mediated inhibition of A2AR signaling (4) and leading to a decrease in the excitability of the striatopallidal neuron, which facilitates psychomotor activation. A2AR and D2R activation can also modify gene expression through different mechanisms, including G protein-dependent and independent MAPK activation and activation of the transcription factor Elk-1 (see text). In **(B,C)**, schematic slice-representation viewed from the extracellular side of the minimal functional unit of the A2AR-D2R heterotetramer in complex with AC5 (see text), in the absence **(B)** and presence **(C)** of agonists, which induce a rearrangement of the heterotetramer-AC5 interfaces (modified from Navarro et al., 2018).

to allosterically modulate the GTP-independent D2R ligand-mediated MAPK activation, while binding of NCS-1 also counteracts the A2AR-mediated allosteric modulation of D2R-ligand-mediated G protein signaling (and therefore the canonical interaction). This provides a mechanism by which co-activation of A2AR and D2R in the heteromer promotes and counteracts MAPK activation upon low and high concentrations of Ca^{2+}, respectively (Navarro et al., 2014).

The question is how two apparently simultaneous reciprocal interactions between A2AR- and D2R signaling (allosteric and canonical interactions) can take place in the same cell. Based on some studies obtained with the A2AR antagonist SCH 442416, we initially hypothesized the existence of two populations of A2AR in striatopallidal neurons (Orrú et al., 2011b). One population would be forming heteromers with D2R and would mediate the allosteric interaction, while another population would not be forming heteromers with D2R and would allow the antagonistic interaction at the second messenger level, cAMP (Ferré et al., 2011; Orrú et al., 2011b). However, we recently hypothesized that the putative heterotetrameric structure of the A2AR-D2R heteromer could sustain both the allosteric and the canonical interactions (Navarro et al., 2014). In addition, based on the emergent view that considers GPCR homodimers as main functional units (Ferré et al., 2014), we postulated that heteromers are constituted by different interacting homodimers (Ferré et al., 2014; Ferré, 2015). This could be of special functional importance with heteromers formed by one homodimer coupled to a Gs/olf protein and another different homodimer coupled to a Gi/o protein. Our hypothesis was that such a GPCR *heterotetramer* would be part of a pre-coupled macromolecular complex that also includes AC5, the predominant AC subtype in the striatum (Lee et al., 2002), a necessary frame for the canonical antagonistic interaction at the AC level (Ferré, 2015). In fact, in mammalian transfected cells, using synthetic peptides with amino acid sequences of all transmembrane domains (TM) of A2AR and D2R and the putative TMs of AC5, we recently provided clear evidence for the existence of functional pre-coupled complexes of A2AR and D2R homodimers, their cognate Golf and Gi proteins and AC5 (Navarro et al., 2018). We first identified a symmetrical TM 6 interface for the A2AR and D2R homodimers and a symmetrical TM 4/TM 5 A2AR-D2R heteromeric interface. Computational analysis provided one minimal solution, a linear arrangement with two internal interacting A2AR and D2R protomers and two external non-interacting A2AR and D2R protomers which interact with the α-subunits of the corresponding Golf and Gi proteins (**Figure 3**). Second, we found asymmetrical interfaces formed by TMs of the receptors and putative TMs of AC5 which rearrange upon agonist exposure. Computational analysis indicated the existence of a minimal functional complex formed by two A2AR-D2R heterotetramers and two AC5 molecules (**Figures 3B,C**). In fact, this quaternary structure suggests the possible formation of zig-zagged arranged high-order oligomeric structures, a higher-order linear arrangement of GPCR heteromers and effectors (Navarro et al., 2018). Finally, we could demonstrate that this macromolecular complex provides the sufficient but necessary condition for the canonical Gs-Gi interactions at the AC level (Navarro et al., 2018). The most demonstrative experiment was that destabilization of the quaternary structure of the A2AR-D2R heterotetramer, with interfering synthetic peptides with the amino acid sequence of the TMs involved in heteromeric interface, blocked the ability of a D2R agonist to counteract AC5 activation by an A2AR agonist in striatal neurons in culture (Navarro et al., 2018).

The A2AR-D2R heterotetramer therefore acts as an integrative molecular device, which allows reciprocal antagonistic interactions between adenosine and dopamine to facilitate a switch in the activation-inhibition of the striatopallidal neuron: A preferential A2AR vs. D2R activation leads to an increase in neuronal activity determined by the A2AR-mediated activation of the AC5/PKA pathway, which is potentiated by the allosteric counteraction of D2R signaling ("1" and "2" in **Figure 3A**); a preferential D2R vs. A2AR activation leads to a decrease in neuronal activity by activation of the PLC/PP2B pathway and switching off the A2A-mediated activation of AC5 through the canonical interaction ("3" in **Figure 3A**), which we have shown depends on the integrity of the A2AR-D2R heterotetramer-AC5 complex (Azdad et al., 2009; Higley and Sabatini, 2010; Navarro et al., 2014, 2018; Bonaventura et al., 2015; Ferré, 2016; Ferré et al., 2016).

The heterotetrameric structure of the A2AR-D2R heteromer provides the framework for allosteric mechanisms of A2AR ligands that could explain recent experimental findings apparently incompatible with classical pharmacology, such as the agonist-like behavior of A2AR antagonists, which includes caffeine, a non-selective adenosine receptor antagonist. The initial unexpected finding came from a human PET study. In this study, the acute administration of caffeine produced an increase in the binding of [^{11}C]raclopride, a D2R antagonist, in the putamen and ventral striatum (Volkow et al., 2015). As a significant additional finding, the caffeine-dependent increase in D2R antagonist binding in the ventral striatum correlated with an increase in alertness (Volkow et al., 2015). Considering that previous studies demonstrated antagonistic allosteric interactions between A2AR and D2R agonists, caffeine should have induced the opposite effect, a decrease in [^{11}C]raclopride binding, due to an increase in the affinity of endogenous dopamine. We therefore studied the possibility of a direct allosteric modulation of caffeine on D2R agonist binding. Both the A2AR agonist CGS 21680 and caffeine significantly decreased the binding of the D2R agonist [^{3}H]quinpirole in membrane preparations from sheep striatum and mammalian cells transfected with A2AR and D2R. We could also demonstrate that both agonist-agonist and antagonist-agonist allosteric modulations were dependent on heteromerization, since they were not observed when transfecting a mutated A2AR with impaired ability to heteromerize with D2R (Bonaventura et al., 2015). Therefore, we initially assumed that the caffeine-induced increase in [^{11}C]raclopride binding demonstrated in PET experiments could be explained by a caffeine-induced decrease in the affinity of endogenous dopamine. However, the observation that both A2AR agonists and A2AR antagonists can produce the same allosteric interaction in the A2AR-D2R heteromer, a reduction in the affinity of agonists for the D2R, contradicts the hypothesis of a key role of allosteric interactions within the A2AR-D2R heteromer as a main mechanism involved in the opposite behavioral effects of A2AR agonists and antagonists (Ferré, 2008, 2016). Nevertheless, a biphasic effect was observed when analyzing the effect of increasing concentrations of caffeine or the selective A2AR antagonists SCH 58261 and KW 6002 on the ability of a single concentration of CGS 21680 to decrease [^{3}H]quinpirole binding. Low concentrations of caffeine and the A2AR antagonists significantly counteracted the effect of CGS 21680, while high concentrations further decreased [^{3}H]quinpirole binding (Bonaventura et al., 2015). Therefore, the results implied that orthosteric A2AR agonists and antagonists produce the same allosteric modulation of D2R agonist binding within the A2AR-D2R heteromer when applied individually, but, when co-applied, they cancel out each other's effect. This could be explained by the existence of two A2AR protomers in the A2AR-D2R heteromer and allosteric interactions between orthosteric agonists and antagonists, by which simultaneous occupation of the A2AR homodimer by an agonist and an antagonist would "freeze" the ability of either ligand to allosterically modulate D2R agonist binding. The existence of allosteric interactions between orthosteric A2AR agonists and antagonists could be confirmed through binding kinetics experiments with the A2AR antagonist [^{3}H]ZM 241385. Thus, when analyzing the effect of CGS 21680, caffeine and SCH 58261, only CGS 21680 modified the dissociation rate of [^{3}H]ZM 241385 (Bonaventura et al., 2015). Considering that CGS 21680 and [^{3}H]ZM 241385 bind to the same orthosteric site (Lebon et al., 2011), the effect of CGS 21680 could be explained by co-occupation of both ligands of the two orthosteric sites in an A2AR homodimer.

The same allosteric effects on D2R agonist binding demonstrated by A2AR agonists and antagonists were also shown in functional experiments. By measuring ERK1/2 phosphorylation in transfected cells, we could demonstrate that CGS 21680 counteracts quinpirole-induced MAPK activation, that this effect of CGS 21680 can be counteracted by low concentrations of caffeine or the A2AR antagonist SCH 58261 and that high concentration of the antagonists induce the opposite effect (Bonaventura et al., 2015). We should therefore expect that in the experimental animal A2AR antagonists behave as A2AR agonists under specific conditions. In fact, in patch-clamp experiments, we could demonstrate that the A2AR antagonist SCH 58261 counteracts the D2R antagonist-like properties of CGS 21680, but it reproduces the effect of the A2AR agonist when administered alone (Bonaventura et al., 2015). These results challenge the traditional view of competitive antagonism as the mechanism of the psychostimulant effects of caffeine (and selective A2AR antagonists). According to our model, the psychostimulant effect of caffeine can be explained by the counteraction of the allosteric interaction by co-occupation of the A2AR homodimer with caffeine and endogenous adenosine in the A2AR-D2R heterotetramer.

However, these allosteric interactions between A2AR agonists and antagonists and D2R agonists do not yet explain the increase in striatal [^{11}C]raclopride binding in human PET experiments induced by caffeine. Again, counteraction by caffeine of the inhibitory effect of endogenous adenosine on the binding of endogenous dopamine should lead to a decrease of [^{11}C]raclopride binding. It was then demonstrated that CGS 21680 and caffeine also inhibit the binding of [^{3}H]raclopride binding in membrane preparations from striatum or transfected cells (Bonaventura et al., 2015). That these results imply allosteric interactions within the A2AR-D2R heteromer was demonstrated by their disappearance upon transfection of a mutated A2AR with impaired ability to heteromerize with D2R and by using a synthetic peptide that disrupts A2AR-D2R heteromerization (Bonaventura et al., 2015). Therefore, within the A2AR-D2R heteromer, any orthosteric A2AR ligand, agonist or antagonist, exerts a negative allosteric modulation on the affinity of any orthosteric D2R ligand, agonist or antagonist. Finally, the same as with [^{3}H]quinpirole binding, we could also demonstrate a biphasic effect of caffeine on CGS 21680-mediated decrease of [^{3}H]raclopride binding (Bonaventura et al., 2015). These results would at last provide a plausible mechanism for the effect of caffeine on [^{11}C]raclopride binding in humans, by its ability to antagonize the effect of endogenous adenosine on the binding of the exogenous D2R antagonist. An alternative explanation could still be that caffeine blocks an adenosine-mediated internalization of A2AR-D2R heteromers (Hillion et al., 2002; Huang et al., 2013), thus leading to higher D2R availability along with higher [^{11}C]raclopride binding. The positive association between caffeine-induced increases in D2R availability and caffeine-induced increases in alertness (Volkow et al., 2015) would support this interpretation, since increased D2R signaling contributes to alertness (Isaac and Berridge, 2003). Irrespective of the mechanism involved, the effect of caffeine on [^{11}C]raclopride binding in human PET experiments implies its dependence on the A2AR-D2R heteromer and, therefore, that a significant proportion of striatal [^{11}C]raclopride binding visualized with PET labels A2AR-D2R heteromers. Furthermore, these results call for the need to control caffeine intake when evaluating the effect of D2R ligands in humans, not only when using them as probes for imaging studies, but also when using them as therapeutic agents in neuropsychiatric disorders.

Very different qualitative differences between several A2AR antagonists emerged when evaluating their potencies and efficacies on different *in vitro* and *in vivo* techniques. Particularly significant was the demonstration of different binding properties of the A2AR antagonist SCH 442416 depending on the presence and absence of D2R, when forming or not forming heteromers with D2R (Orrú et al., 2011a). In cells expressing A2AR and D2R, competitive-inhibition curves of the A2AR antagonist [^{3}H]ZM 241388 binding vs. increasing concentrations of SCH 442416 were clearly biphasic. On the other hand, in cells expressing only A2AR, or A1R and A2AR, the curves were monophasic. When analyzing the radioligand binding experiments with the two-state dimer model (Casadó et al., 2007; Ferré et al., 2014), the data indicated a negative cooperativity of SCH 442416 binding to the A2AR (Orrú et al., 2011b; Ferré et al., 2014), an additional demonstration of A2AR homomerization. This, in fact, was the first indication that the A2AR-D2R comprises at least two A2AR protomers, in agreement with a tetrameric structure of the A2AR-D2R heteromer. We have now been able to reproduce these findings in striatal tissue, comparing the results of competitive-inhibition experiments of [^{3}H]ZM 241388 binding vs. increasing concentrations of SCH 442416 in striatal membrane preparations of wild-type (WT) and striatal D2R knockout mice with a CRE-mediated deletion of D2R expression in A2AR-expressing neurons. The same as with mammalian transfected cells, the curves were biphasic or monophasic in the presence or absence of the D2R, respectively (**Figure 4**). The demonstration of the same binding properties of SCH 442416 in striatal tissue than in A2AR-D2R transfected cells implies that the A2AR-D2R heterotetramer represents the predominant population of A2AR and D2R in the striatum. Nevertheless, as mentioned below, striatal A2AR are also localized presynaptically, in glutamatergic terminals, where most probably do not form heteromers with D2R. These receptors, although playing a significant role in the modulation of striatal glutamate release, represent a very small fraction of the total of striatal A2AR, as compared to the postsynaptic A2AR.

REVISITING THE BEHAVIORAL EFFECTS OF ADENOSINE RECEPTOR LIGANDS IN THE FRAME OF ONE MAIN POPULATION OF STRIATAL A2AR AND D2R FORMING HETEROMERS

Considering that increases or decreases in the activity of the GABAergic striatopallidal neuron lead to the respective opposite effect on psychomotor activity and using a model that considers the A2AR-D2R heteromer as a key modulator of striatopallidal neuronal function, we could recently explain most psychomotor effects of caffeine (Ferré, 2016). This included the enigmatic caffeine-induced rotational behavior in rats with unilateral striatal dopamine denervation (Fuxe and Ungerstedt, 1974; Herrera-Marschitz et al., 1988; Casas et al., 1989; Garrett and Holtzman, 1995) and the ability of caffeine to significantly counteract the adipsic-aphagic syndrome in rodents with 6-hydroxy-dopamine-induced or genetic-induced dopamine deficiency (Casas et al., 2000; Kim and Palmiter, 2003, 2008). According to the model, under resting conditions there is a tonic activation of A2AR and D2R by the endogenous neurotransmitters which results in a predominant A2AR vs. D2R signaling and a predominant allosteric interaction (**Figure 5A**),

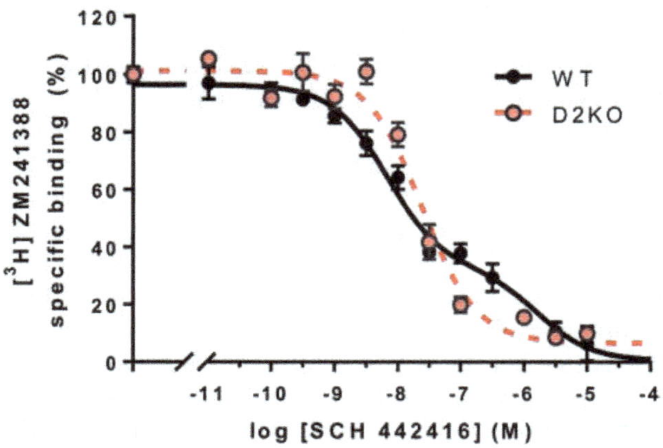

FIGURE 4 | Specific A2AR-D2R heteromer-dependent properties of SCH 442416 in mouse striatum. Transgenic conditional knockout striatopallidal neuron-Drd2-KO mice were generated by crossing mice expressing Cre driven by regulatory elements of the A2AR gene (Adora2a) [B6.FVB(Cg)-Tg(Adora2a-Cre)KG139Gsat/Mmucd; GENSAT; 036158-UCD] with mice carrying conditional D2R gene (Drd2) null alleles B6.129S4(FVB)-Drd2tm1.1Mrub/J,JAX020631 (Bello et al., 2017). Membrane preparations from the striatum of striatopallidal-Drd2-KO (red) and their CRE negative littermates (WT, black) were incubated with [^{3}H]ZM 241385 (2 nM) and increasing concentrations of SCH 442416 as described elsewhere (Bonaventura et al., 2015). Data points were fit to the two-state dimer receptor model (Casadó et al., 2007; Ferré et al., 2014), showing a biphasic curve due to negative cooperativity of SCH 442416 in WT mice (DCB = −1.8), but a monophasic curve in the conditional D2R null mice, thus reproducing the same behavior of SCH 442416 previously demonstrated in mammalian cells co-expressing A2AR and D2R and only A2AR, respectively (Orrú et al., 2011a).

which results in low psychomotor activity. Reward-related stimuli and, particularly a "better than expected" rewarding stimulus (positive reward prediction error), leads to striatal dopamine release with a predominant D2R vs. A2AR signaling, potentiated by the canonical interaction (**Figure 5B**), leading to psychomotor activation. Aversive-related stimuli or a "worse than expected" rewarding stimuli (negative reward prediction error) leads to inhibition of dopamine release, to the weakest D2R and strongest A2AR signaling, which is potentiated by the canonical interaction (**Figure 5C**), leading to psychomotor arrest.

A pathogenic hallmark of akinesia in Parkinson's disease is a pronounced hyperactivity of the striatopallidal neuron associated with the dopamine deficiency and pronounced decrease in the tonic D2R signaling. The discoveries on A2AR localization and function in striatopallidal neurons gave the rational for the recently implemented A2AR antagonists in this disease (Müller and Ferré, 2007; Morelli et al., 2009; Armentero et al., 2011). It was initially suggested that the value of A2AR antagonists as antiparkinsonian agents would depend mostly on the allosteric interaction, on the ability of A2AR antagonists to potentiate D2R signaling by concomitant administration of L-dopa or a selective D2R agonist (Ferré et al., 1991b, 1992). This was followed by behavioral studies with genetic inactivation of A2AR and D2R, which stressed the value of the canonical interaction, which was assumed to be independent of intermolecular interactions between A2AR and D2R (Chen et al., 2001). As mentioned above, the existence of the two apparently incompatible simultaneous allosteric and canonical interactions led to the hypothesis of the existence of two populations of A2AR in the striatopallidal neuron, one population forming heteromers with D2R and sustaining the allosteric interaction and another population not forming heteromers with D2R and sustaining the canonical interaction (Ferré et al., 2011; Orrú et al., 2011b). The unique pharmacological properties of SCH 442416, with its specific reduced affinity for the A2AR-D2R heteromer, due to negative cooperativity, were then exploited to attempt a pharmacological dissection of the two populations of postsynaptic A2AR. In fact, we previously used this strategy to dissect postsynaptic from presynaptic A2AR, which forms heteromers with A1R in the striatal glutamatergic terminals, where they play an important role in the modulation of glutamate release (Ciruela et al., 2006; Quiroz et al., 2009). A correlation had been shown with the higher potency of SCH 442416 to block presynaptic A1R-A2AR heteromers vs. postsynaptic A2AR-D2R heteromers and its higher potency to inhibit corticostriatal glutamate release than to produce locomotor activation (Orrú et al., 2011a). The preferential presynaptic profile of SCH 442416 was confirmed by other studies including other research groups (Hobson et al., 2013; O'Neill et al., 2014) and was suggested to provide a therapeutic approach for conditions with increased corticostriatal transmission, such as cannabinoid use disorder (Justinová et al., 2014). An apparently stronger potency of SCH 442416 to counteract locomotor depression induced by the D2R antagonist raclopride, as compared to that produced by the A2AR agonist CGS 2160, was then interpreted as the ability of SCH 442416 to also dissect the two putative postsynaptic populations of A2AR. The more sensitive population to SCH 442416 would be A2AR that do not form heteromers with D2R and that would sustain the canonical interaction (Orrú et al., 2011b). However, as mentioned before, we now know that the canonical interaction requires receptor heteromerization (Navarro et al., 2018). Therefore, we recently performed new studies on the behavioral effects of SCH 442416 upon genetic blockade of A2AR or D2R and upon administration of the A2AR agonist CGS 21680 and the D2R antagonist haloperidol, to reevaluate if they could all be explained within the framework of a predominant population of striatal postsynaptic A2AR-D2R heteromers (Taura et al., 2017).

To control strain-dependent behavioral differences and differences in drug responses, using CRISPR-Cas9 technology, we generated a D2R deficient mouse with the same genetic background as the CD-1 A2AR$^{-/-}$ mouse (Ledent et al., 1997). CD-1 D2R$^{-/-}$ mice showed a significant but relatively small reduction in spontaneous locomotor activity (Taura et al., 2017), as previously reported in D2R$^{-/-}$ C57BL/6 mice (Baik et al., 1995). This is in contrast with the pronounced akinesia and catalepsy that characterize pharmacological D2R blockade (Ferré et al., 1990; Kanda et al., 1994; Shiozaki et al., 1999). Therefore, genetic D2R blockade is associated with neuroadaptations that counteract the loss of a D2R-mediated tonic stimulatory effect of endogenous dopamine on psychomotor activity. Indeed, a recent study in inducible D2R knockout adult mice that obviated developmental compensations reported that the loss of D2R was

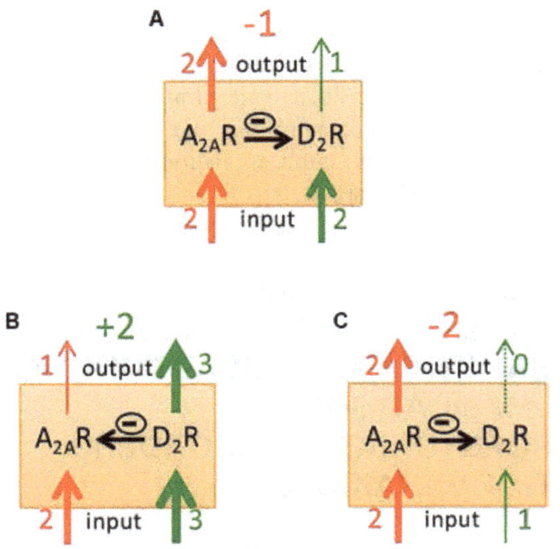

FIGURE 5 | Model of the striatal A2AR-D2R receptor heteromer as a main modulator of the excitability of the striatopallidal neuron. The relative thickness (and close number) of the red and green input arrows represents the degree of activation of the A2AR and the D2R that depends on the concentration of the corresponding neurotransmitter or exogenous ligands. The thickness (and close number) of the red and green output arrows represents the intensity of A2AR and D2R signaling, respectively, which depends on the input signal for each receptor and on the predominance of either the antagonistic or the canonical interaction (represented by horizontal arrows with a minus enclosed sign). Predominant psychomotor activation or depression will result when subtraction of the A2AR signaling from the D2R receptor signaling gives a positive or negative value (also in green or red, respectively). In **(A)**, resting condition. In **(B,C)**, processing of a positive or a negative reward prediction error, respectively.

associated with severe hypolocomotion and catalepsy (Bello et al., 2017). Likewise, the spontaneous locomotor activity of A2AR$^{-/-}$ mice was also significantly reduced, as previously reported in the A2AR C57BL/6 mouse (Yang et al., 2009). Since pharmacological blockade leads to significant locomotor activation (see below and Karcz-Kubicha et al., 2003; Orrú et al., 2011a), the reduced activity of A2AR$^{-/-}$ mice indicates the development of neuroadaptations that counteract the loss of an A2AR-mediated tonic inhibitory effect of endogenous adenosine on psychomotor activity. We also assessed sensorimotor processing of A2AR$^{-/-}$ and D2R$^{-/-}$ CD-1 mice by monitoring pre-pulse inhibitory responses (PPI) (Taura et al., 2017). As compared with WT mice, D2R$^{-/-}$ mice did not show significant differences, while A2AR$^{-/-}$ mice showed a significantly reduced PPI as previously reported (Wang et al., 2003; Moscoso-Castro et al., 2016), demonstrating a significant dependence on A2AR, but not D2R, signaling for a normal PPI. We also evaluated drug-induced catalepsy in A2AR$^{-/-}$ and D2R$^{-/-}$ mice. Our results showed that haloperidol-induced catalepsy was abolished and partially but significantly reduced in D2R$^{-/-}$ and A2AR$^{-/-}$ mice, respectively, as compared with WT mice (Taura et al., 2017), which is in agreement with previous work (Usiello et al., 2000; Chen et al., 2001; El Yacoubi et al., 2001). The results support the dependence on A2AR signaling in the catalepsy induced by pharmacological blockade of D2R, which would agree with the existence of the tonic inhibition of A2AR signaling by endogenous dopamine driven by the canonical interaction in the A2AR-D2R heteromer. Neuroadaptations occurring in the A2AR$^{-/-}$ mouse should explain the partial effect of genetic blockade of A2AR on D2R antagonist-induced catalepsy, which contrasts with the very effective blockade with A2AR antagonists (see below and Kanda et al., 1994; Shiozaki et al., 1999; Morelli and Wardas, 2001). We also assessed catalepsy induced by the A2AR agonist CGS 21680 (Ferré et al., 1991a; Kanda et al., 1994; Hauber and Münkle, 1997) in A2AR$^{-/-}$ and D2R$^{-/-}$ mice. As expected, CGS 21680 failed to induce catalepsy in A2AR$^{-/-}$ mice, but its effect was partially but significantly reduced in D2R$^{-/-}$ mice (Taura et al., 2017). Again, these results might reflect a functional antagonism related to neuroadaptations associated with genetic D2R blockade, which would tend to counteract the loss of the D2R-mediated tonic stimulatory effect of endogenous dopamine on psychomotor activity.

We then reevaluated the effect of SCH 442416 on locomotion, PPI and drug-induced catalepsy in WT, but also in A2AR$^{-/-}$ and D2R$^{-/-}$ mice. In WT CD-1 mice, SCH 442416 produced a significant and effective locomotor activation at 1 mg/kg (i.p.) (Taura et al., 2017), a dose three times lower than the minimal effective dose in Sprague-Dawley rats (Orrú et al., 2011a). As expected, SCH 44241 was unable to alter the locomotor activity in A2AR$^{-/-}$ mice and it only moderately, but significantly, increased the activity in D2R$^{-/-}$ mice (Taura et al., 2017). The decrease in the effect of the A2AR antagonist in D2R$^{-/-}$ mice would agree with a dependence on D2R signaling in the locomotor activation induced by pharmacological blockade of A2AR, due to the tonic inhibition of D2R signaling by endogenous adenosine driven by the allosteric interaction in the A2AR-D2R heteromer. In agreement with the dependence on A2AR for PPI, SCH 442416 (at the minimal dose of 3 mg/kg, i.p.) induced a blockade of PPI in WT mice (Taura et al., 2017). This is also in agreement with a previous study in rats with intracranial infusion of another A2AR antagonist (MSX-3) in the NAc (Nagel et al., 2003). SCH 442416 was obviously ineffective on the already disrupted PPI in A2AR$^{-/-}$ mice, but its disruptive effect was reduced in D2R$^{-/-}$ mice (Taura et al., 2017). This could be related to the competing effect of endogenous adenosine by the released tonic inhibition of A2AR signaling by endogenous dopamine driven by the canonical interaction in the A2AR-D2R heteromer. Finally, SCH 442416 significantly reduced haloperidol-induced catalepsy, as previously reported for other A2AR antagonists (Kanda et al., 1994; Shiozaki et al., 1999; Morelli and Wardas, 2001), but with a higher minimal dose than the one needed to produce locomotor activation (3 vs. 1 mg/kg, i.p., respectively; Taura et al., 2017). To confirm the preferential pre- vs. postsynaptic profile of SCH 442416 in mice, we also performed dose-response experiments in C57BL/6 mice on locomotor activity and counteraction of corticostriatal glutamate release using a recently introduced optogenetic-microdialysis technique (Quiroz et al., 2016; Bonaventura et al., 2017). Different to previous experiments in rats, SCH 442416 showed the same potency and efficiency as the selective A2AR antagonist KW 6002 at eliciting locomotor activation. Both drugs produced significant activation at 1 mg/kg (i.p.) but were inefficient at 0.1 mg/kg (**Figure 6A**). At this moment, we do not have an explanation for the lower potency and efficacy of SCH 442416 in rats as compared to mice. On the other hand, SCH 442416 was able to block optogenetically induced striatal glutamate release at 0.1 mg/kg, while KW 6002 was ineffective at 1 mg/kg (**Figure 6B**). This confirmed the experimental findings in rats, demonstrating a predominant striatal presynaptic and postsynaptic A2AR blocking properties of SCH 442416 and KW 6002, respectively (Orrú et al., 2011a).

Altogether, the results with genetic and pharmacological blockade of A2AR and D2R agree with a main role of A2AR-D2R heteromers in the striatopallidal neuron in conveying locomotor activation and PPI disruption induced by A2AR antagonists and D2R agonists and catalepsy mediated by A2AR agonists and D2R antagonists. More specifically, they also agree with A2AR-D2R heteromers in striatopallidal neurons mediating all postsynaptic pharmacological effects of SCH 442416, locomotor activation, blockade of PPI and counteraction of D2R antagonist-induced catalepsy. As shown in the scheme of **Figure 3A**, the A2AR-D2R heteromer explains the qualitatively different behavioral outputs depending on direct A2AR-Golf-AC-PKA-mediated increase in excitability or indirect D2R-Gi-PLC-PP2B-mediated disinhibition of the excitability of the striatopallidal neuron, leading to catalepsy and PPI (more related to the direct activation of the PKA-DARPP-32-CREB signaling; Bateup et al., 2010; Berger et al., 2011) or just psychomotor depression, respectively. In fact, it is well known that catalepsy, with its rigidity component, is not qualitatively equivalent to a high degree of locomotor depression. Finally, and as mentioned before, depending on the intracellular concentrations of Ca^{2+}, A2AR and D2R activation and co-activation lead to differential MAPK and Elk-1 activation, with implications for gene expression and synaptic plasticity (**Figure 3A**).

A2AR-D2R HETEROMER-MEDIATED CONTROL OF THE VENTRAL VS. DORSAL STRIATOPALLIDAL FUNCTION AND IMPLICATIONS FOR NEUROPSYCHIATRIC DISORDERS. 'APATHY' VS. 'AKINESIA'

Dysfunction of the central dopamine system is involved in a variety of disorders, including Parkinson's disease, schizophrenia, and substance use disorders (SUD). The functional separation of striatal compartments in ventral, rostral-dorsal and caudal-dorsal striata allows a more syndromic sub-classification of those disorders with potentially significant new therapeutic approaches. Parkinson's disease and non-human primate models of Parkinson's disease provide the clearest illustration. The cardinal motor symptoms of Parkinson's disease, bradykinesia, rigidity and tremor (Jankovic, 2008), have been classically attributed to dysfunction of the skeletomotor system, the brain

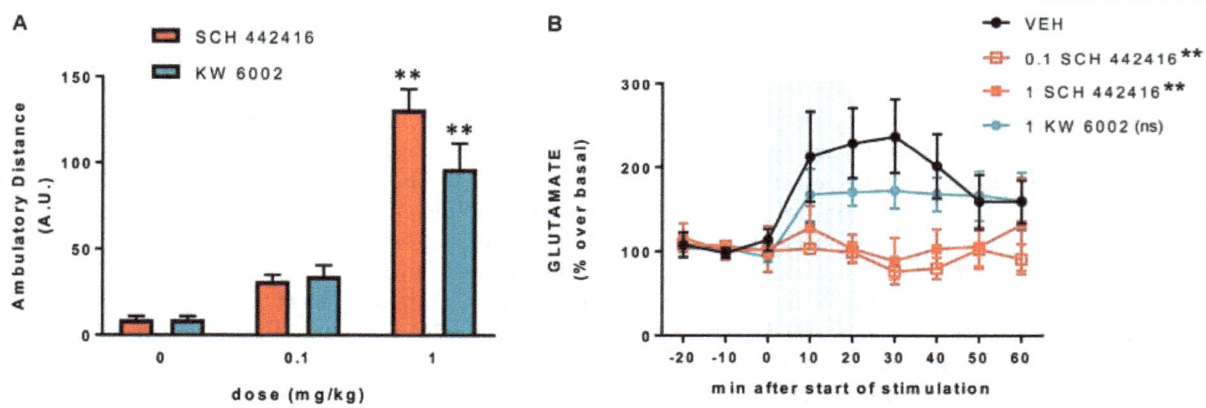

FIGURE 6 | Preferential presynaptic profile of SCH 442416 in C57BL/6 mice. **(A)** SCH 442416 shows similar potency and efficacy to KW 6002 at producing locomotor activation. Locomotor activity was measured in an open field arena as described elsewhere (Bonaventura et al., 2015); animals were injected intraperitoneally (i.p.) with vehicle (saline with 10% DMSO and 10% Tween-80) and the indicated concentrations of SCH 442416 or KW 6002 and the locomotor activity was measured for 2 h in activity chambers with 42.0 cm × 42.0 cm open fields (Coulbourn Instruments); values are mean ± SEM of the traveled distance (arbitrary units, A.U.); two-way ANOVA with Newman–Keuls *post hoc* test did not demonstrate significant differences between the two A2AR antagonists and, for both drugs, it only showed significant differences with the dose of 1 mg/kg as compared to the corresponding vehicle-treated groups (**$p < 0.01$ compared to vehicle; $n = 8$–11). **(B)** Optogenetic-microdialysis experiments were performed as described elsewhere (Bonaventura et al., 2017); briefly, C57BL/6 mice received a unilateral injection of an AAV encoding ChR2 (ChR2/H134R) fused to EYFP under control of the CaMKIIa neuronal promoter [AAV-CaMKIIa-hChR2(H134R)-EYFP] in the motor cortex. One month later, an optogenetic-microdialysis probe (Quiroz et al., 2016; Bonaventura et al., 2017) was implanted in the dorsal striatum, and glutamate in the dialysate was measured at 10-min intervals before, during, and after optogenetic stimulation of the corticostriatal terminals. Vehicle (black plot, see above) or the indicated doses of SCH 442416 (red plot) or KW 6002 (blue plot) were administered (i.p.) 10 min before the start of the stimulation. Values (in % over basal) represent mean ± SEM, normalized to the mean of the concentration of GLU present in the three samples preceding stimulation; one-way ANOVA with Newman–Keuls *post hoc* test showed a significant decrease of the transformed values (area under the curve, data from min 0 to min 60) from both groups treated with SCH 442416 (1 and 0.1 mg/kg), but not from the group treated with KW 6002, compared to the vehicle group (**$p < 0.01$ compared to vehicle; ns, non-significant; $n = 7$–8).

circuits involved in the execution and coordination of body movements. Contemporary theories embracing parallel cortical-striatal-thalamic-cortical circuits in the pathogenesis of this disorder emphasize the particular involvement of the "motor circuit," which includes motor cortical areas (DeLong and Wichmann, 2015). In fact, in Parkinson's disease, dopamine cell degeneration tends to occur initially and predominantly in the lateral part of the SNpc, which projects mainly to the caudal-dorsal striatum. Thus, there is a predominant deficit of the more "automatic" vs. "volitional" action skills and most sequential psychomotor responses need to be performed with full attention (Kim and Hikosaka, 2015). Nevertheless, with more advanced stages of Parkinson's disease the function of the more rostral striatum becomes also compromised, with deficits in "volitional" actions skills (Kim and Hikosaka, 2015). With further (or preferential) ventral degeneration of the dopamine mesencephalic nuclei (VTA) we move to the pathology of the ventral striatum, to apathy (Tremblay et al., 2015), as it has also been demonstrated experimentally in the non-human primate (Brown et al., 2012; Tian et al., 2015).

Initial studies on the psychomotor-activating effects of caffeine or selective A2AR antagonists dealt with general locomotor activity and were translationally applied to the treatment of akinesia in Parkinson's disease (see above and Müller and Ferré, 2007; Morelli et al., 2009; Armentero et al., 2011). Those initial studies implicitly considered A2AR-D2R heteromers in the dorsal striatum, but a large number of studies indicated that not only dorsal but also ventral striatopallidal neurons express A2R and A2AR-D2R heteromers (Ferré et al., 1994; Ferré, 1997; Hauber and Münkle, 1997; Pinna et al., 1997; Svenningsson et al., 1997; Ishiwari et al., 2007). More recent studies have also analyzed the effect of caffeine and A2AR antagonists on more specific reward-oriented behaviors, showing that they can increase the responsiveness to food-related stimuli, sucrose solutions, stimuli that elicit maternal behavior and self-administration (Pereira et al., 2011; Randall et al., 2011; Sheppard et al., 2012; Nunes et al., 2013; Lazenka et al., 2015). The work by Salamone's group has specifically addressed the role of adenosine and A2AR in effort-related choice behavior. Direct administration of A2AR agonists in the NAc altered effort-related choice behavior in a manner closely resembling the effects of interference with ventral striatal dopamine neurotransmission, decreasing the degree of responsiveness ("effort") to reward-associated stimuli. Furthermore, A2AR antagonists reversed the effort discounting effects of D2R antagonists (Salamone et al., 2012; Nunes et al., 2013).

Clinically, apathy has been defined as "a syndrome consisting of loss of motivation not attributable to disturbances in emotion, intellect or consciousness" (Marin, 1991). However, it is becoming obvious that apathy is a multifaceted concept that includes dissociable constructs that should correspond to dissociable neurobiological correlates (Sinha et al., 2013). We hypothesize that some if not all those dissociable correlates correspond to corticostriatal circuits involving the different functional striatal compartments and their "Go" and "NoGo" pathways. In fact, attuned with the role of dopamine in reward-associated behavior in all striatal compartments, recent studies even allow conceptualizing Parkinson's disease bradykinesia in a motivational framework (Mazzoni et al., 2007; Chong et al., 2015). Nevertheless, as defined clinically, apathy is a common non-motor symptom of Parkinson's disease (den Brok et al., 2015) that correlates negatively with dopamine innervation in the ventral striatum (Remy et al., 2005; Chaudhuri et al., 2006; Brown et al., 2012). In fact, a deficit in the dopamine modulation of the ventral striatum should translate, first, in a deficit in responsiveness, with a global inability to respond to reward- and punishment-associated stimuli (attuned with the "whether to respond" vs. "how to respond" functions of ventral vs. dorsal striatum). Second, it should lead to dysfunction of reward valuation, in alterations (increase) in DD, ED and LPD (attuned with the ventral striatum as forming part of corticostriatal circuits involved in reward valuation tasks). Indeed, non-medicated patients with Parkinson's disease have shown increases in DD and ED (Al-Khaled et al., 2015; Chong et al., 2015).

Interestingly, apathy is also a major negative symptom of schizophrenia, classically considered as a disorder associated with central hyperdopaminergic tone. Several studies have found evidence for selective dysfunction of the ventral striatum in schizophrenia, specifically hypoactivation with reward-associated stimuli (Simon et al., 2010, 2015; Strauss et al., 2015; Kirschner et al., 2016). Ventral striatal activation during reward anticipation was in fact found to be selectively and inversely correlated with apathy but not with other negative symptoms (Simon et al., 2010; Kirschner et al., 2016). Two additional findings give a clue for the mechanisms of apathy in schizophrenia, which seem to be dopamine-independent or at least not related to a decrease in the dopamine tone. First, there is a reduced functional connectivity between the orbito-frontal cortex (OFC) and the ventral striatum (Simon et al., 2015); second, there is consistent evidence that schizophrenic patients suffer from selective deficits in learning from positive outcomes, with intact learning from negative outcomes (Strauss et al., 2015). Therefore, the apathetic schizophrenic patient seems to have a selective decreased activation of the "Go" pathway, a reduction in the ratio of activation of "Go" vs. "NoGo" pathways secondary to impaired cortical-ventral striatal connectivity (Strauss et al., 2015). A similar situation would also be present in the patient with SUD, a decreased "Go"/"NoGo" pathway activation, also with reduced ventral striatal activation to reward stimuli (which can basically only be activated by the addictive drugs) (Volkow et al., 2011). Apathy is a well-known symptom in SUD, although it has been scarcely addressed experimentally (Verdejo-García et al., 2006; Verdejo-García and Pérez-García, 2008; Gjini et al., 2014). The SUD patient is motivated to procure the drug but tends to be withdrawn and apathetic when exposed to non-drug-related activities (Verdejo-García et al., 2006). In this case, however, the pathogenesis seems to follow from an initial reduction in D2R density (maybe with a concomitant relative increase of A2AR which would not be opposed by D2R forming heteromers), leading to an increased activity of the ventral striatopallidal neuronal function, of the

"NoGo" pathway. The tonic decrease in feedback activation of the ventromedial prefrontal cortex, orbitofrontal cortex and anterior cingulate cortex leads to additional dysfunction of the decision-making cortical-ventral striatal circuits (Volkow et al., 2011; Belcher et al., 2014). These changes lead to a similar situation than the non-motor symptoms in patients with Parkinson's disease, to apathy and choice impulsivity, as demonstrated by several studies indicating increase DD in patients with SUD (Belcher et al., 2014; Hamilton et al., 2015). In summary, for all types of apathy, the relative increase in the ventral striopallidal vs. striatonigral neuronal function should benefit from the treatment with A2AR antagonists, targeting A2AR-D2R heterotetramer-AC5 complexes.

CONCLUSION

A significant amount of experimental and clinical evidence demonstrates that A2AR and D2R localized in the ventral and dorsal striatopallidal neurons cannot be considered anymore as single functional units, but as forming part of complexes of the A2AR-D2R heterotetramer-AC5 complexes, which exert a fine-tuned integration of adenosine and dopamine neurotransmission. The current accumulated knowledge of the biochemical properties of the A2AR-D2R heteromer offer new therapeutic possibilities for Parkinson's disease, schizophrenia, SUD and other neuropsychiatric disorders with dysfunction of dorsal or ventral striatopallidal neurons. More generally, this knowledge implies we should modify classical views of GPCR physiology and pharmacology and include GPCR heteromers as main targets for drug development. The understanding of the biochemical properties of GPCR heteromers specifically localized in neuronal elements that form part of neuronal circuits involved in the pathophysiology of specific neuropsychiatric disorders should provide new selective pharmacological approaches with less unwanted side effects.

AUTHOR CONTRIBUTIONS

JB, WZ, CH-S, and KT performed the experiments and analyzed the data. SF, JB, KT, AK, VC, DL, and DZ designed the experiments. SF, JB, JT, CQ, N-SC, EM, VC-A, AK, DT, GN, AC, LP, CL, CWD, NV, VC, FC, DL, and DZ wrote the manuscript.

FUNDING

This work was supported by the intramural funds of the National Institute on Drug Abuse, "Ministerio de Economía y Competitividad", MINECO/FEDER (SAF2017-87349-R, SAF2014-54840-R, and PIE14/00034), Generalitat de Catalunya (2017 SRG 1604 and 2014-SGR-1236), and Fundació la Marató de TV3 (20140610 and 20152031).

ACKNOWLEDGMENTS

The authors apologize if they unwittingly omitted other relevant studies about the interactions between A2AR and D2R in the functional control of striatopallidal neurons.

REFERENCES

Al-Khaled, M., Heldmann, M., Bolstorff, I., Hagenah, J., and Münte, T. F. (2015). Intertemporal choice in Parkinson's disease and restless legs syndrome. *Parkinsonism Relat. Disord.* 21, 1330–1335. doi: 10.1016/j.parkreldis.2015.09.026

Armentero, M. T., Pinna, A., Ferré, S., Lanciego, J. L., Müller, C. E., and Franco, R. (2011). Past, present and future of A(2A) adenosine receptor antagonists in the therapy of Parkinson's disease. *Pharmacol. Ther.* 132, 280–299. doi: 10.1016/j.pharmthera.2011.07.004

Azdad, K., Gall, D., Woods, A. S., Ledent, C., Ferré, S., and Schiffmann, S. N. (2009). Dopamine D2 and denosine A2A receptors regulate NMDA-mediated excitation in accumbens neurons through A2A-D2 receptor heteromerization. *Neuropsychopharmacology* 34, 972–986. doi: 10.1038/npp.2008.144

Baik, J. H., Picetti, R., Saiardi, A., Thiriet, G., Dierich, A., Depaulis, A., et al. (1995). Parkinsonian-like locomotor impairment in mice lacking dopamine D2 receptors. *Nature* 377, 424–428. doi: 10.1038/377424a0

Balleine, B. W., and O'Doherty, J. P. (2010). Human and rodent homologies in action control: corticostriatal determinants of goal-directed and habitual action. *Neuropsychopharmacology* 35, 48–69. doi: 10.1038/npp.2009.131

Bateup, H. S., Santini, E., Shen, W., Birnbaum, S., Valjent, E., Surmeier, D. J., et al. (2010). Distinct subclasses of medium spiny neurons differentially regulate striatal motor behaviors. *Proc. Natl. Acad. Sci. U.S.A.* 107, 14845–14850. doi: 10.1073/pnas.1009874107

Belcher, A. M., Volkow, N. D., Moeller, F. G., and Ferré, S. (2014). Personality traits and vulnerability or resilience to substance use disorders. *Trends Cogn. Sci.* 18, 211–217. doi: 10.1016/j.tics.2014.01.010

Bello, E. P., Casas-Cordero, R., Galiñanes, G. L., Casey, E., Belluscio, M. A., Rodríguez, V., et al. (2017). Inducible ablation of dopamine D2 receptors in adult mice impairs locomotion, motor skill learning and leads to severe parkinsonism. *Mol. Psychiatry* 22, 595–604. doi: 10.1038/mp.2016.105

Berger, A. K., Green, T., Siegel, S. J., Nestler, E. J., and Hammer, R. P. Jr. (2011). cAMP response element binding protein phosphorylation in nucleus accumbens underlies sustained recovery of sensorimotor gating following repeated D_2-like receptor agonist treatment in rats. *Biol. Psychiatry* 69, 288–294. doi: 10.1016/j.biopsych.2010.08.032

Bertran-Gonzalez, J., Bosch, C., Maroteaux, M., Matamales, M., Hervé, D., Valjent, E., et al. (2008). Opposing patterns of signaling activation in dopamine D1 and D2 receptor-expressing striatal neurons in response to cocaine and haloperidol. *J. Neurosci.* 28, 5671–5685. doi: 10.1523/jneurosci.1039-08.2008

Besnard, A., Galan-Rodriguez, B., Vanhoutte, P., and Caboche, J. (2011). Elk-1 a transcription factor with multiple facets in the brain. *Front. Neurosci.* 5:35. doi: 10.3389/fnins.2011.00035

Boegman, R. J., and Vincent, S. R. (1996). Involvement of adenosine and glutamate receptors in the induction of c-fos in the striatum by haloperidol. *Synapse*

22, 70–77. doi: 10.1002/(SICI)1098-2396(199601)22:1<70::AID-SYN8>3.0.CO;2-F

Bonaventura, J., Navarro, G., Casadó-Anguera, V., Azdad, K., Rea, W., Moreno, E., et al. (2015). Allosteric interactions between agonists and antagonists within the adenosine A2A receptor-dopamine D2 receptor heterotetramer. *Proc. Natl. Acad. Sci. U.S.A.* 112, E3609–E3618. doi: 10.1073/pnas.1507704112

Bonaventura, J., Quiroz, C., Cai, N. S., Rubinstein, M., Tanda, G., and Ferré, S. (2017). Key role of the dopamine D(4) receptor in the modulation of corticostriatal glutamatergic neurotransmission. *Sci. Adv.* 3:e1601631. doi: 10.1126/sciadv.1601631

Bromberg-Martin, E. S., Matsumoto, M., and Hikosaka, O. (2010). Dopamine in motivational control: rewarding, aversive, and alerting. *Neuron* 68, 815–834. doi: 10.1016/j.neuron.2010.11.022

Brown, C. A., Campbell, M. C., Karimi, M., Tabbal, S. D., Loftin, S. K., Tian, L. L., et al. (2012). Dopamine pathway loss in nucleus accumbens and ventral tegmental area predicts apathetic behavior in MPTP-lesioned monkeys. *Exp. Neurol.* 236, 190–197. doi: 10.1016/j.expneurol.2012.04.025

Casadó, V., Cortés, A., Ciruela, F., Mallol, J., Ferré, S., Lluis, C., et al. (2007). Old and new ways to calculate the affinity of agonists and antagonists interacting with G-protein-coupled monomeric and dimeric receptors: the receptor-dimer cooperativity index. *Pharmacol. Ther.* 116, 343–354. doi: 10.1016/j.pharmthera.2007.05.010

Casas, M., Ferré, S., Cobos, A., Grau, J. M., and Jané, F. (1989). Relationship between rotational behaviour induced by apomorphine and caffeine in rats with unilateral lesion of the nigrostriatal pathway. *Neuropharmacology* 28, 407–409. doi: 10.1016/0028-3908(89)90037-3

Casas, M., Prat, G., Robledo, P., Barbanoj, M., Kulisevsky, J., and Jané, F. (2000). Methylxanthines reverse the adipsic and aphagic syndrome induced by bilateral 6-hydroxydopamine lesions of the nigrostriatal pathway in rats. *Pharmacol. Biochem. Behav.* 66, 257–263. doi: 10.1016/S0091-3057(00)00189-1

Chang, C. Y., Esber, G. R., Marrero-Garcia, Y., Yau, H. J., Bonci, A., and Schoenbaum, G. (2016). Brief optogenetic inhibition of dopamine neurons mimics endogenous negative reward prediction errors. *Nat. Neurosci.* 19, 111–116. doi: 10.1038/nn.4191

Chaudhuri, K. R., Martinez-Martin, P., Schapira, A. H., Stocchi, F., Sethi, K., Odin, P., et al. (2006). International multicenter pilot study of the first comprehensive self-completed nonmotor symptoms questionnaire for Parkinson's disease: the NMSQuest study. *Mov. Disord.* 21, 916–923. doi: 10.1002/mds.20844

Chen, J. F., Moratalla, R., Impagnatiello, F., Grandy, D. K., Cuellar, B., Rubinstein, M., et al. (2001). The role of the D(2) dopamine receptor (D(2)R) in A(2A) adenosine receptor (A(2A)R)-mediated behavioral and cellular responses as revealed by A(2A) and D(2) receptor knockout mice. *Proc. Natl. Acad. Sci. U.S.A.* 98, 1970–1975. doi: 10.1073/pnas.98.4.1970

Chong, T. T., Bonnelle, V., Manohar, S., Veromann, K. R., Muhammed, K., Tofaris, G. K., et al. (2015). Dopamine enhances willingness to exert effort for reward in Parkinson's disease. *Cortex* 69, 40–46. doi: 10.1016/j.cortex.2015.04.003

Ciruela, F., Casadó, V., Rodrigues, R. J., Luján, R., Burgueño, J., Canals, M., et al. (2006). Presynaptic control of striatal glutamatergic neurotransmission by adenosine A1-A2A receptor heteromers. *J. Neurosci.* 26, 2080–2087. doi: 10.1523/JNEUROSCI.3574-05.2006

Danjo, T., Yoshimi, K., Funabiki, K., Yawata, S., and Nakanishi, S. (2014). Aversive behavior induced by optogenetic inactivation of ventral tegmental area dopamine neurons is mediated by dopamine D2 receptors in the nucleus accumbens. *Proc. Natl. Acad. Sci. U.S.A.* 111, 6455–6460. doi: 10.1073/pnas.1404323111

DeLong, M. R., and Wichmann, T. (2015). Basal ganglia circuits as targets for neuromodulation in Parkinson disease. *JAMA Neurol.* 72, 1354–1360. doi: 10.1001/jamaneurol.2015.2397

den Brok, M. G., van Dalen, J. W., van Gool, W. A., Moll van Charante, E. P., de Bie, R. M., and Richard, E. (2015). Apathy in Parkinson's disease: a systematic review and meta-analysis. *Mov. Disord.* 30, 759–769. doi: 10.1002/mds.26208

Dreyer, J. K., Herrik, K. F., Berg, R. W., and Hounsgaard, J. D. (2010). Influence of phasic and tonic dopamine release on receptor activation. *J. Neurosci.* 30, 14273–14283. doi: 10.1523/jneurosci.1894-10.2010

Durieux, P. F., Bearzatto, B., Guiducci, S., Buch, T., Waisman, A., Zoli, M., et al. (2009). D2R striatopallidal neurons inhibit both locomotor and drug reward processes. *Nat. Neurosci.* 12, 393–395. doi: 10.1038/nn.2286

El Yacoubi, M., Ledent, C., Parmentier, M., Costentin, J., and Vaugeois, J. M. (2001). Adenosine A2A receptor knockout mice are partially protected against drug-induced catalepsy. *Neuroreport* 12, 983–986. doi: 10.1097/00001756-200104170-00024

Ferré, S. (1997). Adenosine-dopamine interactions in the ventral striatum. Implications for the treatment of schizophrenia. *Psychopharmacology* 133, 107–120. doi: 10.1007/s002130050380

Ferré, S. (2008). An update on the mechanisms of the psychostimulant effects of caffeine. *J. Neurochem.* 105, 1067–1079. doi: 10.1111/j.1471-4159.2007.05196.x

Ferré, S. (2015). The GPCR heterotetramer: challenging classical pharmacology. *Trends Pharmacol. Sci.* 36, 145–152. doi: 10.1016/j.tips.2015.01.002

Ferré, S. (2016). Mechanisms of the psychostimulant effects of caffeine: implications for substance use disorders. *Psychopharmacology* 233, 1963–1979. doi: 10.1007/s00213-016-4212-2

Ferré, S. (2017). "Adenosine control of striatal function. Implications for the treatment of apathy in basal ganglia disorders," in *Adenosine Receptors in Degenerative Diseases*, eds D. Blum and L. V. Lopes (Amsterdam: Elsevier), 231–255. doi: 10.1016/B978-0-12-803724-9.00012-0

Ferré, S., Bonaventura, J., Tomasi, D., Navarro, G., Moreno, E., Cortés, A., et al. (2016). Allosteric mechanisms within the adenosine A2A-dopamine D2 receptor heterotetramer. *Neuropharmacology* 104, 154–160. doi: 10.1016/j.neuropharm.2015.05.028

Ferré, S., Casadó, V., Devi, L. A., Filizola, M., Jockers, R., Lohse, M. J., et al. (2014). G protein-coupled receptor oligomerization revisited: functional and pharmacological perspectives. *Pharmacol. Rev.* 66, 413–434. doi: 10.1124/pr.113.008052

Ferré, S., Fredholm, B. B., Morelli, M., Popoli, P., and Fuxe, K. (1997). Adenosine-dopamine receptor-receptor interactions as an integrative mechanism in the basal ganglia. *Trends Neurosci.* 20, 482–487. doi: 10.1016/S0166-2236(97)01096-5

Ferré, S., Fuxe, K., von Euler, G., Johansson, B., and Fredholm, B. B. (1992). Adenosine-dopamine interactions in the brain. *Neuroscience* 51, 501–512. doi: 10.1016/0306-4522(92)90291-9

Ferré, S., Guix, T., Prat, G., Jane, F., and Casas, M. (1990). Is experimental catalepsy properly measured? *Pharmacol. Biochem. Behav.* 35, 753–757. doi: 10.1016/0091-3057(90)90354-K

Ferré, S., O'Connor, W. T., Fuxe, K., and Ungerstedt, U. (1993). The striopallidal neuron: a main locus for adenosine-dopamine interactions in the brain. *J. Neurosci.* 13, 5402–5406.

Ferré, S., O'Connor, W. T., Snaprud, P., Ungerstedt, U., and Fuxe, K. (1994). Antagonistic interaction between adenosine A2A receptors and dopamine D2 receptors in the ventral striopallidal system. *Implications for the treatment of schizophrenia. Neuroscience* 63, 765–773. doi: 10.1016/0306-4522(94)90521-5

Ferré, S., Quiroz, C., Orru, M., Guitart, X., Navarro, G., Cortés, A., et al. (2011). Adenosine A(2A) receptors and A(2A) receptor heteromers as key players in striatal function. *Front. Neuroanat.* 5:36. doi: 10.3389/fnana.2011.00036

Ferré, S., Rubio, A., and Fuxe, K. (1991a). Stimulation of adenosine A2 receptors induces catalepsy. *Neurosci. Lett.* 130, 162–164.

Ferré, S., von Euler, G., Johansson, B., Fredholm, B. B., and Fuxe, K. (1991b). Stimulation of high-affinity adenosine A2 receptors decreases the affinity of dopamine D2 receptors in rat striatal membranes. *Proc. Natl. Acad. Sci. U.S.A.* 88, 7238–7241.

Frank, M. J. (2005). Dynamic dopamine modulation in the basal ganglia: a neurocomputational account of cognitive deficits in medicated and nonmedicated Parkinsonism. *J. Cogn. Neurosci.* 17, 51–72. doi: 10.1162/0898929052880093

Frank, M. J., Seeberger, L. C., and O'Reilly, R. C. (2004). By carrot or by stick: cognitive reinforcement learning in parkinsonism. *Science* 306, 1940–1943.

Frederick, A. L., Yano, H., Trifilieff, P., Vishwasrao, H. D., Biezonski, D., Mészáros, J., et al. (2015). Evidence against dopamine D1/D2 receptor heteromers. *Mol. Psychiatry* 20, 1373–1385. doi: 10.1038/mp.2014.166

Freeze, B. S., Kravitz, A. V., Hammack, N., Berke, J. D., and Kreitzer, A. C. (2013). Control of basal ganglia output by direct and indirect pathway projection neurons. *J. Neurosci.* 33, 18531–18539. doi: 10.1523/JNEUROSCI.1278-13.2013

Fuxe, K., and Ungerstedt, U. (1974). Action of caffeine and theophyllamine on supersensitive dopamine receptors: considerable enhancement of receptor response to treatment with DOPA and dopamine receptor agonists. *Med. Biol.* 52, 48–54.

Garrett, B. E., and Holtzman, S. G. (1995). Does adenosine receptor blockade mediate caffeine-induced rotational behavior? *J. Pharmacol. Exp. Ther.* 274, 207–214.

Gerfen, C. R. (2004). "Basal ganglia," in *The Rat Nervous System*, ed. G. Paxinos (Amsterdam: Elsevier), 445–508.

Gjini, K., Qazi A., Greenwald, M. K., Sandhu, R., Gooding, D. C., and Boutros, N. N. (2014). Relationships of behavioral measures of frontal lobe dysfunction with underlying electrophysiology in cocaine-dependent patients. *Am. J. Addict.* 23, 265–271. doi: 10.1111/j.1521-0391.2014.12095.x

Haber, S. N. (2014). The place of dopamine in the cortico-basal ganglia circuit. *Neuroscience* 282, 248–257. doi: 10.1016/j.neuroscience.2014.10.008

Haber, S. N., and Behrens, T. E. (2014). The neural network underlying incentive-based learning: implications for interpreting circuit disruptions in psychiatric disorders. *Neuron* 83, 1019–1039. doi: 10.1016/j.neuron.2014.08.031

Håkansson, K., Galdi, S., Hendrick, J., Snyder, G., Greengard, P., and Fisone, G. (2006). Regulation of phosphorylation of the GluR1 AMPA receptor by dopamine D2 receptors. *J. Neurochem.* 96, 482–488. doi: 10.1111/j.1471-4159.2005.03558.x

Hamilton, K. R., Mitchell, M. R., Wing, V. C., Balodis, I. M., Bickel, W. K., Fillmore, M., et al. (2015). Choice impulsivity: definitions, measurement issues, and clinical implications. *Personal. Disord.* 6, 182–198. doi: 10.1037/per0000099

Hauber, W., and Münkle, M. (1997). Motor depressant effects mediated by dopamine D2 and adenosine A2A receptors in the nucleus accumbens and the caudate-putamen. *Eur. J. Pharmacol.* 323, 127–131. doi: 10.1016/S0014-2999(97)00040-X

Hernandez-Lopez, S., Tkatch, T., Perez-Garci, E., Galarraga, E., Bargas, J., Hamm, H., et al. (2000). D2 dopamine receptors in striatal medium spiny neurons reduce L-type Ca^{2+} currents and excitability via a novel PLC[beta]1-IP3-calcineurin-signaling cascade. *J. Neurosci.* 20, 8987–8995.

Herrera-Marschitz, M., Casas, M., and Ungerstedt, U. (1988). Caffeine produces contralateral rotation in rats with unilateral dopamine denervation: comparisons with apomorphine-induced responses. *Psychopharmacology* 94, 38–45. doi: 10.1007/BF00735878

Higley, M. J., and Sabatini, B. L. (2010). Competitive regulation of synaptic Ca2+ influx by D2 dopamine and A2A adenosine receptors. *Nat. Neurosci.* 13, 958–966. doi: 10.1038/nn.2592

Hikida, T., Kimura, K., Wada, N., Funabiki, K., and Nakanishi, S. (2010). Distinct roles of synaptic transmission in direct and indirect striatal pathways to reward and aversive behavior. *Neuron* 66, 896–907. doi: 10.1016/j.neuron.2010.05.011

Hikida, T., Yawata, S., Yamaguchi, T., Danjo, T., Sasaoka, T., Wang, Y., et al. (2013). Pathway-specific modulation of nucleus accumbens in reward and aversive behavior via selective transmitter receptors. *Proc. Natl. Acad. Sci. U.S.A.* 110, 342–347. doi: 10.1073/pnas.1220358110

Hikosaka, O. (2007). Basal ganglia mechanisms of reward-oriented eye movement. *Ann. N. Y. Acad. Sci.* 1104, 229–249. doi: 10.1196/annals.1390.012

Hillion, J., Canals, M., Torvinen, M., Casado, V., Scott, R., Terasmaa, A., et al. (2002). Coaggregation, cointernalization, and codesensitization of adenosine A2A receptors and dopamine D2 receptors. *J. Biol. Chem.* 277, 18091–18097. doi: 10.1074/jbc.M107731200

Hobson, B. D., O'Neill, C. E., Levis, S. C., Monteggia, L. M., Neve, R. L., Self, D. W., et al. (2013). Adenosine A1 and dopamine d1 receptor regulation of AMPA receptor phosphorylation and cocaine-seeking behavior. *Neuropsychopharmacology* 38, 1974–1983. doi: 10.1038/npp.2013.96

Huang, L., Wu, D. D., Zhang, L., and Feng, L. Y. (2013). Modulation of A_2a receptor antagonist on D_2 receptor internalization and ERK phosphorylation. *Acta Pharmacol. Sin.* 34, 1292–1300. doi: 10.1038/aps.2013.87

Isaac, S. O., and Berridge, C. W. (2003). Wake-promoting actions of dopamine D1 and D2 receptor stimulation. *J. Pharmacol. Exp. Ther.* 307, 386–394. doi: 10.1124/jpet.103.053918

Ishiwari, K., Madson, L. J., Farrar, A. M., Mingote, S. M., Valenta, J. P., DiGianvittorio, M. D., et al. (2007). Injections of the selective adenosine A2A antagonist MSX-3 into the nucleus accumbens core attenuate the locomotor suppression induced by haloperidol in rats. *Behav. Brain Res.* 178, 190–199. doi: 10.1016/j.bbr.2006.12.020

Jankovic, J. (2008). Parkinson's disease: clinical features and diagnosis. *J. Neurol. Neurosurg. Psychiatry* 79, 368–376. doi: 10.1136/jnnp.2007.131045

Justinová, Z., Redhi, G. H., Goldberg, S. R., and Ferré, S. (2014). Differential effects of presynaptic versus postsynaptic adenosine A2A receptor blockade on Δ9-tetrahydrocannabinol (THC) self-administration in squirrel monkeys. *J. Neurosci.* 34, 6480–6484. doi: 10.1523/jneurosci.5073-13.2014

Kable, J. W., and Glimcher, P. W. (2009). The neurobiology of decision: consensus and controversy. *Neuron* 63, 733–745. doi: 10.1016/j.neuron.2009.09.003

Kanda, T., Shiozaki, S., Shimada, J., Suzuki, F., and Nakamura, J. (1994). KF17837: a novel selective adenosine A2A receptor antagonist with anticataleptic activity. *Eur. J. Pharmacol.* 256, 263–268. doi: 10.1016/0014-2999(94)90551-7

Karcz-Kubicha, M., Antoniou, K., Terasmaa, A., Quarta, D., Solinas, M., Justinova, Z., et al. (2003). Involvement of adenosine A1 and A2A receptors in the motor effects of caffeine after its acute and chronic administration. *Neuropsychopharmacology* 28, 1281–1291. doi: 10.1038/sj.npp.1300167

Kim, D. S., and Palmiter, R. D. (2003). Adenosine receptor blockade reverses hypophagia and enhances locomotor activity of dopamine-deficient mice. *Proc. Natl. Acad. Sci. U.S.A.* 100, 1346–1351. doi: 10.1073/pnas.252753799

Kim, D. S., and Palmiter, R. D. (2008). Interaction of dopamine and adenosine receptor function in behavior: studies with dopamine-deficient mice. *Front. Biosci.* 13,2311–2318.

Kim, H. F., and Hikosaka, O. (2015). Parallel basal ganglia circuits for voluntary and automatic behaviour to reach rewards. *Brain* 138, 1776–1800. doi: 10.1093/brain/awv134

Kirschner, M., Hager, O. M., Bischof, M., Hartmann, M. N., Kluge, A., Seifritz, E., et al. (2016). Ventral striatal hypoactivation is associated with apathy but not diminished expression in patients with schizophrenia. *J. Psychiatry Neurosci.* 41, 152–161. doi: 10.1503/jpn.140383

Kravitz, A. V., Freeze, B. S., Parker, P. R., Kay, K., Thwin, M. T., Deisseroth, K., et al. (2010). Regulation of parkinsonian motor behaviours by optogenetic control of basal ganglia circuitry. *Nature* 466, 622–626. doi: 10.1038/nature09159

Kravitz, A. V., Tye, L. D., and Kreitzer, A. C. (2012). Distinct roles for direct and indirect pathway striatal neurons in reinforcement. *Nat. Neurosci.* 15, 816–818. doi: 10.1038/nn.3100

Kull, B., Ferré, S., Arslan, G., Svenningsson, P., Fuxe, K., Owman, C., et al. (1999). Reciprocal interactions between adenosine A2A and dopamine D2 receptors in Chinese hamster ovary cells co-transfected with the two receptors. *Biochem. Pharmacol.* 58, 1035–1045. doi: 10.1016/S0006-2952(99)00184-7

Lazenka, M. F., Moeller, F. G., and Negus, S. S. (2015). Effects of caffeine and its metabolite paraxanthine on intracranial self-stimulation in male rats. *Exp. Clin. Psychopharmacol.* 23, 71–80. doi: 10.1037/pha0000012

Lebon, G., Warne, T., Edwards, P. C., Bennett, K., Langmead, C. J., Leslie, A. G., et al. (2011). Agonist-bound adenosine A2A receptor structures reveal common features of GPCR activation. *Nature* 474, 521–525. doi: 10.1038/nature10136

Ledent, C., Vaugeois, J. M., Schiffmann, S. N., Pedrazzini, T., El Yacoubi, M., Vanderhaeghen, J. J., et al. (1997). Aggressiveness, hypoalgesia and high blood pressure in mice lacking the adenosine A2a receptor. *Nature* 388, 674–678. doi: 10.1038/41771

Lee, K. W., Hong, J. H., Choi, I. Y., Che, Y., Lee, J. K., Yang, S. D., et al. (2002). Impaired D2 dopamine receptor function in mice lacking type 5 adenylyl cyclase. *J. Neurosci.* 22, 7931–7940.

Lindskog, M., Svenningsson, P., Fredholm, B. B., Greengard, P., and Fisone, G. (1999). Activation of dopamine D2 receptors decreases DARPP-32 phosphorylation in striatonigral and striatopallidal projection neurons via different mechanisms. *Neuroscience* 88, 1005–1008. doi: 10.1016/S0306-4522(98)00411-4

Macpherson, T., Morita, M., and Hikida, T. (2014). Striatal direct and indirect pathways control decision-making behavior. *Front. Psychol.* 5:1301. doi: 10.3389/fpsyg.2014.01301

Marin, R. S. (1991). Apathy: a neuropsychiatric syndrome. *J. Neuropsychiatry Clin. Neurosci.* 3, 243–254. doi: 10.1176/jnp.3.3.243

Mazzoni, P., Hristova, A., and Krakauer, J. W. (2007). Why don't we move faster? Parkinson's disease, movement vigor, and implicit motivation. *J. Neurosci.* 27, 7105–7116. doi: 10.1523/JNEUROSCI.0264-07.2007

Mogenson, G. J., Jones, D. L., and Yim, C. Y. (1980). From motivation to action: functional interface between the limbic system and the motor system. *Prog. Neurobiol.* 14, 69–97. doi: 10.1016/0301-0082(80)90018-0

Morelli, M., Carta, A. R., and Jenner, P. (2009). Adenosine A2A receptors and Parkinson's disease. *Handb. Exp. Pharmacol.* 193, 589–615. doi: 10.1007/978-3-540-89615-9_18

Morelli, M., and Wardas, J. (2001). Adenosine A(2a) receptor antagonists: potential therapeutic and neuroprotective effects in Parkinson's disease. *Neurotox. Res.* 3, 545–556. doi: 10.1007/BF03033210

Moscoso-Castro, M., Gracia-Rubio, I., Ciruela, F., and Valverde, O. (2016). Genetic blockade of adenosine A2A receptors induces cognitive impairments and anatomical changes related to psychotic symptoms in mice. *Eur. Neuropsychopharmacol.* 26, 1227–1240. doi: 10.1016/j.euroneuro.2016.04.003

Müller, C. E., and Ferré, S. (2007). Blocking striatal adenosine A2A receptors: a new strategy for basal ganglia disorders. *Recent Pat. CNS Drug Discov.* 2, 1–21. doi: 10.2174/157488907779561772

Nagel, J., Schladebach, H., Koch, M., Schwienbacher, I., Müller, C. E., and Hauber, W. (2003). Effects of an adenosine A2A receptor blockade in the nucleus accumbens on locomotion,feeding, and prepulse inhibition in rats. *Synapse* 49, 279–286. doi: 10.1002/syn.10240

Nakamura, K., and Hikosaka, O. (2006). Role of dopamine in the primate caudate nucleus in reward modulation of saccades. *J. Neurosci.* 26, 5360–5369. doi: 10.1523/JNEUROSCI.4853-05.2006

Navarro, G., Aguinaga, D., Moreno, E., Hradsky, J., Reddy, P. P., Cortés, A., et al. (2014). Intracellular calcium levels determine differential modulation of allosteric interactions within G protein-coupled receptor heteromers. *Chem. Biol.* 21, 1546–1556. doi: 10.1016/j.chembiol.2014.10.004

Navarro, G., Cordomí, A., Casadó-Anguera, V., Moreno, E., Cai, N.-S., Cortés, A., et al. (2018). Evidence for functional pre-coupled complexes of receptor heteromers and adenylyl cyclase. *Nat. Commun.* 9:1242. doi: 10.1038/s41467-018-03522-3

Nunes, E. J., Randall, P. A., Podurgiel, S., Correa, M., and Salamone, J. D. (2013). Nucleus accumbens neurotransmission and effort-related choice behavior in food motivation: effects of drugs acting on dopamine, adenosine, and muscarinic acetylcholine receptors. *Neurosci. Biobehav. Rev.* 37, 2015–2025. doi: 10.1016/j.neubiorev.2013.04.002

O'Neill, C. E., Hobson, B. D., Levis, S. C., and Bachtell, R. K. (2014). Persistent reduction of cocaine seeking by pharmacological manipulation of adenosine A1 and A 2A receptors during extinction training in rats. *Psychopharmacology* 231, 3179–3188. doi: 10.1007/s00213-014-3489-2

Orrú, M., Bakešová, J., Brugarolas, M., Quiroz, C., Beaumont, V., Goldberg, S. R., et al. (2011a). Striatal pre- and postsynaptic profile of adenosine A(2A) receptor antagonists. *PLoS One* 6:e16088. doi: 10.1371/journal.pone.0016088

Orrú, M., Quiroz, C., Guitart, X., and Ferré, S. (2011b). Pharmacological evidence for different populations of postsynaptic adenosine A2A receptors in the rat striatum. *Neuropharmacology* 61, 967–974. doi: 10.1016/j.neuropharm.2011.06.025

Pereira, M., Farrar, A. M., Hockemeyer, J., Müller, C. E., Salamone, J. D., and Morrell, J. I. (2011). Effect of the adenosine A2A receptor antagonist MSX-3 on motivational disruptions of maternal behavior induced by dopamine antagonism in the early postpartum rat. *Psychopharmacology* 213, 69–79. doi: 10.1007/s00213-010-2015-4

Pinna, A., Wardas, J., Cristalli, G., and Morelli, M. (1997). Adenosine A2A receptor agonists increase Fos-like immunoreactivity in mesolimbic areas. *Brain Res.* 759, 41–49. doi: 10.1016/S0006-8993(97)00214-X

Prévost, C., Pessiglione, M., Météreau, E., Cléry-Melin, M. L., and Dreher, J. C. (2010). Separate valuation subsystems for delay and effort decision costs. *J. Neurosci.* 30, 14080–14090. doi: 10.1523/jneurosci.2752-10.2010

Quiroz, C., Luján, R., Uchigashima, M., Simoes, A. P., Lerner, T. N., Borycz, J., et al. (2009). Key modulatory role of presynaptic adenosine A2A receptors in cortical neurotransmission to the striatal direct pathway. *ScientificWorldJournal* 9, 1321–1344. doi: 10.1100/tsw.2009.143

Quiroz, C., Orrú, M., Rea, W., Ciudad-Roberts, A., Yepes, G., Britt, J. P., et al. (2016). Local control of extracellular dopamine levels in the medial nucleus accumbens by a glutamatergic projection from the infralimbic cortex. *J. Neurosci.* 36, 851–859. doi: 10.1523/jneurosci.2850-15.2016

Randall, P. A., Nunes, E. J., Janniere, S. L., Stopper, C. M., Farrar, A. M., Sager, T. N., et al. (2011). Stimulant effects of adenosine antagonists on operant behavior: differential actions of selective A2A and A1 antagonists. *Psychopharmacology* 216, 173–186. doi: 10.1007/s00213-011-2198-3

Remy, P., Doder, M., Lees, A., Turjanski, N., and Brooks, D. (2005). Depression in Parkinson's disease: loss of dopamine and noradrenaline innervation in the limbic system. *Brain* 128, 1314–1322. doi: 10.1093/brain/awh445

Roitman, M. F., Wheeler, R. A., Wightman, R. M., and Carelli, R. M. (2008). Real-time chemical responses in the nucleus accumbens differentiate rewarding and aversive stimuli. *Nat. Neurosci.* 11, 1376–1377. doi: 10.1038/nn.2219

Root, D. H., Melendez, R. I., Zaborszky, L., and Napier, T. C. (2015). The ventral pallidum: subregion-specific functional anatomy and roles in motivated behaviors. *Prog. Neurobiol.* 130, 29–70. doi: 10.1016/j.pneurobio.2015.03.005

Salamone, J. D., Correa, M., Nunes, E. J., Randall, P. A., and Pardo, M. (2012). The behavioral pharmacology of effort-related choice behavior: dopamine, adenosine and beyond. *J. Exp. Anal. Behav.* 97, 125–146. doi: 10.1901/jeab.2012.97-125

Schiffmann, S. N., Fisone, G., Moresco, R., Cunha, R. A., and Ferré, S. (2007). Adenosine A2A receptors and basal ganglia physiology. *Prog. Neurobiol.* 83, 277–292. doi: 10.1016/j.pneurobio.2007.05.001

Shen, W., Flajolet, M., Greengard, P., and Surmeier, D. J. (2008). Dichotomous dopaminergic control of striatal synaptic plasticity. *Science* 321, 848–851. doi: 10.1126/science.1160575

Sheppard, A. B., Gross, S. C., Pavelka, S. A., Hall, M. J., and Palmatier, M. I. (2012). Caffeine increases the motivation to obtain non-drug reinforcers in rats. *Drug Alcohol Depend.* 124, 216–222. doi: 10.1016/j.drugalcdep.2012.01.008

Shiozaki, S., Ichikawa, S., Nakamura, J., Kitamura, S., Yamada, K., and Kuwana, Y. (1999). Actions of adenosine A2A receptor antagonist KW-6002 on drug-induced catalepsy and hypokinesia caused by reserpine or MPTP. *Psychopharmacology* 147, 90–95. doi: 10.1007/s002130051146

Simon, J. J., Biller, A., Walther, S., Roesch-Ely, D., Stippich, C., Weisbrod, M., et al. (2010). Neural correlates of reward processing in schizophrenia–relationship to apathy and depression. *Schizophr. Res.* 118, 154–161. doi: 10.1016/j.schres.2009.11.007

Simon, J. J., Cordeiro, S. A., Weber, M. A., Friederich, H. C., Wolf, R. C., Weisbrod, M., et al. (2015). Reward system dysfunction as a neural substrate of symptom expression across the general population and patients with schizophrenia. *Schizophr. Bull.* 41, 1370–1378. doi: 10.1093/schbul/sbv067

Sinha, N., Manohar, S., and Husain, M. (2013). Impulsivity and apathy in Parkinson's disease. *J. Neuropsychol.* 7, 255–283. doi: 10.1111/jnp.12013

Steinberg, E. E., Keiflin, R., Boivin, J. R., Witten, I. B., Deisseroth, K., and Janak, P. H. (2013). A causal link between prediction errors, dopamine neurons and learning. *Nat. Neurosci.* 16, 966–973. doi: 10.1038/nn.3413

Stopper, C. M., and Floresco, S. B. (2011). Contributions of the nucleus accumbens and its subregions to different aspects of risk-based decision making. *Cogn. Affect. Behav. Neurosci.* 11, 97–112. doi: 10.3758/s13415-010-0015-9

Strauss, G. P., Morra, L. F., Sullivan, S. K., and Gold, J. M. (2015). The role of low cognitive effort and negative symptoms in neuropsychological impairment in schizophrenia. *Neuropsychology* 29, 282–291. doi: 10.1037/neu0000113

Svenningsson, P., Fourreau, L., Bloch, B., Fredholm, B. B., Gonon, F., and Le Moine, C. (1999). Opposite tonic modulation of dopamine and adenosine on c-fos gene expression in striatopallidal neurons. *Neuroscience* 89, 827–837. doi: 10.1016/S0306-4522(98)00403-5

Svenningsson, P., Le Moine, C., Kull, B., Sunahara, R., Bloc, H. B., and Fredholm, B. B. (1997). Cellular expression of adenosine A2A receptor messenger RNA in the rat central nervous system with special reference to dopamine innervated areas. *Neuroscience* 80, 1171–1185. doi: 10.1016/S0306-4522(97)00180-2

Svenningsson, P., Lindskog, M., Rognoni, F., Fredholm, B. B., Greengard, P., and Fisone, G. (1998). Activation of adenosine A2A and dopamine D1 receptors stimulates cyclic AMP-dependent phosphorylation of DARPP-32 in distinct populations of striatal projection neurons. *Neuroscience* 84, 223–228. doi: 10.1016/S0306-4522(97)00510-1

Taura, J., Valle-León, M., Sahlholm, K., Watanabe, M., Van Craenenbroeck, K., Fernández-Dueñas, V., et al. (2017). Behavioral control by striatal adenosine A_{2A}-dopamine D_2 receptor heteromers. *Genes Brain Behav.* e12432. doi: 10.1111/gbb.12432 [Epub ahead of print].

Tian, L., Xia, Y., Flores, H. P., Campbell, M. C., Moerlein, S. M., and Perlmutter, J. S. (2015). Neuroimaging analysis of the dopamine basis for apathetic behaviors in an MPTP-lesioned primate model. *PLoS One* 10:e0132064. doi: 10.1371/journal.pone.0132064

Tremblay, L., Worbe, Y., Thobois, S., Sgambato-Faure, V., and Féger, J. (2015). Selective dysfunction of basal ganglia subterritories: from movement to behavioral disorders. *Mov. Disord.* 30, 1155–1170. doi: 10.1002/mds.26199

Usiello, A., Baik, J. H., Rougé-Pont, F., Picetti, R., Dierich, A., LeMeur, M., et al. (2000). Distinct functions of the two isoforms of dopamine D2 receptors. *Nature* 408, 199–203. doi: 10.1038/35041572

Valjent, E., Bertran-Gonzalez, J., Hervé, D., Fisone, G., and Girault, J. A. (2009). Looking BAC at striatal signaling: cell-specific analysis in new transgenic mice. *Trends Neurosci.* 32, 538–547. doi: 10.1016/j.tins.2009.06.005

Verdejo-García, A., Bechara, A., Recknor, E. C., and Pérez-García, M. (2006). Executive dysfunction in substance dependent individuals during drug use and abstinence: an examination of the behavioral, cognitive and emotional correlates of addiction. *J. Int. Neuropsychol. Soc.* 12, 405–415. doi: 10.1017/S1355617706060486

Verdejo-García, A., and Pérez-García, M. (2008). Substance abusers' self-awareness of the neurobehavioral consequences of addiction. *Psychiatry Res.* 158, 172–180. doi: 10.1016/j.psychres.2006.08.001

Volkow, N. D., Wang, G. J., Fowler, J. S., Tomasi, D., and Telang, F. (2011). Addiction: beyond dopamine reward circuitry. *Proc. Natl. Acad. Sci. U.S.A.* 108, 15037–15042. doi: 10.1073/pnas.1010654108

Volkow, N. D., Wang, G. J., Logan, J., Alexoff, D., Fowler, J. S., Thanos, P. K., et al. (2015). Caffeine increases striatal dopamine D_2/D_3 receptor availability in the human brain. *Transl. Psychiatry* 5:e549. doi: 10.1038/tp.2015.46

Voon, V., Pessiglione, M., Brezing, C., Gallea, C., Fernandez, H. H., Dolan, R. J., et al. (2010). Mechanisms underlying dopamine-mediated reward bias in compulsive behaviors. *Neuron* 65, 135–142. doi: 10.1016/j.neuron.2009.12.027

Voorn, P., Vanderschuren, L. J., Groenewegen, H. J., Robbins, T. W., and Pennartz, C. M. (2004). Putting a spin on the dorsal-ventral divide of the striatum. *Trends Neurosci.* 27, 468–474. doi: 10.1016/j.tins.2004.06.006

Wang, J. H., Short, J., Ledent, C., Lawrence, A. J., and van den Buuse, M. (2003). Reduced startle habituation and prepulse inhibition in mice lacking the adenosine A2A receptor. *Behav. Brain Res.* 143, 201–207. doi: 10.1016/S0166-4328(03)00036-6

Wise, R. A. (2004). Dopamine, learning and motivation. *Nat. Rev. Neurosci.* 5, 483–494. doi: 10.1038/nrn1406

Wise, R. A., and Bozarth, M. A. (1987). A psychomotor stimulant theory of addiction. *Psychol. Rev.* 94, 469–492. doi: 10.1037/0033-295X.94.4.469

Yang, J. N., Chen, J. F., and Fredholm, B. B. (2009). Physiological roles of A1 and A2A adenosine receptors in regulating heart rate, body temperature, and locomotion as revealed using knockout mice and caffeine. *Am. J. Physiol. Heart Circ. Physiol.* 296, H1141–H1149. doi: 10.1152/ajpheart.00754.2008

Yin, H. H., and Knowlton, B. J. (2006). The role of the basal ganglia in habit formation. *Nat. Rev. Neurosci.* 7, 464–476. doi: 10.1038/nrn1919

Zwilling, D., Zhu, W., Lee, H., Gallager, I., Braithwaite, S. P., and Thompson, K. R. (2014). *An optogenetic Model to Study Motor and Psychiatric Symptoms of Parkinson's Disease. 2014 Neuroscience Meeting Planner.* Washington, DC: Society for Neuroscience.

17

Uridine Adenosine Tetraphosphate-Induced Coronary Relaxation is Blunted in Swine With Pressure Overload: A Role for Vasoconstrictor Prostanoids

*Zhichao Zhou[1,2,3], Inge M. Lankhuizen[1,2], Heleen M. van Beusekom[1,2], Caroline Cheng[1,2,4], Dirk J. Duncker[1,2] and Daphne Merkus[1,2]**

[1] Division of Experimental Cardiology, Department of Cardiology, Thoraxcenter, Erasmus Medical Center, University Medical Center Rotterdam, Rotterdam, Netherlands, [2] Cardiovascular Research School Erasmus University Rotterdam, Erasmus Medical Center, University Medical Center Rotterdam, Rotterdam, Netherlands, [3] Division of Cardiology, Department of Medicine, Karolinska University Hospital, Karolinska Institutet, Solna, Sweden, [4] Department of Nephrology and Hypertension, University Medical Center Utrecht, Utrecht, Netherlands

***Correspondence:**
Daphne Merkus
d.merkus@erasmusmc.nl

Plasma levels of the vasoactive substance uridine adenosine tetraphosphate (Up_4A) are elevated in hypertensive patients and Up_4A-induced vascular contraction is exacerbated in various arteries isolated from hypertensive animals, suggesting a potential role of Up_4A in development of hypertension. We previously demonstrated that Up_4A produced potent and partially endothelium-dependent relaxation in the porcine coronary microvasculature. Since pressure-overload is accompanied by structural abnormalities in the coronary microvasculature as well as by endothelial dysfunction, we hypothesized that pressure-overload blunts the coronary vasodilator response to Up_4A, and that the involvement of purinergic receptors and endothelium-derived factors is altered. The effects of Up_4A were investigated using wire-myography in isolated coronary small arteries from Sham-operated swine and swine with prolonged (8 weeks) pressure overload of the left ventricle induced by aortic banding (AoB). Expression of purinergic receptors and endothelium-derived factors was assessed in isolated coronary small arteries using real-time PCR. Up_4A (10^{-9} to 10^{-5} M) failed to produce contraction in isolated coronary small arteries from either Sham or AoB swine, but produced relaxation in preconstricted arteries, which was significantly blunted in AoB compared to Sham. Blockade of purinergic P1, and P2 receptors attenuated Up_4A-induced coronary relaxation more, while the effect of $P2X_1$-blockade was similar and the effects of A_{2A}- and $P2Y_1$-blockade were reduced in AoB as compared to Sham. mRNA expression of neither A1, A2, A3, nor $P2X_1$, $P2X_7$, $P2Y_1$, $P2Y_2$, nor $P2Y_6$-receptors was altered in AoB as compared to Sham, while $P2Y_{12}$ expression was higher in AoB. eNOS inhibition attenuated Up_4A-induced coronary relaxation in both Sham and AoB. Additional blockade of cyclooxygenase enhanced Up_4A-induced coronary relaxation in AoB but not Sham swine, suggesting the involvement of vasoconstrictor prostanoids. In endothelium-denuded coronary small arteries from normal swine, thromboxane synthase (TxS) inhibition enhanced relaxation to Up_4A compared to endothelium-intact arteries, to a similar extent as $P2Y_{12}$ inhibition, while the combination inhibition of $P2Y_{12}$ and TxS had no additional effect. In conclusion, Up_4A-induced coronary relaxation is blunted in swine with AoB, which appears to be due to the production of a vasoconstrictor prostanoid, likely thromboxane A_2.

Keywords: Up_4A, coronary, microcirculation, purinergic receptor, hypertension, prostanoid

INTRODUCTION

Hypertension and aortic stenosis result in chronic pressure-overload of the left ventricle, producing left ventricular hypertrophy, and are considered risk factors for the development of heart failure (Khatibzadeh et al., 2013). Prolonged pressure-overload has also been shown to cause structural and functional adaptations in the coronary vasculature. Coronary flow reserve is decreased and minimal coronary resistance is increased (Duncker et al., 1993; Hamasaki et al., 2000; Galderisi et al., 2001), due to increased extravascular compression of the arterioles, decreased capillary density and vascular remodeling (Breisch et al., 1986; Tomanek et al., 1986; Bache, 1988; Hamasaki et al., 2000; van den Heuvel et al., 2001; Urbieta-Caceres et al., 2011). Functional changes in the coronary vasculature mainly result from an increase in oxidative stress and endothelial dysfunction (Rodriguez-Porcel et al., 2003; Lavi et al., 2008; Alexánderson et al., 2012) resulting in an imbalance between endothelium-derived vasodilators such as Nitric Oxide (NO) and prostacyclin and endothelium-derived vasoconstrictors like endothelin and reactive oxygen species (Vanhoutte, 1996).

Uridine adenosine tetraphosphate (Up4A) was initially identified as an endothelium-derived vasoconstrictor. A role for Up_4A in the pathogenesis of hypertension has been suggested by the observation that Up_4A-induced vascular contraction in the renal, femoral and basilar artery is potentiated in hypertension (Matsumoto et al., 2011b). In addition, the Up_4A plasma concentration in hypertensive subjects is significantly higher as compared to healthy subjects and positively correlates with blood pressure (Jankowski et al., 2007). Up_4A contains both purine and pyrimidine moieties and, like other extracellular nucleotides, exerts its vasoactive influence by binding to purinergic receptors (Matsumoto et al., 2011a; Zhou et al., 2013b), a class of receptors comprising P1 (adenosine receptors) and P2 receptors, that can be further subdivided into P2X and P2Y subtypes (Ralevic and Burnstock, 1998). Subsequent studies found that the vasoactive effect of Up_4A is not only dependent on the vascular bed but also on the species studied. Thus, Up_4A produces potent relaxation in the healthy porcine coronary vasculature (Zhou et al., 2013b) whereas vasoconstriction is observed in response to Up_4A in the murine coronary microcirculation (Teng et al., 2017). Interestingly, Up_4A-induced relaxation is attenuated in the remote coronary vasculature after myocardial infarction via downregulation of P1 receptors (Zhou et al., 2013a). Although Up_4A-induced coronary relaxation is maintained in swine with metabolic derangement, the purinergic signaling and endothelium-derived factors involved in Up_4A responses are markedly altered (Zhou et al., 2017). Altogether, these findings indicate that the effects of Up_4A in the porcine coronary vasculature change in cardiovascular disease.

Consequently, the first aim of the present study was to investigate whether prolonged pressure overload induced by AoB alters the response to Up_4A in isolated porcine coronary small arteries, and to determine the purinergic receptors and endothelium-derived factors mediating this altered vascular response to Up_4A. Interestingly, we found evidence for release of a vasoconstrictor prostanoid in response to Up_4A in AoB. As the vasoconstrictor prostanoid thromboxane A_2 (TxA_2) was recently shown to be released in response to Up_4A in renal arteries and aortas (Matsumoto et al., 2014; Zhou et al., 2015b), we further investigated whether Up_4A can induce production of TxA_2 in the porcine coronary microvasculature.

MATERIALS AND METHODS

Animals

Studies were performed in accordance with the "Guiding Principles in the Care and Use of Laboratory Animals" as approved by the Council of the American Physiological Society, and with approval of the Animal Care Committee at Erasmus Medical Center Rotterdam. Fifteen Crossbred Yorkshire X Landrace swine (2 to 3-month-old, 18.5 ± 0.3 kg at the time of surgery) of either sex entered the study. Swine were housed in the animal facility in cages with a 12/12 h light/dark cycle, *ad libitum* access to water and were fed twice per day. After 1 week of daily adaptation to laboratory conditions, animals underwent either AoB ($n = 7$) or a sham procedure (Sham; $n = 8$).

Surgery

After overnight fasting, swine were sedated with an intramuscular injection of Zoletil (Tiletamine/Zolazepam; 5 mg kg^{-1}), Xylazine (2.25 mg kg^{-1}), and Atropine (1 mg), and a small catheter was placed in an earvein for subsequent administration of fluid. Swine were intubated and ventilated with a mixture of oxygen and nitrogen (1:2 vol/vol), to which 2% (vol/vol) isoflurane was added to maintain anesthesia (Haitsma et al., 2001; Kappers et al., 2012). Under sterile conditions, the chest was opened via the fourth left intercostal space and fluid-filled polyvinylchloride

Abbreviations: AoB, aortic banding; BW, body weight; CO, cardiac output; HR, heart rate; LNAME, N^{ω}-nitro-L-arginine methyl ester HCl; LVSP, left ventricular systolic pressure measured proximal to the band; LVW, left ventricular weight at end of follow-up; MAP, mean arterial pressure measured in the descending aorta; NO, nitric oxide; PAP, pulmonary arterial pressure; PGI2, prostacyclin; PGI2S, prostacyclin synthase; PPADS, pyridoxalphosphate-6-azophenyl-2′,4′-disulfonic acid; P1-receptors, purinergic type 1 receptors; P2-receptors, purinergic type 2 receptors; SAP, systolic artery pressure measured in the descending aorta; TxS, thromboxane synthase; Up_4A, uridine adenosine tetraphosphate; U46619, 9,11-dideoxy-9α,11α-methanoepoxy Prostaglandin F2α; 8PT, 8-phenyltheophylline.

TABLE 1 | Primer information.

Receptors	Sequence		Size (bp)
A_1	5′-CCTGGCCATGCTGGCAATTGC-3′	5′-GAAGGAGAGAACCCAGCAGCC-3′	251
A_{2A}	5′-ATGTTGGGCTGGAATAGCTG-3′	5′-CACGGAGTTGGTGTGAGAGA-3′	426
A_3	5′-TACCTGCGGGTCAAGCTCACG-3′	5′-CCAGGAATGACACCAGCCAGC-3′	97
$P2X_1$	5′-TTGAACCCCATTTCTTCCTG-3′	5′-AGTGCACCACACATCTGCTC-3′	248
$P2X_4$	5′-TGTCCCCAGGCTACAATTTC-3′	5′-GGCAGCTTTTTCTCCCTTCT-3′	373
$P2X_7$	5′-CTTTTGCACCTTGAGCTTCC-3′	5′-TCCATGCTAAGGGATTCTGG-3′	152
P2Y1	5′-TTCCTGACTTGCATCAGTGC-3′	5′-CAGTGCCCGAGTAGAAGAGG-3′	157
$P2Y_2$	5′-GTGGCCTACAGCTTGGTCAT-3′	5′-GCGTGCGGAAGGAGTAGTAG-3′	235
$P2Y_4$	5′-GACTGCCGGTTTAATGAGGA-3′	5′-AGGAAAAGGACGCTGCAGTA-3′	302
$P2Y_6$	5′-CTGCTCTTGCCACCTGTGTA-3′	5′-AGGTTGGCGTAGAACAGGAA-3′	251
$P2Y_{12}$	5′-AGTGATGCCAAACTGGGAAC-3′	5′-TGAATGCCCAGATAACCACA-3′	208
COX1	5′-GGAGTTTGTCAATGCCACCT-3′	5′-GCAACTGCTTCTTCCCTTTG-3′	215
COX2	5′-GGCTGCGGGAACATAATAGA-3′	5′-GCAGCTCTGGGTCAAACTTC-3′	183
PGIS	5′-CATGCGTGCTCTGATTCACT-3′	5′-AAGCTGATGCAAAGGCAAGT-3′	233
TxS	5′-AGCAAGCAGCAGAAGAGAGG-3′	5′-TCAGAGGCTTGGACAGAGGT-3′	180
eNOS	5′-CTCTCCTGTTGGCCTGACCA-3′	5′-CCGGTTACTCAGACCCAAGG-3′	151
GAPDH	5′-TCGGAGTGAACGGATTTG-3′	5′-CCTGGAAGATGGTGATGG-3′	219

catheters were inserted into the left ventricle (LV), only in AoB swine, and in the aortic arch (Ao) of both Sham and AoB swine, for the measurement of the pressure and blood sampling for the determination of PO_2, PCO_2, pH, O_2 saturation, and hemoglobin concentration. The ascending aorta was exposed in all swine, a sterile plastic band was placed around the ascending aorta in AoB animals and gradually tightened until the systolic pressure gradient between distal aorta and proximal LV catheters reached approximately 80 mmHg. Then, the chest was closed and animals were allowed to recover, receiving analgesia (0.3 mg buprenorphine i.m.) for 2 days and antibiotic prophylaxis (25 mg kg^{-1} amoxicillin and 5 mg kg^{-1} gentamycin i.v.) for 5 days. Pressure in the proximal and distal catheters were recorded at the time of surgery, as well as 1 and 3 weeks after surgery, and the systolic pressure gradient was calculated. Due to malfunctioning of the catheters in a number of animals, pressures could not be obtained 8 weeks after the initial surgery.

Eight weeks after initial Sham and AoB surgery, animals were re-anesthetized, intubated and ventilated as described above. Pentobarbital (20 mg kg^{-1} h^{-1}) was infused to induce and maintain anesthesia. A catheter was introduced via the femoral artery into the descending aorta for measurement of mean arterial pressure. A Swan Ganz catheter was inserted via the jugular vein and advanced into the pulmonary artery for measurement of PAP and CO (via thermodilution) (van Kats et al., 2000). Following thoracotomy, hearts were arrested and immediately excised and placed in cold, oxygenated Krebs bicarbonate buffer solution.

Myograph Studies

Coronary small arteries (diameter: ~150 μm) were dissected out from the apex of eight Sham-operated and seven AoB swine and stored overnight in cold, oxygenated Krebs bicarbonate solution of the following composition (mM): NaCl 118, KCl 4.7, $CaCl_2$ 2.5, $MgSO_4$ 1.2, KH_2PO_4 1.2, $NaHCO_3$ 25, and glucose 8.3; pH 7.4. The next day, coronary small arteries were cut into segments of ~2 mm length and mounted in microvascular myographs (Danish Myo Technology) with separated organ baths containing 6 ml Krebs bicarbonate solution aerated with 95%O_2/5%CO_2 and maintained at 37°C (Batenburg et al., 2004; Zhou et al.,

TABLE 2 | Anatomic and hemodynamic variables.

		Sham N = 8	AoB N = 7
MAP (mmHg)	Surgery	84 ± 6	56 ± 3*
	Week 1	92 ± 2	83 ± 2*
	Week 3	88 ± 2	90 ± 3
LVSP (mmHg)	Surgery	–	155 ± 5
	Week 1	–	176 ± 8
	Week 3	–	188 ± 14
SAP (mmHg)	Surgery	99 ± 6	67 ± 4*
	Week 1	112 ± 2	100 ± 2*
	Week 3	105 ± 2	104 ± 3
Pressure gradient (mmHg)	Surgery	–	88 ± 2
	Week 1	–	82 ± 8
	Week 3	–	98 ± 6
At end of follow-up			
BW (kg)		45 ± 0.9	42 ± 1.1
LVW/BW (g kg^{-1})		2.3 ± 0.1	3.6 ± 0.1*
HR (beats min^{-1})		109 ± 3	108 ± 4
MAP (mmHg)		98 ± 5	104 ± 3
CO (L min^{-1})		4.0 ± 0.2	4.2 ± 0.1
PAP (mmHg)		19 ± 1	23 ± 1*

*AoB, aortic banding; MAP, mean arterial pressure measured in the descending aorta; LVSP, left ventricular systolic pressure measured proximal to the band; SAP, systolic artery pressure measured in the descending aorta; BW, body weight; LVW, left ventricular weight; HR, heart rate; CO, cardiac output; PAP, pulmonary arterial pressure. Those values were obtained under anesthesia at the end of follow-up. Values are mean ± SEM; *$P < 0.05$ vs. Sham.*

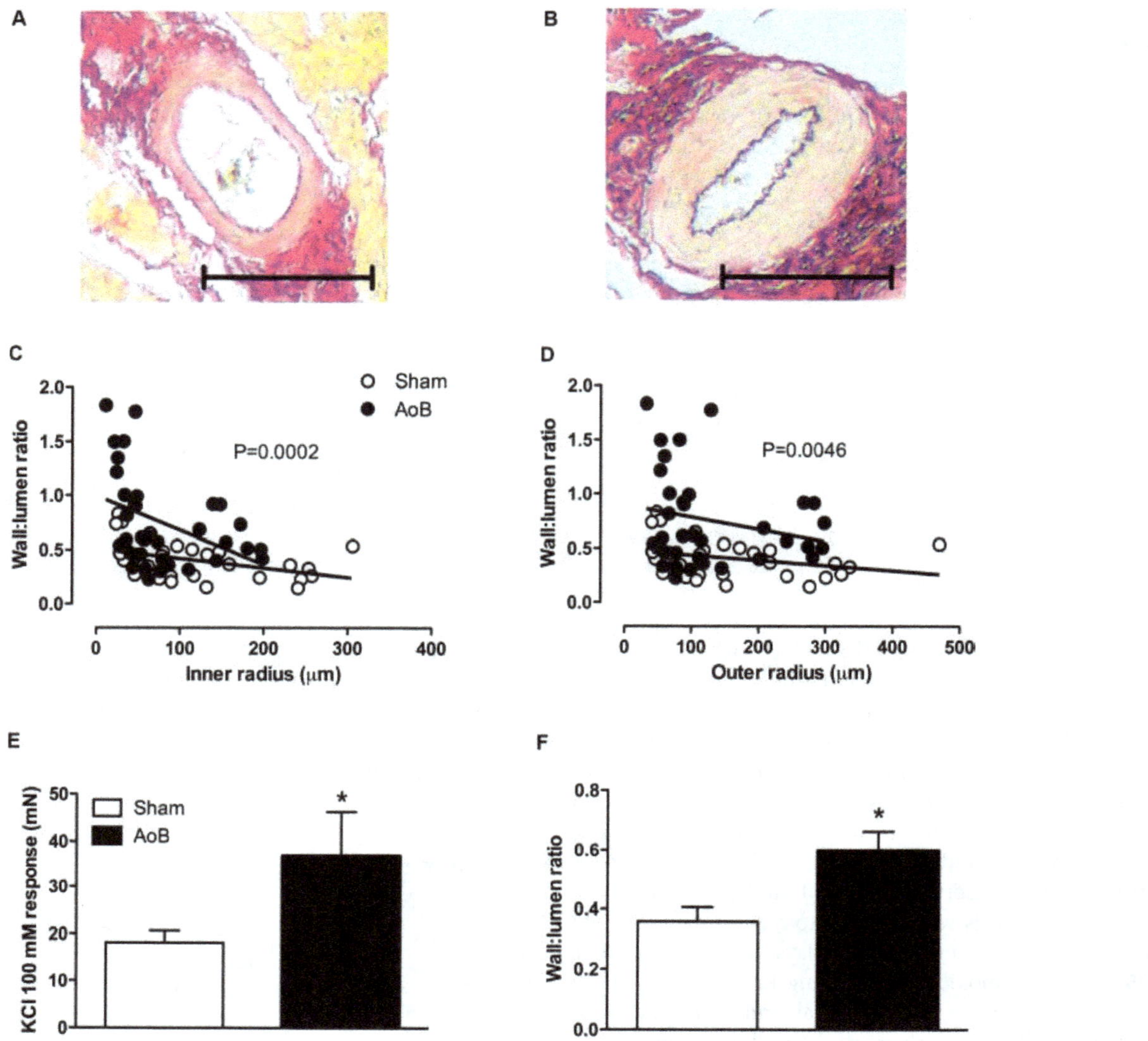

FIGURE 1 | Typical examples of coronary small arteries within the myocardium of Sham-operated swine **(A)** and swine with AoB **(B)**. The scale bar denotes 100 μm. The wall to lumen ratio both as a function of inner **(C)** and outer **(D)** was significantly increased in myocardium from swine with AoB. Shown are 34 vessels from 4 Sham-operated swine and 36 vessels from 5 AoB swine. The vasoconstrictor response to 100 mM KCl was significantly increased in vessels from AoB ($n = 6$) as compared to Sham ($n = 8$), **(E)**. The wall to lumen ratio in vessels with inner diameters ranging from 100 to 200 μm was increased in AoB as compared to Sham **(F)**. *$P < 0.05$ AoB vs. Sham.

2013b, 2017). Changes in contractile force were recorded with a Harvard isometric transducer. Following a 30 min stabilization period, the internal diameter was set to a tension equivalent to 0.9 times the estimated diameter at 100 mmHg effective transmural pressure (Batenburg et al., 2004; Zhou et al., 2013b, 2017). At the end of the stabilization period, the vessels were exposed to 30 mM KCl twice to check the contractility. Endothelial integrity was verified by observing dilation to 10 nM substance P after preconstriction with 100 nM of the stable TxA_2 analog U46619. Then vessels were subjected to 100 mM KCl to determine maximal vascular contraction. Thereafter, vessels were allowed to equilibrate in fresh organ bath fluid for 30 min before initiating different experimental protocols (Batenburg et al., 2004; Zhou et al., 2013b). In experiments where the effect of an antagonist on the response to Up_4A was assessed, antagonists were added to the organ baths 30 min before preconstriction with U46619 and were present throughout the experiments. Only one protocol was executed per vessel and, within one protocol, all vessels were obtained from different animals.

Experimental Protocols

Coronary small arteries from both Sham and AoB swine were subjected to Up_4A in incremental concentrations ranging from 10^{-9} to 10^{-5} M in the absence and presence of preconstriction with U46619 (Zhou et al., 2013b). To assess the involvement of different purinergic receptors in the vasodilator response to Up_4A, coronary small arteries from Sham and AoB swine were pre-incubated with non-selective P1 receptor antagonist 8PT (10^{-5} M), non-selective P2 receptor antagonist PPADS (10^{-5} M), adenosine A_{2A} receptor antagonist SCH58261 (10^{-8}

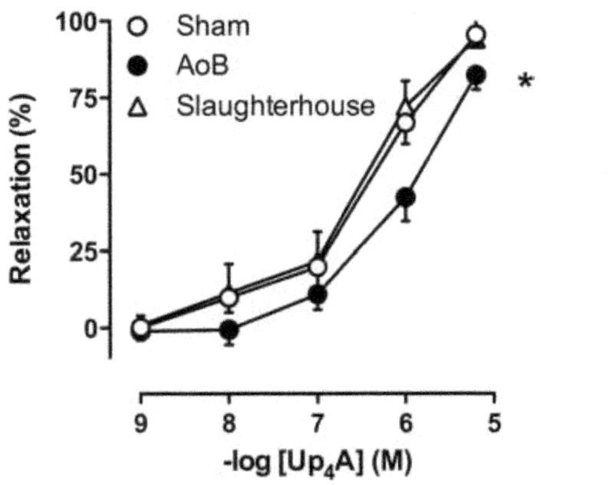

FIGURE 2 | Reduced vasodilator responses to Up4A in coronary small arteries from swine with AoB (n = 6) as compared to Sham-operated (n = 8) or Slaughterhouse (n = 5) swine. *P < 0.05 AoB vs. Sham or Slaughterhouse.

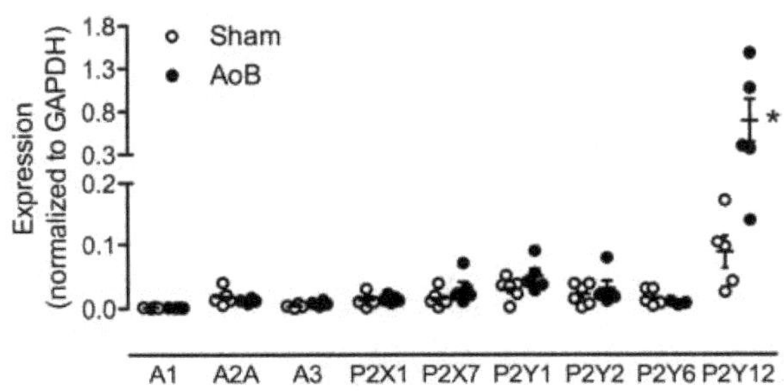

FIGURE 3 | mRNA expression of various P receptor subtypes in coronary small arteries from Sham-operated swine and swine with AoB. mRNA expression was normalized to expression of GAPDH. *P < 0.05 vs. Sham.

M), $P2X_1$ receptor antagonist MRS2159 (3×10^{-5} M), and $P2Y_1$ receptor antagonist MRS2179 (10^{-6} M) followed by preconstriction with U46619 (100 nM) (Zhou et al., 2013b) and exposed to Up_4A (10^{-9} to 10^{-5} M). To investigate if the role of endothelium-derived factors in the vasodilator response to Up_4A was altered after AoB, vessels from both Sham and AoB were exposed to Up_4A (10^{-9} to 10^{-5} M) in the absence and presence of nitric oxide synthase (NOS) inhibitor LNAME (10^{-4} M) alone or in combination with cyclooxygenase (COX) inhibitor indomethacin (10^{-5} M) (Zhou et al., 2013b). A potential role for TxA_2 in the response to Up_4A was assessed using coronary small arteries from porcine hearts (n = 5) obtained from a local slaughterhouse. The response to Up_4A of coronary small arteries of slaughterhouse pigs was similar to that of Sham-operated pigs (**Figure 2**). A subset of these vessels was de-endothelialized to mimic endothelial dysfunction of cardiovascular disease condition and exposed to the TxS inhibitor ozagrel (10^{-5} M), the $P2Y_{12}$ receptor antagonist clopidogrel (10^{-6} M), that can be converted to its active metabolites by cytochrome P450 enzymes shown to be present in the heart (Chaudhary et al., 2009; Sangkuhl et al., 2010) or a combination of ozagrel and clopidogrel prior to exposure to Up_4A.

Histology

Fresh sections of anterior wall of the left ventricle were fixed by 4% buffered formaldehyde and paraffin-embedded for histological analysis of remodeling of coronary small arteries. Sections were stained with resorcin-fuchsin as an elastin stain, photographed and inner and outer area of the coronary small arteries was assessed by planimetry (Sorop et al., 2016). Only transversely cut vessels with an inner radius below 200 μm were analyzed. Assuming circularity of the vessels, inner and outer radius were calculated as $r = \sqrt{(area/\pi)}$. Wall to lumen ratio was calculated as (outer–inner diameter)/inner diameter.

Quantitative Real-Time PCR Analysis

Following dissection, coronary small arteries (diameter: ~150 μm) were snap-frozen in liquid nitrogen to be used for detection of purinergic receptor subtypes A_1, A_{2A}, A_3, $P2X_1$, $P2X_4$, $P2X_7$, $P2Y_1$, $P2Y_2$, $P2Y_4$, $P2Y_6$, and $P2Y_{12}$ mRNA. In addition, the expression of endothelial NOS (eNOS), cyclooxygenase (COX) 1, COX2, prostacyclin synthase (PGIS), and TxS were measured (Rondelet et al., 2003). Total RNA was extracted from 5 to 7 frozen samples per group using a Qiagen RNA kit. cDNA was synthesized from 100 ng of total RNA with iScript Reverse Transcriptase (Bio-Rad). Quantitative real-time PCR (MyIQ, Bio-Rad) was performed with SYBR Green (Bio-Rad) (Zhou et al., 2013b). Target gene mRNA levels were expressed relative to the housekeeping gene glyceraldehyde-3-phosphate dehydrogenase (GAPDH) as an endogenous control (Martino et al., 2011). The primer sequences are shown in **Table 1**.

Data Analysis and Statistics

Hemodynamic data were averaged over a time period of at least 10 s. Vascular contractions were normalized to the response to 100 mM KCl, while vascular relaxation to Up_4A was expressed as percentage of contraction to U46619 (Zhou et al., 2013b). Statistical comparison of hemodynamic data, purinergic receptor expression, vascular response to KCl and comparison of wall to lumen ratio of vessels < 200 μm between Sham and AoB swine were performed using unpaired t-tests. The effect of AoB on wall to lumen ratio was analyzed with ANCOVA, using inner or outer radius as covariant. The effects of AoB as well as drug treatment on the Up_4A response were assessed using two-way ANOVA for repeated measures. Statistical significance was accepted when P < 0.05 (two-tailed). Data are presented as means ± SEM.

RESULTS

Characteristics of AoB Animals

Aortic banding of the ascending aorta resulted in a systolic pressure gradient of 88 ± 2 mmHg as measured during surgery (**Table 2**). The systolic pressure gradient was stable over the time course of the experiment, as evidenced by a systolic pressure gradient of 82 ± 8 and 98 ± 6 mmHg at week 1 and week 3 after AoB (**Table 2**). Mean arterial pressure distal to the band

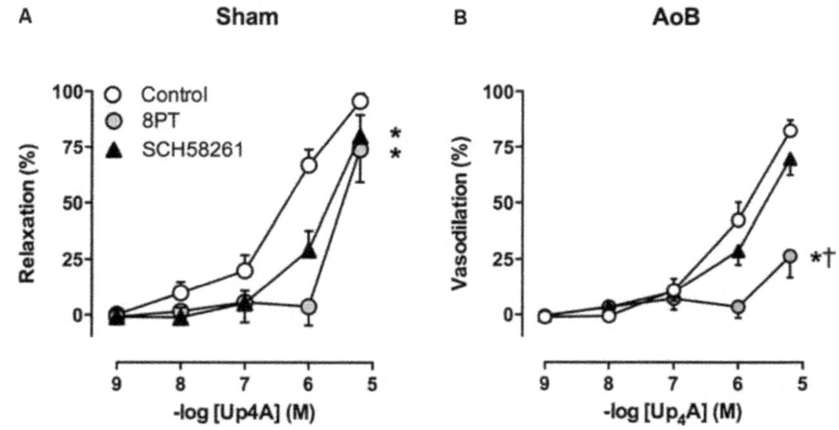

FIGURE 4 | P1 receptor blockade with 8PT attenuated relaxation to Up_4A less in coronary small arteries from Sham-operated swine (**A**, $n = 6$) as compared to coronary small arteries from swine with AoB (**B**, $n = 6$). A_{2A} receptor blockade with SCH58261 attenuated Up_4A-induced relaxation in coronary small arteries from Sham ($n = 5$), but not AoB ($n = 5$). Control data are the same as in **Figure 2** ('Sham' and 'AoB'). $^{*}P < 0.05$ effect of 8PT vs. corresponding control. $^{\dagger}P < 0.05$ effect of 8PT vs. corresponding SCH58261.

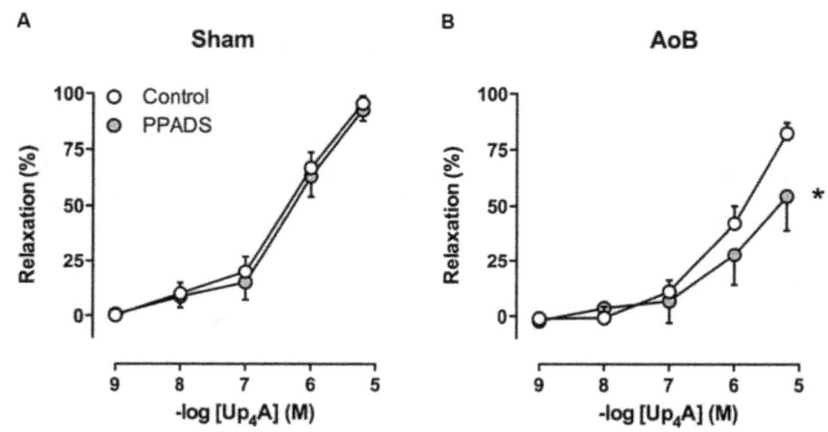

FIGURE 5 | P2 receptor blockade with PPADS had no effect on relaxation to Up_4A in coronary small arteries from Sham-operated swine (**A**, $n = 8$) but attenuated relaxation in coronary small arteries from swine with AoB (**B**, $n = 7$). Control data are the same as in **Figure 2** ('Sham' and 'AoB'). $^{*}P < 0.05$ effect of PPADS vs. corresponding control.

was lower in AoB as compared to Sham during surgery and 1 week after surgery, but was similar to mean arterial pressure in Sham-operated swine 3 weeks after surgery. At end of follow-up, the HR, mean arterial pressure, and CO were comparable between Sham and AoB swine, while the PAP was slightly increased in AoB (**Table 2**). Eight weeks of AoB resulted in left ventricular hypertrophy as evidenced by a 56% increase in left ventricle weight to BW ratio (**Table 2**). The wall to lumen ratio of coronary small arteries was also increased (**Figures 1A,B** for typical examples, **Figures 1C,D** for all results, **Figure 1F** for vessels with an inner diameter ranging from 100 to 200 μm) and the vascular response to 100 mM KCl in the coronary small arteries from AoB was significantly greater as compared to that from Sham (**Figure 1E**). These observations indicate that during 8 weeks of AoB, swine develop left ventricular hypertrophy as well as medial hypertrophy of the coronary microvessels.

Up_4A-Induced Coronary Relaxation Is Blunted in AoB

Cumulative concentrations of Up_4A (10^{-9} to 10^{-5} M) failed to induce vascular contraction in coronary small arteries from either Sham or AoB swine. The vasoconstrictor effect of U46619 (normalized to 100 mM KCl) was not significantly different between Sham and AoB (89 ± 15 vs. 61 ± 9%, $P = 0.16$). In these preconstricted vessels, Up_4A produced concentration-dependent relaxation, but the relaxation was significantly less in vessels from AoB as compared to Sham (**Figure 2**).

Involvement of Purinergic Receptor Subtypes

Despite unaltered expression of the A_1, A_{2A}, and A_3 receptor (**Figure 3**), P1 receptor blockade with 8PT attenuated Up_4A-induced relaxation in coronary small arteries from AoB more

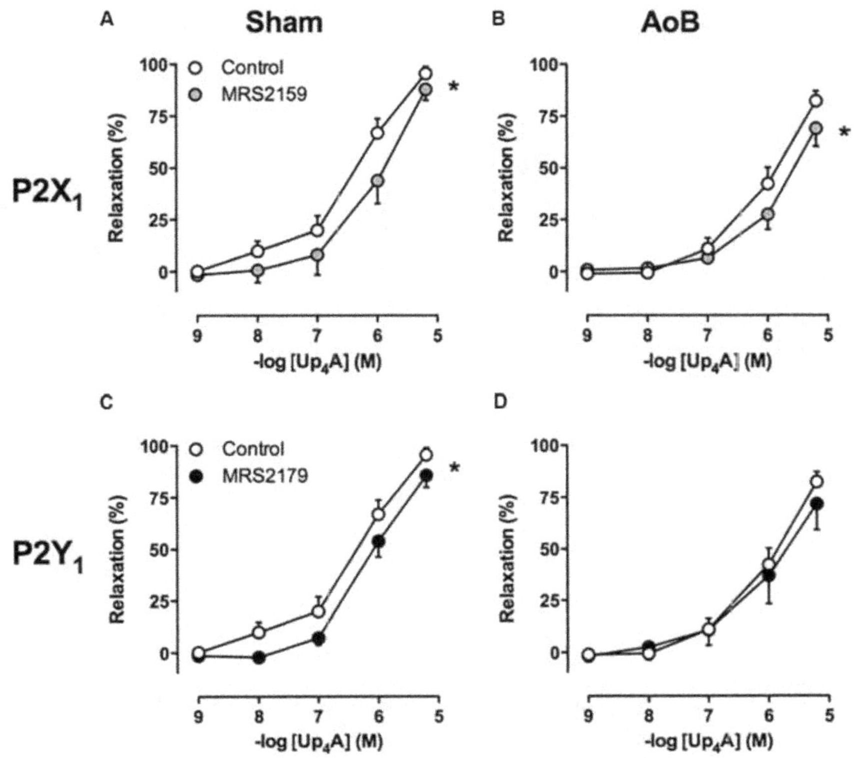

FIGURE 6 | $P2X_1$ receptor blockade with MRS2159 attenuated relaxation to Up_4A to the same extent in coronary small arteries from Sham-operated swine (**A**, $n = 8$) and from swine with AoB (**B**, $n = 6$), whereas and $P2Y_1$ receptor blockade with MRS2179 attenuated relaxation to Up_4A in coronary small arteries from Sham-operated swine (**C**, $n = 7$) but not from swine with AoB (**D**, $n = 5$). Control data are the same as in **Figure 2** ('Sham' and 'AoB').*$P < 0.05$ effect of MRS2159 or MRS2179 vs. corresponding control.

than in Sham (**Figures 4A,B**). Conversely, A_{2A} receptor blockade with SCH58261 attenuated Up_4A-induced relaxation to the same extent as 8PT in coronary small arteries from Sham, but had no effect on Up_4A-induced relaxation in AoB (**Figures 4A,B**). Non-selective P2 receptor blockade with PPADS had no effect on Up_4A-induced relaxation in coronary small arteries from Sham (**Figure 5A**), but did attenuate Up_4A-induced relaxation in vessels from AoB (**Figure 5B**). $P2X_1$ receptor blockade with MRS2159 attenuated Up_4A-induced relaxation in coronary small arteries from Sham (**Figure 6A**) and AoB swine (**Figure 6B**) to a similar extent, whereas $P2Y_1$ receptor blockade with MRS2179 attenuated Up_4A-induced relaxation in coronary small arteries from Sham (**Figure 6C**), but not AoB swine (**Figure 6D**). $P2X_1$, $P2X_7$, $P2Y_1$, $P2Y_2$ and $P2Y_6$ receptors were expressed, but no differences in expression in coronary small arteries between Sham and AoB were found (**Figure 3**). Expression of $P2Y_{12}$ receptors was higher in coronary small arteries from AoB (**Figure 3**), while expression of $P2X_4$ and $P2Y_4$ could not be detected (data not shown).

Involvement of Endothelium-Derived Factors in the Response to Up_4A

To investigate the contribution of alterations in endothelial function to the attenuated response to Up_4A after AoB, the effects of eNOS and COX inhibition on Up_4A-induced relaxation were assessed. eNOS inhibition with LNAME attenuated Up_4A-induced relaxation to the same extent in coronary small arteries from Sham and AoB swine (**Figures 7A,B**), which was corroborated by similar eNOS expression level in vessels from AoB and Sham (**Figure 8**).

In Sham-operated swine, combined inhibition of eNOS and COX (LNAME+indomethacin) attenuated Up_4A-induced relaxation to the same extent as LNAME alone (**Figure 7C**). In contrast, combined inhibition of eNOS and COX in vessels from AoB swine significantly enhanced Up_4A-induced relaxation compared to LNAME alone (**Figure 7D**), although COX1, COX2, and PGIS expression were not different in coronary small arteries between Sham and AoB (**Figure 8**). The observation that COX-inhibition enhanced the vasodilator effect of Up_4A suggests the production of a vasoconstrictor prostanoid(s). There is some evidence linking TxA_2 production to $P2Y_{12}$ receptor activation (Bhavaraju et al., 2010). Given the increased $P2Y_{12}$ receptor expression in coronary small arteries of AoB (**Figure 3**), we further investigated if TxA_2 could be the vasoconstrictor prostanoid produced in response to Up_4A, as well as the functional involvement of $P2Y_{12}$ receptor in this process. Coronary small arteries were denuded to mimic endothelial dysfunction in hypertension. Subsequently, endothelium-intact and -denuded vessels were exposed to Up_4A in the presence of the TxS inhibitor ozagrel, the $P2Y_{12}$ receptor antagonist

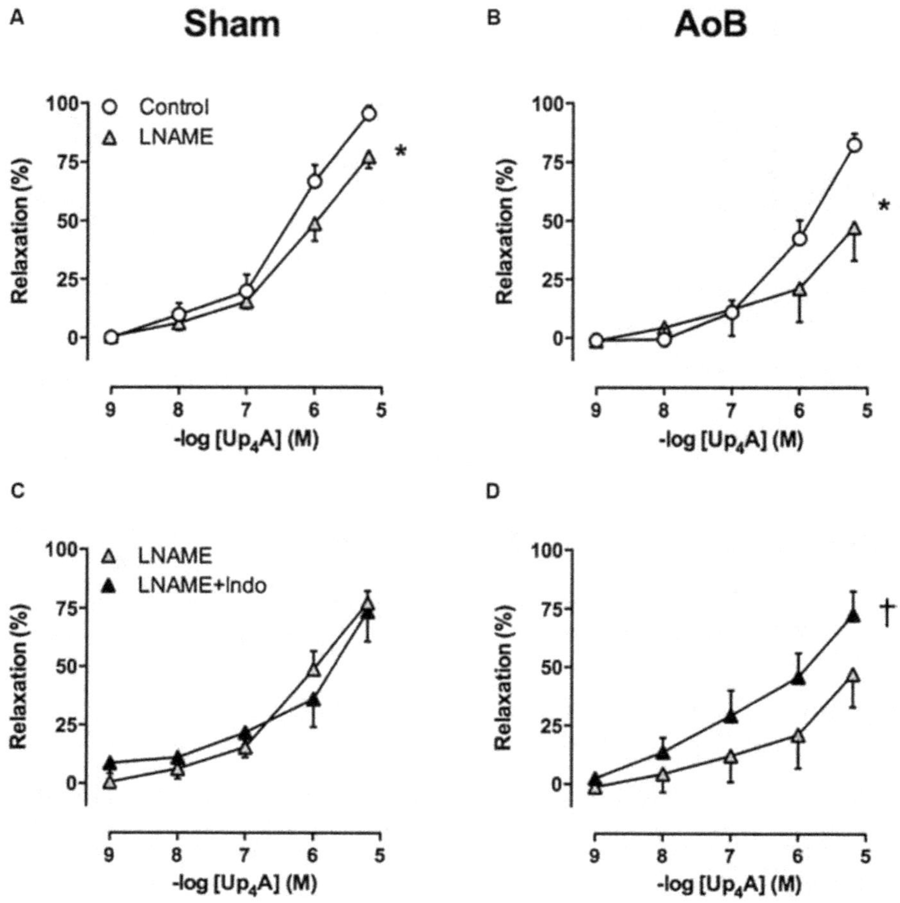

FIGURE 7 | eNOS inhibition with LNAME attenuated the response to Up_4A to a similar extent in coronary small arteries from Sham-operated swine (**A**, $n = 8$) and swine with AoB (**B**, $n = 7$). Subsequent inhibition of cyclooxygenase with indomethacin (Indo) had no effect in vessels from Sham (**C**, $n = 7$), but enhanced relaxation to Up_4A in vessels from swine with AoB (**D**, $n = 6$). Control data are the same as in **Figure 2** ('Sham' and 'AoB'). *$P < 0.05$ effect of LNAME vs. corresponding control; $^{\dagger}P < 0.05$ effect of LNAME + indomethacin vs. LNAME alone.

clopidogrel or their combination. Ozagrel had no effect on the response to Up_4A in coronary small arteries with intact endothelium (**Figure 9A**), but enhanced the vasodilator response to Up_4A in denuded coronary small arteries (**Figure 9B**). Similarly, clopidogrel enhanced the vasodilator response to Up_4A in denuded coronary small arteries (**Figure 9B**), but not in coronary small arteries with intact endothelium (**Figure 9A**). As the effect of the combination of ozagrel and clopidogrel was identical to the effect of either ozagrel or clopidogrel alone (**Figure 9B**), these data are consistent with the concept that $P2Y_{12}$ receptor activation may induce TxA_2 production.

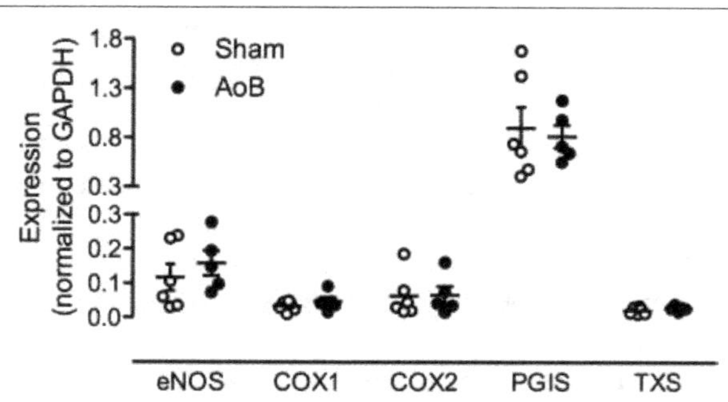

FIGURE 8 | mRNA expression of eNOS, cyclooxygenase (COX) 1 and COX2, prostacycline synthase (PGIS) and TxS in coronary small arteries from Sham-operated swine and swine with AoB. mRNA expression was normalized to expression of GAPDH.

DISCUSSION

The main findings of the present study were that (i) AoB resulted in medial hypertrophy of coronary small arteries as evidenced by an increase in wall-to-lumen ratio and an increased KCl-induced contractile force. (ii) Up_4A-induced relaxation was reduced in coronary small arteries from AoB as compared to Sham. (iii) Blockade of P1 receptors attenuated Up_4A-induced relaxation less in coronary small arteries from Sham as compared to AoB, but the contribution of the A_{2A} receptor was reduced. (iv) P2 receptor blockade with PPADS attenuated Up_4A-induced relaxation in AoB but not Sham. (v) The response to $P2X_1$

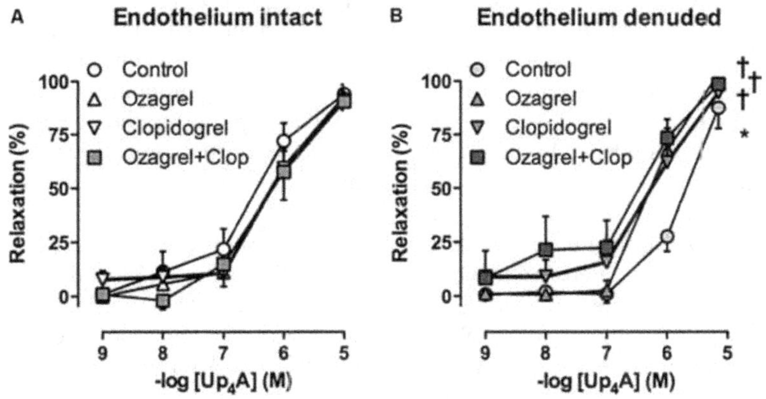

FIGURE 9 | Neither TxS inhibition with ozagrel, nor $P2Y_{12}$ receptor blockade with clopidogrel (Clop), nor the combination affected the response to Up_4A in coronary small arteries from slaughterhouse swine with intact endothelium (**A**, $n = 5$). Ozagrel and clopidogrel enhanced vasodilator response to Up_4A in denuded coronary small arteries, while the effect of the combination of ozagrel and clopidogrel was similar to the effect of either inhibitor alone (**B**, $n = 5$). Control data are the same as in **Figure 2** 'Slaughterhouse.' $^*P < 0.05$ effect of denudation; $^\dagger P < 0.05$ effect of ozagrel and/or clopidogrel vs. corresponding control.

blockade was similar in coronary small arteries from AoB and Sham. (vi) $P2Y_1$ receptor blockade attenuated Up_4A-induced relaxation in Sham, but not AoB. (vii) Expression of the $P2Y_{12}$ receptor was increased in coronary small arteries from AoB, while expression of other purinergic receptor subtypes involved in vascular tone regulation was not altered. (viii) eNOS inhibition attenuated Up_4A-induced relaxation to the same extent in Sham and AoB, whereas additional COX inhibition had no effect in Sham, but enhanced Up_4A-induced relaxation in AoB. (ix) $P2Y_{12}$ receptor blockade and/or TxS inhibition enhanced the vasodilator response to Up_4A in denuded coronary small arteries. The implications of these findings are discussed below.

Consistent with previous reports (Desjardins et al., 2005; Aubin et al., 2007), 8 weeks of AoB resulted in left ventricular hypertrophy and coronary microvascular remodeling, as evidenced by doubling of wall to lumen ratio of the coronary small arteries and doubling of the contractile response to KCl. The vasodilator response to Up_4A was blunted in coronary small arteries from swine with AoB. Up_4A exerts its vasoactive effect through interaction with purinergic receptors. In accordance with previous studies from our laboratory (Zhou et al., 2013b), coronary relaxation induced by Up_4A in swine was mediated primarily by the P1 receptors. Although the expression of the A_1, A_{2A}, and A_3 receptors was unaltered after AoB, the overall contribution of the P1 receptors to Up_4A-induced vasorelaxation was increased, while contribution of the A_{2A} receptor was reduced. These findings are different from our findings in the porcine coronary vasculature after MI (Zhou et al., 2013a) and metabolic derangement (Zhou et al., 2017), in which the reduced response to Up_4A was not due to functional loss of A_{2A} receptors. Although studies in mice (Zhou et al., 2015a) and swine (Long et al., 2010) showed that the main vasoactive effect of adenosine was mediated through A_{2A}, rather than A_{2B} receptor, we cannot exclude that altered expression of the A_{2B} receptor could explain the increased contribution of P1 receptors to the vasorelaxation to Up_4A in coronary small arteries from AoB as compared to Sham.

The assessment of the contribution of the P2 receptors to the response to Up_4A is difficult due to lack of selective antagonists of many of the P2 receptor subtypes. In general, activation of P2 receptors on endothelial cells is thought to result in vasodilation, whereas activation of P2 receptors on vascular smooth muscle cells results in vasoconstriction (Matsumoto et al., 1997; Burnstock, 2010; Zhou et al., 2013b). The non-selective P2 antagonist PPADS attenuated Up_4A-induced relaxation in coronary small arteries from swine with AoB, but not from Sham-operated swine, indicating that the contribution of P2 receptors blocked by PPADS is altered. PPADS has been shown to block $P2X_2$, $P2X_3$, $P2X_5$ (Burnstock, 2007), $P2X_7$ (Mezzaroma et al., 2011), $P2Y_1$ (Ju et al., 2003), $P2Y_2$, $P2Y_4$ (Rayment et al., 2007), and $P2Y_6$ (Schreiber and Kunzelmann, 2005) receptors. In contrast to the altered effect of PPADS, blockade of $P2X_1$ receptors attenuated the vasodilator response to Up_4A to the same extent in coronary small arteries from AoB and Sham-operated swine, which is in accordance with its unaltered expression. Conversely, despite unaltered expression of the $P2Y_1$ receptor, its vasodilator effect in response to Up_4A that was present in coronary small arteries from Sham disappeared after AoB. The observation that, in vessels from Sham-operated swine, $P2Y_1$ blockade attenuated the response to Up_4A, whereas PPADS, that has also been shown to block the $P2Y_1$ receptor, does not, suggests that PPADS also blocks a P2 vasoconstrictor receptor. The exact identity of this receptor remains to be elucidated. Interestingly, expression of the $P2Y_{12}$ receptor was increased in coronary small arteries from swine with AoB. As activation of the $P2Y_{12}$ receptor on vascular smooth muscle cells results in vasoconstriction (Wihlborg et al., 2004), increased expression of this receptor could explain the reduced vasodilator effect of Up_4A in coronary small arteries from swine with AoB. A role for the $P2Y_{12}$ receptor in the reduced vasodilator response to Up_4A is further substantiated by our observation that $P2Y_{12}$ blockade with clodipogrel enhanced the vasodilator response to Up_4A in denuded vessels, although it had no effect on the vasodilator response in vessels with intact endothelium. Altogether, our data indicate that Up_4A-mediated activation of the $P2Y_{12}$ receptor on the vascular smooth muscle cells results in vascular contraction, while the presence of healthy endothelium prevents such response.

Since several studies have shown endothelial dysfunction in the porcine coronary vasculature following AoB (Malo et al., 2003a,b; Desjardins et al., 2005; Aubin et al., 2007), we further investigated whether the contribution of endothelial vasodilator pathways to Up_4A-induced relaxation was altered. The blunted response to Up_4A was not due to a decreased contribution of NO, as both the effect of eNOS-inhibition with LNAME and eNOS expression were similar in coronary small arteries from Sham-operated swine and swine with AoB. The unaltered expression of eNOS is consistent with another study in isolated coronary arteries from swine with AoB (Malo et al., 2003b). Also, the contribution of eNOS to bradykinin-induced relaxation was maintained (Aubin et al., 2007), despite the presence of eNOS uncoupling (Malo et al., 2003b).

Cyclooxygenase-inhibition with indomethacin potentiated the vasodilator response to Up_4A in vessels from AoB, but not Sham-operated animals, suggesting that the reduced responsiveness to Up_4A was, at least in part, due to production of a vasoconstrictor prostanoid(s). A shift in the balance from vasodilator prostanoids to vasoconstrictor prostanoids has been implicated in the pathogenesis of cardiovascular disease (Kawabe et al., 2010). A potential mechanism behind such shift may be that oxidative stress and/or endothelial dysfunction result in eNOS uncoupling, which subsequently leads to the production of peroxynitrite, that is capable of inactivating PGIS thereby causing a shift in production from prostacyclin to TxA_2 (Zou et al., 2004; Nie et al., 2006). Indeed, TxA_2 levels were increased in the myocardium of hypercholesterolemic swine with endothelial dysfunction (Chu et al., 2012). Furthermore, the presence of a healthy endothelium in the present study prevented production of TxA_2, as inhibition of TxS with ozagrel enhanced the vasodilator response to Up_4A in denuded coronary small arteries, but not in those with intact endothelium. A link between the vasoconstrictor effect of Up_4A and TxA_2 production is further supported by a recent study demonstrating that Up_4A stimulates TxA_2 production leading to vascular contraction in mouse aortas (Zhou et al., 2015b). Moreover, an enhanced contraction in response to Up_4A is mediated through activation of COX2 and production of TxA_2 in the renal vasculature of diabetic rats (Matsumoto et al., 2014). Although mRNA levels of COX1, COX2, PGIS, and TxS were unaltered in coronary small arteries from swine with AoB in the present study, it is possible that the *activity* of COX2 and/or TxS was increased following stimulation with Up_4A. Preliminary data from coronary small arteries from two swine with AoB show that inhibition of TxS with ozagrel after LNAME has a similar effect as indomethacin, suggesting that indeed, TxS activity is increased. An increased production of TxA_2 in the coronary vasculature in AoB is not unique to Up_4A, but has also been shown in response to bradykinin and serotonin (Desjardins et al., 2005). It is unlikely that the response of the coronary microvasculature to TxA_2 receptor activation was altered, as the response to the TxA_2 analog U46619 was identical in vessels from Sham and AoB swine.

There is some evidence linking TxA_2 production to activation of the $P2Y_{12}$ receptor. Thus, TxA_2 levels were reduced in human serum treated with $P2Y_{12}$ inhibitors, $P2Y_{12}$ inhibition reduced serum TxA_2 in mice, and serum TxA_2 levels were reduced in $P2Y_{12}$ knockout mice (Bhavaraju et al., 2010). Consistent with these observations, in the present study, $P2Y_{12}$ blockade enhanced the vasodilator response to Up_4A to a similar extent as TxS inhibition, and combined inhibition of $P2Y_{12}$ receptor and TxS had no additional effect as compared to each treatment alone.

A role for Up_4A in the pathogenesis of hypertension has been suggested by the observation that Up_4A-induced vascular contraction in the renal, femoral, and basilar artery is potentiated in hypertension (Matsumoto et al., 2011b), while the Up_4A plasma concentration in hypertensive subjects is significantly higher as compared to that in healthy subjects and correlates with blood pressure (Jankowski et al., 2007). The present study shows that pressure overload-induced coronary vascular remodeling results in attenuation of the vasodilator effect of Up_4A, which is accompanied by increased expression of $P2Y_{12}$ receptor. Activation of the $P2Y_{12}$ receptor on vascular smooth muscle likely results in activation of TxS and TxA_2 production in response to Up_4A, thereby blunting its vasodilator effect in the coronary microcirculation. Future experiments are required to investigate if indeed the $P2Y_{12}$ receptor is a key factor in activation of TxS in AoB animals, as well as the signal transduction pathway involved.

AUTHOR CONTRIBUTIONS

ZZ: designed and performed the experiments, interpreted the data, drafted the manuscript. IL: performed the experiments, drafted the manuscript. HvB and CC: interpreted the data, revised the manuscript. DD and DM: designed the experiments, interpreted the data, revised the manuscript.

FUNDING

This work was supported by the China Scholarship Council 2009624027 (to ZZ) and CTMM-TRIUMPH (to DD and DM) as well as by the Netherlands CardioVascular Research Initiative CVON-RECONNECT 2014-11 (to DD and DM).

REFERENCES

Alexánderson, E., Jacome, R., Jimenez-Santos, M., Ochoa, J. M., Romero, E., Cabral, M. A., et al. (2012). Evaluation of the endothelial function in hypertensive patients with 13N-ammonia PET. *J. Nucl. Cardiol.* 19, 979–986. doi: 10.1007/s12350-012-9584-z

Aubin, M. C., Gendron, M. E., Lebel, V., Thorin, E., Tardif, J. C., Carrier, M., et al. (2007). Alterations in the endothelial G-protein coupled receptor pathway in epicardial arteries and subendocardial arterioles in compensated left ventricular hypertrophy. *Basic Res. Cardiol.* 102, 144–153. doi: 10.1007/s00395-006-0626-z

Bache, R. J. (1988). Effects of hypertrophy on the coronary circulation. *Prog. Cardiovasc. Dis.* 30, 403–440. doi: 10.1016/0033-0620(88)90005-9

Batenburg, W. W., Popp, R., Fleming, I., de Vries, R., Garrelds, I. M., Saxena, P. R., et al. (2004). Bradykinin-induced relaxation of coronary microarteries: S-nitrosothiols as EDHF? *Br. J. Pharmacol.* 142, 125–135. doi: 10.1038/sj.bjp.0705747

Bhavaraju, K., Georgakis, A., Jin, J., Gartner, T. K., Tomiyama, Y., Nurden, A., et al. (2010). Antagonism of P2Y12 reduces physiological thromboxane levels. *Platelets* 21, 604–609. doi: 10.3109/09537104.2010.511684

Breisch, E. A., White, F. C., Nimmo, L. E., and Bloor, C. M. (1986). Cardiac vasculature and flow during pressure-overload hypertrophy. *Am. J. Physiol.* 251(5 Pt 2), H1031–H1037. doi: 10.1152/ajpheart.1986.251.5.H1031

Burnstock, G. (2007). Purine and pyrimidine receptors. *Cell. Mol. Life Sci.* 64, 1471–1483. doi: 10.1007/s00018-007-6497-0

Burnstock, G. (2010). Control of vascular tone by purines and pyrimidines. *Br. J. Pharmacol.* 161, 527–529. doi: 10.1111/j.1476-5381.2010.00937.x

Chaudhary, K. R., Batchu, S. N., and Seubert, J. M. (2009). Cytochrome P450 enzymes and the heart. *IUBMB Life* 61, 954–960. doi: 10.1002/iub.241

Chu, L. M., Robich, M. P., Bianchi, C., Feng, J., Liu, Y., Xu, S. H., et al. (2012). Effects of cyclooxygenase inhibition on cardiovascular function in a hypercholesterolemic swine model of chronic ischemia. *Am. J. Physiol. Heart Circ. Physiol.* 302, H479–H488. doi: 10.1152/ajpheart.00146.2011

Desjardins, F., Aubin, M. C., Carrier, M., and Perrault, L. P. (2005). Decrease of endothelin receptor subtype ETB and release of COX-derived products contribute to endothelial dysfunction of porcine epicardial coronary arteries in left ventricular hypertrophy. *J. Cardiovasc. Pharmacol.* 45, 499–508. doi: 10.1097/01.fjc.0000159641.36900.14

Duncker, D. J., Zhang, J., and Bache, R. J. (1993). Coronary pressure-flow relation in left ventricular hypertrophy. Importance of changes in back pressure versus changes in minimum resistance. *Circ. Res.* 72, 579–587. doi: 10.1161/01.RES.72.3.579

Galderisi, M., Cicala, S., De Simone, L., Caso, P., Petrocelli, A., Pietropaolo, L., et al. (2001). Impact of myocardial diastolic dysfunction on coronary flow reserve in hypertensive patients with left ventricular hypertrophy. *Ital. Heart J.* 2, 677–684.

Haitsma, D. B., Bac, D., Raja, N., Boomsma, F., Verdouw, P. D., and Duncker, D. J. (2001). Minimal impairment of myocardial blood flow responses to exercise in the remodeled left ventricle early after myocardial infarction, despite significant hemodynamic and neurohumoral alterations. *Cardiovasc. Res.* 52, 417–428. doi: 10.1016/S0008-6363(01)00426-6

Hamasaki, S., Al Suwaidi, J., Higano, S. T., Miyauchi, K., Holmes, D. R. Jr., and Lerman, A. (2000). Attenuated coronary flow reserve and vascular remodeling in patients with hypertension and left ventricular hypertrophy. *J. Am. Coll. Cardiol.* 35, 1654–1660. doi: 10.1016/S0735-1097(00)00594-5

Jankowski, V., Meyer, A. A., Schlattmann, P., Gui, Y., Zheng, X. L., Stamcou, I., et al. (2007). Increased uridine adenosine tetraphosphate concentrations in plasma of juvenile hypertensives. *Arterioscler. Thromb. Vasc. Biol.* 27, 1776–1781. doi: 10.1161/ATVBAHA.107.143958

Ju, Y. K., Huang, W., Jiang, L., Barden, J. A., and Allen, D. G. (2003). ATP modulates intracellular Ca^{2+} and firing rate through a P2Y1 purinoceptor in cane toad pacemaker cells. *J. Physiol.* 552(Pt 3), 777–787. doi: 10.1113/jphysiol.2003.052258

Kappers, M. H., de Beer, V. J., Zhou, Z., Danser, A. H., Sleijfer, S., Duncker, D. J., et al. (2012). Sunitinib-induced systemic vasoconstriction in swine is endothelin mediated and does not involve nitric oxide or oxidative stress. *Hypertension* 59, 151–157. doi: 10.1161/HYPERTENSIONAHA.111.182220

Kawabe, J., Ushikubi, F., and Hasebe, N. (2010). Prostacyclin in vascular diseases. - Recent insights and future perspectives. *Circ. J.* 74, 836–843. doi: 10.1253/circj.CJ-10-0195

Khatibzadeh, S., Farzadfar, F., Oliver, J., Ezzati, M., and Moran, A. (2013). Worldwide risk factors for heart failure: A systematic review and pooled analysis. *Int. J. Cardiol.* 168, 1186–1194. doi: 10.1016/j.ijcard.2012.11.065

Lavi, S., Yang, E. H., Prasad, A., Mathew, V., Barsness, G. W., Rihal, C. S., et al. (2008). The interaction between coronary endothelial dysfunction, local oxidative stress, and endogenous nitric oxide in humans. *Hypertension* 51, 127–133. doi: 10.1161/HYPERTENSIONAHA.107.099986

Long, X., Mokelke, E. A., Neeb, Z. P., Alloosh, M., Edwards, J. M., and Sturek, M. (2010). Adenosine receptor regulation of coronary blood flow in Ossabaw miniature swine. *J. Pharmacol. Exp. Ther.* 335, 781–787. doi: 10.1124/jpet.110.170803

Malo, O., Carrier, M., Shi, Y. F., Tardif, J. C., Tanguay, J. F., and Perrault, L. P. (2003a). Specific alterations of endothelial signal transduction pathways of porcine epicardial coronary arteries in left ventricular hypertrophy. *J. Cardiovasc. Pharmacol.* 42, 275–286. doi: 10.1097/00005344-200308000-00018

Malo, O., Desjardins, F., Tanguay, J. F., Tardif, J. C., Carrier, M., and Perrault, L. P. (2003b). Tetrahydrobiopterin and antioxidants reverse the coronary endothelial dysfunction associated with left ventricular hypertrophy in a porcine model. *Cardiovasc. Res.* 59, 501–511. doi: 10.1016/S0008-6363(03)00390-0

Martino, A., Cabiati, M., Campan, M , Prescimone, T., Minocci, D., Caselli, C., et al. (2011). Selection of reference genes for normalization of real-time PCR data in minipig heart failure model and evaluation of TNF-alpha mRNA expression. *J. Biotechnol.* 153, 92–99. doi: 10.1016/j.jbiotec.2011.04.002

Matsumoto, T., Nakane, T., and Chiba, S. (1997). Pharmacological analysis of responses to ATP in the isolated and perfused canine coronary artery. *Eur. J. Pharmacol.* 334, 173–180.

Matsumoto, T., Tostes, R. C., and Webb, R. C. (2011a). The role of uridine adenosine tetraphosphate in the vascular system. *Adv. Pharmacol. Sci.* 2011:435132. doi: 10.1155/2011/435132

Matsumoto, T., Tostes, R. C., and Webb, R. C. (2011b). Uridine adenosine tetraphosphate-induced contraction is increased in renal but not pulmonary arteries from DOCA-salt hypertensive rats. *Am. J. Physiol. Heart Circ. Physiol.* 301, H409–H417. doi: 10.1152/ajpheart.00084.2011

Matsumoto, T., Watanabe, S., Kawamura, R., Taguchi, K., and Kobayashi, T. (2014). Enhanced uridine adenosine tetraphosphate-induced contraction in renal artery from type 2 diabetic Goto-Kakizaki rats due to activated cyclooxygenase/thromboxane receptor axis. *Pflugers Arch.* 466, 331–342. doi: 10.1007/s00424-013-1330-0

Mezzaroma, E., Toldo, S., Farkas, D., Seropian, I. M., Van Tassell, B. W., Salloum, F. N., et al. (2011). The inflammasome promotes adverse cardiac remodeling following acute myocardial infarction in the mouse. *Proc. Natl. Acad. Sci. U.S.A.* 108, 19725–19730. doi: 10.1073/pnas.1108586108

Nie, H., Wu, J. L., Zhang, M., Xu, J., and Zou, M. H. (2006). Endothelial nitric oxide synthase-dependent tyrosine nitration of prostacyclin synthase in diabetes in vivo. *Diabetes Metab. Res. Rev.* 55, 3133–3141. doi: 10.2337/db06-0505

Ralevic, V., and Burnstock, G. (1998). Receptors for purines and pyrimidines. *Pharmacol. Rev.* 50, 413–492.

Rayment, S. J., Latif, M. L., Ralevic, V., and Alexander, S. P. (2007). Evidence for the expression of multiple uracil nucleotide-stimulated P2 receptors coupled to smooth muscle contraction in porcine isolated arteries. *Br. J. Pharmacol.* 150, 604–612. doi: 10.1038/sj.bjp.0707120

Rodriguez-Porcel, M., Lerman, L. O., Herrmann, J., Sawamura, T., Napoli, C., and Lerman, A. (2003). Hypercholesterolemia and hypertension have synergistic deleterious effects on coronary endothelial function. *Arterioscler. Thromb. Vasc. Biol.* 23, 885–891. doi: 10.1161/01.ATV.0000069209.26507.BF

Rondelet, B., Kerbaul, F., Motte, S., van Beneden, R., Remmelink, M., Brimioulle, S., et al. (2003). Bosentan for the prevention of overcirculation-induced experimental pulmonary arterial hypertension. *Circulation* 107, 1329–1335. doi: 10.1161/01.CIR.0000053443.27512.33

Sangkuhl, K., Klein, T. E., and Altman, R. B. (2010). Clopidogrel pathway. *Pharmacogenet. Genomics* 20, 463–465. doi: 10.1097/FPC.0b013e3283385420

Schreiber, R., and Kunzelmann, K. (2005). Purinergic P2Y6 receptors induce Ca^{2+} and Cftr dependent Cl^- secretion in mouse trachea. *Cell Physiol. Biochem.* 16, 99–108. doi: 10.1159/000087736

Sorop, O., van den Heuvel, M., van Ditzhuijzen, N. S., de Beer, V. J., Heinonen, I., van Duin, R. W., et al. (2016). Coronary microvascular dysfunction after long-term diabetes and hypercholesterolemia. *Am. J. Physiol. Heart Circ. Physiol.* 311, H1339–H1351. doi: 10.1152/ajpheart.00458.2015

Teng, B., Labazi, H., Sun, C., Yang, Y., Zeng, X., Mustafa, S. J., et al. (2017). Divergent coronary flow responses to uridine adenosine tetraphosphate in atherosclerotic ApoE knockout mice. *Purinergic Signal.* 13, 591–600. doi: 10.1007/s11302-017-9586-z

Tomanek, R. J., Palmer, P. J , Peiffer, G. L., Schreiber, K. L., Eastham, C. L., and Marcus, M. L. (1986). Morphometry of canine coronary arteries, arterioles, and capillaries during hypertension and left ventricular hypertrophy. *Circ. Res.* 58, 38–46. doi: 10.1161/01.RES.58.1.38

Urbieta-Caceres, V. H., Zhu, X. Y., Gibson, M. E., Favreau, F. D., Jordan, K., Lerman, A., et al. (2011). Reversal of experimental renovascular hypertension restores coronary microvascular function and architecture. *Am. J. Hypertens.* 24, 458–465. doi: 10.1038/ajh.2010.259

van den Heuvel, A. F., Blanksma, P. K., Siebelink, H. M., van Wijk, L. M., Boomsma, F., Vaalburg, W., et al. (2001). Impairment of myocardial blood flow reserve in patients with asymptomatic left ventricular dysfunction: effects of ACE-inhibition with perindopril. *Int. J. Cardiovasc. Imag.* 17, 353–359. doi: 10.1023/A:1011971800052

van Kats, J. P., Duncker, D. J., Haitsma, D. B., Schuijt, M. P., Niebuur, R., Stubenitsky, R., et al. (2000). Angiotensin-converting enzyme inhibition and angiotensin II type 1 receptor blockade prevent cardiac remodeling in pigs after myocardial infarction: role of tissue angiotensin II. *Circulation* 102, 1556–1563. doi: 10.1161/01.CIR.102.13.1556

Vanhoutte, P. M. (1996). Endothelium-dependent responses in congestive heart failure. *J. Mol. Cell Cardiol.* 28, 2233–2240. doi: 10.1006/jmcc.1996.0215

Wihlborg, A. K., Wang, L., Braun, O. O., Eyjolfsson, A., Gustafsson, R., Gudbjartsson, T., et al. (2004). ADP receptor P2Y12 is expressed in vascular smooth muscle cells and stimulates contraction in human blood vessels. *Arterioscler. Thromb. Vasc. Biol.* 24, 1810–1815. doi: 10.1161/01.ATV.0000142376.30582.ed

Zhou, Z., de Wijs-Meijler, D., Lankhuizen, I., Jankowski, J., Jankowski, V., Jan Danser, A. H., et al. (2013a). Blunted coronary vasodilator response to uridine adenosine tetraphosphate in post-infarct remodeled myocardium is due to reduced P1 receptor activation. *Pharmacol. Res.* 77, 22–29. doi: 10.1016/j.phrs.2013.08.007

Zhou, Z., Merkus, D., Cheng, C., Duckers, H. J., Jan Danser, A. H., and Duncker, D. J. (2013b). Uridine adenosine tetraphosphate is a novel vasodilator in the coronary microcirculation which acts through purinergic P1 but not P2 receptors. *Pharmacol. Res.* 67, 10–17. doi: 10.1016/j.phrs.2012.09.011

Zhou, Z., Rajamani, U., Labazi, H., Tilley, S. L., Ledent, C., Teng, B., et al. (2015a). Involvement of NADPH oxidase in A2A adenosine receptor-mediated increase in coronary flow in isolated mouse hearts. *Purinergic Signal.* 11, 263–273. doi: 10.1007/s11302-015-9451-x

Zhou, Z., Sorop, O., de Beer, V. J., Heinonen, I., Cheng, C., Jan Danser, A. H., et al. (2017). Altered purinergic signaling in uridine adenosine tetraphosphate-induced coronary relaxation in swine with metabolic derangement. *Purinergic Signal.* 13, 319–329. doi: 10.1007/s11302-017-9563-6

Zhou, Z., Sun, C., Tilley, S. L., and Mustafa, S. J. (2015b). Mechanisms underlying uridine adenosine tetraphosphate-induced vascular contraction in mouse aorta: Role of thromboxane and purinergic receptors. *Vascul. Pharmacol.* 73, 78–85. doi: 10.1016/j.vph.2015.04.009

Zou, M. H., Cohen, R., and Ullrich, V. (2004). Peroxynitrite and vascular endothelial dysfunction in diabetes mellitus. *Endothelium* 11, 89–97. doi: 10.1080/10623320490482619

18

The Ionotropic P2X4 Receptor has Unique Properties in the Heart by Mediating the Negative Chronotropic Effect of ATP While Increasing the Ventricular Inotropy

Bruno Bragança[1,2], Sílvia Nogueira-Marques[1], Fátima Ferreirinha[1], Ana Patrícia Fontes-Sousa[1] and Paulo Correia-de-Sá[1]*

[1] Laboratório de Farmacologia e Neurobiologia, Center for Drug Discovery and Innovative Medicines (MedInUP), Instituto de Ciências Biomédicas de Abel Salazar, Universidade do Porto, Porto, Portugal, [2] Hospital Pedro Hispano, ULS Matosinhos, Matosinhos, Portugal

***Correspondence:**
Paulo Correia-de-Sá
farmacol@icbas.up.pt

Background: Mounting evidence indicate that reducing the sinoatrial node (SAN) activity may be a useful therapeutic strategy to control of heart failure. Purines, like ATP and its metabolite adenosine, consistently reduce the SAN spontaneous activity leading to negative cardiac chronotropy, with variable effects on the force of myocardial contraction (inotropy). Apart from adenosine A_1 receptors, the human SAN expresses high levels of ATP-sensitive ionotropic P2X4 receptors (P2X4R), yet their cardiac role is unexplored.

Methods: Here, we investigated the activity of P2 purinoceptors on isolated spontaneously beating atria (chronotropy) and on 2 Hz-paced right ventricular (RV, inotropy) strips from Wistar rats.

Results: ATP ($pEC_{50} = 4.05$) and its stable analogue ATPγS ($pEC_{50} = 4.69$) concentration-dependently reduced atrial chronotropy. Inhibition of ATP breakdown into adenosine by NTPDases with POM-1 failed to modify ATP-induced negative chronotropy. The effect of ATP on atrial rate was attenuated by a broad-spectrum P2 antagonist, PPADS, as well as by 5-BDBD, which selectively blocks the P2X4R subtype; however, no effect was observed upon blocking the A_1 receptor with DPCPX. The P2X4R positive allosteric modulator, ivermectin, increased the negative chronotropic response of ATP. Likewise, CTP, a P2X agonist that does not generate adenosine, replicated the P2X4R-mediated negative chronotropism of ATP. Inhibition of the Na^+/Ca^{2+} exchanger (NCX) with KB-R7943 and ORM-10103, but not blockage of the HCN channel with ZD7288, mimicked the effect of the P2X4R blocker, 5-BDBD. In paced RV strips, ATP caused a mild negative inotropic effect, which magnitude was 2 to 3-fold increased by 5-BDBD and KB-R7943. Immunofluorescence confocal microscopy studies confirm that cardiomyocytes of the rat SAN and RV co-express P2X4R and NCX1 proteins.

Conclusions: Data suggest that activation of ATP-sensitive P2X4R slows down heart rate by reducing the SAN activity while increasing the magnitude of ventricular contractions. The mechanism underlying the dual effect of ATP in the heart may involve inhibition of intracellular Ca^{2+}-extrusion by bolstering NCX function in the reverse mode. Thus, targeting the P2X4R activation may create novel well-tolerated heart-rate lowering drugs with potential benefits in patients with deteriorated ventricular function.

Keywords: ATP, P2X4 receptor, Na^+/Ca^{2+} exchanger, sinoartrial node, spontaneously beating atria, paced right ventricle

INTRODUCTION

Heart rate is primarily set in the right atria by spontaneous generation of rhythmic actions potentials in the sinoatrial node (SAN) (Boyett et al., 2000). The autonomous activity of SAN cardiomyocytes is orchestrated by activation of several ion channels and regulating proteins, which interplay to generate effective action potentials in a regular time basis (Yaniv et al., 2015; Fabbri et al., 2017). The unstable resting membrane potential characteristic of SAN cardiomyocytes is mainly due to mutual influence of intracellular Ca^{2+} "clocks" and membrane potential oscillations. The unstable resting membrane potential and the spontaneous firing of SAN cardiomyocytes are mainly attributed to "funny" currents carried by hyperpolarization-activated cyclic nucleotide-gated channels (HCN) and by the electrogenic Na^+/Ca^{2+} exchanger (NCX) functioning in the forward Ca^{2+}-extrusion mode (Tsutsui et al., 2018; Vinogradova et al., 2018). NCX operates as an integrator of intracellular Ca^{2+} with the membrane potential, in a way that it is responsible by a slow depolarizing current that drives the diastolic depolarization phase in response to calcium leakage from sarcoplasmatic reticulum and other subsidiary Ca^{2+} stores (Bogdanov et al., 2001; Sanders et al., 2006; Groenke et al., 2013; Herrmann et al., 2013). The NCX dynamically fluctuates between forward and reverse modes, thereby extruding or importing Ca^{2+} to subcellular regions, respectively (Samanta et al., 2018). Impairment of the NCX forward-mode by genetic ablation, pharmacological inhibition or even by simply changing its electrochemical gradient consistently induces bradycardia, supporting NCX as a key element in SAN pacemaker activity (Kurogouchi et al., 2000; Bogdanov et al., 2001; Sanders et al., 2006; Groenke et al., 2013; Herrmann et al., 2013).

The SAN, like other regions of the heart, is under control of countless number of signaling molecules, including adenosine triphosphate (ATP) and its derivatives, namely adenosine (Erlinge and Burnstock, 2008; Mangoni and Nargeot, 2008; Burnstock and Pelleg, 2015). Since the pioneering work of Drury and Szent-Gyorgyi almost a century ago (1929), the protective role of purine nucleotides and nucleosides as retaliatory mediators released in response to hypoxia and stressful stimuli in the vascular system has been expanded to the myocardium (Forrester and Williams, 1977), where purines engage energy-saving negative chronotropic, dromotropic and inotropic actions (Versprille and van Duyn, 1966; Lundberg et al., 1984; Pelleg et al., 1987; Belardinelli et al., 1995). Apart from cellular damage, ATP release is not stochastic but rather a fine regulated process (Lazarowski, 2012), involving (1) electrodiffusional movement through membrane ion channels, including pannexin- and connexin-containing hemichannels; (2) facilitated diffusion by nucleotide-specific ATP-binding cassette (ABC) transporters; and (3) cargo-vesicle trafficking and exocytotic granule secretion (Clarke et al., 2009; Pinheiro et al., 2013a; Pinheiro et al., 2013b; Timoteo et al., 2014).

Once in the extracellular milieu, ATP builds up its effects through activation of P2 purinoceptors, which comprise seven ionotropic (P2X1-7) and eight metabotropic ($P2Y_{1,2,4,6,11,12,13,14}$) receptors. Extracellular ATP can also indirectly activate purinoceptors of the P1 family (A_1, A_{2A}, A_{2B}, and A_3) after its conversion into adenosine by cascade of ectonucleoside triphosphate diphosphohydrolases (NTPDases) (Yegutkin, 2008). Intravenous ATP produces negative chronotropy, as well as several other acute cardiovascular effects that resembles adenosine application, almost neglecting ATP-sensitive receptors as active and functional regulators of the cardiac function (Pelleg and Belhassen, 2010). Apart from a massive presence of adenosine A_1 receptors (Braganca et al., 2016), the SAN from both rodents and humans expresses several P2 purinoceptor subtypes, including ionotropic P2X4, P2X7, and metabotropic $P2Y_1$, $P2Y_2$, and $P2Y_{14}$ (Musa et al., 2009), yet their role is still largely unknown. Besides species differences, the type and relative abundance of P2 purinoceptors in the heart varies with location and disease conditions (Musa et al., 2009).

Relatively recent evidence called our attention showing that the highly expressed ionotropic P2X4 in the human SAN may be an important modulator of NCX function (Shen et al., 2014). Activation of ionotropic P2X receptors, including the P2X4, triggers the influx of Na^+ that is subsequently exchanged by Ca^{2+} *via* the NCX (Jarvis and Khakh, 2009). Using various models of heart failure in rodents, it has been demonstrated that reversion of the NCX function by P2X4 activation may lead to improvements of ventricular performance and clinical outcome (Hu et al., 2001; Mei and Liang, 2001; Yang et al., 2004; Yang et al., 2014; Yang et al., 2015). Indeed, pharmacological inhibition of Na^+/K^+-ATPase with digitalis interferes with cardiac NCX function, resulting in both negative chronotropy and positive inotropy, thus explaining the rationale for usage of digitalis-like drugs in the management of patients with tachyarrhythmias and ventricular contractile incompetence (Blomstrom-Lundqvist et al., 2003; Ponikowski et al., 2016).

In this study, we aimed at characterizing the effect of the P2X4 on heart rate using isolated spontaneously beating rat atria strips. Taking into consideration that most currently available negative chronotropic drugs are associated with a negative inotropic impact as a major drawback (Ponikowski et al., 2016), experiments were designed to assess the effect of the P2X4 on the magnitude of paced ventricular contractions.

MATERIALS AND METHODS

Animals

Animals care and experimental procedures were conducted in strict accordance with the recommendations of the European Convention for the Protection of Vertebrate Animals used for Experimental and Other Scientific Purposes (ETS 123), Directive 2010/63/EU and Portuguese rules (DL 113/2013). All experimental protocols involving animals were approved by the competent national authority Direção Geral de Alimentação e Veterinária, and by the ICBAS Animal Ethical Committee (No. 224/2017). All efforts were made to minimize animal suffering and to reduce the number of animals used according to the ARRIVE guidelines. Wistar rats (*Rattus norvegicus*; 250–300 g; Charles River, Barcelona, Spain) of either sex were kept at a constant temperature (21 °C) and a regular light (06:30–19:30 h) - dark (19:30–06:30 h) cycle, with food and water provided *ad libitium*.

Isolated Spontaneously Beating Atria

Isolated spontaneously beating atria were prepared using a previously described method (Braganca et al., 2016), with some modifications. In brief, hearts were rapidly excised after decapitation followed by exsanguination (Rodent guillotine, Stoelting 51330), and placed in a physiological solution (Tyrode's solution) composed of (mM): NaCl 137; KCl 4.7; $CaCl_2$ 1.8; $MgCl_2$ 1; NaH_2PO_4 0.4; $NaHCO_3$ 11.9; glucose 11.2 and gassed with 95% O_2 + 5% CO_2 (at pH 7.4). Hearts were allowed to beat freely for a few seconds at room temperature, to empty its blood content. The paired rat atria with the SAN region were dissected out, cleaned of fatty tissues, and suspended in a 14-ml organ bath containing gassed Tyrode's solution at 37 °C. Each auricular appendage was tied and connected with thread to the organ bath wall and to an isometric force transducer (MLT050/D; AD Instruments, Colorado Springs, CO, USA). Changes in isometric tension were recorded continuously using a PowerLab data acquisition system (Chart 5, version 4.2; AD Instruments, Colorado Springs, CO, USA). The preparations were allowed to equilibrate for 30–40 min. During this time, the preparations were continuously superfused with Tyrode's solution (1 ml/min) and the tension was adjusted to 9.8 mN. This procedure allows atria (with intact SA node) to progressively recover rhythmic spontaneous beatings (average of 247 ± 5 beats min^{-1} at the beginning of the experimental protocol, n = 79); preparations with spontaneous atrial rate below 200 beats min^{-1} or exhibiting rhythm variations above 10 beats min^{-1} during equilibrium were discarded to ensure measurements were made in atria with intact primary pacemaker SAN activity. None of the preparations exhibited noticeable signs of ectopic-activity caused by secondary pacemakers, usually related to asynchronous and abnormal contractions.

Under these experimental conditions, spontaneously beating rat atria respond to muscarinic and β-adrenergic stimulation, but are unaffected by the application of atropine or atenolol alone used in concentrations high enough (1 μM and 3 μM, respectively) to prevent the effects of acetylcholine (100 μM) and isoproterenol (30 nM), respectively (data not shown). Thus, myographic recordings reported in this study include rate (chronotropic effect) and contractile force (inotropic effect) of spontaneously beating atria measured in the absence of cholinergic and/or adrenergic tone.

Isolated Paced Right Ventricle Strips

Following the isolation procedures described above for spontaneously beating atria, we also obtained right ventricular (RV) strips (2 mm wide, 8–10 mm long and 1.5 mm thick) by cutting RV-free wall longitudinally to its surface. A pair of ventricular strips was used from each right ventricle. RV strip ends were tied and connected with thread to the 14-ml organ bath hook and to an isometric force transducer (MLT050/D; AD Instruments, Colorado Springs, CO, USA). Changes in the isometric tension of RV strips, measured both by the active tension (mN/mg of wet tissue weight) and by the derivative of developed force over time (+dF/dt, mN/s), were tested at a fixed frequency of 120 beats per min commanded by electric field stimulation of the preparations, so that inotropy was measured without being affected by concurrent changes in chronotropy. Electric pacing (2 Hz, +50% voltage above threshold, 2 ms) was generated by independent Grass S48 stimulators (Quincy, MA, USA) and delivered *via* two platinum electrodes positioned on each side of the preparations. Equilibrium of the preparations was performed as described above for spontaneously beating atria. Only ventricular preparations exhibiting rhythmic contractions with similar amplitude were used.

Experimental Design

After reaching a steady-state, the Tyrode's solution flow through the organ bath was stopped and the preparations were incubated for an additional period of 15 min before drug applications. The concentration–response curves for ATP and related nucleotides were performed by non-cumulative application of increasing concentrations of the nucleotides during 5 min followed by a washout period with Tyrode's solution (15 ml/min) to avoid biases resulting from accumulation of their metabolites and to prevent receptors desensitization. To shorten the experimental duration and, thus, to increase results reproducibility, the majority of the preparations were incubated for 5 min with a fixed concentration (near the EC_{50} value) of the nucleotide either in the absence and in the presence of drug modulator (e.g. receptor antagonist, channel inhibitor); the latter contacted with the preparations at least for 15 min before application of the nucleotide and we kept 2-h washout intervals between testing again the same nucleotide to exclude biases related to P2 purinoceptors desensitization (controls not shown). To avoid damage of RV strips performance by prolonged pacing at 2 Hz, parallel experiments were performed using the two strips coming from the same animal to test the effect of ATP in the absence and in the presence of any modulator.

Immunofluorescence Staining and Confocal Microscopy Studies

Rat hearts were excised (see above) and placed in oxygenated Tyrode's solution at 33–34°C. Following heart excision, the right atrium (RA) containing the SAN region and RV were accurately isolated through the interauricular and interventricular septa and cleaned from tissue debris. Tissue fragments were placed over a small lung lobule fragment with the endocardial layer facing down, stretched to all directions, pinned flat onto cork slices and embedded in Shandon cryomatrix (Thermo Scientific) before frozen in a liquid nitrogen–isopentane; frozen samples were stored at −80°C until use. Frozen sections with 8 μm thickness were cut perpendicular to the crista terminalis of the RA and parallel to the long axis in the case of RV (see Braganca et al., 2016). Following fixation, the preparations were washed three times for 10 min each using 0.1 M PBS and incubated with a blocking buffer, consisting in fetal bovine serum 10%, bovine serum albumin 1%, Triton X-100 0.3% in PBS, for 2 h. After blocking and permeabilization, samples were incubated with selected primary antibodies (**Table 1**) diluted in incubation buffer (fetal bovine serum 5%, serum albumin 1%, Triton X-100 0.3% in PBS), overnight at 4°C. For double immunostaining, antibodies were combined before application to tissue samples. Following the washout of primary antibodies with PBS (3 cycles of 10 min) tissue samples were incubated with species-specific secondary antibodies (**Table 1**) in the dark for 2 h, at room temperature. Finally, VectaShield mounting medium with 4′-6-diamidino-2-phenylindole (DAPI) to stain the nuclei (H-1200; Vector Labs) was used, before cover-slipping the glass slides. Observations were performed and analyzed with a laser-scanning confocal microscope (Olympus Fluo View, FV1000, Tokyo, Japan).

The SAN was characterized as described in a previous study from our group (Braganca et al., 2016). SAN identification was also facilitated by observation of the sinus node artery surrounded by small-size cardiomyocytes positive for the hyperpolarization-activated cyclic nucleotide-gated channel 4 (HCN4) and negative against connexin-43 (Cx43), a gap junction protein ubiquitously expressed in the heart apart from in nodal tissue. In some of the experiments, the existence of a large number of neurofilament 160 (NF-160) positive neuronal fibers was also used to identify the SAN region (Tellez et al., 2006; Braganca et al., 2016).

Solutions and Chemicals

Adenosine-5′-triphosphate (ATP); adenosine 5′-[γ-thio]-triphosphate(ATPγS); cytidine-5′-triphosphate(CTP); 1,3-dipropyl-8-cyclopentyl-xanthine (DPCPX); 22,23-dihydroavermectin B1 (ivermectin); and 2-[(3,4-dihydro-2-phenyl-2H-1-benzopyran-6-yl)oxy]-5-nitro-pyridine (ORM-10103) were obtained from Sigma (Poole, U.K.). 5-(3-bromophenyl)-1,3-dihydro-2H-benzofuro[3,2-e]-1,4-diazepin-2-one (5-BDBD); 3-[[5-(2,3-dichlorophenyl)-1H-tetrazol-1-yl]methyl]pyridine hydrochloride (A438079); 2-[2-[4-(4-nitrobenzyloxy)phenyl]ethyl]isothiourea mesylate (KR-R7943) and sodium metatungstate (POM-1) were from Tocris Cookson Inc. (Bristol, UK). Pyridoxalphosphate-6-azophenyl-2′,4′-disulphonic acid (PPADS) and ZD7288 were from Ascent Scientific (Bristol, UK). Dimethylsulfoxide (DMSO), serum albumin and Triton X-100 were from Merck (Darmstadt, Germany). DPCPX was made up in 99% DMSO/1% NaOH 1 mM (v/v); 5-BDBD, A438079, Ivermectin, ORM-10103, KB-R7943 were made up in DMSO. Other drugs were prepared in distilled water. All stock solutions were stored as frozen aliquots at −20°C. Dilutions of these stock solutions were made daily and kept protected from the light to prevent photodecomposition. No statistically significant differences between control experiments, made in the absence or in the presence of the solvents at the maximal concentrations used (0.5% v/v), were observed. The pH of the Tyrode's solution did not change by the addition of the drugs in the maximum concentrations applied to the preparations.

Presentation of Data and Statistical Analysis

The isometric contractions were recorded and analyzed before and after the addition of each drug at the desired concentration. Results were presented as percentages of variation compared to baseline (% Δ baseline), obtained before application of the test drug. Data are expressed as mean ± SEM, with *n* indicating the number of animals used for a particular group of experiments. Graphical data are expressed as box-and-whiskers plots, with whiskers ranging from minimum to maximum values calculated as a percentage of variation from baseline. Since modulation of ATP-mediated responses were unpredictable, we did not apply any power calculations to pre-determine sample size, thus we pre-specified a number of 4–7 experiments for each condition. Concentration–response curves were analyzed by fitting four-parameter logistic sigmoidal functions to the experimental data to estimate pEC_{50} for negative chronotropy and inotropy of the nucleotides. All curve fitting procedures, graphical, and

TABLE 1 | List of primary and secondary antibodies used in immunohistochemistry experiments.

Antigen	Code	Host	Dilution	Supplier
Primary antibodies				
Cx43	Ab11370	Rabbit (rb)	1:700	Abcam
NF-160	Ab7794	Mouse (ms)	1:1,000	Abcam
HCN4	Agp-004	Guinea-pig (gp)	1:150	Alomone
P2X4 (C-terminus)	Apr-002	Rabbit (rb)	1:200	Alomone
P2X4 (extracell. loop)	Apr-024	Rabbit (rb)	1:200	Alomone
NCX1	Anx-011	Rabbit (rb)	1:50	Alomone
Secondary antibodies				
Alexa Fluor 488 anti-rb	A-21206	Donkey	1:1,500	Molecular probes
Alexa Fluor 568 anti-ms	A-10037	Donkey	1:1,500	Molecular probes
TRITC 568 anti-gp	706-025-148	Donkey	1:150	Jackson Immuno Res.

statistical analyses were carried out using GraphPad Prism 7.04 for Windows software (La Jolla, USA). Spontaneous or electrically-evoked mechanical tension (inotropic effect) and contraction rate (chronotropic effect) were evaluated using the Student's *t*-test for paired samples assuming a Gaussian distribution of data. Given that significant variability (ranging from 15 to 35%) was observed amongst animals for the negative chronotropic action of ATP (100 μM), changes on the nucleotide effect in the presence of a modulator was always compared to its absence in the same animal or preparation to make differences between paired values consistent. A value of $p < 0.05$ was considered to represent a significant difference.

RESULTS

Effects of ATP on Sinoatrial Chronotropy and Right Ventricular Inotropy

Non-cumulative application of ATP (0.001–1 mM) concentration-dependently decreased atrial chronotropy and right ventricular inotropy (**Figure 1**). The onset of ATP response was readily visible in about 30 s for both myocardial preparations; it reached a sustained maximal effect roughly 1 min after application and lasted while the nucleotide was kept in the incubation fluid, *i.e.* at least for 5 min. Spontaneously beating atria were slightly more sensitive ($p < 0.05$) to the inhibitory effect of ATP compared to paced RV strips (**Figure 1C**). The estimated pEC_{50} for the negative chronotropic and inotropic ATP responses were 4.05 and 3.45, respectively. Of note, ATP exhibited a biphasic effect on atrial inotropy, which was characterized by an initial decrease in the magnitude of atrial contractions followed by a gradual recovery to levels above the baseline (**Figure 1A**), as reported by other authors (Froldi et al., 1994; Gergs et al., 2008).

The Negative Chronotropic Effect of ATP Depends of P2 Purinoceptors Activation

The negative chronotropic effect of ATP following intravenous application of the nucleotide resembles that obtained after administration of adenosine (Pelleg and Belhassen, 2010), the end product of ATP hydrolysis by the ectonucleotidase cascade (Cardoso et al., 2015). To know whether ATP is acting directly on P2 purinoceptors or indirectly *via* P1 receptors after its extracellular conversion into adenosine, we tested the effect of ATPγS, an enzymatically-stable ATP analogue. ATPγS (100 μM) decreased sinoatrial chronotropy (−19 ± 5%, n = 6) by a similar extent to that observed for ATP (100 μM, −18 ± 5%, n = 6) (**Figure 2A**); the estimated pEC_{50} for the negative chronotropic effect of ATPγS was 4.69 (**Supplementary Figure S1A**). Moreover, the broad-spectrum P2 receptor antagonist PPADS (10 μM) significantly attenuated the negative chronotropic response of ATP (−20 ± 2% vs −11 ± 4%, n = 7, $p < 0.001$) (**Figure 2B**); the blocking effect of PPADS was more evident upon increasing the concentration of the P2 receptor antagonist to 100 μM (−17 ± 4% vs −2 ± 2%, n = 4) (see **Supplementary Figure S1D**).

Blockage of ATP breakdown by NTPDases with POM-1 (100 μM) significantly ($p < 0.05$) potentiated the negative chronotropic response of ATP (100 μM) (−19 ± 6% vs −35 ± 8%, n = 5, $p < 0.05$) (**Figure 2C**), whereas the selective adenosine A_1 receptor antagonist, DPCPX (3 nM) (Lohse et al., 1987), was ineffective (−19 ± 3% vs −21 ± 4%, n = 5; $p > 0.05$) (**Figure 2D**). Indeed, the NTPDase inhibitor, POM-1 (100 μM), shifted to the left ($pEC_{50} = 5.10$; $p < 0.05$) the concentration-response curve of ATP (0.001–1 mM) without significantly modifying the Hill slope (see **Supplementary Figure S1B**).

On their own, PPADS (10 μM and 100 μM), POM-1 (100 μM) and DPCPX (3 nM) were virtually devoid of effect on spontaneous atrial beating rate (see **Supplementary Figure S2**). It is also worth noting that blockage of muscarinic acetylcholine

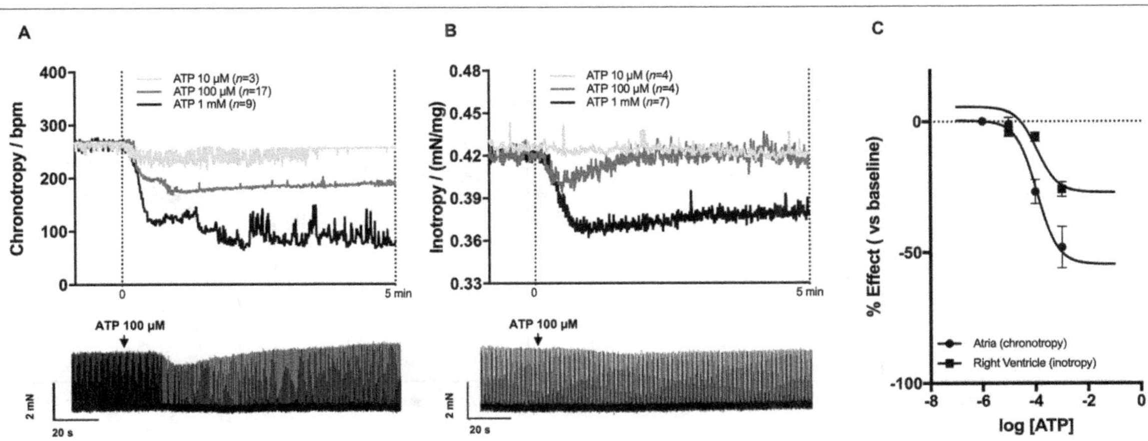

FIGURE 1 | Effects of ATP on spontaneously beating atria (**A**, chronotropy, beats min^{-1}) and 2 Hz-paced right ventricular (**B**, inotropy, mN/mg of tissue) strips from Wistar rats. ATP (0.01–1 mM) was applied non-cumulatively for 5 min followed by a washout period to avoid biases resulting from bath accumulation of metabolites and from receptors desensitization. Upper panels **(A)** and **(B)** show average values; bottom panels show typical myographical recordings of atrial and ventricular preparations challenged with ATP (100 μM). Panel **(C)** shows the concentration-response curves for ATP (0.001–1 mM) fitted by four-parameter logistic sigmoidal functions used to estimate pEC_{50} values for the negative chronotropic and inotropic effects of the nucleotide. Data are expressed as mean ± SEM from an *n* number of animals indicated in upper panels **(A)** and **(B)**, respectively.

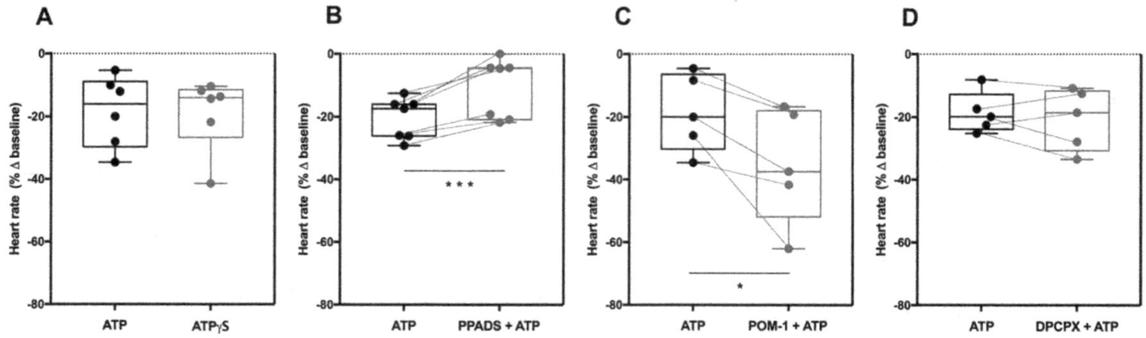

FIGURE 2 | The negative chronotropic effect of ATP depends of P2 purinoceptors activation. The negative chronotropic effect of ATP (100 μM) was tested either in the absence or in the presence of the non-selective P2 receptor antagonist, PPADS (10 μM, **B**), the NTPDase inhibitor, POM-1 (100 μM, **C**), and the selective adenosine A_1 receptor antagonist, DPCPX (3 nM, **D**). The negative chronotropic effect of the enzymatically stable ATP analogue, ATPγS (100 μM, **A**), is also shown for comparison. Represented are box-and-whiskers plots, with whiskers ranging from minimum to maximum values calculated as a percentage (%) of variation from baseline; horizontal lines inside boxes indicate the corresponding medians. Each data point represents the result of a single experiment; data from the same experiment are connected by lines. *p < 0.05, ***p < 0.001 (Student's *t*-test for paired samples) represent significant differences when compared to the effect of ATP alone.

receptors with atropine (1 μM) did not modify the negative chronotropic effect of ATP (100 μM) (data not shown), ruling out putative changes in the cholinergic tone operated by ATP.

The Negative Chronotropic Effect of ATP Is Mediated by P2X4 Receptors Activation

The P2 purinoceptors expression in the SAN is species specific. For instance, in humans the rank order of expression of ionotropic P2X receptors is the following: P2X4 > P2X7> > P2X1 > P2X5 (P2X2 and P2X3 are absent), while in rats it is P2X5> > P2X7> > P2X4~P2X1~P2X2 > P2X3 (Musa et al., 2009). Regrettably, there are no specific pharmacologic agonists or antagonists to the P2X5 receptor. It is worth noting that the P2X7 receptor is negatively modulated by extracellular Ca^{2+} and shows low affinity (0.1–1mM) for ATP. This contrasts with the estimated EC_{50} values in the low micromolar range for ATP and ATPγS that is characteristic of the most abundant P2X4 receptor in the human SAN (Soto et al., 1996; Michel et al., 1997). Interestingly, both P2X4 and P2X7 receptor pores are able to translocate extensive amounts of Na^+ into the cells. These premises prompted us to test whether these receptors could be involved in the negative chronotropic effect of ATP.

Selective blockage of the P2X7 receptor with A438079 (3 μM, **Figure 3A**) failed to modify the negative chronotropy effect of ATP (100 μM) (−31 ± 5% vs −26 ± 9%, n = 6, $p > 0.05$), whereas the potent and selective P2X4 receptor antagonist, 5-BDBD (10 μM) (Coddou et al., 2019), significantly attenuated ATP-induced negative chronotropism (−31 ± 7% vs −17 ± 5%, n = 6, $p < 0.05$) (**Figure 3B**). The negative chronotropic action of ATP (100 μM) was potentiated by ivermectin (30 μM) (−16 ± 3% vs −25 ± 3%, n = 5, $p < 0.05$) (**Figure 3C**), a drug that acts as positive allosteric

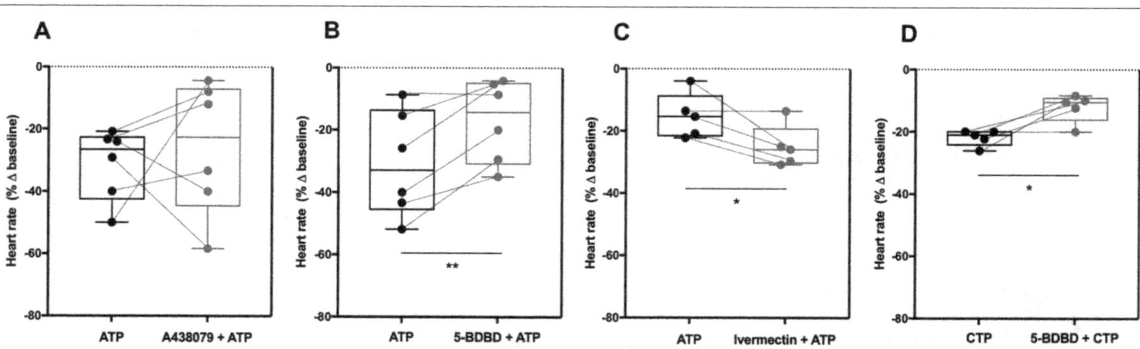

FIGURE 3 | The negative chronotropic effect of ATP is mediated by activation of P2X4. The negative chronotropic effect of ATP (100 μM) was tested either in the absence or in the presence of the P2X7 receptor antagonist, A438079 (3 μM, **A**), the P2X4 receptor antagonist, 5-BDBD (10 μM, **B**) and the positive allosteric modulator of the P2X4 receptor, ivermectin (30 μM, **C**). The negative chronotropic effect of CTP (1 mM, **D**) either in the absence or in the presence of 5-BDBD (10 μM), is also shown for comparison. Represented are box-and-whiskers plots, with whiskers ranging from minimum to maximum values calculated as a percentage (%) of variation from baseline; horizontal lines inside boxes indicate the corresponding medians. Each data point represents the result of a single experiment; data from the same experiment are connected by lines. *p < 0.05, **p < 0.01 (Student's *t*-test for paired samples) represent significant differences when compared to the effects of ATP or CTP alone, respectively.

modulator of the P2X4 receptor *via* a dual mechanism that involves potentiation and delayed inactivation of its currents, exhibiting selectivity over other P2X receptors (Khakh et al., 1999). The concentration-response curve of ATP (0.001–1 mM) was shifted to the left ($pEC_{50} = 4.99$; $p < 0.05$) by ivermectin (30 μM) compared to the effect of ATP alone (see **Supplementary Figure S1C**). Please note that, on their own, A438079 (3 μM, −5 ± 3%, n = 6), 5-BDBD (10 μM, −8 ± 9%, n = 5) and ivermectin (30 μM, 3 ± 3%, n = 5) were virtually devoid of effect on the spontaneous atrial frequency (see **Supplementary Figure S2**).

In order to further explore the potential involvement of the P2X4 receptor, we used CTP as a preferential P2X receptor agonist whose hydrolysis does not directly generate adenosine or other adenine nucleotides. Despite the fact that the P2X4 receptor exhibits low affinity for CTP compared to ATP (Soto et al., 1996; Kasuya et al., 2017), CTP (1 mM) decreased the spontaneous atrial rate by 22 ± 1% (n = 5) and this effect was also antagonized by 5-BDBD (10 μM, −12 ± 2%, n = 5, $p < 0.05$) (**Figure 3D**).

The P2X4-Mediated Negative Chronotropic Effect of ATP Involves NCX, But Not HCN

ATP binding to the P2X4 receptor dramatically increases Na^+ and Ca^{2+} influx through the receptor pore, which may interfere with NCX function as one of the sarcolemma controllers of the SAN pacemaker activity (Shen et al., 2014). Besides NCX, the normal sinus rhythm also depends on HCN channels mediating I_f currents (Bogdanov et al., 2001; Sanders et al., 2006; Groenke et al., 2013; Herrmann et al., 2013). Therefore, we thought it was relevant to evaluate the P2X4 receptor influence on downstream activation of NCX and/or HCN membrane transporters, which are essential to control heart rate. To this end, we used two different compounds known to inhibit NCX activity, namely KB-R7943 and the recently developed ORM-10103 (Jost et al., 2013). Since both inhibitors have putative negative chronotropic actions, we performed concentration–response curves to determine the minimal concentration beyond that reduction of chronotropy would be a problem in interaction experiments (data not shown). Incubations of KB-R7943 and ORM-10103 for 15 min at a final concentration of 3 μM had no effect on spontaneously beating atria strips (−3 ± 3%, n = 6, $p > 0.05$ vs baseline; −1 ± 2%, n = 5, $p > 0.05$ vs baseline; respectively) (**Supplementary Figure S2**).

The negative chronotropic effect of ATP (100 μM) was attenuated by KB-R7943 (3 μM; −19 ± 4% vs −8 ± 3%, n = 6, $p < 0.05$) and by ORM-10103 (3 μM; −29 ± 4% vs −17 ± 5%, n = 5, $p < 0.05$) (**Figures 4A, B**); the inhibitory effect of these compounds had a similar magnitude to that observed with the P2X4 antagonist, 5-BDBD (10 μM) (see **Figure 3B**). Pre-incubation with the ivabradine-like HCN channel inhibitor ZD7288 (300 nM) did not significantly modify the chronotropic effect of ATP (100 μM) (−12 ± 2% vs −11 ± 3%, n = 5, $p > 0.05$) (**Figure 4C**). On its own, ZD7288 (300 nM) decreased the spontaneous atrial rate only by 6 ± 2% below the control (n = 5, $p < 0.05$) (**Supplementary Figure S2**).

P2X4-Induced NCX Transport Reversal Counteracts the Negative Inotropic Effect of ATP in Paced Ventricular Strips

Apart from digitalis, heart rate slowing drugs used in clinical practice decrease cardiac inotropism as a major drawback (Ponikowski et al., 2016). As shown in **Figure 1B**, ATP (0.001–1 mM) concentration-dependently decreased the amplitude of paced RV contractions. **Figure 5** shows that blockage of P2X4 receptors with 5-BDBD (10 μM) augmented the negative inotropic effect of ATP (100 μM) measuring the percent variation of the active tension (−6 ± 2% vs −19 ± 5%, n = 5, $p < 0.05$; **Figure 5A**) or of the derivative of developed force over time (+dF/dt) (−4 ± 2% vs −18 ± 6%, n = 5, $p < 0.05$; **Figure 5B**) in paced RV strips. The effect of 5-BDBD (10 μM) was mimicked by KB-R7943 (3 μM), *i.e.* inhibition of NCX

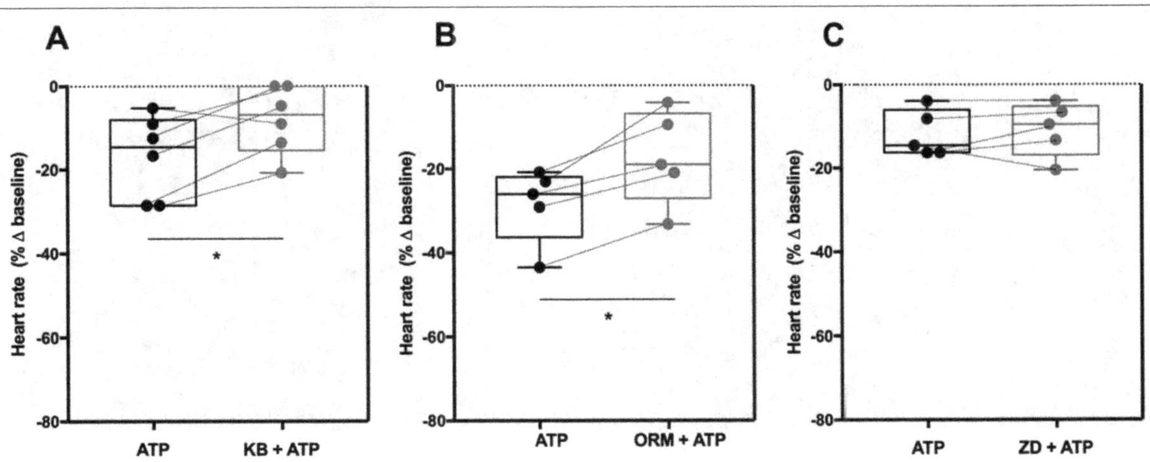

FIGURE 4 | The negative chronotropic effect of ATP involves ion exchange *via* pacemaker NCX, but not HCN. ATP (100 μM)-induced negative chronotropism was tested either in the absence or in the presence of two NCX inhibitors, KB-R7943 (3 μM, **A**) and ORM-10103 (3 μM, **B**), and of a HCN channel inhibitor, ZD7288 (300 nM, **C**). Represented are box-and-whiskers plots, with whiskers ranging from minimum to maximum values calculated as a percentage (%) of variation from baseline; horizontal lines inside boxes indicate the corresponding medians. Each data point represents the result of a single experiment; data from the same experiment are connected by lines. *p < 0.05 (Student's *t*-test for paired samples) represent significant differences when compared to the effect of ATP alone.

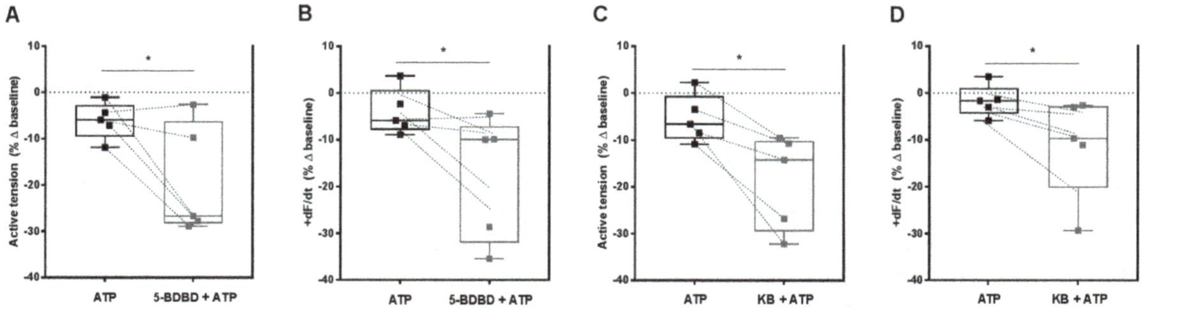

FIGURE 5 | Selective blockage of P2X4 and of NCX transporter partially offsets the negative inotropic effect of ATP in paced rat ventricular strips. The negative inotropic effect of ATP (100 μM) was tested either in the absence or in the presence of the P2X4 receptor antagonist, 5-BDBD (10 μM, **A** and **B**) and of the NCX inhibitor, KB-R7943 (3 μM, **C** and **D**). Represented are box-and-whiskers plots, with whiskers ranging from minimum to maximum values calculated as a percentage (%) of variation from the baseline isometric tension of RV strips, measured as the active tension (mN/mg of wet tissue weight, panels **A** and **C**) and the derivative of developed force over time (+dF/dt, mN/s, panels **B** and **D**); horizontal lines inside boxes indicate the corresponding medians. Each data point represents the result of a single experiment; data from the same experiment are connected by lines. *p < 0.05 (Student's *t*-test for paired samples) represent significant differences when compared to the effect of ATP alone.

sensitized RV strips to the negative inotropic effect of ATP (100 μM) calculated also measuring the percent variation of the active tension (−5 ± 2% vs −19 ± 5%, n = 5, $p < 0.05$; **Figure 5C**) or of the derivative of developed force over time (+dF/dt) (−2 ± 2% vs −12 ± 4%, n = 5, $p < 0.05$; **Figure 5D**). On their own, 5-BDBD (10 μM) and KB-R7943 (3 μM) marginally reduced ventricular inotropy by 14 ± 4% (n = 5, $p < 0.05$) and by 11 ± 19% (n = 5, $p > 0.05$), respectively (**Supplementary Figure S3**). These findings suggest that activation of the P2X4 partially counteracts the negative inotropic effect of ATP probably by reversing the NCX electrogenic current to pump Na^+ out and Ca^{2+} into ventricular cardiomyocytes.

Localization of P2X4, NCX1, and HCN4 Proteins in the Rat Heart

Confocal micrographs shown in **Figure 6** demonstrate that P2X4 receptor protein is expressed in the plasma membrane of cardiomyocytes of all assayed regions of the rat heart; in these experiments we used a knock-out validated antibody targeting the amino acid residues 370–388 of the C-terminus of the rat P2X4 receptor (Apr-002 from Alomone). Using tissues prepared in identical conditions and visualized with the same acquisition settings, one may conclude that the P2X4 receptor expression is higher in the SAN followed by the RV and RA. This regional

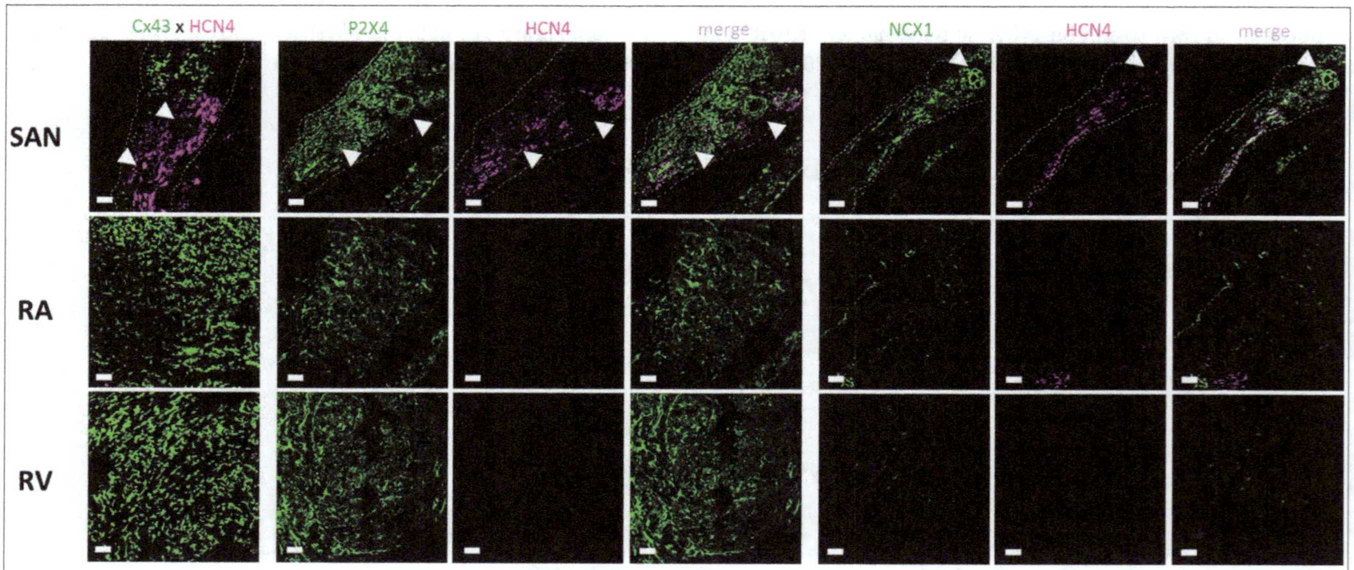

FIGURE 6 | Representative confocal micrographs showing the immunolocalization of the P2X4 receptor (Apr-002, C-terminus, Alomone) and NCX1 (Anx-011, Alomone) protein in the sinoatrial node (SAN), right atria (RA) and right ventricle (RV). The SAN was identified based on its low Cx43 (green) and high HCN4 (magenta) protein expression (left hand-side images). Images were taken from whole-mount heart preparations including the three analyzed regions, SAN, RA and RV. Dashed lines represent boundaries of the SAN. The pulmonary parenchyma was used as a structural support to facilitate immunostaining of myocardial sections and it is visible in the bottom right quadrant of each SAN image. White arrows indicate blood vessels including the SAN artery. Scale bar 30 μm. Images are representative of three different individuals.

difference was confirmed using a distinct antibody targeting amino acid residues 301–313 of the extracellular loop of the rat P2X4 receptor (Apr-024 from Alomone) (**Supplementary Figure S4**).

The immunoreactivity against NCX1 protein followed the same staining pattern to that found for the P2X4 receptor; the strongest immunofluorescence signal was also found in the SAN followed by other regions of the rat heart (**Figure 6**). Cardiomyocytes of the SAN region staining positively against NCX1 also exhibit immunoreactivity against the HCN4 protein. The same occurred regarding co-localization of P2X4 and HCN4. Taking this into consideration, even though double immunolabelling against P2X4 and NCX1 was not possible because available antibodies were raised in the same species (rabbit), it looks like that the staining pattern obtained with both P2X4 and NCX1 antibodies indicates that they may co-localize in HCN4 positive cardiomyocytes of the SAN (**Figure 6**). Please note that the smooth muscular layer of SAN blood vessels also exhibits strong immunoreactivity against P2X4 and NCX proteins (**Figure 6**, arrow heads). Likewise, these two proteins also co-localize with neurofilament 160 (NF160) in neuronal fibers of the SAN region (**Supplementary Figure S5**).

DISCUSSION

Data suggest that activation of ATP-sensitive P2X4 receptors plays a major contribution in decreasing the spontaneous activity of the SAN while partially offsetting the negative inotropic effect of the nucleotide by downstream reversing the electrogenic NCX mode of function (**Figure 7**).

ATP-Sensitive P2X4 Receptors Decrease Sinoatrial Pacemaker Activity

Extracellular ATP is an endogenous regulator of the cardiovascular function by acting either directly on P2 receptors or indirectly on P1 receptors after its breakdown to adenosine by NTPDases

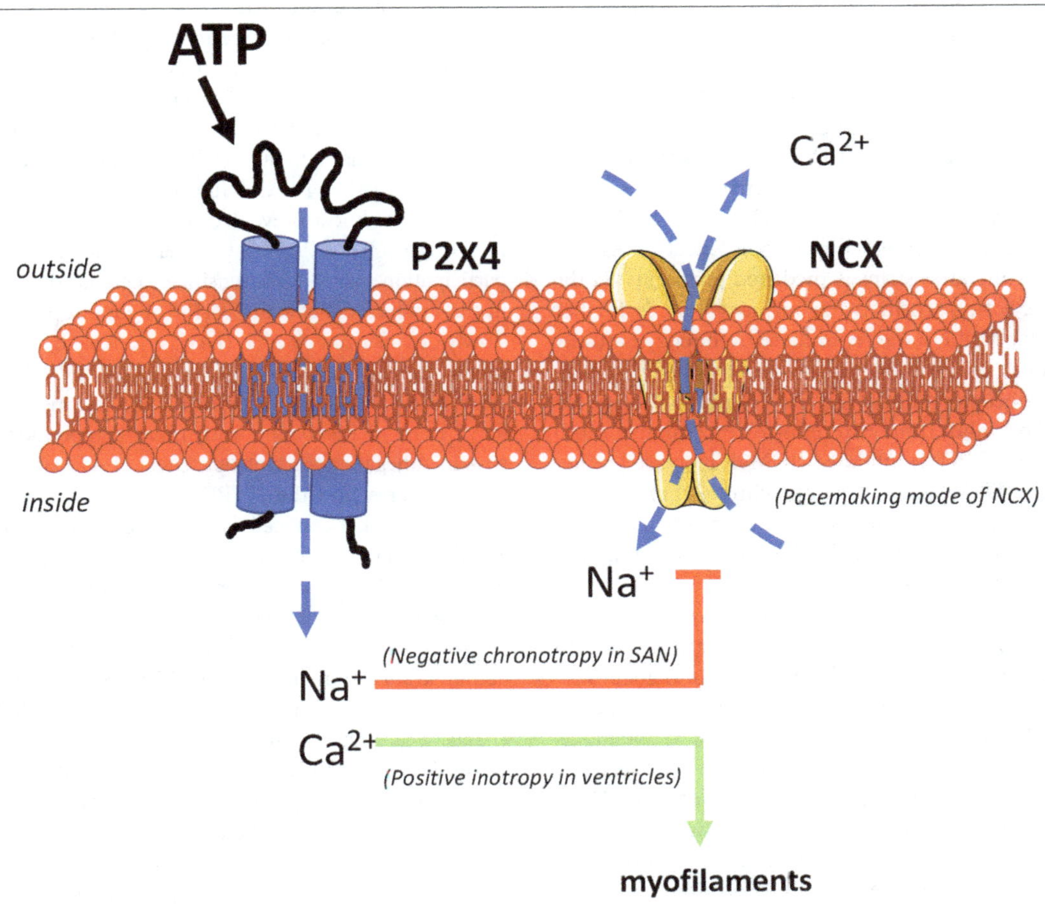

FIGURE 7 | The mechanism underlying the dual P2X4 receptor-mediated effects on cardiac chronotropy and inotropy implicates downstream modulation of NCX activity (digitalis-like phenomenon). Besides ion fluxes carried by pacemaker HCN channels (not represented), the unstable resting membrane potential and the spontaneous firing of SAN cardiomyocytes are attributed mainly to the electrogenic NCX transport operating in the forward Ca^{2+}-extrusion mode. Na^+ influx through the P2X4 receptor pore dissipates the electrochemical gradient of this ion across the plasma membrane leading to inhibition and/or reversion of the NCX pacemaker current. This may justify slowing down of SAN cells depolarizations and the negative chronotropic effect of ATP. Likewise, intracellular Ca^{2+} accumulation due both (1) to Ca^{2+} influx through the P2X4 receptor pore, and (2) to reversal of NCX activity may explain the positive inotropic effect of the P2X4 receptor in paced ventricular cardiomyocytes. Figure composition used elements from *Servier Medical Art*.

(Yegutkin, 2008; Headrick et al., 2013; Burnstock and Pelleg, 2015). Although the mammalian myocardium expresses multiple purinoceptors (Musa et al., 2009), the adenosine A_1 receptor has received most attention due to its relative abundance and well characterized functional role in the acute regulation of the heart (Musa et al., 2009; Chandrasekera et al., 2010; Headrick et al., 2013). Adenosine A_1 receptors activation decreases cardiac chronotropy, dromotropy, inotropy and counteracts adrenergic stimulation by a dual mechanism involving inhibition of adenylyl cyclase and opening of potassium channels (Belardinelli and Lerman, 1991; Burnstock and Pelleg, 2015; Braganca et al., 2016). Despite ATP effects may be mediated by breakdown to adenosine, the negative chronotropic action of ATP was insensitive to blockage of adenosine A_1 receptors with DPCPX used in a 6-fold higher concentration (3 nM) than that required to block this receptor (K_i~0.45 nM) (Lohse et al., 1987). However, one cannot exclude ATP conversion into adenosine during incubation with the nucleotide, yet even if this had occurred in our experimental conditions the amount of adenosine falls below the threshold to activate A_1 receptors in the SAN. These findings contrast with those obtained by Camara et al. (2015); these authors concluded that the negative chronotropic effect of ATP was dependent on A_1 receptors activation by using DPCPX in a concentration (1 μM) that is more than 2,000-fold higher than the K_i value for this antagonist to block the A_1 receptor (Camara et al., 2015). Under such conditions, off-target effects of DPCPX may appear, which include inhibition of phosphodiesterases that may explain reversal of the negative chronotropic effect of ATP (Camara et al., 2018).

Our theory that the negative chronotropic effect of ATP in spontaneously beating atria strips is mediated primarily *via* the activation of nucleotide-sensitive P2 purinoceptors is further supported by the fact that 1) it was reproduced by the enzymatically stable ATP analogue, ATPγS, 2) it was blocked by PPADS, a non-selective P2 purinoceptors antagonist exhibiting no affinity for adenosine receptors, and 3) prevention of ATP breakdown into adenosine with the NTPDase inhibitor, POM-1, increased rather than decreased ATP-induced negative chronotropism. Our findings agree with previous reports in the literature about the role of ATP and related adenine nucleotides on cardiac function (Versprille and van Duyn, 1966; Lundberg et al., 1984; Camara et al., 2015) and questions the most accepted hypothesis that the negative chronotropic action of ATP is most likely due to A_1 receptors activation after its rapid conversion into adenosine (Pelleg and Belhassen, 2010). While this hypothesis neglected the pivotal role of P2 purinoceptors in the control of spontaneous activity of the SAN, it has been demonstrated that ATP was more potent than adenosine in reducing heart rate (Pelleg et al., 1985; Sharma and Klein, 1988), which was interpreted as being due to an additional vagal reflex of ATP *via* sensory P2X2 and/or P2X3 receptors (Pelleg et al., 1987; Xu et al., 2005). This idea is difficult to admit in the present experimental conditions due to the fact that blockage of muscarinic acetylcholine receptors with atropine (1μM) failed to affect the rate and tension of spontaneous atrial contractions and did not modify ATP-induced effects, thus indicating that the cholinergic vagal tone is irrelevant for the P2-mediated effects of the nucleotide.

To the best of our knowledge, this is the first study demonstrating a role for the P2X4 receptor in the regulation of sinoatrial node automatism. Despite limited availability of selective drugs acting on the P2X4 receptor, it may be pharmacologically characterized by comparing agonists rank order of potency: ATP > 2-methylthioATP > CTP > α, β-methyleneATP (Soto et al., 1996), as well as by the use of selective antagonists and allosteric modulators (reviewed in Stokes et al., 2017). The potent and selective P2X4 receptor antagonist, 5-BDBD, with an IC_{50} value of about 1 μM, attenuated the negative chronotropic effect of ATP on spontaneously beating atria, while the positive allosteric modulator of the P2X4 receptor, ivermectin, potentiated the nucleotide response. Furthermore, we show here that besides ATP and its stable analogue, ATPγS, also the P2X4 agonist, CTP, whose hydrolysis does not directly yield adenosine, decreased the spontaneous atrial rate in a 5-BDBD-sensitive manner, but with a weaker potency comparing with adenine nucleotides (Soto et al., 1996; Kasuya et al., 2017). In this study we used 5-BDBD at a concentration (10 μM) that might also interfere with P2X1- and P2X3-mediated actions (Coddou et al., 2019), but we are confident that this is irrelevant in this case because very low amounts of these receptors are expressed in the SAN (Musa et al., 2009).

The P2X4 receptor shares structural and functional properties with other P2X receptors. For instance, it is known that the rat P2X4 receptor is relatively insensitive to PPADS (IC_{50}~100 μM), in contrast to mouse and human P2X4 orthologs (IC_{50}~10 μM; Jones et al., 2000). Although exhibiting a weaker potency for the rat P2X4 receptor, we almost prevented the negative chronotropic effect of ATP using 100 μM PPADS. One cannot, however, exclude a minor participation of PPADS-sensitive metabotropic P2Y receptors in the bradycardic effect of ATP. The ionotropic P2X4 receptor is slowly desensitized by ATP (Jarvis and Khakh, 2009). This feature might explain the relatively sustained negative chronotropic effect of ATP and its analogue, ATPγS, during the time (at least for 5 min) of incubation with these compounds. However, the sustained negative chronotropic effect of ATP does not explain the potentiating action the NTPDase inhibitor, POM-1, unless one hypothesizes that extracellular ATP accumulation also contributes to reduce adenosine formation by feed-forwardly inhibiting ecto-5'-nucleotidase/CD73, as demonstrated in other studies (Magalhães-Cardoso et al., 2003; Duarte-Araújo et al., 2009; Vieira et al., 2014).

Notwithstanding our observations, other studies failed to demonstrate the involvement of P2X receptors in the control of heart rate. For instance, infusion of 2-methylthioATP did not change heart rate in the Langendorff-perfused heart (Mei and Liang, 2001), most probably because the used concentration (100 nM) of the ATP analogue falls below the threshold (1 μM) required to activate the P2X4 in the SAN (Jarvis and Khakh, 2009). The same group also failed to find any difference in the spontaneous heart rate when comparing wild-type with mice overexpressing or missing the P2X4 receptor (Hu et al., 2001; Yang et al., 2014). One must, however, emphasize that these studies were designed to evaluate the P2X4 receptor tone under basal conditions, *i.e.* in the absence of any P2X4 agonist, which is a different situation from the present report. Thus, future studies are required to elucidate the role of the P2X4 receptor in the *in vivo* control of heart rate.

In the rat heart, the P2X4 receptor is the third most abundant P2X receptor after P2X7 and P2X5 receptors, while in the human heart it is considered the most expressed P2X receptor subtype (Musa et al., 2009). Also the regional distribution of the P2X4 receptor in the heart displays some differences among species. Using immunofluorescence confocal microscopy, we show here that the P2X4 protein is slightly more expressed in the plasma membrane of SAN cells (mostly cardiomyocytes, but also blood vessels and nerve fibers) followed by the RV and RA of the rat. This is slightly different from data obtained in humans where the P2X4 receptor mRNA seems to be evenly expressed through the myocardium (Musa et al., 2009).

P2X4-Induced Negative Chronotropism Requires Reversal of the NCX Activity Mode

Interestingly, the distribution of the P2X4 receptor in SAN cardiomyocytes matches the immunofluorescence staining pattern of NCX1 and HCN4 in the rat. This led us to hypothesize that the P2X4 receptor-mediated negative chronotropic effect of ATP could involve downstream modulation of NCX and/ or HCN pacemaker activities. Crosstalk between P2X4- and NCX-mediated effects has been demonstrated (Shen et al., 2014). Opening of the P2X4 ion pore mediates the influx of positive charges, mainly Na^+ and Ca^{2+} in a 1:4 ratio (Jarvis and Khakh, 2009), in the proximity of NCX carriers, which might affect their operation mode. Indeed, the ATP analogue, 2-methylthioATP (3 μM), inhibited the electrogenic forward mode of NCX in ventricular myocytes *via* an increase (by about 1 mM) in the intracellular Na^+ concentration (Shen et al., 2014), which represents a net increase of 7–25% considering the resting intracellular Na^+ concentration (Despa and Bers, 2013). Increases in intracellular Na^+ may be even more relevant in cells with limited pathways for Na^+ entry due to low expression levels of voltage-sensitive Na^+ channels, like the SAN cardiomyocytes (Remme and Bezzina, 2010). Likewise, it has been demonstrated that persistent Na^+ currents evoked by veratridine triggers intracellular calcium transients by reversing the operation mode of NCX in CA1 pyramidal cells (Fekete et al., 2009). Although speculative, reversal of the NCX function mode by the influx of Na^+ represents an alternative mechanism for dysrhythmias (including bradycardia) in some inherited cardiac sodium channelopathies, such as the type 3 long QT syndrome associated with SCN5A mutations and persistent sodium currents (Remme and Bezzina, 2010). In agreement with our theory that Na^+ influx *via* the P2X4 receptor pore might affect the NCX mode of function to decrease heart rate (**Figure 7**), we showed here for the first time that partial blockage of NCX, but not HCN channel, with two distinct inhibitors, KR-R7943 or ORM-10103, turned the spontaneously beating atria less sensitive to the negative chronotropic effect of ATP. Although beyond the scope of the present work, the interplay between P2X4 and NCX deserves further investigations using highly-demanding electrophysiology patch-clamp techniques in acutely isolated SAN cardiomyocytes from both rats and humans (ongoing research project).

Co-localization of P2X4 and NCX1 immunoreactivity in NF160 positive neuronal fibers was also detected. The presence of the P2X4 receptor in neuronal structures is widely accepted, but its function remains to be explored (Stokes et al., 2017). The SAN and the surrounding myocardium are regulated by a dense network of autonomic fibers, which are mainly parasympathetic followed by a sympathetic origin (Crick et al., 1994; Crick et al., 1999; Pauza et al., 2013; Zarzoso et al., 2013; Rajendran et al., 2019). Interestingly, some intracardiac neurons within atria contain ATP stored in vesicles (Crowe and Burnstock, 1982), which upon activation may represent an important source of extracellular ATP (Burnstock, 1972; Fredholm et al., 1982; Tokunaga et al., 1995). Reversion of NCX forward activity during ischemic conditions contributes to increase the magnitude of Ca^{2+} transients and, thus, the release of neurotransmitters from presynaptic nerve terminals (Lee and Kim, 2015). Given the co-localization and putative interplay between the P2X4 receptor and NCX in NF160-positive nerve fibers, one may speculate that these players may also interact to control the activity of cardiac neurons (Griffioen et al., 2007). This is even more relevant taking into consideration that cardiac ischemia is accompanied by P2X4 overexpression, particularly in the SAN (Musa et al., 2009). Thus, ATP released from autonomic cardiac nerves may trigger a positive feedback loop involving the NCX leading to an increase in the purinergic control of atrial cardiomyocyte function at both pre- and post-junctional levels.

ATP-Induced Negative Inotropism Is Partially Offset by P2X4 Activation and NCX Transport Reversal

The inotropic effect of ATP was investigated in paced RV strips; the nucleotide decreased ventricular inotropy in a concentration-dependent manner, yet changes in paced ventricular tension were less potent than the recorded ATP-induced negative chronotropic actions in spontaneously beating atria. This raised the possibility for the existence of a yet unraveled ATP-induced negative inotropic offsetting mechanism. Although we did not fully characterized the receptors involved in the negative inotropic effect of ATP, previous studies agree that P2 purinoceptors activation may be necessary, also taking into consideration that adenosine plays a minor (if any) role on ventricular inotropy (Burnstock and Meghji, 1983; Belardinelli et al., 1995; Balogh et al., 2005). There is, however, a contention regarding to whether ATP exerts a positive or a negative inotropic effect on ventricular contractions. In contrast to our findings, most reports in the literature suggest that ATP exerts a predominant positive inotropic effect in the heart. Nonetheless, it is worth to emphasize that the vast majority of these studies were performed in isolated ventricular myocytes (Danziger et al., 1988; De Young and Scarpa, 1989; Christie et al., 1992; Podrasky et al., 1997; Mei and Liang, 2001; Balogh et al., 2005). These findings attenuate the theory that ATP-induced positive inotropism could be mediated by P2X4 receptors facilitating noradrenaline release from sympathetic nerve terminals in paced ventricular strips. Only three studies were performed in more complex tissue preparations, namely in rat papillary muscles (Legssyer et al., 1988; Scamps et al., 1990) and in the frog ventricle (Flitney and Singh, 1980). Interestingly, the

Legssyer's and Flitney's studies reported a dual and opposing role of ATP in cardiac tissues. In support of a negative inotropic role for ATP, a recent study performed in intact isolated hearts, as well as in ventricular fragments and acutely isolated myocytes proposed that diadenosine tetraphosphate decreased ventricular inotropy probably *via* the activation of P2Y purinoceptors (Pakhomov et al., 2018).

Notwithstanding the conflicting results regarding the nature of the inotropic role of ATP, the use of ATP analogues and more selective P2 receptor modulators, in combination with genetic and other advanced biochemical techniques, provided strong evidence that several P2X and P2Y receptors may be positive ventricular inotropic mediators (reviewed in Erlinge and Burnstock, 2008; Burnstock and Pelleg, 2015). Regarding the P2Y receptor family, positive inotropy is generally attributed to stimulation of Gs and Gq-protein coupled receptors (Erlinge and Burnstock, 2008). Among them, ATP preferentially activates the $P2Y_{11}$ receptor (Abbracchio et al., 2006). The selective $P2Y_{11}$ agonist, AR-C67085, increased contraction in isolated cardiomyocytes as well as in isolated trabecular preparations. In that study, $P2Y_{12}$ and $P2Y_{13}$ receptors were excluded by the lack of effect of the stable ADP analogue, 2-methylthioADP, in cardiomyocytes contractile activity, which also nearly exclude any involvement of ATP-sensitive Gi-protein coupled P2Y receptor (Balogh et al., 2005). Of note, it is likely that these authors performed their studies in a mixed population of ventricular and atrial cardiomyocytes, as these cells were not separated by the enzymatic digestion of the heart. The putative involvement of P2Y receptors in the negative inotropic effect of ATP in paced ventricular strips was not assessed here, which is a limitation of our study that certainly deserves further investigations along with the corresponding effects in the *in vivo* animal.

Given the involvement of the P2X4 receptor in the negative control of sinoatrial automatism (see above), we focused our interest at investigating the role of this ionotropic receptor on ventricular contractile activity (Erlinge and Burnstock, 2008; Burnstock and Pelleg, 2015). This question was raised because heart rate slowing drugs devoid of effect or with a moderate positive inotropic action on ventricular contraction may be relevant to treat heart failure. Our findings show that selective blockage of the P2X4 receptor activation with 5-BDBD significantly increased the negative inotropic effect of ATP in paced RV strips, thus suggesting that the P2X4 receptor may exert a counteracting positive inotropic action that is responsible for partially offsetting ATP-induce downsizing of ventricular contractions. As a matter of fact, the ATP analogues, 2-methylthioATP and α,β-methyleneATP, increased contractions of isolated ventricular cells, as well as of ventricular strips and isolated working hearts in rodents (Burnstock and Meghji, 1983; Hu et al., 2001; Mei and Liang, 2001). Overexpression of the P2X4 receptor 1) enhances ATP-induced cardiac contractility in the intact heart, and 2) rescues the systolic function and increase survival of animals with cardiomyopathy (Yang et al., 2004; Shen et al., 2009). The beneficial effects of the P2X4 receptor on cardiac function were attributed to activation of calcium-dependent endothelial-type nitric oxide synthase (Blaustein and Lederer, 1999; Yang et al., 2015). Ca^{2+} influx through the P2X4 receptor pore may itself account for the positive inotropic action of ATP analogues. On the other hand, Na^+ influx through the P2X4 receptor also contributes to inhibit or, even revert, the electrogenic transport of NCX in the forward mode (Ca^{2+} extrusion mode) leading to an additional increase in the amplitude and duration of Ca^{2+} transients inside cardiomyocytes, which boosts their contractile activity (Shen et al., 2014; see **Figure 7**).

This concept may also explain the biphasic effect of ATP on atrial inotropy reported in this study and by other authors (Froldi et al., 1994; Gergs et al., 2008), which consisted of a transient decrease followed by a gradual recovery of the amplitude of atrial contractions while the preparations were still in contact with the nucleotide. Even though atrial inotropy represents an important reserve to maintain cardiac output in demanding conditions and in the setting of ventricular diastolic dysfunction, this phenomenon was not further evaluated in spontaneously beating rat atria due to significant bias introduced by changes in the rate of contractions.

Another relevant aspect of the P2X4 receptor regulation with potential implications for cardiac pathophysiology is its sensitivity to pH; in acidotic conditions, as it occurs in ischemia/hypoxia or renal failure, the P2X4 receptor activity significantly decreases, whereas the opposite occurs alkaline conditions (Wildman et al., 1999). Growing evidence exist demonstrating that the P2X4 receptor is overexpressed in ventricles under stressful conditions, namely in pulmonary hypertension and ischemia-induced heart failure (Sonin et al., 2008; Musa et al., 2009; Ohata et al., 2011). Altogether these findings strengthen the potential involvement of the P2X4 receptor in cardiac normal physiology and diseases progression.

CONCLUSION

Overall, data suggest that ATP-sensitive P2X4 ionotropic receptors play a major role in decreasing the spontaneous activity of the SAN while partially offsetting the negative inotropic effect of the nucleotide in paced rat ventricles. The mechanism underlying the dual P2X4 receptor-mediated effects on cardiac chronotropy and inotropy involves downstream interaction with the activity of NCX. Na^+ influx *via* the P2X4 receptor pore may inhibit and/or revert the electrogenic forward current of the NCX, thus decreasing chronotropy. Likewise, intracellular Ca^{2+} accumulation due to interference with NCX might explain the positive inotropic effect attributed to the P2X4 receptor activation on paced RV strips (**Figure 7**). Regional differences observed for the distribution of the P2X4 receptor, along with its biophysical properties, bring new therapeutic opportunities for P2X4 activation with potential to create novel well-tolerated heart-rate lowering drugs with promising benefits in patients with deteriorated ventricular function.

AUTHOR CONTRIBUTIONS

PC-S supervised the project. BB and PC-S designed the experiments and wrote the manuscript. BB and SN-M carried out myographic recordings. BB and FF performed immunofluorescence confocal microscopy experiments. BB, FF, AF-S, and PC-S interpreted data, discussed the clinical implications, and commented on the manuscript at all stages.

FUNDING

This work was supported by Foundation for Science and Technology (FCT) (FCOMP-01-0124-FEDER-028726-FEDER, COMPETE-FCT PTDC/DTP-FTO/0802/2012, PEst-OE/SAU/UI0215/2014, UID/BIM/4308/2016 and UID/BIM/4308/2019). The funders had no role in study design, data collection and analysis, decision to publish, or preparation of the manuscript. BB is in receipt of a PhD studentship from FCT (FEDER funding SFRH/BD/104114/2014).

ACKNOWLEDGMENTS

We are grateful to Catarina Pereira and Nádia Oliveira-Monteiro for their collaboration in some of the experiments. The authors wish to thank Mrs. Helena Costa e Silva and Belmira Silva for their valuable technical assistance.

SUPPLEMENTARY MATERIAL

FIGURE S1 | ATP (0.1 μM–1 mM) concentration-dependently decrease the spontaneous atrial rate. The negative chronotropic effect of ATP was mimicked by its enzymatically stable analogue, ATPγS (0.001–0.1 mM, A), and its potency was increased after pretreatment of the preparations with POM-1 (100 μM, a non-selective NTPDase inhibitor, B) and with ivermectin (30 μM, a positive allosteric modulator of the P2X4 receptor, C). For comparison purposes, we show in panel D that ATP (100 μM)-induced negative chronotropy was fully blocked by PPADS (100 μM). In panels A–C, data are expressed as mean ± SEM from an *n* number of animals. In panel D, represented are box-and-whiskers plots, with whiskers ranging from minimum to maximum values calculated as a percentage (%) of variation from baseline; horizontal lines inside boxes indicate the corresponding medians; each data point represents the result of a single experiment; data from the same experiment are connected by lines. $^*p < 0.05$ (Student's *t*-test for paired samples) represent significant differences when compared to the effect of ATP alone.

FIGURE S2 | Effects of receptor antagonists/allosteric modulators, NTPDase inhibitor and ion transport blockers on spontaneously beating rat atria (A–J). POM-1 (100 μM, A), PPADS (10 μM B; 100 μM, C), DPCPX (3 nM, D), A438079 (3 μM, E), 5-BDBD (10 μM, F), ivermectin (30 μM, G), KB-R7943 (3 μM, H), ORM-10103 (3 μM, I), and ZD7288 (300nM, J) contacted with the preparations at least for 15 min; the rate of spontaneous atrial contractions (beats min^{-1}) was measured immediately before ATP applications (see Figures 2–4) and compared to baseline conditions in the absence of any drug. Each data point represents the result of a single experiment; points from the same experiment are connected by lines. On the right hand-side of each panel, represented are box-and-whiskers plots, with whiskers ranging from minimum to maximum values calculated as a percentage (%) of variation from baseline; horizontal lines inside boxes indicate the corresponding medians. $^*p < 0.05$ (Student's *t*-test for paired samples) represent significant differences when compared to baseline.

FIGURE S3 | Effects of the P2X4 receptor antagonist, 5-BDBD (10 μM, A and B) and of the NCX inhibitor, KB-R7943 (3 μM, C and D) on paced right ventricular contractions. Drugs contacted with the preparations at least for 15 min; the amplitude of 2 Hz-paced ventricular contractions measured as active tension (mN/mg of wet tissue weight, panels A and C) and as the derivative of developed force over time (+dF/dt, mN/s, panels B and D) was measured immediately before ATP applications (see **Figure 5**) and compared to baseline conditions in the absence of any drug. Each data point represents the result of a single experiment; points from the same experiment are connected by lines. On the right hand-side of each panel, represented are box-and-whiskers plots, with whiskers ranging from minimum to maximum values calculated as a percentage (%) of variation from baseline; horizontal lines inside boxes indicate the corresponding medians. $^*p < 0.05$ (Student's *t*-test for paired samples) represent significant differences when compared to baseline.

FIGURE S4 | Representative confocal micrographs showing the immunolocalization of the P2X4 receptor (Apr-024, extracellular loop, Alomone) and of the HCN4 channel (Agp-004, Alomone) in the rat sinoatrial node (SAN); images obtained in right atria (RA) and right ventricle (RV) are also shown for comparison. It is worth noting that while the SAN was positive for both markers, RA and RV were positive for the P2X4 receptor (green) but negative for the HCN4 (magenta). Images were taken from one whole-mount preparation of the rat heart including the three regions, SAN, RA and RV. Dashed lines represent boundaries of the SAN region. White arrows indicate blood vessels including the SAN artery. Scale bar 30 μm.

FIGURE S5 | Representative confocal micrographs of SAN showing positive immunoreactivity against P2X4 (Apr-002, Alomone), NCX1 (Anx-011, Alomone), and NF160 (Ab7794, Abcam) proteins. The upper three panels show lower magnification confocal images of the SAN identified by the enrichment in NF160-positive nerve fibers; images also show surrounding atrial cardiomyocytes characterized as being NF160-negative and Cx43-positive. Images were taken from only one atrial preparation. Dashed lines represent boundaries of the SAN region. White arrows indicate blood vessels including the SAN artery. Scale bar 30 μm.

REFERENCES

Abbracchio, M. P., Burnstock, G., Boeynaems, J. M., Barnard, E. A., Boyer, J. L., Kennedy, C., et al. (2006). International Union of Pharmacology LVIII: update on the P2Y G protein-coupled nucleotide receptors: from molecular mechanisms and pathophysiology to therapy. *Pharmacol. Rev.* 58 (3), 281–341. doi: 10.1124/pr.58.3.3

Balogh, J., Wihlborg, A. K., Isackson, H., Joshi, B. V., Jacobson, K. A., Arner, A., et al. (2005). Phospholipase C and cAMP-dependent positive inotropic effects of ATP in mouse cardiomyocytes *via* P2Y11-like receptors. *J. Mol. Cell Cardiol.* 39 (2), 223–230. doi: 10.1016/j.yjmcc.2005.03.007

Belardinelli, L., and Lerman, B. B. (1991). Adenosine: cardiac electrophysiology. *Pacing. Clin. Electrophysiol.* 14 (11 Pt 1), 1672–1680. doi: 10.1111/j.1540-8159.1991.tb02742.x

Belardinelli, L., Shryock, J. C., Song, Y., Wang, D., and Srinivas, M. (1995). Ionic basis of the electrophysiological actions of adenosine on cardiomyocytes. *FASEB J.* 9 (5), 359–365. doi: 10.1096/fasebj.9.5.7896004

Blaustein, M. P., and Lederer, W. J. (1999). Sodium/calcium exchange: its physiological implications. *Physiol. Rev.* 79 (3), 763–854. doi: 10.1152/physrev.1999.79.3.763

Blomstrom-Lundqvist, C., Scheinman, M. M., Aliot, E. M., Alpert, J. S., Calkins, H., Camm, A. J., et al. (2003). ACC/AHA/ESC guidelines for the management of patients with supraventricular arrhythmias—executive summary: a report of the American College of Cardiology/American Heart Association Task Force on Practice Guidelines and the European Society of Cardiology Committee for Practice Guidelines (Writing Committee to Develop Guidelines for the Management of Patients With Supraventricular Arrhythmias). *Circulation* 108 (15), 1871–1909. doi: 10.1161/01.CIR.0000091380.04100.84

Bogdanov, K. Y., Vinogradova, T. M., and Lakatta, E. G. (2001). Sinoatrial nodal cell ryanodine receptor and Na(+)-Ca(2+) exchanger: molecular partners in pacemaker regulation. *Circ. Res.* 88 (12), 1254–1258. doi: 10.1161/hh1201.092095

Boyett, M. R., Honjo, H., and Kodama, I. (2000). The sinoatrial node, a heterogeneous pacemaker structure. *Cardiovasc. Res.* 47 (4), 658–687. doi: 10.1016/S0008-6363(00)00135-8

Braganca, B., Oliveira-Monteiro, N., Ferreirinha, F., Lima, P. A., Faria, M., Fontes-Sousa, A. P., et al. (2016). Ion fluxes through KCa2 (SK) and Cav1 (L-type) channels contribute to chronoselectivity of adenosine A1 receptor-mediated actions in spontaneously beating rat atria. *Front. Pharmacol.* 7, 45. doi: 10.3389/fphar.2016.00045

Burnstock, G. (1972). Purinergic nerves. *Pharmacol. Rev.* 24 (3), 509–581.

Burnstock, G., and Meghji, P. (1983). The effect of adenyl compounds on the rat heart. *Br. J. Pharmacol.* 79 (1), 211–218. doi: 10.1111/j.1476-5381.1983.tb10514.x

Burnstock, G., and Pelleg, A. (2015). Cardiac purinergic signalling in health and disease. *Purinergic Signal.* 11 (1), 1–46. doi: 10.1007/s11302-014-9436-1

Camara, H., da Silva Junior, E. D., Garcia, A. G., Jurkiewicz, A., and Rodrigues, J. Q. D. (2018). Cardiac arrest induced by muscarinic or adenosine receptors agonists is reversed by DPCPX through double mechanism. *Eur. J. Pharmacol.* 819, 9–15. doi: 10.1016/j.ejphar.2017.09.030

Camara, H., Rodrigues, J. Q., Alves, G. A., da Silva Junior, E. D., Caricati-Neto, A., Garcia, A. G., et al. (2015). Would calcium or potassium channels be responsible for cardiac arrest produced by adenosine and ATP in the right atria of Wistar rats? *Eur. J. Pharmacol.* 768, 199–206. doi: 10.1016/j.ejphar.2015.10.054

Cardoso, A. M., Schetinger, M. R., Correia-de-Sa, P., and Sevigny, J. (2015). Impact of ectonucleotidases in autonomic nervous functions. *Auton. Neurosci.* 191, 25–38. doi: 10.1016/j.autneu.2015.04.014

Chandrasekera, P. C., McIntosh, V. J., Cao, F. X., and Lasley, R. D. (2010). Differential effects of adenosine A2a and A2b receptors on cardiac contractility. *Am. J. Physiol. Heart. Circ. Physiol.* 299 (6), H2082–H2089. doi: 10.1152/ajpheart.00511.2010

Christie, A., Sharma, V. K., and Sheu, S. S. (1992). Mechanism of extracellular ATP-induced increase of cytosolic Ca2+ concentration in isolated rat ventricular myocytes. *J. Physiol.* 445, 369–388. doi: 10.1113/jphysiol.1992.sp018929

Clarke, T. C., Williams, O. J., Martin, P. E., and Evans, W. H. (2009). ATP release by cardiac myocytes in a simulated ischaemia model: inhibition by a connexin mimetic and enhancement by an antiarrhythmic peptide. *Eur. J. Pharmacol.* 605 (1–3), 9–14. doi: 10.1016/j.ejphar.2008.12.005

Coddou, C., Sandoval, R., Hevia, M. J., and Stojilkovic, S. S. (2019). Characterization of the antagonist actions of 5-BDBD at the rat P2X4 receptor. *Neurosci. Lett.* 690, 219–224. doi: 10.1016/j.neulet.2018.10.047

Crick, S. J., Sheppard, M. N., Ho, S. Y., and Anderson, R. H. (1999). Localisation and quantitation of autonomic innervation in the porcine heart I: conduction system. *J. Anat.* 195 (Pt 3), 341–357. doi: 10.1046/j.1469-7580.1999.19530341.x

Crick, S. J., Wharton, J., Sheppard, M. N., Royston, D., Yacoub, M. H., Anderson, R. H., et al. (1994). Innervation of the human cardiac conduction system. A quantitative immunohistochemical and histochemical study. *Circulation* 89 (4), 1697–1708. doi: 10.1161/01.CIR.89.4.1697

Crowe, R., and Burnstock, G. (1982). Fluorescent histochemical localisation of quinacrine-positive neurones in the guinea-pig and rabbit atrium. *Cardiovasc. Res.* 16 (7), 384–390. doi: 10.1093/cvr/16.7.384

Danziger, R. S., Raffaeli, S., Moreno-Sanchez, R., Sakai, M., Capogrossi, M. C., Spurgeon, H. A., et al. (1988). Extracellular ATP has a potent effect to enhance cytosolic calcium and contractility in single ventricular myocytes. *Cell Calcium* 9 (4), 193–199. doi: 10.1016/0143-4160(88)90023-1

De Young, M. B., and Scarpa, A. (1989). ATP receptor-induced Ca2+ transients in cardiac myocytes: sources of mobilized Ca2+. *Am. J. Physiol.* 257 (4 Pt 1), C750–C758. doi: 10.1152/ajpcell.1989.257.4.C750

Despa, S., and Bers, D. M. (2013). Na(+) transport in the normal and failing heart — remember the balance. *J. Mol. Cell Cardiol.* 61, 2–10. doi: 10.1016/j.yjmcc.2013.04.011

Duarte-Araújo, M., Nascimento, C., Timóteo, M. A., Magalhães-Cardoso, MT., and Correia-de-Sá, P. (2009). Relative contribution of ecto-ATPase and ecto-ATPDase pathways to the biphasic effect of ATP on acetylcholine release from myenteric motoneurons. *Br. J. Pharmacol.* 156 (3), 519–33. doi: 10.1111/j.1476-5381.2008.00058.x.

Erlinge, D., and Burnstock, G. (2008). P2 receptors in cardiovascular regulation and disease. *Purinergic Signal.* 4 (1), 1–20. doi: 10.1007/s11302-007-9078-7

Fabbri, A., Fantini, M., Wilders, R., and Severi, S. (2017). Computational analysis of the human sinus node action potential: model development and effects of mutations. *J. Physiol.* 595 (7), 2365–2396. doi: 10.1113/JP273259

Fekete, A., Franklin, L., Ikemoto, T., Rozsa, B., Lendvai, B., Sylvester Vizi, E., et al. (2009). Mechanism of the persistent sodium current activator veratridine-evoked Ca elevation: implication for epilepsy. *J. Neurochem.* 111 (3), 745–756. doi: 10.1111/j.1471-4159.2009.06368.x

Flitney, F. W., and Singh, J. (1980). Inotropic responses of the frog ventricle to adenosine triphosphate and related changes in endogenous cyclic nucleotides. *J. Physiol.* 304, 21–42. doi: 10.1113/jphysiol.1980.sp013307

Forrester, T., and Williams, C. A. (1977). Release of adenosine triphosphate from isolated adult heart cells in response to hypoxia. *J. Physiol.* 268 (2), 371–390. doi: 10.1113/jphysiol.1977.sp011862

Fredholm, B. B., Hedqvist, P., Lindstrom, K., and Wennmalm, M. (1982). Release of nucleosides and nucleotides from the rabbit heart by sympathetic nerve stimulation. *Acta Physiol. Scand.* 116 (3), 285–295. doi: 10.1111/j.1748-1716.1982.tb07142.x

Froldi, G., Pandolfo, L., Chinellato, A., Ragazzi, E., Caparrotta, L., and Fassina, G. (1994). Dual effect of ATP and UTP on rat atria: which types of receptors are involved? *Naunyn. Schmiedebergs. Arch. Pharmacol.* 349 (4), 381–386. doi: 10.1007/BF00170884

Gergs, U., Boknik, P., Schmitz, W., Simm, A., Silber, R. E., and Neumann, J. (2008). A positive inotropic effect of ATP in the human cardiac atrium. *Am. J. Physiol. Heart. Circ. Physiol.* 294 (4), H1716–H1723. doi: 10.1152/ajpheart.00945.2007

Griffioen, K. J., Gorini, C., Jameson, H., and Mendelowitz, D. (2007). Purinergic P2X receptors mediate excitatory transmission to cardiac vagal neurons in the nucleus ambiguus after hypoxia. *Hypertension* 50 (1), 75–81. doi: 10.1161/HYPERTENSIONAHA.106.086140

Groenke, S., Larson, E. D., Alber, S., Zhang, R., Lamp, S. T., Ren, X., et al. (2013). Complete atrial-specific knockout of sodium-calcium exchange eliminates sinoatrial node pacemaker activity. *PLoS One* 8 (11), e81633. doi: 10.1371/journal.pone.0081633

Headrick, J. P., Ashton, K. J., Rose'meyer, R. B., and Peart, J. N. (2013). Cardiovascular adenosine receptors: expression, actions and interactions. *Pharmacol. Ther.* 140 (1), 92–111. doi: 10.1016/j.pharmthera.2013.06.002

Herrmann, S., Lipp, P., Wiesen, K., Stieber, J., Nguyen, H., Kaiser, E., et al. (2013). The cardiac sodium-calcium exchanger NCX1 is a key player in the initiation and maintenance of a stable heart rhythm. *Cardiovasc. Res.* 99 (4), 780–788. doi: 10.1093/cvr/cvt154

Hu, B., Mei, Q. B., Yao, X. J., Smith, E., Barry, W. H., and Liang, B. T. (2001). A novel contractile phenotype with cardiac transgenic expression of the human P2X4 receptor. *FASEB J.* 15 (14), 2739–2741. doi: 10.1096/fj.01-0445fje

Jarvis, M. F., and Khakh, B. S. (2009). ATP-gated P2X cation-channels. *Neuropharmacology* 56 (1), 208–215. doi: 10.1016/j.neuropharm.2008.06.067

Jones, C. A., Chessell, I. P., Simon, J., Barnard, E. A., Miller, K. J., Michel, A. D., et al. (2000). Functional characterization of the P2X(4) receptor orthologues. *Br. J. Pharmacol.* 129 (2), 388–394. doi: 10.1038/sj.bjp.0703059

Jost, N., Nagy, N., Corici, C., Kohajda, Z., Horvath, A., Acsai, K., et al. (2013). ORM-10103, a novel specific inhibitor of the Na+/Ca2+ exchanger, decreases early and delayed afterdepolarizations in the canine heart. *Br. J. Pharmacol.* 170 (4), 768–778. doi: 10.1111/bph.12228

Kasuya, G., Fujiwara, Y., Tsukamoto, H., Morinaga, S., Ryu, S., Touhara, K., et al. (2017). Structural insights into the nucleotide base specificity of P2X receptors. *Sci. Rep.* 7, 45208. doi: 10.1038/srep45208

Khakh, B. S., Proctor, W. R., Dunwiddie, T. V., Labarca, C., and Lester, H. A. (1999). Allosteric control of gating and kinetics at P2X(4) receptor channels. *J. Neurosci.* 19 (17), 7289–7299. doi: 10.1523/JNEUROSCI.19-17-07289.1999

Kurogouchi, F., Furukawa, Y., Zhao, D., Hirose, M., Nakajima, K., Tsuboi, M., et al. (2000). A Na+/Ca2+ exchanger inhibitor, KB-R7943, caused negative inotropic responses and negative followed by positive chronotropic responses in isolated, blood-perfused dog heart preparations. *Jpn J. Pharmacol.* 82 (2), 155–163. doi: 10.1254/jjp.82.155

Lazarowski, E. R. (2012). Vesicular and conductive mechanisms of nucleotide release. *Purinergic Signal.* 8 (3), 359–373. doi: 10.1007/s11302-012-9304-9

Lee, S. Y., and Kim, J. H. (2015). Mechanisms underlying presynaptic Ca2+ transient and vesicular glutamate release at a CNS nerve terminal during *in vitro* ischaemia. *J. Physiol.* 593 (13), 2793–2806. doi: 10.1113/JP270060

Legssyer, A., Poggioli, J., Renard, D., and Vassort, G. (1988). ATP and other adenine compounds increase mechanical activity and inositol trisphosphate production in rat heart. *J. Physiol.* 401, 185–199. doi: 10.1113/jphysiol.1988.sp017157

Lohse, M. J., Klotz, K. N., Lindenborn-Fotinos, J., Reddington, M., Schwabe, U., and Olsson, R. A. (1987). 8-Cyclopentyl-1,3-dipropylxanthine (DPCPX)—a selective high affinity antagonist radioligand for A1 adenosine receptors. *Naunyn. Schmiedebergs. Arch. Pharmacol.* 336 (2), 204–210. doi: 10.1007/BF00165806

Lundberg, J. M., Hua, Y., and Fredholm, B. B. (1984). Capsaicin-induced stimulation of the guinea-pig atrium. Involvement of a novel sensory transmitter or a direct action on myocytes? *Naunyn. Schmiedebergs. Arch. Pharmacol.* 325 (2), 176–182. doi: 10.1007/BF00506198

Magalhães-Cardoso, MT., Pereira, M. F., Oliveira, L., Ribeiro, J. A., Cunha, R. A., and Correia-de-Sá, P. (2003). Ecto-AMP deaminase blunts the ATP-derived adenosine A2A receptor facilitation of acetylcholine release at rat motor nerve endings. *J. Physiol.* 549 (Pt 2), 399–408. doi: 10.1113/jphysiol.2003.040410

Mangoni, M. E., and Nargeot, J. (2008). Genesis and regulation of the heart automaticity. *Physiol. Rev.* 88 (3), 919–982. doi: 10.1152/physrev.00018.2007

Mei, Q., and Liang, B. T. (2001). P2 purinergic receptor activation enhances cardiac contractility in isolated rat and mouse hearts. *Am. J. Physiol. Heart. Circ. Physiol.* 281 (1), H334–H341. doi: 10.1152/ajpheart.2001.281.1.H334

Michel, A. D., Miller, K. J., Lundstrom, K., Buell, G. N., and Humphrey, P. P. (1997). Radiolabeling of the rat P2X4 purinoceptor: evidence for allosteric interactions of purinoceptor antagonists and monovalent cations with P2X purinoceptors. *Mol. Pharmacol.* 51 (3), 524–532.

Musa, H., Tellez, J. O., Chandler, N. J., Greener, I. D., Maczewski, M., Mackiewicz, U., et al. (2009). P2 purinergic receptor mRNA in rat and human sinoatrial node and other heart regions. *Naunyn Schmiedebergs Arch. Pharmacol.* 379 (6), 541–549. doi: 10.1007/s00210-009-0403-2

Ohata, Y., Ogata, S., Nakanishi, K., Kanazawa, F., Uenoyama, M., Hiroi, S., et al. (2011). Expression of P2X4R mRNA and protein in rats with hypobaric hypoxia-induced pulmonary hypertension. *Circ. J.* 75 (4), 945–954. doi: 10.1253/circj.CJ-09-0575

Pakhomov, N., Pustovit, K., Potekhina, V., Filatova, T., Kuzmin, V., and Abramochkin, D. (2018). Negative inotropic effects of diadenosine tetraphosphate are mediated by protein kinase C and phosphodiesterases stimulation in the rat heart. *Eur. J. Pharmacol.* 820, 97–105. doi: 10.1016/j.ejphar.2017.12.024

Pauza, D. H., Saburkina, I., Rysevaite, K., Inokaitis, H., Jokubauskas, M., Jalife, J., et al. (2013). Neuroanatomy of the murine cardiac conduction system: a combined stereomicroscopic and fluorescence immunohistochemical study. *Auton. Neurosci.* 176 (1-2), 32–47. doi: 10.1016/j.autneu.2013.01.006

Pelleg, A., and Belhassen, B. (2010). The mechanism of the negative chronotropic and dromotropic actions of adenosine 5'-triphosphate in the heart: an update. *J. Cardiovasc. Pharmacol.* 56 (1), 106–109. doi: 10.1097/FJC.0b013e3181e0f8b2

Pelleg, A., Belhassen, B., Ilia, R., and Laniado, S. (1985). Comparative electrophysiologic effects of adenosine triphosphate and adenosine in the canine heart: influence of atropine, propranolol, vagotomy, dipyridamole and aminophylline. *Am. J. Cardiol.* 55 (5), 571–576. doi: 10.1016/0002-9149(85)90249-8

Pelleg, A., Mitsuoka, T., Michelson, E. L., and Menduke, H. (1987). Adenosine mediates the negative chronotropic action of adenosine 5'-triphosphate in the canine sinus node. *J. Pharmacol. Exp. Ther.* 242 (3), 791–795.

Pinheiro, A. R., Paramos-de-Carvalho, D., Certal, M., Costa, C., Magalhaes-Cardoso, M. T., Ferreirinha, F., et al. (2013a). Bradykinin-induced Ca2+ signaling in human subcutaneous fibroblasts involves ATP release *via* hemichannels leading to P2Y12 receptors activation. *Cell Commun. Signal.* 11, 70. doi: 10.1186/1478-811X-11-70

Pinheiro, A. R., Paramos-de-Carvalho, D., Certal, M., Costa, M. A., Costa, C., Magalhaes-Cardoso, M. T., et al. (2013b). Histamine induces ATP release from human subcutaneous fibroblasts, *via* pannexin-1 hemichannels, leading to Ca2+ mobilization and cell proliferation. *J. Biol. Chem.* 288 (38), 27571–27583. doi: 10.1074/jbc.M113.460865

Podrasky, E., Xu, D., and Liang, B. T. (1997). A novel phospholipase C- and cAMP-independent positive inotropic mechanism *via a* P2 purinoceptor. *Am. J. Physiol.* 273 (5), H2380–H2387. doi: 10.1152/ajpheart.1997.273.5.H2380

Ponikowski, P., Voors, A. A., Anker, S. D., Bueno, H., Cleland, J. G. F., Coats, A. J. S., et al. (2016). 2016 ESC Guidelines for the diagnosis and treatment of acute and chronic heart failure: the task force for the diagnosis and treatment of acute and chronic heart failure of the European Society of Cardiology (ESC)Developed with the special contribution of the Heart Failure Association (HFA) of the ESC. *Eur. Heart. J.* 37 (27), 2129–2200. doi: 10.1093/eurheartj/ehw128

Rajendran, P. S., Challis, R. C., Fowlkes, C. C., Hanna, P., Tompkins, J. D., Jordan, M. C., et al. (2019). Identification of peripheral neural circuits that regulate heart rate using optogenetic and viral vector strategies. *Nat. Commun.* 10 (1), 1944. doi: 10.1038/s41467-019-09770-1

Remme, C. A., and Bezzina, C. R. (2010). Sodium channel (dys)function and cardiac arrhythmias. *Cardiovasc. Ther.* 28 (5), 287–294. doi: 10.1111/j.1755-5922.2010.00210.x

Samanta, K., Mirams, G. R., and Parekh, A. B. (2018). Sequential forward and reverse transport of the Na(+) Ca(2+) exchanger generates Ca(2+) oscillations within mitochondria. *Nat. Commun.* 9 (1), 156. doi: 10.1038/s41467-017-02638-2

Sanders, L., Rakovic, S., Lowe, M., Mattick, P. A., and Terrar, D. A. (2006). Fundamental importance of Na+-Ca2+ exchange for the pacemaking mechanism in guinea-pig sino-atrial node. *J. Physiol.* 571 (Pt 3), 639–649. doi: 10.1113/jphysiol.2005.100305

Scamps, F., Legssyer, A., Mayoux, E., and Vassort, G. (1990). The mechanism of positive inotropy induced by adenosine triphosphate in rat heart. *Circ. Res.* 67 (4), 1007–1016. doi: 10.1161/01.RES.67.4.1007

Sharma, A. D., and Klein, G. J. (1988). Comparative quantitative electrophysiologic effects of adenosine triphosphate on the sinus node and atrioventricular node. *Am. J. Cardiol.* 61 (4), 330–335. doi: 10.1016/0002-9149(88)90939-3

Shen, J. B., Shutt, R., Agosto, M., Pappano, A., and Liang, B. T. (2009). Reversal of cardiac myocyte dysfunction as a unique mechanism of rescue by P2X4 receptors in cardiomyopathy. *Am. J. Physiol. Heart. Circ. Physiol.* 296 (4), H1089–H1095. doi: 10.1152/ajpheart.01316.2008

Shen, J. B., Yang, R., Pappano, A., and Liang, B. T. (2014). Cardiac P2X purinergic receptors as a new pathway for increasing Na(+) entry in cardiac myocytes. *Am. J. Physiol. Heart. Circ. Physiol.* 307 (10), H1469–H1477. doi: 10.1152/ajpheart.00553.2014

Sonin, D., Zhou, S. Y., Cronin, C., Sonina, T., Wu, J., Jacobson, K. A., et al. (2008). Role of P2X purinergic receptors in the rescue of ischemic heart failure. *Am. J. Physiol. Heart. Circ. Physiol.* 295 (3), H1191–H1197. doi: 10.1152/ajpheart.00577.2008

Soto, F., Garcia-Guzman, M., Gomez-Hernandez, J. M., Hollmann, M., Karschin, C., and Stuhmer, W. (1996). P2X4: an ATP-activated ionotropic receptor cloned from rat brain. *Proc. Natl. Acad. Sci. U.S.A.* 93 (8), 3684–3688. doi: 10.1073/pnas.93.8.3684

Stokes, L., Layhadi, J. A., Bibic, L., Dhuna, K., and Fountain, S. J. (2017). P2X4 Receptor function in the nervous system and current breakthroughs in pharmacology. *Front. Pharmacol.* 8, 291. doi: 10.3389/fphar.2017.00291

Tellez, J. O., Dobrzynski, H., Greener, I. D., Graham, G. M., Laing, E., Honjo, H., et al. (2006). Differential expression of ion channel transcripts in atrial muscle and sinoatrial node in rabbit. *Circ. Res.* 99 (12), 1384–1393. doi: 10.1161/01.RES.0000251717.98379.69

Timoteo, M. A., Carneiro, I., Silva, I., Noronha-Matos, J. B., Ferreirinha, F., Silva-Ramos, M., et al. (2014). ATP released *via* pannexin-1 hemichannels mediates bladder overactivity triggered by urothelial P2Y6 receptors. *Biochem. Pharmacol.* 87 (2), 371–379. doi: 10.1016/j.bcp.2013.11.007

Tokunaga, T., Katsuragi, T., Sato, C., and Furukawa, T. (1995). ATP release evoked by isoprenaline from adrenergic nerves of guinea pig atrium. *Neurosci. Lett.* 186 (2-3), 95–98. doi: 10.1016/0304-3940(95)11290-D

Tsutsui, K., Monfredi, O. J., Sirenko-Tagirova, S. G., Maltseva, L. A., Bychkov, R., Kim, M. S., et al. (2018). A coupled-clock system drives the automaticity of human sinoatrial nodal pacemaker cells. *Sci. Signal* 11 (534), eaap 7608. doi: 10.1126/scisignal.aap7608

Versprille, A., and van Duyn, C. D. (1966). The negative chronotropic effect of adenine derivatives and acetylcholine on frog and rat hearts. *Pflugers Arch. Gesamte Physiol. Menschen Tiere* 292 (4), 288–296. doi: 10.1007/BF00363197

Vieira, C., Magalhães-Cardoso, M. T., Ferreirinha, F., Silva, I., Dias, A. S., Pelletier, J., et al. (2014). Feed-forward inhibition of CD73 and upregulation of adenosine deaminase contribute to the loss of adenosine neuromodulation in postinflammatory ileitis. *Mediators Inflamm.* 2014, 254640. doi: 10.1155/2014/254640.

Vinogradova, T. M., Tagirova Sirenko, S., and Lakatta, E. G. (2018). Unique Ca(2+)-cycling protein abundance and regulation sustains local Ca(2+) releases and spontaneous firing of rabbit sinoatrial node cells. *Int. J. Mol. Sci.* 19 (8), E2173. doi: 10.3390/ijms19082173

Wildman, S. S., King, B. F., and Burnstock, G. (1999). Modulation of ATP-responses at recombinant rP2X4 receptors by extracellular pH and zinc. *Br. J. Pharmacol.* 126 (3), 762–768. doi: 10.1038/sj.bjp.0702325

Xu, J., Kussmaul, W., Kurnik, P. B., Al-Ahdav, M., and Pelleg, A. (2005). Electrophysiological-anatomic correlates of ATP-triggered vagal reflex in the dog. V. Role of purinergic receptors. *Am. J. Physiol. Regul. Integr. Comp. Physiol.* 288 (3), R651–R655. doi: 10.1152/ajpregu.00553.2004

Yang, A., Sonin, D., Jones, L., Barry, W. H., and Liang, B. T. (2004). A beneficial role of cardiac P2X4 receptors in heart failure: rescue of the calsequestrin overexpression model of cardiomyopathy. *Am. J. Physiol. Heart. Circ. Physiol.* 287 (3), H1096–H1103. doi: 10.1152/ajpheart.00079.2004

Yang, R., Beqiri, D., Shen, J. B., Redden, J. M., Dodge-Kafka, K., Jacobson, K. A., et al. (2015). P2X4 receptor-eNOS signaling pathway in cardiac myocytes as a novel protective mechanism in heart failure. *Comput. Struct. Biotechnol. J.* 13, 1–7. doi: 10.1016/j.csbj.2014.11.002

Yang, T., Shen, J. B., Yang, R., Redden, J., Dodge-Kafka, K., Grady, J., et al. (2014). Novel protective role of endogenous cardiac myocyte P2X4 receptors in heart failure. *Circ. Heart Fail* 7 (3), 510–518. doi: 10.1161/CIRCHEARTFAILURE.113.001023

Yaniv, Y., Lakatta, E. G., and Maltsev, V. A. (2015). From two competing oscillators to one coupled-clock pacemaker cell system. *Front. Physiol.* 6, 28. doi: 10.3389/fphys.2015.00028

Yegutkin, G. G. (2008). Nucleotide- and nucleoside-converting ectoenzymes: important modulators of purinergic signalling cascade. *Biochim. Biophys. Acta* 1783 (5), 673–694. doi: 10.1016/j.bbamcr.2008.01.024

Zarzoso, M., Rysevaite, K., Milstein, M. L., Calvo, C. J., Kean, A. C., Atienza, F., et al. (2013). Nerves projecting from the intrinsic cardiac ganglia of the pulmonary veins modulate sinoatrial node pacemaker function. *Cardiovasc. Res.* 99 (3), 566–575. doi: 10.1093/cvr/cvt081

Permissions

All chapters in this book were first published by Frontiers; hereby published with permission under the Creative Commons Attribution License or equivalent. Every chapter published in this book has been scrutinized by our experts. Their significance has been extensively debated. The topics covered herein carry significant findings which will fuel the growth of the discipline. They may even be implemented as practical applications or may be referred to as a beginning point for another development.

The contributors of this book come from diverse backgrounds, making this book a truly international effort. This book will bring forth new frontiers with its revolutionizing research information and detailed analysis of the nascent developments around the world.

We would like to thank all the contributing authors for lending their expertise to make the book truly unique. They have played a crucial role in the development of this book. Without their invaluable contributions this book wouldn't have been possible. They have made vital efforts to compile up to date information on the varied aspects of this subject to make this book a valuable addition to the collection of many professionals and students.

This book was conceptualized with the vision of imparting up-to-date information and advanced data in this field. To ensure the same, a matchless editorial board was set up. Every individual on the board went through rigorous rounds of assessment to prove their worth. After which they invested a large part of their time researching and compiling the most relevant data for our readers.

The editorial board has been involved in producing this book since its inception. They have spent rigorous hours researching and exploring the diverse topics which have resulted in the successful publishing of this book. They have passed on their knowledge of decades through this book. To expedite this challenging task, the publisher supported the team at every step. A small team of assistant editors was also appointed to further simplify the editing procedure and attain best results for the readers.

Apart from the editorial board, the designing team has also invested a significant amount of their time in understanding the subject and creating the most relevant covers. They scrutinized every image to scout for the most suitable representation of the subject and create an appropriate cover for the book.

The publishing team has been an ardent support to the editorial, designing and production team. Their endless efforts to recruit the best for this project, has resulted in the accomplishment of this book. They are a veteran in the field of academics and their pool of knowledge is as vast as their experience in printing. Their expertise and guidance has proved useful at every step. Their uncompromising quality standards have made this book an exceptional effort. Their encouragement from time to time has been an inspiration for everyone.

The publisher and the editorial board hope that this book will prove to be a valuable piece of knowledge for researchers, students, practitioners and scholars across the globe.

List of Contributors

Marçal Pastor-Anglada and Sandra Pérez-Torras
Molecular Pharmacology and Experimental Therapeutics, Department of Biochemistry and Molecular Biomedicine, Institute of Biomedicine, University of Barcelona, Barcelona, Spain
Oncology Program, National Biomedical Research Institute on Liver and Gastrointestinal Diseases - CIBER ehd, Institut de Recerca Sant Joan de Déu, Barcelona, Spain

Clara Quintas
Laboratory of Pharmacology, Department of Drug Sciences, Faculty of Pharmacy, University of Porto, Porto, Portugal
REQUIMTE/LAQV, University of Porto, Porto, Portugal

Nuno Vale
Laboratory of Pharmacology, Department of Drug Sciences, Faculty of Pharmacy, University of Porto, Porto, Portugal
REQUIMTE/UCIBIO, University of Porto, Porto, Portugal

Jorge Gonçalves and Glória Queiroz
Laboratory of Pharmacology, Department of Drug Sciences, Faculty of Pharmacy, University of Porto, Porto, Portugal
MedInUP, University of Porto, Porto, Portugal

Irene Fusco, Elisabetta Coppi, Ilaria Dettori, Lisa Gaviano, Federica Cherchi, Felicita Pedata and Anna M. Pugliese
Department of Neuroscience, Psychology, Drug Research and Child Health, NEUROFARBA, Section of Pharmacology and Toxicology, University of Florence, Florence, Italy

Filippo Ugolini, Daniele Lana and Maria G. Giovannini
Department of Health Sciences, Section of Clinical Pharmacology and Oncology, University of Florence, Florence, Italy

Daniele Nosi
Department of Experimental and Clinical Medicine, University of Florence, Florence, Italy

Tiziana Pietrangelo, Ester S. Di Filippo and Stefania Fulle
Dipartimento Neuroscienze Imaging and Scienze Cliniche, Università degli Studi "G. d'Annunzio" Chieti-Pescara, Chieti, Italy

Marcello Locatelli
Dipartimento di Farmacia, Università degli Studi "G. d'Annunzio" Chieti-Pescara, Chieti, Italy

Francesco Piacenza and Mauro Provinciali
IRCCS-Istituto Nazionale di Riposo e Cura per Anziani, Polo Scientifico e Tecnologico, Centro di Tecnologie Avanzate nell'Invecchiamento, Ancona, Italy

Marco Farina and Eleonora Pavoni
Dipartimento di Ingegneria dell'Informazione, Università Politecnica delle Marche, Ancona, Italy

Andrea Di Donato
Harvard John A. Paulson School of Engineering and Applied Sciences, Harvard University, Cambridge, MA, United States

Denise Innosa
Facoltà di Bioscienze e Tecnologie Agro-Alimentari e Ambientali, Università di Teramo, Teramo, Italy

Alberto L. Horenstein, Antonella Chillemi, Valeria Quarona and Fabio Malavasi
Laboratory of Immunogenetics and CeRMS, Department of Medical Sciences, University of Torino, Torino, Italy

Roberta Zini and Rossella Manfredini
Centre for Regenerative Medicine "Stefano Ferrari," Department of Life Sciences, University of Modena and Reggio Emilia, Modena, Italy

Nicoletta Bianchi, Roberto Gambari and Davide Ferrari
Department of Life Science and Biotechnology, Section of Microbiology and Applied Pathology, University of Ferrara, Ferrara, Italy

Helena Pinheiro, Rita Gaspar and Filipa I. Baptista
Coimbra Institute for Clinical and Biomedical Research, Faculty of Medicine, University of Coimbra, Coimbra, Portugal
Center for Innovation in Biomedicine and Biotechnology, University of Coimbra, Coimbra, Portugal

Carlos A. Fontes-Ribeiro, António F. Ambrósio and Catarina A. Gomes
Coimbra Institute for Clinical and Biomedical Research, Faculty of Medicine, University of Coimbra, Coimbra, Portugal
Center for Innovation in Biomedicine and Biotechnology, University of Coimbra, Coimbra, Portugal
Faculty of Medicine, University of Coimbra, Coimbra, Portugal

Laura López-Cruz
Àrea de Psicobiologia, Universitat Jaume I, Castellón de la Plana, Spain

John D. Salamone
Behavioral Neuroscience Division, University of Connecticut, Storrs, CT, United States

Mercè Correa
Àrea de Psicobiologia, Universitat Jaume I, Castellón de la Plana, Spain
Behavioral Neuroscience Division, University of Connecticut, Storrs, CT, United States

Wennan Lu, Ann O'Brien-Jenkins, Néstor M. Gómez, Jason C. Lim, Erin E. Coffey, Keith E. Campagno and Stuart A. McCaughey
Department of Anatomy and Cell Biology, University of Pennsylvania, Philadelphia, PA, United States

Sonia Guha
Department of Anatomy and Cell Biology, University of Pennsylvania, Philadelphia, PA, United States
Jules Stein Eye Institute, University of California, Los Angeles, Los Angeles, CA, United States

Alan M. Laties
Jules Stein Eye Institute, University of California, Los Angeles, Los Angeles, CA, United States

Leif G. Carlsson
Department of Bioscience Heart Failure, Cardiovascular, Renal and Metabolic Diseases, IMED Biotech Unit, AstraZeneca, Gothenburg, Sweden

Claire H. Mitchell
Department of Anatomy and Cell Biology, University of Pennsylvania, Philadelphia, PA, United States
Department of Ophthalmology, University of Pennsylvania, Philadelphia, PA, United States
Department of Physiology, University of Pennsylvania, Philadelphia, PA, United States

Yan Li, Zhe Wang and Xiong Zhang
Department of Neurology, The Second Affiliated Hospital and Yuying Children's Hospital of Wenzhou Medical University,Wenzhou, China

Xinran Pan, Yan He, Yang Ruan, Linshan Huang, Yuling Zhou, Zhidong Hou and Chaoxiang He
School of Optometry and Ophthalmology and Eye Hospital, The Institute of Molecular Medicine, Wenzhou Medical University, Wenzhou, China

Robert D. Lasley
Department of Physiology, Wayne State University School of Medicine, Detroit, MI, United States

Jiang-Fan Chen
School of Optometry and Ophthalmology and Eye Hospital, The Institute of Molecular Medicine, Wenzhou Medical University, Wenzhou, China
Department of Neurology, School of Medicine, Boston University, Boston, MA, United States

Ana M. Sebastião, Nádia Rei and Joaquim A. Ribeiro
Instituto de Farmacologia e Neurociências, Faculdade de Medicina, Universidade de Lisboa, Lisbon, Portugal, Instituto de Medicina Molecular, Universidade de Lisboa, Lisbon, Portugal

Josep Tomàs, Neus Garcia, Maria A. Lanuza, Manel M. Santafé, Marta Tomàs, Laura Nadal, Erica Hurtado, Anna Simó-Ollé, Víctor Cilleros-Mañé and Laia Just-Borràs
Unitat d'Histologia i Neurobiologia, Facultat de Medicina i Ciències de la Salut, Universitat Rovira i Virgili, Reus, Spain

Stephan Menzel, Nicole Schwarz, Friedrich Haag and Friedrich Koch-Nolte
Institute of Immunology, University Medical Center Hamburg-Eppendorf, Hamburg, Germany

Ágatha Oliveira-Giacomelli, Yahaira Naaldijk, Laura Sardá-Arroyo, Juliana Corrêa-Velloso, Micheli M. Pillat, Héllio D. N. de Souza and Henning Ulrich
Department of Biochemistry, Institute of Chemistry, University of São Paulo, São Paulo, Brazil

Maria C. B. Gonçalves
Department of Neurology and Neuroscience, Medical School, Federal University of São Paulo, São Paulo, Brazil

A. J. Timmerman, Tim S. Heistek and Huibert D. Mansvelder
Department of Integrative Neurophysiology, Center for Neurogenomics and Cognitive Research, VU University, Amsterdam, Netherlands

Amber Kerkhofs
Department of Integrative Neurophysiology, Center for Neurogenomics and Cognitive Research, VU University, Amsterdam, Netherlands
Center for Neuroscience and Cell Biology, University of Coimbra, Coimbra, Portugal

Paula M. Canas, Joana I. Real, Carolina Xavier and Samira G. Ferreira
Center for Neuroscience and Cell Biology, University of Coimbra, Coimbra, Portugal

Rodrigo A. Cunha
Center for Neuroscience and Cell Biology, University of Coimbra, Coimbra, Portugal
Faculty of Medicine, University of Coimbra, Coimbra, Portugal

Sergi Ferré, Jordi Bonaventura, Candice Hatcher-Solis, César Quiroz and Ning-Sheng Cai
Integrative Neurobiology Section, National Institute on Drug Abuse, Intramural Research Program, National Institutes of Health, Baltimore, MD, United States

Wendy Zhu, Daniel Zwilling and Kimberly R. Thompson
Circuit Therapeutics, Inc., Menlo Park, CA, United States

Jaume Taura and Francisco Ciruela
Unitat de Farmacologia, Departament de Patologia i Terapèutica Experimental, Facultat de Medicina i Ciències de la Salut, IDIBELL, Universitat de Barcelona, Barcelona, Spain
Institut de Neurociències, Universitat de Barcelona, Barcelona, Spain

Estefanía Moreno, Verónica Casadó-Anguera, Carme Lluís and Vicent Casadó
Center for Biomedical Research in Neurodegenerative Diseases Network, Department of Biochemistry and Molecular Biomedicine, Faculty of Biology, Institute of Biomedicine of the University of Barcelona, University of Barcelona, Barcelona, Spain

Alexxai V. Kravitz
Eating and Addiction Section, Diabetes, Endocrinology and Obesity Branch, National Institute of Diabetes and Digestive and Kidney Diseases, Intramural Research Program, National Institutes of Health, Bethesda, MD, United States

Dardo G. Tomasi and Nora D. Volkow
Laboratory of Neuroimaging, National Institute on Alcohol Abuse and Alcoholism, Intramural Research Program, National Institutes of Health, Rockville, MD, United States

Gemma Navarro
Department of Biochemistry and Physiology, Faculty of Pharmacy, University of Barcelona, Barcelona, Spain

Arnau Cordomí and Leonardo Pardo
Laboratory of Computational Medicine, School of Medicine, Autonomous University of Barcelona, Bellaterra, Spain

Carmen W. Dessauer
Department of Integrative Biology and Pharmacology, McGovern Medical School, University of Texas Health Science Center at Houston, Houston, TX, United States

Diomedes E. Logothetis
Department of Pharmaceutical Sciences, Bouvé College of Health Sciences, Northeastern University, Boston, MA, United States

Inge M. Lankhuizen, Heleen M. van Beusekom, Dirk J. Duncker and Daphne Merkus
Division of Experimental Cardiology, Department of Cardiology, Thoraxcenter, Erasmus Medical Center, University Medical Center Rotterdam, Rotterdam, Netherlands
Cardiovascular Research School Erasmus University Rotterdam, Erasmus Medical Center, University Medical Center Rotterdam, Rotterdam, Netherlands

Zhichao Zhou
Division of Experimental Cardiology, Department of Cardiology, Thoraxcenter, Erasmus Medical Center, University Medical Center Rotterdam, Rotterdam, Netherlands
Cardiovascular Research School Erasmus University Rotterdam, Erasmus Medical Center, University Medical Center Rotterdam, Rotterdam, Netherlands
Division of Cardiology, Department of Medicine, Karolinska University Hospital, Karolinska Institutet, Solna, Sweden

Caroline Cheng
Division of Experimental Cardiology, Department of Cardiology, Thoraxcenter, Erasmus Medical Center, University Medical Center Rotterdam, Rotterdam, Netherlands
Cardiovascular Research School Erasmus University Rotterdam, Erasmus Medical Center, University Medical Center Rotterdam, Rotterdam, Netherlands
Department of Nephrology and Hypertension, University Medical Center Utrecht, Utrecht, Netherlands

Sílvia Nogueira-Marques, Fátima Ferreirinha, Ana Patrícia Fontes-Sousa and Paulo Correia-de-Sá
Laboratório de Farmacologia e Neurobiologia, Center for Drug Discovery and Innovative Medicines (MedInUP), Instituto de Ciências Biomédicas de Abel Salazar, Universidade do Porto, Porto, Portugal

Bruno Bragança
Hospital Pedro Hispano, ULS Matosinhos, Matosinhos, Portugal

Index

www.ingramcontent.com/pod-product-compliance
Lightning Source LLC
LaVergne TN
LVHW082151200926
848484LV00008B/2140